VITAMINS
IN
ANIMAL
AND
HUMAN
NUTRITION

Lee Russell McDowell

VITAMINS

IN

ANIMAL

AND

HUMAN

NUTRITION

SECOND EDITION

Iowa State University Press / Ames

Lee Russell McDowell, PhD, is a professor of animal science in the Department of Animal Science, University of Florida, Gainesville. His research interests center primarily on minerals for grazing livestock, vitamins for livestock, and feed composition. Dr. McDowell also collaborates with numerous animal nutritionists in tropical countries of Latin America, Africa, and Southeast Asia.

© 2000 Iowa State University Press; 1989 Academic Press

Iowa State University Press
2121 South State Avenue, Ames, Iowa 50014

Orders:	1-800-862-6657
Office:	1-515-292-0140
Fax:	1-515-292-3348
Web site:	www.isupress.edu

Authorization to photocopy items for internal or personal use, or the internal or personal use of specific clients, is granted by Iowa State University Press, provided that the base fee of $.10 per copy is paid directly to the Copyright Clearance Center, 222 Rosewood Drive, Danvers, MA 01923. For those organizations that have been granted a photocopy license by CCC, a separate system of payments has been arranged. The fee code for users of the Transactional Reporting Service is 0-8138-2630-6/2000 $.10.

♾ Printed on acid-free paper in the United States of America

First edition, 1989 (© Academic Press)
Second edition, 2000

Library of Congress Cataloging-in-Publication Data
McDowell, L. R.
    Vitamins in animal and human nutrition/Lee Russell McDowell—2nd ed.
        p.   cm.
    Includes bibliographical references and index.
    ISBN 0-8138-2630-6
        1. Vitamins in human nutrition. 2. Vitamins in animal nutrition.
    3. Avitaminosis. I. Title.

QP771.M396 2000
613.2′86—dc21   00-027082

The last digit is the print number: 9   8   7   6   5   4   3   2   1

This book is dedicated, with appreciation, to my parents; my wife, Lorraine; my daughters, Suzannah, Joanna, and Teresa and their husbands and children; and to Tony J. Cunha (deceased), the former head of the Department of Animal Science at the University of Florida, for his practical knowledge of the livestock industry and for his support and encouragement to write books.

CONTENTS

PREFACE

Vitamins in Animal and Human Nutrition contains 19 chapters of concise, up-to-date information on vitamin nutrition for both animals and humans. The first chapter deals with the definition of vitamins, general considerations, and the fascinating history of these nutrients. Chapters 2 through 16 discuss the 15 established vitamins in relation to history; chemical structure, properties, and antagonists; analytical procedures; metabolism; functions; requirements; sources; deficiency; supplementation; and toxicity. Chapter 17 deals with other vitamin-like substances, and Chapter 18 reviews the importance of essential fatty acids. The final chapter discusses vitamin supplementation considerations.

An earlier edition of this book with a somewhat similar title was published by Academic Press in 1989. The present book has been completely and vigorously revised with one additional chapter. In the last 10 years, a great deal of new information has been generated in the field of vitamins; this is reflected by the fact that more than half of all the references have been published since the first edition. It is hoped that this book will be of worldwide use and will continue, as the first edition, to be used as a textbook and as an authoritative reference book for use by research and extension specialists, feed manufacturers, teachers, students, and others. An attempt has been made to provide a balance between animal nutrition and clinical human nutrition. Likewise, a comparison between the balance of chemical, metabolic, and functional aspects of vitamins and their practical and applied considerations has been made.

A unique feature is the description of the practical implications of vitamin deficiencies and excesses and the conditions that might occur with various animal species and humans. A large number of photographs illustrate vitamin deficiencies in farm livestock, laboratory animals, and humans. Unlike other textbooks, this one places strong emphasis on vitamin supplementation in each chapter and devotes the last chapter to this subject.

In preparing this book, I have obtained numerous suggestions from eminent scientists both in the United States and in other countries. I wish to express my sincere appreciation to them and to those who supplied photographs and other material used. I am especially grateful to the following: L.B. Bailey, R.B. Becker, B.J. Bock, H.L. Chapman, J.H. Conrad, G.L. Ellis (deceased), R.H. Harms, J.F. Hentges, J.K. Loosli, R. Miles, R.L. Shirley, R.R Streiff, and W.B. Weaver (Florida); R.T. Lovell and H.E. Sauberlich (Alabama); O. Balbuena, B.J. Carillo, and B. Ruksan (Argentina); H. Heitman (California); J.M. Bell, M. Hidiroglou, and N. Hidiroglou (Canada); N. Ruiz (Colombia); N. Comben (England); M. Sandholm (Finland); L.S. Jensen (Georgia); T.B. Keith (deceased) (Idaho); A.H. Jensen (Illinois); V. Ramadas Murthy (India); A. Prabowo (Indonesia); V. Catron (deceased) and V.C. Speer (Iowa); G.L. Cromwell (Kentucky); G.F. Combs (Maryland); F.J. Stare (Massachusetts); D.K. Beede, R.W. Luecke, E.R. Miller, R.C. Piper, J.W. Thomas, and D.E. Ullrey (Michigan); R.T. Holman and T.W. Sullivan (Minnesota); V. Herbert, L.E. Kook, M.C. Latham, and M.L. Scott (deceased) (New York); A. Helgebostad and H. Rimeslatten (Norway); D.E. Becker (Ohio); P.R. Cheeke, D.C. Church, O.H. Muth, and J.E. Oldfield (Oregon); D.S. McLaren (Scotland); J.R. Couch and T.M. Ferguson (deceased) (Texas); D.C. Dobson (Utah); J.P. Fontenot, M.D. Lindemann, and L.M. Potter (Virginia); J.R. Carlson, J.A. Froseth, and L.L. Madsen (deceased) (Washington); and M.L. Sunde (Wisconsin). Appreciation is expressed to company representatives, including G. Patterson (Chas. Pfizer Co); J.C. Bauernfeind, T.M. Fry, E.L. MacDonald, L.A. Peterson, William Seymour, and S.N. Williams (Hoffmann-LaRoche, Inc.); C.H. McGinnis (Rhône-Poulenc, Inc.); A.T. Forrester (The Upjohn Co.); and M.B. Coelho (BASF Co.). Special thanks go to J.P. Fontenot for the preliminary planning of the first edition, and to P.R. Cheeke and J.E. Oldfield for editing and providing useful suggestions for the first edition of this book.

I am particularly grateful to Nancy Wilkinson and Lorraine M. McDowell for their useful suggestions and assistance in the editing of the entire book. Likewise, I wish to acknowledge with thanks and appreciation the skill and care of Patricia French for overseeing the typing and proofreading of chapters, and also thank Vanessa Carbia and Mary Schemear for their valuable assistance. Also, I am indebted to the Animal Science Department of the University of Florida for providing the opportunity and support for this undertaking. Finally, I thank Tony J. Cunha (deceased) for encouraging me to undertake the responsibility of writing nutrition books and for his expertise on vitamins.

VITAMINS
IN
ANIMAL
AND
HUMAN
NUTRITION

INTRODUCTION AND HISTORICAL CONSIDERATIONS

DEFINITION OF VITAMINS

Vitamins are defined as a group of complex organic compounds present in minute amounts in natural foodstuffs that are essential to normal metabolism and lack of which in the diet causes deficiency diseases. Vitamins consist of a mixed group of chemical compounds and are not related to each other as are proteins, carbohydrates, and fats. Their classification together depends not on chemical characteristics but on function. Vitamins are differentiated from the trace elements, also present in the diet in small quantities, by their organic nature.

Vitamins are required in trace amounts (micrograms to milligrams per day) in the diet for health, growth, and reproduction. Omission of a single vitamin from the diet of a species that requires it will produce deficiency signs and symptoms. Many of the vitamins function as coenzymes (metabolic catalysts); others have no such role, but perform certain essential functions.

Some vitamins deviate from the preceding definition in that they do not always need to be constituents of food. Certain substances that are considered to be vitamins are synthesized by intestinal tract bacteria in quantities that are often adequate for body needs. However, a clear distinction is made between vitamins and substances that are synthesized in tissues of the body. Ascorbic acid, for example, can be synthesized by most species of animals, except when they are young or under stress conditions. Likewise, in most species, niacin can be synthesized from the amino acid tryptophan and vitamin D from action of ultraviolet light on precursor compounds in the skin. Thus, under certain conditions and for specific species, vitamin C, niacin, and vitamin D would not always fit the classic definition of a vitamin.

1

3

CLASSIFICATION OF VITAMINS

Classically, vitamins have been divided into two groups based on their solubilities in fat solvents or in water. Thus, fat-soluble vitamins include A, D, E, and K, while vitamins of the B-complex and C are classified water soluble. Fat-soluble vitamins are found in foodstuffs in association with lipids. The fat-soluble vitamins are absorbed along with dietary fats, apparently by mechanisms similar to those involved in fat absorption. Conditions favorable to fat absorption, such as adequate bile flow and good micelle formation, also favor absorption of the fat-soluble vitamins (Scott et al., 1982). Water-soluble vitamins are not associated with fats, and alterations in fat absorption do not affect their absorption. Three of the four fat-soluble vitamins (vitamins A, D, and E) are well stored in appreciable amounts in the animal body. Except for vitamin B_{12}, water-soluble vitamins are not well stored, and excesses are rapidly excreted. A continual dietary supply of the water-soluble vitamins and vitamin K is needed to avoid deficiencies. Fat-soluble vitamins are excreted primarily in the feces via the bile, whereas water-soluble vitamins are excreted mainly in the urine. Water-soluble vitamins are relatively nontoxic, but excesses of fat-soluble vitamins A and D can cause serious problems. Fat-soluble vitamins consist only of carbon, hydrogen, and oxygen, whereas some of the water-soluble vitamins also contain nitrogen, sulfur, or cobalt.

Table 1.1 lists 14 vitamins classified as either fat or water soluble. The number of compounds justifiably classified as vitamins is controversial. The term vitamin has been applied to many substances that do not meet the definition or criteria for vitamin status. Of the 14 vitamins listed, choline is only tentatively classified as one of the B-complex vitamins. Unlike other B vitamins, choline can be synthesized in the body, is required in larger amounts, and apparently functions as a structural constituent rather than as a coenzyme. *Myo*-inositol and carnitine are not listed in Table 1.1 even though they could fit the vitamin category but apparently for only several species. Chapters 2 through 15 in this book concern the 14 vitamins listed in Table 1.1; Chapter 16 is about carnitine; Chapter 17 concerns vitamin-like substances; and Chapter 18 considers essential fatty acids. The essential fatty acids are not vitamins, but a deficiency disease does result that is similar to vitamin deficiency. The final chapter deals with vitamin supplementation considerations.

■ Table 1.1   Fat- and Water-Soluble Vitamins with Synonym Names

Vitamin	Synonym
Fat soluble	
Vitamin A_1	Retinol, retinal, retinoic acid
Vitamin A_2	Dehydroretinol
Vitamin D_2	Ergocalciferol
Vitamin D_3	Cholecalciferol
Vitamin E	Tocopherol, tocotrienols
Vitamin K_1	Phylloquinone
Vitamin K_2	Menaquinone
Vitamin K_3	Menadione[a]
Water soluble	
Thiamin	Vitamin B_1
Riboflavin	Vitamin B_2
Niacin	Vitamin pp, vitamin B_3
Vitamin B_6	Pyridoxol, pyridoxal, pyridoxamine
Pantothenic acid	Vitamin B_5
Biotin	Vitamin H
Folacin	Folic acid, folate, vitamin M, vitamin B_c
Vitamin B_{12}	Cobalamin
Choline	Gossypine
Vitamin C	Ascorbic acid

[a]The synthetic form is water soluble.

VITAMIN NOMENCLATURE

When the vitamins were originally discovered, they were isolated from certain foods. During these early years, the chemical composition of the essential factors was unknown; therefore, these factors were assigned letters of the alphabet. The system of alphabetizing became complicated when it was discovered that activity attributed to a single vitamin was instead the result of several of the essential factors. In this way, the designation of groups of vitamins appeared (e.g., the vitamin "B" group). Additional chemical studies showed that variations in chemical structure occurred within compounds having the same vitamin activity but in different species. To overcome this, a system of suffixes was adopted (e.g., vitamin D_2 and D_3). The original letter system of designation thus became excessively complicated.

With the determination of the chemical structure of the individual vitamins, letter designations were sometimes replaced with chemical-structure names (e.g., thiamin, riboflavin, and niacin). Vitamins have also been identified by describing a function or its source. The term vitamin H (biotin) was used because the factor protected the *haut*, the

German word for skin. Likewise, vitamin K was derived from the Danish word *koagulation* (coagulation). The vitamin pantothenic acid refers to its source, as it is derived from the Greek word *pantos*, meaning "found everywhere."

The Committee on Nomenclature of the American Institute of Nutrition (CNAIN, 1981) has provided definite rules for the nomenclature of the vitamins. This nomenclature is used in this book. The official and major synonym names of vitamins are given in Table 1.1 and in the respective vitamin chapters.

VITAMIN REQUIREMENTS

Vitamin requirements for animals and humans are listed in the Appendix tables at the end of this book and in the appropriate chapter. While metabolic needs are similar, dietary needs for vitamins differ widely among species. Some vitamins are metabolic essentials, but not dietary essentials, for certain species, because they can be synthesized readily from other food or metabolic constituents.

Poultry, swine, and other monogastric animals are dependent on their diet for vitamins to a much greater degree than are ruminants. Tradition has it that ruminants in which the rumen is fully functioning cannot suffer from a deficiency of B vitamins. It is generally assumed that ruminants can always satisfy their needs from the B vitamins naturally present in their feed, plus that synthesized by symbiotic microorganisms. However, under specific conditions relating to stress and high productivity, ruminants have more recently been shown to have requirements, particularly for the B vitamins thiamin (see Chapter 6) and niacin (see Chapter 8). Likewise, vitamin B_{12} cannot be synthesized in the rumen if the essential building block cobalt is lacking in the diet.

The rumen does not become functional with respect to vitamin synthesis for some time after birth. For the first few days of life, the young ruminant resembles a nonruminant in requiring dietary sources of the B vitamins. Beginning as early as 8 days, and certainly by 2 months of age, ruminal flora have developed to the point of contributing significant amounts of the B vitamins (Smith, 1970). Production of these vitamins at the proximal end of the gastrointestinal tract is indeed fortunate for they become available to the host as they pass down the tract through areas of efficient digestion and absorption.

In monogastric animals, including humans, intestinal synthesis of many B vitamins is considerable (Mickelsen, 1956) though not as extensive or as efficiently utilized as in ruminants. Low efficiency of utilization is probably related to several factors. Intestinal synthesis in non-ruminants occurs in the lower intestinal tract, an area of poor absorption. The horse, with a large production of B vitamins in the large intestine, is apparently able to meet most of its requirements for these vitamins in spite of the poor absorption from this area. Intestinally produced vitamins are more available to those animals (rabbit, rat, and others) that habitually practice coprophagy and thus recycle products of the lower gut. This behavior yields significant amounts of B vitamins to the host animal.

VITAMIN OCCURRENCE

Vitamins originate primarily in plant tissues and are present in animal tissue only as a consequence of consumption of plants, or because the animal harbors microorganisms that synthesize them. Vitamin B_{12} is unique in that it occurs in plant tissues as a result of microbial synthesis. Two of the four fat-soluble vitamins, A and D, differ from the water-soluble B vitamins in that they occur in plant tissue in the form of a provitamin (a precursor of the vitamin), which can be converted into a vitamin in the animal body. No provitamins are known for any water-soluble vitamin. However, the amino acid tryptophan can be converted to niacin for most species. In addition, fat- and water-soluble vitamins differ in that water-soluble B vitamins are universally distributed in all living tissues, whereas fat-soluble vitamins are completely absent from some tissues.

HISTORY OF THE VITAMINS

The history of the discovery of the vitamins is an inspirational and exciting reflection of the ingenuity, dedication, and self-sacrifice of many individuals. Excellent reviews of vitamin history with appropriate references include Funk (1922), McCollum (1957), Wagner and Folkers (1962), Maynard et al. (1979), Scott et al. (1982), Widdowson (1986), and Loosli (1991). Important books that describe the historical discovery of three specific vitamin deficiency diseases include the following: Eijkman, 1890–1896; Funk, 1911; Williams, 1961 (beriberi); Hess, 1920; Carpenter, 1986 (scurvy); Harris, 1919; and Carpenter, 1981 (pellagra). A brief sketch of important events emphasizing early history of vitamins is outlined in Table 1.2.

The existence of nutritive factors, such as vitamins, was not recognized until about the start of the twentieth century. The word "vitamin"

2697 B.C.	Beriberi was recognized in China and is probably the earliest documented deficiency disorder.
1500 B.C.	Scurvy, night blindness, and xerophthalmia were described in ancient Egypt. Liver consumption was found to be curative for night blindness and xerophthalmia.
130–200 A.D	Soranus Ephesius provided classical descriptions of rickets.

1492-1600	World exploration threatened by scurvy:
	    Magellan lost four-fifths of his crew.
	    Vasco da Gama lost 100 of his 160 men.

1747	Lind performed controlled shipboard experiments on the preventive effect of oranges and lemons on scurvy. He also developed a method of preserving citrus juice by evaporation and conserving in acid form.
1768–1771	Captain Cook demonstrated that prolonged sea voyages were possible without ravages of scurvy.
1816	Magendie described xerophthalmia in dogs fed carbohydrate and olive oil.
1824	Combe described a fatal anemia (pernicious anemia) and suggested that it could be related to a disorder of the digestive tract.
1849	Choline was isolated by Streker from the bile of pigs.
1881	Lunin reported that animals did not survive on diets composed solely of purified fat, protein, carbohydrate, salts, and water.
1880s	Japanese physician Takaki prevented beriberi in the Japanese Navy by substituting other foods for polished rice.
1897	Eijkman showed that beriberi (thiamin deficiency) from polished rice consumption could be cured by adding rice polishings back into the diet.
1901	Grijins concluded that beriberi was caused by a vitally important food constituent.
1906	Hopkins suggested that substances in natural foods, termed "accessory food factors," were indispensable and did not fall into the categories of carbohydrate, fat, protein, or mineral.
1907	Holst and Frolich produced experimental scurvy in guinea pigs by feeding a deficient diet, with pathological changes resembling those in humans.
1909	Hopkins reported a rat growth factor in some fats.
1910	Vedder was convinced that beriberi was caused by a nutritional deficiency and saved many lives in the Philippines by feeding rice polishings.
1911	The term "vitamine" was first used by the Polish biochemist Funk to describe an accessory food factor.
1913	McCollum and Davis discovered fat-soluble A in butter that was associated with growth.
1919	Steenbock reported that the yellow color (carotene) of vegetables was vitamin A.
1919	Mellanby produced rickets in dogs, which responded to a fat-soluble vitamin in cod liver oil.
1920	Goldberger reported that pellagra was not caused by bacterial infection, but rather was an ill-balanced diet high in corn.
1922	McCollum established vitamin D as independent of vitamin A by preventing rickets after destroying vitamin A activity when bubbling oxygen through cod liver oil.
1923	Evans and Bishop discovered vitamin E. The deficiency caused female rats to abort, while male rats became sterile.
1926	Jansen and Donath isolated thiamin in crystalline form from rice bran.
1926	Minot and Murphy showed that large amounts of raw liver given by mouth daily would alleviate pernicious anemia.

1926	Steenbock showed that irradiation of foods as well as animals produced vitamin D.
1926	Goldberger and Lillie described a rat syndrome, later shown to be riboflavin deficiency.
1928	Bechtel and coworkers established that rumen bacteria of cattle synthesized B vitamins.
1928	Szent-Györgyi isolated hexuronic acid (ascorbic acid, vitamin C) from orange juice, cabbage juice, and cattle adrenal glands.
1929	Moore proved that the animal body converts carotene to vitamin A.
1929	Norris and coworkers reported a curled-toe paralysis (riboflavin deficiency) in chicks.
1929	Castle showed that pernicious anemia resulted from the interaction of a dietary (extrinsic) factor and an intrinsic factor produced by the stomach.
1930	Norris and Ringrose described a pellagra-like dermatitis in the chick, later established as a pantothenic acid deficiency.
1931	Pappenheimer and Goettsch showed that vitamin E is required for prevention of encephalomalacia of chicks and nutritional muscular dystrophy in rabbits and guinea pigs.
1931	Willis demonstrated that a factor from yeast was active in treating a tropical macrocytic anemia seen in women of India.
1932	Choline was discovered to be the active component of pure lecithin previously shown to prevent fatty livers in rats.
1933	Williams and associates fractionated a growth factor from yeast and named it pantothenic acid.
1934	György named a factor that would cure dermatitis in young rats, vitamin B_6.
1934	Dam and Schönheyder described a nutritional disease of chickens characterized by bleeding, thus a new fat-soluble vitamin was discovered (vitamin K).
1935	Wald demonstrated the relation of vitamin A to night blindness and vision.
1935	Kuhn in Germany and Karrer in Switzerland synthesized riboflavin.
1935	Warburg and coworkers first demonstrated a biochemical function for nicotinic acid when they isolated it from an enzyme (NADP).
1935–1937	Cobalt, the central ion in vitamin B_{12}, was shown to be a dietary essential for cattle and sheep by Underwood and coworkers in Australia and in Florida by Becker and associates.
1936	Biotin was the name given to a substance isolated from egg yolk by Kogl and Tonnis that was necessary for the growth of yeast.
1936	Williams and colleagues determined the structure of thiamin and synthesized the vitamin.
1937	Elvehjem and associates found that nicotinic acid cured black tongue in dogs. It was quickly shown to be effective for pellagra in humans.
1939	Vitamin K was isolated by Dam and Karrer of Europe and a few months later in the U.S. from three different laboratories.
1940	Harris and associates completed the first synthesis of biotin.
1942	Baxter and Robeson crystallized vitamin A.
1943–1946	Chemists from the Lederle group crystallized and later synthesized folacin.
1948	Rickes and coworkers in the U.S. and Smith in England isolated vitamin B_{12}.
1951	Smith and coworkers showed that cobalt deficiency in sheep could be prevented by vitamin B_{12} injection.

had not been coined yet. However, what were to be later known as vitamin-deficiency diseases, such as scurvy, beriberi, night blindness, xerophthalmia, and pellagra, had plagued the world at least since the existence of written records. Records of medical science from antiquity attesting to human association of certain foods with either the cause or prevention of disease and infirmity are considered the nebulous beginnings of the concept of essential nutrients (Wagner and Folkers, 1962). Even so, at the beginning of the twentieth century, the value of food in human nutrition was expressed solely in terms of its ability to provide energy and basic building units necessary for life.

In the late 1800s and early 1900s, some scientists believed that life could be supported with chemically defined diets. In 1860, Louis Pasteur reported that yeast could grow on a medium of sugar, ammonium salts, and ash of yeast. Justus von Liebig observed that certain yeasts were unable to grow at all under these conditions, while others grew only very slowly. The ensuing arguments between Liebig and Pasteur did not solve the question. Pasteur's (1822–1895) research showing that bacteria caused disease led scientists trained in medicine to be reluctant to believe the "vitamin theory" that certain diseases resulted from a shortage of specific nutrients in foods (Loosli, 1991). Guggenheim (1995) suggested that the immensely successful germ theory of disease, with the related toxin theory and success of using antisepsis and vaccination, occupied the thoughts of scientists at that time with the idea that only a positive agent could cause a disease.

The first phase leading to the "vitamin hypothesis" began with gradual recognition that the cause of diseases such as night blindness, scurvy, beriberi, and rickets could be related to diet. Although the true cause, nutritional deficiency, was not suspected, these results marked the first uncertainty in the germ and infection theories of origin for these diseases. Finally, in the early 1900s, many scientists in the field of nutrition almost simultaneously began to realize that a diet could not be adequately defined in terms of carbohydrate, fat, protein, and salts. At that time, it became evident that other organic compounds had to be present in the diet if health was to be maintained.

Beriberi was probably the earliest documented deficiency disorder, being recognized in China as early as 2600 B.C. Scurvy, night blindness, and xerophthalmia were described in the ancient Egyptian literature around 1500 B.C. Substances rich in vitamin A as remedies for night blindness were used very early by the Chinese, and livers were recommended as curative agents for night blindness and xerophthalmia by

Hippocrates around 400 B.C. In 1536, Canadian Indians cured Jacques Cartier's men of scurvy with a broth of evergreen needles. In 1747, James Lind, a British naval surgeon, showed that the juice of citrus fruits was a cure for scurvy, but its routine use was not started in the British Navy until 1795. Cod liver oil was used as a specific treatment for rickets long before anything was known about the cause of this disease, and was fed to farm animals as early as 1824. In the 1880s, the Japanese physician Takaki recognized the cause of beriberi in the Japanese Navy as stemming from an unbalanced white rice diet, and virtually eliminated this condition by increasing the consumption of vegetables, fish, and meat and by substituting barley for rice.

The period before the close of the nineteenth century was characterized by the discovery of diseases of nutritional origin in animals, which opened the way for controlled experimental studies of nutritional causes and cures for diseases that were common to both humans and the lower animals. The rat undoubtedly contributed most to the discovery of vitamins from 1900 through the 1920s, although chickens, pigeons, guinea pigs, mice, and dogs also played their part (Widdowson, 1986). In 1890, Christiaan Eijkman, a Dutch physician working in a military hospital in Java, found that chickens fed almost exclusively on polished rice developed polyneuritic signs bearing a marked resemblance to those of beriberi in humans. A new head cook at the hospital discontinued the supply of "military" rice (polished), and thereafter the birds were fed on whole-grain "civilian" rice, with the result being that they recovered. He also noted that beriberi in prisoners eating polished rice tended to disappear when a less highly milled product was fed. Many great advances in science have started from such chance observations pursued by men and women of inspiration.

Beginning in the middle 1850s, German scientists were recognized as leaders of nutrition. In the late 1800s, Professor C. von Bunge (Dorpat, Estonia, Germany, and then at Basel) had graduate students experimenting with purified diets for small animals (Wolf and Carpenter, 1997). In 1881, N. Lunin, a Russian student studying in von Bunge's laboratory, observed that mice died (16–36 days) when fed a diet composed solely of purified fat, protein, carbohydrate, salts, and water. Lunin proposed that natural foods such as milk contain small quantities of as yet "unknown substances essential to life." Other researchers from von Bunge's school and under his influence had essentially the same results as Lunin; these researchers included C.A. Socin (1891), W.S. Hall (1896), W. Falta (1906), and C.T. Noeggerath (1906).

Von Bunge explained away results of these experiments as he was inclined to disbelieve the existence of unknown nutritional factors. Von Bunge believed that iron and phosphorus must be present in preformed organic combinations, which was his explanation for the deaths of laboratory animals consuming purified diets (Wolf and Carpenter, 1997).

In 1906, Frederick Hopkins in England suggested that unknown nutrients were essential for animal life and used the term "accessory growth factors." Hopkins was responsible for opening up a new field of discovery that largely depended on the use of the rat. When Hopkins later discovered that he was not the first to suggest that unknown nutrients were essential, or to conduct animal experiments, he was anxious to share his Nobel prize with Eijkman in 1929.

In 1911, Casimir Funk proposed the "vitamine theory." He had reviewed the literature and made the important conclusion that beriberi could be prevented or cured by a protective factor present in natural food, which he had isolated from rice by-products (Funk, 1911). Funk named the distinct factor that prevented beriberi a "vitamine." This word was derived from "vital amine." Later, when it became evident that not all "vitamines" contained nitrogen (amine), the term became "vitamin." Funk had not believed that all "vitamines" were amines; rather, the name was chosen as a catchword to create interest in the new emerging field of nutrition.

After reviewing the literature between 1873 and 1906, in which small animals had been fed restricted diets of isolated proteins, fats, and carbohydrates, E.V. McCollum of the United States noted that the animals rapidly failed in health and concluded that the most important problem in nutrition was to discover what was lacking in such diets. By 1915, McCollum and M. Davis of Wisconsin discovered that the rat required at least two essential growth factors: a "fat-soluble A" factor and a "water-soluble B" factor. In addition to being required as factors for normal growth, the "fat-soluble A" factor was found to cure xeropththalmia, and the "water-soluble B" factor cured beriberi. At the same time as their work in Wisconsin, T.B. Osborne and L.B. Mendel of Connecticut also established the importance of what was later named vitamin A.

With the pioneer work of Eijkman, Hopkins, Funk, McCollum, and others, scientists began to seriously consider the new class of essential nutrients. The brilliant research of scientists in the first half of the twentieth century led to the isolation of more than a dozen vitamins as pure chemical substances. The golden age of vitamin research was mainly in the 1930s and 1940s. For vitamin discovery, the general procedure employed was first to study the effects of a deficient diet on a laboratory animal and then to find a food that would prevent the deficiency. Using a variety of chemical manipulations, the particular nutrient involved was gradually concentrated from the food, and its potency was tested at each stage of concentration on further groups of animals (Wagner and Folkers, 1962). This laborious procedure has been simplified in recent years by the discovery that several vitamins are also growth factors for microorganisms that can therefore replace animals for potency testing. By such methods, it is now possible to isolate vitamins and subsequently to identify them chemically. A remarkable achievement has been the direct synthesis by chemists of at least ten vitamins identified in this way. The last vitamin to be discovered was vitamin B_{12} in 1948, which brought the period of vitamin discovery to a close. On the other hand, the possibility that there are still undiscovered vitamins must be recognized (see Chapter 17). More detailed historical considerations for each vitamin are presented in the respective chapters (Chapters 2 through 16).

■ REFERENCES

Carpenter, K.J. (1981). *In* Pellagra, Hutchinson Ross Publishing Company, Stroudsburg, Pennsylvania.

Carpenter, K.J. (1986). *In* The History of Scurvy and Vitamin C. Cambridge University Press, Cambridge, London.

CNAIN. (1981). (Committee on Nomenclature of the American Institute of Nutrition). *J. Nutr. 111*, 8.

Eijkman, C. (1890–1896). Polyneuritis in Chickens, or the Origin of Vitamin Research. Roche, Basel.

Funk, C. (1911). *J. Physiol. 43*, 395.

Funk, C. (1922). The Vitamins, Williams and Wilkins Co., Baltimore.

Guggenheim, K.Y. (1995). *In* Basic Issues of the History of Nutrition, The Magnes Press, Hebrew University, Jerusalem, Israel.

Harris, H.F. (1919). Pellagra, The Macmillan Co., New York.

Hess, A.F. (1920). Scurvy Past and Present, J.B. Lippincott Co., London.

Loosli, J.K. (1991). *In* Handbook of Animal Science (P.A. Putnam, ed.) Academic Press, San Diego.

Maynard, L.A., Loosli, J.K., Hintz, H.F., and Warner, R.G. (1979). Animal Nutrition, 7th Ed., p. 283. McGraw-Hill, New York.

McCollum, E.V. (1957). *In* A History of Nutrition, p. 217. Houghton Mifflin, Boston.

Mickelsen, O. (1956). *Vitam. Horm. 14*, 1.

Scott, M.L., Nesheim, M.C., and Young, R.J. (1982). Nutrition of the Chicken, p. 119. Scott, Ithaca, New York.

Smith, S.E. (1970). *In* Duke's Physiology of Domestic Animals, 8th Ed. p. 634 (M.J. Swenson, ed.), Cornell University Press, Ithaca, New York.

Wagner, A.F., and Folkers, K. (1962). Vitamins and Coenzymes, Wiley (Interscience), New York.

Widdowson, E.M. (1986). *Nutr. Rev. 44,* 221.

Williams, R.R. (1961). Toward the Conquest of Beriberi, Harvard University Press, Cambridge.

Wolf, G., and Carpenter, K.J. (1997). *J. Nutr. 127,* 1255.

VITAMIN A

INTRODUCTION

Although all vitamins are equally important in supporting animal life, vitamin A may be considered the most important vitamin from a practical standpoint. It is important as a dietary supplement for all animals, including ruminants. Vitamin A itself does not occur in plants; however, its precursors (carotenoids) are found in plants, and these can be converted to true vitamin A by a specific enzyme located in the intestinal walls of animals. Prior to the discovery of vitamin A, farmers complained that hogs in dry lot or barns did poorly when fed a ration consisting largely of white corn instead of yellow corn. Agricultural chemists would disagree and explain to farmers that chemical analysis showed that white corn and yellow corn were the same with the exception of color. Then came the vitamin era, which explained what the farmers already knew, that white corn has no carotene, the precursor of vitamin A (Ensminger and Olentine, 1978).

In human nutrition, vitamin A is one of the few vitamins of which both deficiency and excess constitute a serious health hazard. Deficiency occurs in endemic proportions in many developing countries and is considered to be the most common cause of blindness in young children throughout the world. McLaren (1986) lists 73 countries and territories that are considered to have potentially serious vitamin A deficiency problems. Vitamin A toxicity usually arises from abuse of vitamin supplementation.

HISTORY

For thousands of years humans and animals have suffered from vitamin A deficiency, typified by night blindness and xerophthalmia (a condition named for the Latin words for dry eye, a manifestation of vitamin A deficiency in which the conjunctiva [covering of the eye] dries out, the cornea becomes inflamed, and the eye becomes ulcerated). The cause was unknown, but it was recognized that consumption of animal and fish livers had curative powers according to records and folklore from early civilizations. One of the earliest known reports was from Eber's Papyrus, an ancient Egyptian medical treatise of about 1500 B.C., which recommended the livers of cattle or poultry as curative agents (Arykroyd, 1958). An early reference to vitamin A deficiency in livestock is the Bible (Jeremiah 14:6): "and the asses did stand in high places, their eyes did fail, because there was no grass." Also from the Bible was the cure of the blind Tobias by means of fish bile.

The observation that experimental animals lose weight and die on purified diets was noted by many investigators toward the end of the nineteenth century. However, it was not until early in the twentieth century that vitamin A was discovered. Its history has been reviewed by a number of authorities (Funk, 1922; McCollum, 1957; Sebrell and Harris, 1967; Loosli, 1991). From 1906 through 1912, Hopkins of Great Britain found that a growth-stimulating principle from milk was present in an alcoholic extract of milk rather than in the ash. In 1909, Hopkins and Stepp found that certain fat-soluble substances were necessary for growth of mice and rats. In the years 1913 through 1915, McCollum and Davis described "fat-soluble A," a factor isolated from animal fats (unsaponifiable fraction of milk fat) or fish oils, which they associated with a growth-promoting activity. In their experiments, the growth of rats ceased prematurely when lard was used as the source of fat in the diet, whereas adequate growth was obtained when the dietary fat was either butter or fat extracted from egg yolk. At the same time, Osborne and Mendel also reported that something in butter appeared to be essential for life and growth in rats. Later, Drummond suggested that the "fat-soluble factor A" should be named vitamin A. In 1919, Steenbock called attention to the fact that among vegetable foods, vitamin A potency was associated with yellow color. He suggested that carotene was the source of the vitamin, but later recognized that the vitamin was not carotene itself because certain potent sources of the vitamin were colorless. Ten years later, Von Euler and associates in

Stockholm obtained a definite growth response when carotene was added to vitamin A-deficient diets. In 1929, Moore produced proof that the animal body transformed carotene into vitamin A. Animals fed carotene had vitamin A in livers, whereas controls did not.

Research in the 1920s and 1930s demonstrated that most animal species need dietary vitamin A. The simultaneous use of chemical methods and experimental rats to test metabolic products resulted in the successful demonstration of vitamin A activity, making it the first confirmed vitamin rather than vitamin B or C, which had received earlier attention. Similar testing methods were used to identify most of the other vitamins.

Only a few years after vitamin A was discovered, it was thought that rickets was also a vitamin A deficiency. Proof that rickets was not caused by vitamin A deficiency was provided by McCollum and associates in 1922. This proof was obtained by oxidizing cod liver oil until vitamin A was destroyed, as shown by the inability of the oil to cure xerophthalmia, and then by demonstrating that the oxidized oil was still effective in curing rickets.

Vitamin A deficiency was shown to be responsible for xeropththalmia and certain forms of night blindness. A link between vitamin A and the visual process was demonstrated in 1935 when Wald, in a series of experiments, obtained a specific form of vitamin A (retinal) from bleached retinas. Wagner and coworkers suggested in 1939 that the conversion of β-carotene into vitamin A occurs within the intestinal mucosa. In 1944, Morton suggested that retinal from bleached visual purple (rhodopsin) might be identical with vitamin A aldehyde; he was able to prove this by synthesis.

The isolation of pure vitamin A became possible when a relationship was found between its growth-promoting activity and the intensity of the Carr-Price antimony trichloride color at 620 nm or the light absorption at 328 nm. Karrer and his group were thus able to obtain a pure oily retinol from vitamin A-rich concentrates. From 1930 to 1931, Karrer and coworkers proposed the exact structural formulas for vitamin A and β-carotene. Six years later, the first crystals of vitamin A were obtained, and still another growth-promoting factor-vitamin A_2 was isolated from freshwater fish liver oils.

In 1942, Baxter and Robeson crystallized pure vitamin A and several of its esters; five years later, they also succeeded in isolation and crystallization of the 13-*cis*-vitamin A isomer. Isler and coworkers synthesized the first pure vitamin A in 1947. In 1950, Karrer and Inhoffen reported the synthesis of β–carotene. In the early 1980s, β–carotene and other carotenoids began to be recognized as important factors (independent of provitamin A activity) in potentially reducing the risk of certain cancers and other disease conditions.

CHEMICAL STRUCTURE AND PROPERTIES

Vitamin A itself does not occur in plant products, but its precursor, carotene (Fig. 2.1) occurs in several forms. These compounds are commonly referred to as provitamin A because the body can transform them into the active vitamin. This is how the vitamin A needs of farm animals are met, for the most part, because their rations consist mainly or entirely of foods of plant origin. The combined potency of a feed, represented by its vitamin A and carotene content, is referred to as its vitamin A value. Retinol is the alcohol form of vitamin A (Fig. 2.1). Replacement of the alcohol group by an aldehyde group gives retinal, and replacement by an acid group gives retinoic acid. Esters of retinol are called retinyl esters. Vitamin A in animal products exists in several forms, but principally as long-chain fatty acid esters (e.g., retinyl palmitate).

In addition to retinol, there is another form that is isolated from fish. It was originally distinguished on the basis of a different maximum spectral absorption and named A_2 to differentiate it from the previously isolated form. Vitamin A_2 is closely related to vitamin A_1 but contains an additional double bond in the β–ionone ring (Fig. 2.1). Liver oils of marine fish origin usually average less than 10% vitamin A_2 of the total vitamin A content. The relative biological activity of vitamin A_2 is 40 to 50% that of A_1.

Vitamin A is a nearly colorless, fat-soluble, long-chain, unsaturated alcohol with five double bonds. The vitamin is made up of isoprene units with alternate double bonds, starting with one in the β–ionone ring that is in conjugation with those in the side chain (Fig. 2.1). Since it contains double bonds, vitamin A can exist in different isomeric forms. More common isomeric forms of vitamin A and their relative biological activities are presented in Fig. 2.2.

The most active vitamin A form and that most usually found in mammalian tissues is the all-*trans*-vitamin A. *cis*-Forms can arise from the all-*trans*-forms, and a marked loss of vitamin A potency results. These structural changes in the molecule are promoted by moisture, heat, light, and catalysts. Therefore, conditions present during hay making and ensiling, dehydrating, and storage of crops are detrimental to the biological activity of any carotenoids present.

Precursors of vitamin A, the carotenes, occur as orange-yellow pigments mainly in green leaves and to a lesser extent in corn. Of more than

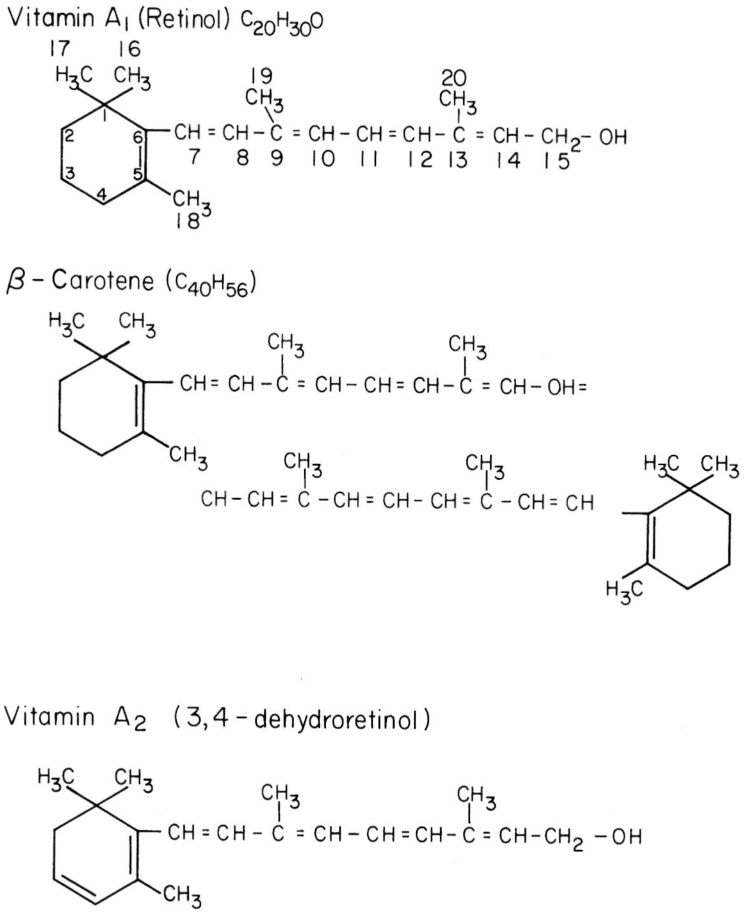

Vitamin A₁ (Retinol) C₂₀H₃₀O

β - Carotene (C₄₀H₅₆)

Vitamin A₂ (3,4 - dehydroretinol)

Fig. 2.1 Chemical structure of vitamin A₁, β-carotene, and vitamin A₂.

500 carotenoids that have been isolated from nature, only 50 to 60 possess biological activity. Structures of some of the important carotenoid pigments and their distribution and relative biological activity are presented in Fig. 2.3. Four of these carotenoids—α-carotene, β–carotene, γ-carotene, and cryptoxanthine (the main carotenoid of corn)—are of particular importance because of their provitamin A activity. Vitamin A activity of β–carotene is substantially greater than that of other carotenoids. Lycopene is an important carotenoid for its antioxidant function but does not possess the β–ionone ring structure, and therefore is not a precursor of vitamin A. In humans, β–carotene and lycopene are

19

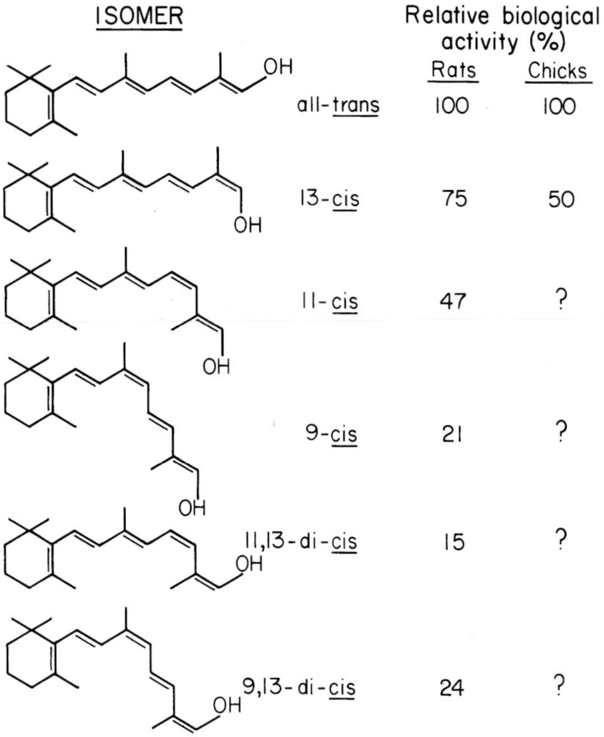

Fig. 2.2 Isomers of vitamin A (retinol). (Adapted from Ullrey, 1972.)

the predominant carotenoids in tissue (Ribaya-Mercado et al., 1995).

Theoretically, 1 mol of β–carotene could be converted (cleavage of the C15=C15′ bond) to yield 2 mol of retinal. However, biological tests have consistently shown that pure vitamin A has twice the potency of β–carotene on a weight-to-weight basis. Thus, only one molecule of vitamin A is formed from one molecule of β–carotene. Loss of potential activity results from inefficient cleavage and intestinal absorption.

Vitamin A activity is expressed in international units (IU) or, less frequently, in United States Pharmacopeia (USP) Units, both of which are of equal value. An IU is defined as the biological activity of 0.300 µg of vitamin A alcohol (retinol) or 0.550 µg of vitamin A palmitate. One IU of provitamin A activity is equal in activity to 0.6 µg of β–carotene, the reference compound. Vitamin A may be expressed as retinol equivalents (RE) instead of IU. By definition, 1 retinol equivalent is equal to 1 µg of

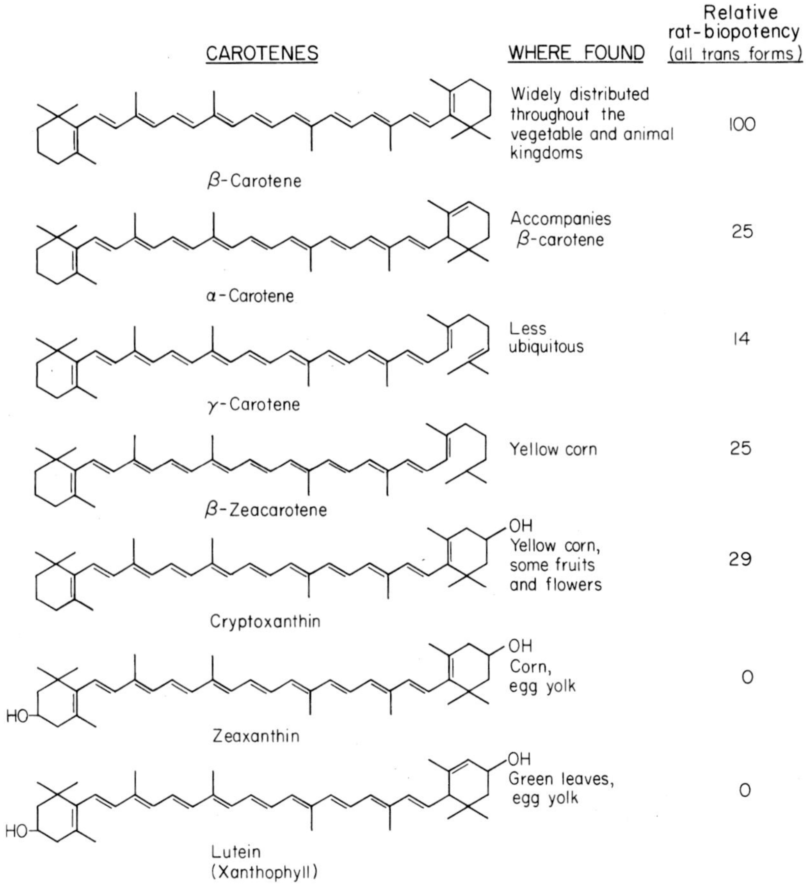

Fig. 2.3 The yellow carotenoids. (Adapted from Ullrey, 1972.)

retinol, 6 µg of β–carotene, or 12 µg of other provitamin A carotenoids. In terms of international units, 1 RE is equal to 3.33 IU of retinol or 10 IU of β–carotene.

ANALYTICAL PROCEDURES

A number of methods are available for carotene and vitamin A determination (Pit, 1985). Biological methods include growth responses of rats or chicks, the storage test (liver), and quantitative evaluations of cell changes in vaginal smears (rats). Physicochemical methods include

21

color reactions with antimony trichloride (Carr-Price method), gas chromatography, thin-layer chromatography, and spectrophotometric procedures. A number of reports (Grace and Bernhard, 1984; Hidiroglou et al., 1986; Horst et al., 1995) indicate excellent results and high recovery rates from high-pressure liquid chromatography (HPLC). The HPLC procedure is the most common method for analyzing carotenoids, vitamin A and its analogs in pharmaceutical preparations, feedstuffs, and tissues combined with an ultraviolet (UV) detector. A procedure for retinol-binding protein is radioimmunoassay (Vallet, 1994).

METABOLISM

Digestion

Vitamin A in animal products and carotenoids are released from proteins by the action of pepsin in the stomach and proteolytic enzymes in the small intestine (Ong, 1993; Ross, 1993). In the duodenum, bile salts break up fatty globules of carotenoids and retinyl esters to smaller lipid congregates, which can be more easily digested by pancreatic lipase, retinyl ester hydrolase, and cholesteryl ester hydrolase.

A number of factors influence digestibility of carotene and vitamin A. Working with lambs, Donoghue et al. (1983) reported that dietary levels of vitamin A ranging from mildly deficient to toxic levels affect digestion and uptake. Percentage transfer from the digestive tract from supplemental dietary levels of 0, 100, and 12,000 µg of retinol per kilogram were 91, 58, and 14%, respectively. Wing (1969) reported that the apparent digestibility of carotene in various forages fed to dairy cattle averaged about 78%. Variables that influenced carotene digestibility included month of forage harvest, type of forage (hay, silage, green-chop, or pasture), species of plant, and plant dry matter. In general, carotene digestibility was higher than average during warmer months and lower than average during winter.

Several reports indicate that appreciable amounts of carotene or vitamin A may be degraded in the rumen. Various studies with different diets have resulted in preintestinal vitamin A disappearance values ranging from 40 to 70% (Ullrey, 1972). Rode et al. (1990) compared microbial degradation of vitamin A (retinyl acetate) from steers fed concentrate, hay, or straw diets. Estimated effective rumen degradation of biologically active vitamin A was 67% for cattle fed concentrates compared to 16 and 19% for animals fed hay and straw diets, respectively.

Absorption and Transport

Much of the conversion of β–carotene to vitamin A takes place in the intestinal mucosa. Provitamin A carotenoids must contain one unsubstituted β–ionone ring to be active. This conversion of β–carotene into vitamin A involves two enzymes. β–Carotene-15,15′-dioxygenase catalyzes the cleavage of β–carotene at the central double bond to yield two molecules of retinal for one molecule of β–carotene. However, extensive evidence exists also for random (eccentric) cleavage, resulting in retinoic acid and retinal, with a preponderance of apocarotenals formed as intermediates (Wolf, 1995). The cleavage enzyme has been found in many vertebrates but is not present in the cat or mink. Therefore, these species cannot utilize carotene as a source of vitamin A. The second enzyme, retinaldehyde reductase, reduces the retinal to retinol.

In most mammals, the product ultimately absorbed from the intestinal tract as a result of feeding carotenoids is mainly vitamin A itself. There is considerable species specificity regarding the ability to absorb dietary carotenoids. In some species, such as the rat, pig, goat, sheep, rabbit, buffalo, and dog, almost all of the carotene is cleaved in the intestine. In humans, cattle, horses, and carp, significant amounts of carotene can be absorbed. Absorbed carotene can be stored in the liver and fatty tissues. Hence, these latter animals have yellow body and milk fat, whereas animals that do not absorb carotene have white fat.

In the case of cattle, there is a strong breed difference in absorption of carotene. The Holstein is an efficient converter, having white adipose tissue and milk fat. The Guernsey and Jersey breeds, however, readily absorb carotene, resulting in yellow fat. The chick, on the other hand, absorbs only hydroxy carotenoids in the unchanged form and stores them in tissues. Hydrocarbon carotenoids with provitamin A activity are converted by the chick intestine and absorbed as vitamin A. Species specificity in vitamin A conversion may be due to presence or absence of suitable receptor proteins or the ability to form suitable micellar solutions in the intestinal lumen.

A number of factors affect absorption of carotenoids. *cis-trans*-isomerism of the carotenoids is important in determining their absorbability, with the *trans*-forms being more efficiently absorbed (Stahl et al., 1995). Among carotenoids there is a differential uptake and clearance of specific carotenoids (Bierer et al., 1995; Johnson et al., 1997; Erdman et al., 1998; Van den Berg, 1999). Dietary fat is important (Roels et al.,

1958; Fichter and Mitchell, 1997; Takyi, 1999). When small supplements of fat were given to vitamin A-deficient boys in a region of Central Africa, the absorption of dietary carotenoids increased remarkably (from less than 5% to about 50%) (Roels et al., 1958). Dietary antioxidants (e.g., vitamin E) also appear to have an important effect on the utilization and perhaps absorption of carotenoids. It is uncertain whether the antioxidants contribute directly to efficient absorption or whether they protect both carotene and vitamin A from oxidative breakdown. Protein deficiency reduces absorption of carotene from the intestine.

Almost no absorption of vitamin A occurs in the stomach. The main site of vitamin A and carotenoid absorption is the mucosa of the proximal jejunum. The absorption of vitamin A in the intestine is believed to be 80 to 90%, while that of β–carotene is about 50 to 60% (Olson, 1991). Vitamin A efficiency of absorption decreases somewhat with very high doses. Intestinal β–carotene cleavage activity was shown to be higher in rats deficient in vitamin A than in rats with a high intake of either vitamin A or β–carotene (Van Vliet et al., 1996). Carotenoids are normally converted to retinol in the intestinal mucosa but may also be converted in the liver and other organs, especially in yellow fat species such as poultry (McGinnis, 1988). Lipid micelles in the intestinal lumen serve as carriers by taking up vitamin A and carotene from emulsified dietary lipid and bringing these lipids into contact with the mucosal cell, where they diffuse from the micelle through the lipid portion of the microvillar membrane.

Vitamin A occurs in food primarily as the palmitate ester. This is hydrolyzed in the small intestine by retinyl ester hydrolase, which is secreted by the pancreas. Bile salts are required both for the activation of this enzyme and for the formation of the lipid micelle, which carries vitamin A from the emulsified dietary lipid to the microvillus. Normally, vitamin A is absorbed almost exclusively as the free alcohol, retinol. Within the mucosal cells, retinol is reesterified mostly to palmitate, is incorporated into the chylomicra of the mucosa, and is secreted into the lymph. A small amount of retinol may be oxidized first to retinal and then to retinoic acid, which may form a glucuronide and pass into the portal blood. A specific transporter in the intestinal brush border for all-*trans*- and 3-dehydroretinol, constituting a process of carrier-facilitated diffusion, was reported, while other retinoids studied were taken up by passive diffusion at a slower rate (Wolf, 1995). At normal intakes, uptake of β–carotene by the rat was linear suggesting passive uptake (Moore et al., 1996).

Vitamin A is transported through the lymphatic system with a low-density lipoprotein in lymph acting as a carrier to the liver, where it is deposited mainly in hepatocytes and stellate and parenchymal cells. When liver stores of vitamin A are adequate, it can be transferred from parenchymal cells to stellate cells, where it is reesterified (Blomhoff et al., 1991).

When vitamin A is mobilized from the liver, stored vitamin A ester is hydrolyzed (retinyl ester hydrolase) prior to its release into the bloodstream, and vitamin A alcohol (retinol) then travels via the bloodstream to the tissues. Retinol is transported by a specific transport and binding protein, retinol-binding protein (RBP). The RBP is synthesized and secreted by hepatic parenchymal cells. Human RBP has a molecular weight of about 21,000 and contains one binding site for one molecule of retinol. Intercellular and intracellular binding proteins belong to a closely related family of retinoid-binding proteins of low molecular weight (Table 2.1).

Retinol is secreted from liver in association with RBP and circulates to peripheral tissues complexed to a thyroxine-binding protein, transthyretin (Blomhoff et al., 1991; Ross, 1993). The retinol-transthyretin complex is transported to target tissues, where the complex binds to a cell-surface receptor and the retinol is transported into cells of target tissue. Metabolism, storage, and release of vitamin A by the liver are under several forms of homeostatic control, with circulating RBP maintained over a wide range of total liver reserves (Blomhoff et al., 1991; Ross, 1993). One factor that specifically regulates RBP secretion from liver is the nutritional vitamin A status of the animal. The secretion of RBP from the liver is regulated by estrogen and nutritional status of vitamin A, protein, and zinc. Retinol deficiency specifically blocks secretion of RBP from the liver so that plasma RBP levels fall and liver RBP levels rise.

Contrary to current knowledge for all other species, vitamin A serum levels in dogs were affected by the daily vitamin A supply as well as the type of food (Schweigert et al., 1990). This was explained by the fact that dogs and other carnivores transport most of their vitamin A in blood as retinyl esters (mainly retinyl stearate) bound to lipoproteins. The differences in the retinyl ester pattern between vitamin A in liver and in blood indicate that the mobilization of vitamin A from the liver involves a selective mechanism.

Once the retinoids are transferred into the cell, they are quickly bound by specific binding proteins in the cell cytosol. The intracellular retinoid-binding proteins bind retinol, retinal, and retinoic acid for pur-

25

■ Table 2.1   Principal Retinoid-Binding Proteins

Name	Abbreviation	Retinoid	Principal Location
INTERCELLULAR TRANSPORT			
Chylomicron		Retinyl esters	Intestine, liver
retinol-binding protein	RBP	Retinol	Liver, extrahepatic organs
Interphotoreceptor retinol-binding protein	IRBP	All-*trans*-retinol/ ll-*cis*-retinol	Retina
INTRACELLULAR TRANSPORT			
Cellular retinol-binding protein (I)	CRBP (I)	Retinol	Most tissues except adrenal, heart, ileum, muscle, serum
Cellular retinoic acid-binding protein (I)	CRABP (I)	Retinoic acid	Seminal vesicle, vas deferens, skin, eye
Cellular retinoic acid-binding protein (II)	CRABP (II)	Retinoic acid	Skin
Epididymal retinoic acid	EBP 1,2	Retinoic acid	Lumen of epididymis
Cellular retinaldehyde-binding protein	CRALBP	ll-*cis*-retinal/ ll-*cis*-retinol	Retina
Nuclear retinoic acid receptors	RAR α, β, γ	All-*trans*-retinoic acid	Most tissues except adult liver
Nuclear retinoic acid X receptors	RXR α, β, γ	9-*cis*-retinoic acid	Most tissues

poses of protection against decomposition, solubilize them in aqueous medium, render them nontoxic, and transport them within cells to their site of action. These binding proteins also function by presenting the retinoids to the appropriate enzymes for metabolism (Wolf, 1991). Some of the principal forms of intracellular (cytoplasmic) retinoid-binding proteins (Table 2.1) are cellular retinol-binding proteins (CRBP I and II), cellular retinoic acid-binding proteins (CRABP I and II), cellular retinaldehyde-binding protein (CRALBP), and six nuclear retinoic acid receptors (RAR α, β, γ and RXR α, β, γ).

The cellular retinol and retinoic acid-binding proteins—CRBP (I, II) and CRABP (I, II)—function in transport and metabolism of retinoids within parenchymal, intestinal, reproductive, and fetal cells and across blood-organ barriers. A different group of retinoid-binding proteins, more related to serum retinol-binding protein, functions in epididymis and uterus. Retinaldehyde-binding protein aids in the oxidation-reduction reaction of 11-*cis*-retinol–11-*cis*-retinaldehyde in the retina, where the interphotoreceptor retinol-binding protein transports retinol between pigment epithelium and photoreceptors (Wolf, 1998). Finally, there are two classes of nuclear receptors: all-*trans*-retinoic acid is the ligand for RAR, and 9-*cis*-retinoic acid is the ligand for RXR.

Receptors for 1,25-dihydroxyvitamin D_3, all-*trans* retinoic acid, and 9-*cis*-retinoic acid are members of the nuclear hormone receptor super family, a gene family having at least 30 members, including receptors for the classic steroid hormones (estrogen, progesterone, glucocorticoids, androgens, thyroid hormone, and several others). The feature common to this class of molecules is that they control gene expression by interacting with specific DNA sequences or regulatory elements in control regions of target genes.

Retinol is readily transferred to the egg in birds, but the transfer of retinol across the placenta is marginal, and mammals are born with very low liver stores of vitamin A. Uterine RBP has been identified in the pig uterus, with the function of delivering retinol to the fetus (Clawitter et al., 1990).

Excretion

Derivatives of vitamin A with an intact carbon chain are generally excreted in feces, whereas acidic chain-shortened products tend to be excreted in urine (Olson, 1991). In the steady state, approximately equal amounts of metabolites are excreted in the feces and urine.

Some vitamin A derivatives are reexcreted into the intestinal lumen via the bile. This is true for much of the retinoic acid and some retinol. The major vitamin A components of the bile are vitamin A glucuronides. An appreciable portion of these glucuronides are reabsorbed, thus creating an enterohepatic circulation for vitamin A derivatives and providing an opportunity for vitamin A conservation (Barua, 1997). Kinetic studies have demonstrated that the retinol molecule cycles several times between liver and extrahepatic tissues before it is degraded (Blomhoff et al., 1991).

Storage

Liver normally contains about 90% of total-body vitamin A. The remainder is stored in the kidneys, lungs, adrenals, and blood, with small amounts also found in other organs and tissues. A large quantity of vitamin A is stored in the kidney as well as the liver in cats and dogs. This high level of vitamin A in the kidney is unique to cats and dogs, and the reasons for the storage are not fully understood (Ralston Purina, 1987; Raila et al., 1997). Vitamin A is highly concentrated in stomach oils of certain seabirds and in the intestinal wall of some fish. The entire vitamin A reserve of certain shrimp is in the eyes. Carotenoids are more evenly distributed in species that have the ability to absorb and store these precursors. Grass-fed cattle have large stores of carotene in their body fat, which is evidenced by a deep yellow color.

The liver can store large amounts of vitamin A; in humans approximately 50 to 80% of the total body vitamin A is stored in the stellate cells in the form of retinyl esters (Blomhoff et al., 1991). Bardos (1991) compared vitamin A content in liver lobes between dogs and other species. Uniformity of liver vitamin A was less for dogs than cattle and chickens. In all species, there was a low correlation between liver and blood retinol. Several studies have shown that liver can store enough vitamin A to protect the animal from long periods of dietary scarcity (McDowell, 1985). This large storage capacity must be considered in studies of vitamin requirements to ensure that intakes that appear adequate for a given function are not being supplemented by reserves stored prior to the period of observation. Measurement of the liver store of vitamin A at slaughter or in samples obtained from a biopsy is a useful technique in the study of vitamin A status and requirements. Fig. 2.4 illustrates a liver biopsy procedure that was adapted from human medicine.

FUNCTIONS

Vitamin A is necessary for support of growth, health, and life of higher animals. In the absence of vitamin A, animals will cease to grow and eventually die. The classic biological assay method is based on measurement of growth responses of weanling rats to graded doses of vitamin A. It is of primary importance in development of young, growing animals.

The metabolic function of vitamin A, explained in biochemical terms, is only now beginning to be understood. Vitamin A deficiency causes at least four different and probably physiologically distinct lesions: loss of vision due to a failure of rhodopsin formation in the retina; defects in bone growth; defects in reproduction (e.g., failure of spermatogenesis in the male and resorption of the fetus in the female); and defects in growth and differentiation of epithelial tissues, frequently resulting in keratinization. Keratinization of these tissues results in loss of function; this occurs in the alimentary, genital, reproductive, respira-

28

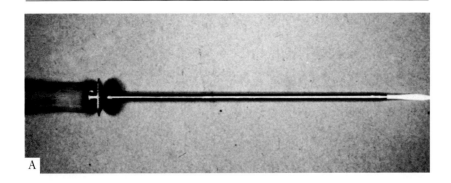

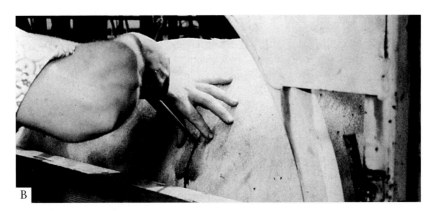

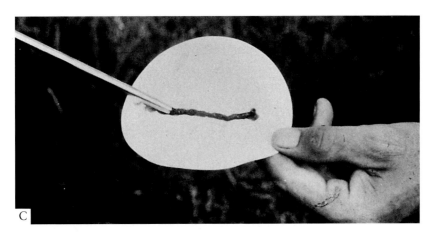

Fig. 2.4 Illustration of liver biopsy sample taken for both vitamin A and mineral analysis. Sample can be taken quickly with a trocar and cannula: (A) Trocar; (B) Insertion of trocar for sampling; (C) Release of sample from the cannula. (Courtesy of H.L. Chapman and L.R. McDowell, University of Florida.)

tory, and urinary tracts. Such altered characteristics make the affected tissue more susceptible to infections. Thus, diarrhea and pneumonia are typical secondary effects of vitamin A deficiency. Retinoic acid is the form of vitamin A that has been shown to perform as a hormone (e.g., all-*trans*-retinoic acid and 9-*cis*-retinoic acid). However, retinoic acid has been found to support growth and tissue differentiation but not vision (Fig. 2.5) or reproduction (Scott et al., 1982). Vitamin A-deficient rats fed retinoic acid were healthy in every respect, with normal estrus and conception, but failed to give birth and resorbed their fetuses. When retinol was given even at a late stage of pregnancy, fetuses were saved. Male rats on retinoic acid were healthy but produced no sperm, and without vitamin A, both sexes were blind (Anonymous, 1977).

Although retinol is needed for normal vision and some aspects of reproduction, discoveries have revealed that most, if not all, actions of vitamin A in development, differentiation, and metabolism are mediated by nuclear receptor proteins that bind retinoic acid, the active form of vitamin A (Anonymous, 1993). A group of retinoic acid binding proteins (receptors) function in the nucleus by attaching to promoter regions in a number of specific genes to stimulate their transcription and thus affect growth, development, and differentiation. Six high-affinity receptor proteins for retinoic acid (RAR α, β, γ and RXR α, β, γ) have been identified. Apparently RAR nuclear receptors bind to all-*trans* retinoic acid, while RXR receptors bind with 9-*cis*-retinoic acid (Kasner et al., 1994; Kliewer et al., 1994). Retinoic acid receptors in cell nuclei are structurally homologous and functionally analogous to the known receptors for steroid hormones, thyroid hormone (triiodothyronine), and vitamin D [1,25-$(OH)_2$D]. Thus, retinoic acid is now recognized to function as a hormone to regulate the transcription activity of a large number of genes (Ross, 1993). As an example, the well-known connection between vitamin A deficiency and hepatic glycogen depletion caused by reduced gluconeogenesis can now be explained at the molecular level by the dependence of phosphoenolpyruvate carboxykinase gene expression on adequate vitamin A (Shin and McGrane, 1997).

Actions of vitamin A in development, differentiation, and metabolism are mediated by nuclear receptor proteins (RARs and RXRs) that bind retinoic acid with steroid and thyroid hormone receptors. The super family of nuclear proteins interact with specific genes and regulate their transcription. Retinoic acid has been found to stimulate, synergistically with thyroid hormone, the production of growth hormone in cultured pituitary cells. The RARs have been found to bind both the gene element responsive to RAR, in addition to the one responsive to tri-

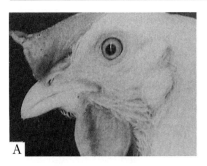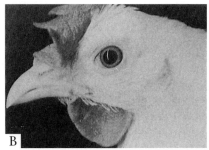

Fig. 2.5 The appearance of (**A**) the eye of a blind hen fed retinoic acid compared with (**B**) the normal eye of a hen fed retinol. (Courtesy of M.L. Scott, Cornell University.)

iodothyronine, suggesting that retinoic acid and the thyroid hormone control overlapping networks of genes. Many proteins appear during retinoic acid-induced cell differentiation.

Retinoids have a wide spectrum of biological activities. Retinoic acid plays an important role in growth and differentiation of embryonic tissues. It also regulates the differentiation of epithelial, connective, and hematopoietic tissues (Safonova et al., 1994). The nature of the growth and differentiation response elicited by retinoic acid depends upon cell type. Retinoic acid can be an inhibitor of many cell types with a potential to reduce adipose tissues in meat-producing animals (Suryawan and Hu, 1997).

Evidence indicates a morphogenic role for retinoic acid and one of its metabolites, 3,4-didehydroretinoic acid (Anonymous, 1991). Morphogens form concentration gradients or morphogenic fields through developing tissues that specify the eventual three-dimensional structure at maturity. Cell differentiation in the developing chick limb bud has been studied where vitamin A morphogens are operative. Cells of the limb bud can differentiate into muscle, cartilage, and bone cells.

Vision

The physiological function of vitamin A that has been most clearly defined on a biochemical basis is its role in vision (Wald, 1968). Vitamin A is an essential component of vision. Retinol is utilized in the aldehyde form (*trans*- form to 11-*cis*-retinal) in the retina of the eye as the prosthetic group in rhodopsin for dim light vision (rods) and as the prosthetic group in iodopsin for bright light and color vision (cones). When 11-*cis*-retinal (aldehyde form of vitamin A) is combined with the protein opsin, rhodopsin (visual purple) is produced. Chemical reactions involved in vision and the roles that *trans*-retinal and 11-*cis*-retinal play in this function are presented in Fig. 2.6. Rhodopsin breaks down in the physiological process of sight as a result of photochemical reaction. The all-*trans*- retinaldehyde cannot form a stable complex with the opsin. Opsin opens through a series of changes that expose reactive groups. Finally, retinaldehyde is hydrolyzed off the opsin. The energy derived from this reaction is transported to the brain via the optic nerve and recorded in various intensities depending on the amount of light entering the eye.

Vitamin A deficiency, in terms of the need for the resynthesis of rhodopsin, results in night blindness (nyctalopia), which is a clinical sign in both animals and humans. During the reactions in the retina, some of the vitamin A is lost and is replaced by vitamin A from blood. If vitamin A blood level is too low, a functional night blindness will result. The deficiency first manifests itself as a slow adaptation to the dark, and progresses to total night blindness. At dusk or in moonlight, livestock with night blindness will bump into obstacles (Fig. 2.7) intentionally placed in their path, or into logs or stumps when driven at night.

In vitamin A deficiency, the outer segments of the rods lose their opsin, leading to their eventual degeneration. The entire structure

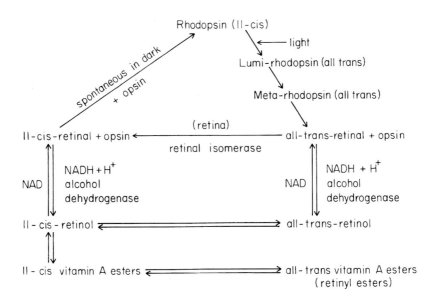

Fig. 2.6 The role of vitamin A in vision. (Adapted from Wald, 1968.)

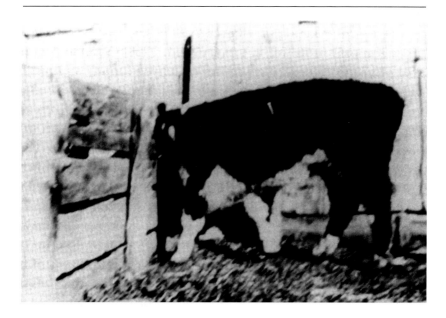

Fig. 2.7 A blind steer with vitamin A deficiency walks into a fence. (Courtesy of T.B. Keith, University of Idaho.)

becomes filled with tubules and vesicles. On a molecular basis, collagenase activity is increased in vitamin A deficiency. Retinoic acid has been shown to inhibit the enzyme collagenase by forming an inactive protein complex with the liganded nuclear retinoic acid receptors (Wolf, 1992). Even at a late stage, it is possible to regenerate rods, but continued deficiency results in disintegration of cones and total blindness. Vitamin A is needed for integrity of the visual cells as well as their normal regeneration.

Other eye clinical signs vary markedly among species, some of which represent secondary infections. Vision also can be impaired in xerophthalmia. Xerophthalmia is an advanced stage of vitamin A deficiency seen in all species. In children, dogs, foxes, and rats, xerophthalmia is characterized by a dry condition of the cornea and conjunctiva, cloudiness, and ulceration. Copious lacrimation is a more prominent eye sign in cows (Fig. 2.8) and horses. In chickens, on the other hand, the secretions of the tear glands dry up and an infection may then occur, resulting in a discharge that causes the lids to stick together. Some of these conditions develop as a result of basic epithelial changes caused by a deficiency of vitamin A (Maynard et al., 1979).

33

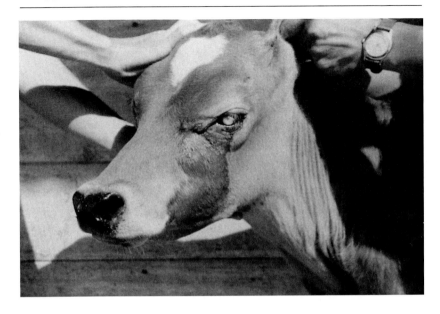

Fig. 2.8 Calf in the Philippines shows vitamin A deficiency characterized by copious lacrimation and blindness. The 6-month-old animal had been fed reconstituted skim milk powder and poor-quality bleached hay (practically devoid of carotene). (Courtesy of J.K. Loosli, University of Florida.)

Maintenance of Normal Epithelium

Vitamin A is required for maintenance of epithelial cells, which form protective linings on many of the body's organs. The respiratory, gastrointestinal, and urogenital tracts, as well as the eye, are protected from environmental influences by mucous membranes. If, however, there is a deficiency of vitamin A, epithelial cells that make up the membrane will change their characteristic structure. It is postulated that vitamin A plays an important role in altering permeability of lipoprotein membranes of cells and of intracellular particles. Vitamin A penetrates lipoprotein membranes and, at optimum levels, may act as a cross-linkage agent between the lipid and protein, thus stabilizing the membrane (Scott et al., 1982).

The normal mucus-secreting cells of epithelium in various locations throughout the body become replaced by a stratified, keratinized epithelium when vitamin A is deficient. Keratinized epithelium allows pathogen entry through the skin, lung, gastrointestinal tract, and urogenital tract surface. Vitamin A deficiency can impair regeneration of normal mucosal epithelium damaged by infection or inflammation (Ahmed et al., 1990; Stephensen et al., 1993) and thus could increase the severity of an infectious episode and/or prolong recovery from that episode. Adequate dietary vitamin A is necessary to help maintain normal resistance to stress and disease.

Studies have shown that the epithelial cells from vitamin A-deficient animals fail to differentiate to mucus-secreting cells, and mesenchymal cells fail to differentiate beyond the blast stage. This occurs in the alimentary, genital, reproductive, respiratory, and urinary tracts. Such altered characteristics make affected tissues more susceptible to infection. Thus, colds and pneumonia are typical secondary effects of vitamin A deficiency. Adequate dietary vitamin A is necessary to help maintain normal resistance to stress and disease. However, greater than optimal intakes of vitamin A will not aid in preventing infections.

There are many noninfective problems due to keratinization of epithelium, such as diarrhea. The formation of kidney and bladder stones is favored when damaged epithelium interferes with normal secretion and elimination of urine, and sloughed keratinized cells may form foci for the formation of stones. There is a specific interference with reproduction caused by altered epithelium that is of great importance. Squamous metaplasia in the parotid gland is an early change in vitamin A-deficient calves and proves useful in diagnosing deficiency. Elevated cerebrospinal fluid pressure observed in vitamin A-deficient animals, a very sensitive measure of the onset of vitamin A deficiency, is the result of cell changes. Increased ground substance in the dura mater surrounding the arachnoid villus and altered epithelial cells cause a decreased absorption of the fluid.

There is evidence that vitamin A is necessary for the formation of large molecules containing glucosamine (Goodman, 1980). These are the mucopolysaccharides occurring in almost all tissues of mammalian organisms but principally in the mucus-secreting epithelia and in the extracellular matrix of cartilage, mainly as chondroitin sulfate. The intimate involvement of vitamin A in the biosynthesis of glycoproteins, which are constitutents of membrane systems in cells, helps explain many biological effects of this vitamin.

In severe vitamin A deficiency, abnormalities in both RNA metabolism and protein synthesis have been reported. These changes in nucleic acid metabolism and protein synthesis may, however, reflect secondary effects of deficiency rather than the primary function of the vitamin.

Reproduction

In most livestock, the absence of vitamin A in the ration will dramatically reduce reproductive ability. Hatchability is significantly reduced when hens are fed a vitamin A-deficient ration. One of the first signs of vitamin A deficiency in rabbits is a reduction in fertility and an increased incidence of abortion in pregnant does.

In a number of species, vitamin A deficiency in the male results in a decline in sexual activity and failure of spermatogenesis, and in the female results in the resorption of the fetus, abortion, or birth of dead offspring. Retained placenta may be a characteristic of vitamin A deficiency in some species. Often the reproductive problems associated with vitamin A deficiency are actually the result of failure to maintain healthy epithelium.

Degeneration of germinal epithelium and seminiferous tubules and cessation of spermatogenesis in vitamin A-deficient rats are not prevented by retinoic acid. However, vitamin A-deficient rats had lowered testosterone levels that were restored by retinoic acid. Since retinoic acid cannot restore the germinal epithelium in vitamin A-deficient rats, these results indicate a role for retinoic acid in testosterone synthesis (Anonymous, 1977).

Bone Development

Vitamin A has a role in the normal development of bone through control exercised over the activity of osteoclasts of the epithelial cartilage. In vitamin A deficiency, osteoclast (reabsorbing bone) activity is reduced, resulting in excessive deposition of periosteal bone by the apparently unchecked function of osteoblasts (depositing bone). Disorganized bone growth and irritation of the joints are two manifestations of vitamin A deficiencies. In some cases, there is a constriction of the openings through which the optic and auditory nerves pass, thereby resulting in blindness and/or deafness.

Bone changes may also be responsible for the muscle incoordination and other nervous symptoms shown by vitamin A-deficient cattle, sheep, and swine. These changes may be involved in the increase in cerebrospinal fluid pressure shown to be characteristic of the deficiency. While the pathological basis is unknown, several studies have shown that a lack of vitamin A causes congenital malformation in certain soft tissues (Maynard et al., 1979). Examples are the birth of pigs without eyeballs and hydrocephalus in rabbits.

Relationship to Immunological Response and Disease Conditions

Animals deficient in vitamin A will show increased frequency and severity of bacterial, protozoal, and viral infections as well as other disease conditions. Part of disease resistance, as a function of vitamin A, is related to maintenance of mucous membranes and normal functioning of the adrenal gland for production of corticosteroids needed to combat disease. An animal's ability to resist disease depends on a responsive immune system, with a vitamin A deficiency causing a reduced immune response (Semba, 1998).

Vitamin A deficiency affects immune function, particularly the antibody response to T-cell–dependent antigens (Ross, 1992). The RAR-α mRNA expression and antigen-specific proliferative responses of T lymphocytes are influenced by vitamin A status in vivo and are directly modulated by retinoic acid (Halevy et al., 1994). Vitamin A deficiency affects a number of cells of the immune system, and that repletion with retinoic acid effectively reestablishes the number of circulating lymphocytes (Zhao and Ross, 1995).

A diminished primary antibody response could also increase the severity and/or duration of an episode of infection, whereas a diminished secondary response could increase the risk of developing a second episode of infection. Vitamin A deficiency causes decreased phagocytic activity in macrophages and neutrophils. The secretory immunoglobulin (Ig) A system is an important first line of defense against infections of mucosal surfaces (McGhee et al., 1992). Several studies in animal models have shown that the intestinal IgA response is impaired by vitamin A deficiency (Davis and Sell, 1989; Wiedermann et al., 1993; Stephensen et al., 1996).

An optimal vitamin A range exists for enhancement of vitamin A responses, because both deficient status and excessive status suppress immune function. In many experiments with laboratory and domestic animals, the effects of both clinical and subclinical deficiencies of vitamin A on the production of antibodies and on the resistance of the different tissues against microbial infection or parasitic infestation have frequently been demonstrated (Kelley and Easter, 1987). Supplemental vitamin A improved the health of animals infected with roundworms, of hens infected with *Capillaria* organisms, and of rats with hookworms (Herrick, 1972). Vitamin A is valuable in treating ringworm (*Trichophyton verrucosum*) infection in cattle.

Vitamin A-deficient chicks showed rapid loss of lymphocytes, and deficient rats showed atrophy of the thymus and spleen and reduced response to diphtheria and tetanus toxoids (Krishnan et al., 1974). Mortality from fowl typhoid (*Salmonella gallinarum*) was reduced in chicks fed vitamin A levels greater than the normal levels in a high-protein diet. Serum antibody levels in chicks were increased twofold to fivefold by high dietary vitamin A concentrations. The immune response to introduced Newcastle disease virus was higher in broiler chicks receiving 2,500 IU of vitamin A than in controls, and was best in those receiving 20,000 IU (Serman and Mazija, 1985). Harmon et al. (1963) studied the effect of a vitamin A deficiency on antibody production by baby pigs and found a high correlation coefficient between serum vitamin A and antibody titer. Baby pigs infected with *Trichuris suis* responded to supplemental vitamin A with an enhanced immunological response compared with controls (Bebravicius et al., 1987).

Vitamin A and β–carotene have important roles in protecting animals against numerous infections, including mastitis. A protective effect of dietary vitamin A supplementation against experimental *Staphylococcus aureus* mastitis in mice has been reported (Chew et al., 1984). Potential pathogens are regularly present in the teat orifice, and under suitable circumstances can invade and initiate clinical mastitis. Any unhealthy state of the epithelium would increase susceptibility of a mammary gland to invasion by pathogens. There are reports of improved mammary health in dairy cows supplemented with β–carotene and vitamin A during the dry (Dahlquist and Chew, 1985) and lactating (Chew and Johnston, 1985) periods.

In vitamin A-deficient animals, incidence of cancer has been shown to be higher than in animals receiving normal vitamin A intakes. In some special cases, administration of toxic doses of vitamin A caused a regression of tumors. Extreme toxicity of natural vitamin A makes it an ineffective drug for treatment of certain types of neoplasms. Synthetic analogs (retinoids) of vitamin A, however, have been successfully used to prevent cancer of the skin, lung, bladder, and breast in experimental animals. This is a pharmacological approach to prevention of cancer by enhancement of intrinsic epithelial defense mechanisms. Synthetic retinoids are superior for this purpose (Goodman, 1980). In humans, studies suggest that diets rich in β–carotene provide a blocking or inhibition of certain types of cancer, including lung cancer (even in people who smoke). Also, skin diseases, including psoriasis, cystic acne, and rosacea have responded exceptionally well to synthetic retinoids.

REQUIREMENTS

Extensive research has been conducted to determine the vitamin A requirements of various species. Requirements have been published in the United States by the Committee on Animal Nutrition of the National Academy of Science-National Research Council. Vitamin A requirements can be expressed on the basis of IU per kilogram of body weight, on a daily basis, or as a unit of diet. In agreement with general practice, the requirements are normally expressed per unit of diet rather than per kilogram of body weight.

Minimum requirements have been determined by various methods, including amounts required to prevent night blindness, amounts required for storage and reproduction, and maintenance of normal pressure in the cerebrospinal fluid. The minimum vitamin A requirement for normal growth may be lower than the amount required for higher growth rates, resistance to various diseases, and normal bone development. It was suggested that calves born with low vitamin A liver stores should receive a minimum of 16,500 IU/100 kg body weight, and that three to five times this level are necessary for adequate vitamin A liver stores in calves during the critical first few months of life.

Table 2.2 summarizes the vitamin A requirements for various species; a more complete listing is provided in Appendix Table A1a. These requirements are deemed sufficient to provide optimal growth; satisfactory reproduction and milk, egg, or wool production; and prevention of deficiency signs. The requirements presented are designed to be adequate for these purposes under practical conditions of feeding and management and to allow for a certain amount of storage. The decision as to the minimum vitamin A requirement of young swine depends upon whether the criterion to determine the requirements is based upon growth and feed utilization or also considers liver vitamin A storage. Storage of vitamin A in the liver certainly appears to be desirable since under conditions of little or no liver storage, stresses and diseases may precipitate vitamin A deficiency. The vitamin A reserves of the sow make it difficult to establish requirements. Braude et al. (1941) reported that mature sows fed diets without supplemental vitamin A completed three pregnancies normally; only in the fourth pregnancy did deficiency signs appear. Gilts receiving adequate vitamin A levels until 9 months of age completed two reproductive cycles without signs of vitamin A deficiency (Selke et al., 1967).

■ Table 2.2 Vitamin A Requirements for Various Animals and for Humans

Animal	Purpose or Class	Requirement[a]	Reference
Beef cattle	Feedlot cattle	2,200 IU/kg	NRC (1996)
	Pregnant heifers and cows	2,800 IU/kg	NRC (1996)
	Lactating cows and bulls	3,900 IU/kg	NRC (1996)
Dairy cattle	Growing	2,200 IU/kg	NRC (1989a)
	Lactating cows and bulls	3,200 IU/kg	NRC (1989a)
	Calf milk replacer	3,800 IU/kg	NRC (1989a)
Goat	All classes	5,000 IU/kg	Morand-Fehr (1981)
Chicken	Leghorn, 0–18 weeks	1,500 IU/kg	NRC (1994)
	Laying (100-g intake)	2,000 IU/kg	NRC (1994)
	Broilers	1,500 IU/kg	NRC (1994)
Geese	Growing	1,500 IU/kg	NRC (1994)
	Breeding	4,000 IU/kg	NRC (1994)
Turkey	Growing and breeding	5,000 IU/kg	NRC (1994)
Sheep	Replacement ewes, 60 kg	1,567 IU/kg	NRC (1985b)
	Pregnancy, 70 kg	3,306 IU/kg	NRC (1985b)
	Lactation, 70 kg	2,380 IU/kg	NRC (1985b)
	Replacement rams, 80–100 kg	1,976 IU/kg	NRC (1985b)
Swine	Growing 5–10 kg	2,200 IU/kg	NRC (1998)
	Growing, 20–120 kg	1,300 IU/kg	NRC (1998)
	Pregnant swine and boars	4,000 IU/kg	NRC (1998)
	Lactating	2,000 IU/kg	NRC (1998)
Horse	Growing, maintenance and working	2,000 IU/kg	NRC (1989b)
	Pregnancy and lactation	3,000 IU/kg	NRC (1989b)
Mink	Growing	5,930 IU/kg	NRC (1982a)
Fox	Growing	2,440 IU/kg	NRC (1982a)
Cat	Gestation	6,000 IU/kg	NRC (1986)
Dog	Growing	3,336 IU/kg	NRC (1985a)
Rabbit	Growing	580 IU/kg	NRC (1977)
	Gestation	1,160 IU/kg	NRC (1977)
Fish	Catfish	1,000–2,000 IU/kg	NRC (1993)
	Common carp	1,000–2,000 IU/kg	NRC (1993)
	Rainbow trout	2,500 IU/kg	NRC (1993)
Rat	Growing and reproduction	2,300 IU/kg	NRC (1995)
Mouse	Growing	2,400 IU/kg	NRC (1995)
Nonhuman primate	All classes	10,000 IU/kg	NRC (1978)
Human	Children	400–700 µg RE[b]	RDA (1989)
	Adults	800–1,000 µg/RE	RDA (1989)
	Lactating	1,200–1,300 µg/RE	RDA (1989)

[a]Expressed as per unit of animal feed either on as-fed (approximately 90% dry matter) or dry basis (see Appendix, Tables A1a,b). Human data are expressed as µg/day.
[b]Retinol equivalent (RE): 1 RE = 1 µg retinol or 6 µg β-carotene.

In establishing a satisfactory vitamin A level for practical diets, it is necessary to consider a number of factors that may alter the vitamin A requirement. Type and level of production are important as greater production rates increase requirements. Pregnancy, lactation, and egg production also lead to higher requirements. Other practical factors are listed in Table 2.3.

■ Table 2.3   Factors Influencing Vitamin A Requirements

Genetic differences (species, breed, strain)

Carryover effect of stored vitamin A (principally in the liver but the kidney is also important for cats)

Conversion efficiency of carotenes to vitamin A

Variations in level, type, and isomerization of carotenoid vitamin A precursors in feedstuffs

Presence of adequate bile in vivo

Destruction of vitamin A in feeds through oxidation, prolonged storage, high pelleting temperatures, catalytic effects of trace minerals, and peroxidizing effects of rancid fats

Presence of disease and/or parasites

Environmental stress and temperature

Adequacy of dietary fat, protein, zinc, phosphorus, and antioxidants (including vitamin E, vitamin C, and selenium)

Pelleting and subsequent storage of feed

Different species of animals convert β–carotene to vitamin A with varying degrees of efficiency. The conversion rate of the rat has been used as the standard value, with 1 μg of β–carotene equal to 1,667 IU of vitamin A. The comparative efficiencies of various species are shown in Table 2.4, based on this standard. Of the species studied, only poultry are equal to rats in vitamin conversion; cattle are only 24% as efficient.

Some factors that influence the rate at which carotenoids are converted to vitamin A are type of carotenoid, class and production level of animal, individual genetic differences in animals, and level of carotene intake (NRC, 1996). Efficiency of vitamin A conversion from β–carotene is decreased with higher levels of intake (Van Vliet et al., 1996) (Table 2.5). As β–carotene level is increased, conversion efficiency drops from a ratio of 2:1 to 5:1 for the chicken and from 8:1 to 16:1 for the calf (Bauernfeind, 1972).

Stress conditions, such as extremely hot weather, viral infection, and altered thyroid function, have also been suggested as causes for reduced conversion efficiency of carotene to vitamin A. Vitamin A requirements are higher under stressful conditions such as abnormal temperatures or exposure to disease. For example, with poultry, coccidiosis not only causes destruction of vitamin A in the gut but also injures the microvilli of the intestinal wall, thereby decreasing absorption of vitamin A and at the same time causing the chickens to stop eating for several days (Scott et al., 1982).

■ Table 2.4   Conversion of β-Carotene to Vitamin A by Different Animals

Animal	Conversion of mg of β-Carotene to IU of Vitamin A (mg) (IU)	IU of vitamin A Activity (Calculated from Carotene) (%)
Standard	1 = 1,667	100
Beef cattle	1 = 400	24
Dairy cattle	1 = 400	24
Sheep	1 = 400–450	24–30
Swine	1 = 500	30
Horse		
Growing	1 = 555	33.3
Pregnant	1 = 333	20
Poultry	1 = 1,667	100
Dog	1 = 833	50
Rat	1 = 1,667	100
Fox	1 = 278	16.7
Cat	Carotene not utilized	—
Mink	Carotene not utilized	—
Human	1 = 556	33.3

Sources: Adapted from Beeson (1965) and United States-Canadian Tables of Feed Composition (NRC, 1982b).

Likewise, other factors may affect metabolism and increase vitamin A requirements. These include free nitrates in feeds, inadequate protein, zinc deficiency, and low dietary phosphorus (Harris, 1975). Considerable work and controversy have been reported on the relationship between nitrates and vitamin A nutrition. In a review of this subject, Rumsey (1975) concluded that although nitrates can be shown to have an adverse effect on vitamin A in vitro, this does not appear to translate into a significant effect under most feeding conditions.

The efficiency of β–carotene in meeting the vitamin A requirement of trout and salmon apparently is dependent on water temperature. Cold-water fish utilize precursors of vitamin A at 12.4 to 14°C but not at 9°C (Poston et al., 1977). Activity of β–carotene-15,15′-dioxygenase, which oxidizes β–carotene to retinal in the intestinal mucosa, may be restricted at cold temperatures.

In humans the recommended allowance for adult females is set at 80% of that for males or 800 retinol equivalents (4,000 IU) (RDA, 1989). The allowance during lactation is increased to 1,200 retinol equivalents to provide for vitamin A secreted in milk. Daily vitamin A requirements for children (10 years or younger) vary between 400 and 700 µg retinol equivalents.

■ Table 2.5   Equivalence of β-Carotene and Retinol at Different Dietary Concentrations in Rats

Dose of β-Carotene (μmol/kg BW)	Relative Molar Biopotency (%)	Moles β-Carotene Equivalent to 1 mol Retinol	μg β-Carotene Equivalent to 1 mol Retinol
< 0.3	100.0	1.0	1.84
1	50.0	2.0	3.75
2	30.0	3.3	6.25
6	15.4	6.5	12.20
12	9.5	10.5	19.70
48	4.3	23.3	43.60

Source: Adapted from Brubacher and Weiser (1985).

NATURAL SOURCES

The richest sources of vitamin A are fish oils. Some swordfish liver oils contain as many as 250,000 IU of vitamin A per gram. Halibut liver oil may contain even more. Thus, both are many times more potent than cod liver oils. Products from the same species, however, may be highly variable in potency; thus, in their manufacture for use as a vitamin A supplement, they are subjected to a biological assay so that the user may be assured of a certain minimum potency. Among the common foods of animal origin, milk fat, egg yolk, and liver are rated as rich sources, but this is not the case if the animal from which they came has been receiving a vitamin A-deficient diet for an extended period. Since the vitamin is present in the fat, skim milk contains very little. The effect of dietary vitamin A on egg yolk concentration was reported by Hill (1961). Vitamin A concentrations of 1,760, 4,400, and 22,000 IU/kg feed resulted in vitamin A yolk levels of 0.9, 6.3, and 16.3 IU/g, respectively.

Sources of supplemental vitamin A are derived primarily from fish liver oils, in which the vitamin occurs largely in esterified form, and from industrial chemical synthesis. Before the era of the chemical production of vitamin A, the principal source of vitamin A concentrates was the liver and/or body oils of marine fish. Since industrial synthesis was developed in 1949, the synthetic form has become the major source of the vitamin to meet the requirements of domestic animals and humans. The synthetic vitamin usually is produced as the all-*trans*-retinyl palmitate or acetate.

Provitamin A carotenoids, mainly β–carotene in green feeds, are the

43

principal source of vitamin A for grazing livestock. All green parts of growing plants are rich in carotene and therefore have a high vitamin A value. In fact, the degree of green color in a roughage is a good index of its carotene content. Although the yellow color of carotenoids is masked by chlorophyll, all green parts of growing plants are rich in carotene and thus have a high vitamin A value. Good pasture always provides a liberal supply, and type of pasture plant—whether grass or legume—appears to be of minor importance. At maturity, however, leaves contain much more than stems, and thus legume hay is richer in vitamin content than grass hay (Maynard et al., 1979). With all hays and other forage, vitamin A value decreases after the bloom stage. Plants at maturity can have 50% or less of the maximum carotenoid value of immature plants.

Both carotene and vitamin A are destroyed by oxidation, and this is the most common cause of any depreciation that may occur in the potency of sources. The process is accelerated at high temperatures, but heat without oxygen has a minor effect. Butter exposed in thin layers in air at 50°C loses all its vitamin A potency in 6 hours, but in the absence of air there is little destruction at 120°C over the same period. Cod liver oil in a tightly corked bottle has shown activity after 31 years, but it may lose all its potency in a few weeks when incorporated in a feed mixture stored under usual conditions (Maynard et al., 1979).

Much of carotene content is destroyed by oxidation in the process of field curing. Russell (1929) found that there may be a loss of more than 80% of the carotene in alfalfa during the first 24 hours of the curing process. This loss occurs chiefly during daylight hours, partly because of photochemical activation of the destructive process. In alfalfa leaves, sunlight-sensitized destruction comprises 7 to 8% of the total pigment destroyed, while enzymatic destruction comprises 27 to 28% (Bauernfeind, 1972). Enzymatic destruction requires oxygen, is greatest at high temperatures, and ceases after complete dehydration.

Hays that are cut in the bloom stage or earlier and cured without exposure to rain or too much sun retain a considerable proportion of their carotene content, while those cut in the seed stage and exposed to rain and sun for extended periods lose most of it. Green hay curing in the swath may lose half its vitamin A activity in one day's exposure to sunlight and almost all of it if left exposed to rain as well as sunlight. Thus, hay usually has only a small proportion of the carotene content of fresh grass. Under similar conditions of curing, alfalfa and other legume hays are much richer than grass hays because of their leafy nature, but a poor grade of alfalfa may have less than a good grade of grass hay (Maynard et al., 1979).

The carotene content of dried or sun-cured forages decreases in storage with the rate of destruction depending on factors such as temperature, exposure to air and sunlight, and length of storage. Under average conditions, carotene content of hay can be expected to decrease by about 6 to 7% per month. In artificial curing of hay with a "hay drier," there is only a slight loss of carotene because of the rapidity of the process and protection against exposure to oxygen, with the final product having 2 to10 times the value of field-cured hay. Severe heating of hay in the mow or stack reduces vitamin content, and there is a gradual loss in storage, so old hay is poorer than new. Aside from yellow corn and its by-products, practically all the concentrates used in feeding animals are devoid of vitamin A value, or nearly so. In addition, yellow corn contains a high proportion of non-β–carotenoids (e.g., cryptoxanthin, lutein, and zeacarotene) that contain much less or no vitamin A value compared to β–carotene.

The potency of yellow corn is only about one-eighth that of good roughage. Roots and tubers as a class supply practically no vitamin A, but carrots are a very rich source, as are sweet potatoes, as might be expected from their yellow color. Pumpkins and squash also supply considerable amounts, and green leafy vegetables used in human nutrition are rich in carotene (Maynard et al., 1979). Tankage, meat scraps, and similar animal by-products have little if any vitamin A potency. Certain fish meals are fair sources, but variation in the raw material and in methods of processing may entirely destroy any potency originally present.

There is evidence that yellow corn may lose carotene rapidly during storage. For instance, a hybrid corn high in carotene lost about half of its carotene in 8 months of storage at 25°C and about three-quarters in 3 years. Less carotene was lost during storage at 7°C (Quackenbush, 1963). Bioavailability of natural β–carotene is less than chemically synthesized forms (Hussein and El-Tohamy, 1990; White et al., 1993). Using ferrets, all-*trans* β–carotene was less bioavailable from carrot juice than from β–carotene beadlet-fortified beverages (White et al., 1993). In calves, a small enhancing effect of mild heat treatment of carrots on serum and tissue accumulation of carotenoids has been reported (Poor et al., 1993).

In forages, carotene in alfalfa hay may be more bioavailable than that in grass hay (NRC, 1989b). A marked discrepancy exists between the carotene content of corn silage and the vitamin A status of ruminants fed corn silage. On the average, corn silage carotenes were found to be about two-thirds as effective as β–carotene for maintaining liver stores in rats (Miller et al., 1969; Rumsey, 1975). Martin et al. (1971) report-ed five times less carotenes in October and November corn silage than in September corn silage. More mature silages were not able to sustain liver vitamin A stores in beef steers, particularly if the ensiled corn plant was finely chopped. Diets high in corn silage harvested after a killing frost and fed to cattle would be marginal in their supply of both vita-mins A and E. Miller et al. (1969) have reported that ethanol, sometimes found in corn silage as a product of fermentation, may reduce liver vita-min A stores as much as 26% by increasing mobilization of vitamin A from liver.

Wing (1969) reported carotene digestibility in plants to be greater during the warmer months. Variations were found in the digestibility of carotenes in plants according to year, species of plant, dry matter con-tent, and form of forage; carotene digestiblity was somewhat lower in silages than in pastures or hay. Table 2.6 presents typical vitamin A val-ues of foods and carotene concentration of feeds. As noted earlier, degree of greenness in a roughage is a good index of its carotene con-tent. The data in Table 2.6 are useful for indicating the order of the dif-ferences found among various roughages differing as to color, kind, and other factors. Average published values of carotene content can serve only as approximate guides in feeding practice because of many factors affecting actual potency of individual samples as fed (NRC, 1982b).

Cooking processes commonly used in human food preparation do not cause much destruction to the vitamin potency. The blanching and freezing process generally causes little loss of carotenoid content in veg-etables and fruits. Heat, however, does isomerize the all-*trans*-carotenoids to *cis*-forms. In a report from Indonesia, isomerization dur-ing traditional cooking caused a loss of up to 9% of vitamin A potency (Van der Pol et al., 1988). Hydrogenation of fats lessens their vitamin A value, while saponification does not destroy the vitamin if oxidation is avoided.

Several factors can influence the loss of vitamin A from feedstuffs during storage. The trace minerals in feeds and supplements, particular-ly copper, are detrimental to vitamin A stability. Dash and Mitchell (1976) reported the vitamin A content of 1,293 commercial feeds over a 3-year period. The loss of vitamin A was over 50% in 1 year's time. Vitamin A loss in commercial feeds was evident even if the commercial feeds contained stabilized vitamin A supplements. The stability of vita-min A in feeds and premixes has been improved tremendously in recent years by chemical stabilization as an ester and by physical protection using antioxidants, emulsifying agents, gelatin, and sugar in spray-dried,

■ **Table 2.6   Vitamin A (Retinol) and β-Carotene Content of Feeds**

Vitamin A Source	Vitamin A (IU/g)
Whale liver oil	400,000
Swordfish liver oil	250,000
Halibut liver oil	240,000
Herring liver oil	211,000
Tuna liver oil	150,000
Shark liver oil	150,000
Bonito liver oil	120,000
White sea bass liver oil	50,000
Barracuda liver oil	40,000
Dogfish liver oil	12,000
Seal liver oil	10,000
Cod liver oil	4,000
Sardine body oil	750
Pilchard body oil	500
Menhaden body oil	340
Butter	35
Cheese	14
Eggs	10
Milk	1.5

Carotene Source	Carotene (mg/kg)
Fresh green legumes and grasses, immature (wet basis)	33–88
Dehydrated alfalfa meal, fresh, dehydrated without field curing, very bright green	242–297
Dehydrated alfalfa meal after considerable time in storage, bright green	110–154
Alfalfa leaf meal, bright green	120–176
Legume hays, including alfalfa, very quickly cured with minimum sun exposure, bright green, leafy	77–88
Legume hays, including alfalfa, good green color, leafy	40–59
Legume hays, including alfalfa, partly bleached, moderate amount of green color	20–31
Legume hays, including alfalfa, badly bleached, or discolored, traces of green color	9–18
Non-legume hays, including timothy, cereal, and prairie hays, well cured, good green color	20–31
Non-legume hays, average quality, bleached, some green color	9–18
Legume silage (wet basis)	11–44
Corn and sorghum silages, medium to good green color (wet basis)	4–22
Grains, mill feeds, protein concentrates, and by-product concentrates, except yellow corn and its by-products	0.02–0.44

Sources: Adapted from Scott et al. (1982) and Maynard et al. (1979).

beaded, or prilled products (Shields et al., 1982). Nevertheless, vitamin A supplements should not be stored for prolonged periods prior to feeding.

Vitamin A and carotene destruction also occurs from processing of feeds with steam and pressure. Pelleting effects on vitamin A in feed are caused by die thickness and hole size, which produce frictional heat and a shearing effect that can break supplemental vitamin A beadlets and expose the vitamin. In addition, steam application exposes feed to heat and moisture. Running fines back through the pellet mill exposes vitamin A to the same factors a second time. Between 30 and 40% of vitamin A present at mixing may be destroyed during pelleting (Shields et al., 1982).

DEFICIENCY

Effects of Deficiency

Vitamin A is necessary for normal vision in animals and humans, maintenance of healthy epithelial or surface tissues, and normal bone development. The vitamin A deficiency signs observed in ruminants vary somewhat, but most relate to these three changes in tissues. Numerous studies have also demonstrated increased frequency and severity of infection in vitamin A-deficient animals. Lack of vitamin A results in decreased antibody production and impaired cell-mediated immune processes against infective agents (Davis and Sell, 1983). Clinical signs may be specific for vitamin A deficiency, or only general signs may be observed, including loss of appetite, loss of weight, unthrifty appearance, thick nasal discharge, and reduced fertility. The normal epithelium in various locations throughout the body becomes replaced by a stratified, keratinized epithelium when vitamin A is deficient. This effect has been noted in the respiratory, alimentary, reproductive, and genitourinary tract as well as in the eye. A wide range of signs of vitamin A deficiency are noted in Table 2.7.

Ruminants

Ruminants lacking vitamin A may be more susceptible to pinkeye or other diseases related to the mucous membranes. Keratinization lowers the resistance of the epithelial tissues to the entrance of infectious organisms. Thus respiratory diseases, such as colds and sinus infections, tend to be more severe when vitamin A is deficient.

Vitamin A deficiency could indirectly result from zinc deficiency. Zinc deficiency, interferes with the synthesis of retinol-binding protein (RBP) in liver, which carries vitamin A (retinol) in plasma. Thus, in zinc deficiency, decreased liver RBP levels may cause low concentrations of plasma vitamin A. Zinc-deficient goats have been observed to have low serum vitamin A despite adequate dietary vitamin A (Chhabra et al., 1980). In calves, serum vitamin A was significantly higher for animals

■ Table 2.7   Signs of Vitamin A Deficiency

General
  Cessation of growth
  Cystic pituitary glands
  Death
  Decline in body weight
  Diarrhea (scours)
  Failure of appetite
  General edema
  Reduced resistance to parasite infections
  Untidy hair or feathers
  Xerosis of membranes
Bone Formation
  Cancellous bone
  Defective modeling
  Narrowing of foramina
  Restriction of brain cavity
Congential Abnormalities
  Anophthalmia
  Aortic arch deformities
  Cleft palate
  Hydrocephalus
  Kidney deformities
  Microophthalmia
Defective Reproduction
  Abnormal estrous cycle
  Dead, weak, or blind offspring
  Degeneration of testes
  Reduced egg production and hatchability
  Resorption of fetuses
Eyes
  Keratomalacia
  Lacrimation
  Night blindness (nyctalopia)
  Xerophthalmia
  Constriction of optic nerve
  Loss of lens
  Opacity of cornea
  Papilledema

Liver
  Degeneration of Kupffer's cells
  Metaplasia of bile ducts
Nervous System
  Constriction at foramina
  Convulsive seizure
  Hydrocephalus
  Incoordination and staggering gait
  Paresis
  Raised cerebrospinal fluid pressure
  Twisting of nerve
Respiratory System
  Lung abscesses
  Metaplasia of nasal passages
  Nasal discharge
  Pneumonia
Urinary System
  Cystitis
  Nephrosis
  Pus in ureters
  Pyelitis
  Thickening of bladder wall
  Urolithiasis

Source: Modified from Bauernfeind and DeRitter (1972).

supplemented with 50 mg/kg zinc (Chhabra and Arora, 1987). Cattle from tropical northern Australia showed a 12% annual mortality in part because of a slow release of liver vitamin A (Guerin, 1981). Apparently, high calcium and low forage zinc concentrations contributed to this slow liver vitamin A release. Since tropical forages have often been shown to be low in zinc (McDowell, 1997), conditioned vitamin A deficiency may result even though liver vitamin A values indicate adequate concentrations of this vitamin.

VITAMIN A DEFICIENCY IN CATTLE

In cattle, signs of vitamin A deficiency (Figs. 2.9–2.11) include reduced feed intake, rough hair coat, edema of the joints and brisket, lacrimation, xerophthalmia, night blindness, slow growth, blindness, low conception rates, abortion, stillbirths, blind calves, abnormal semen, reduced libido, and susceptibility to respiratory and other infections (NRC, 1996). Animals in advanced stages of deficiency may exhibit a staggering gait, convulsive seizures, and papilledema, resulting from elevated cerebrospinal fluid pressure.

The greatest need for vitamin A is during calving and breeding. If it is inadequate, calves may get pinkeye, pneumonia, or other diseases related to the mucous membranes. Vitamin A deficiency lowers reproductive efficiency in both males and females. Reduced libido and sterility in bulls with degeneration of seminiferous tubules has been reported (Larkin and Yates, 1964). Spermatozoa decrease in number and motility, and abnormal forms markedly increase. In cows, key indications of the deficiency are lowered conception rates; shortened pregnancies, either as abortions or reduced gestation length; high incidence of

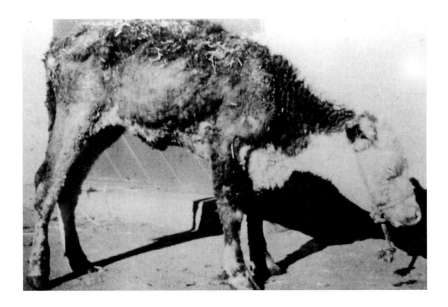

Fig. 2.9 Vitamin A-deficient calf. Note the emaciated appearance and evidence of diarrhea. The calf also shows excessive lacrimation and nasal discharge characteristic of vitamin A deficiency. (Courtesy of G. Patterson, Chas. Pfizer Inc.)

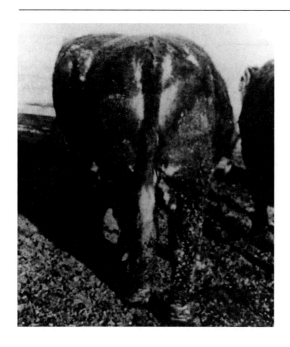

Fig. 2.10 Advanced
stage of anasarca in
hindquarters of vitamin
A-deficient steer.
(Courtesy of L.L.
Madsen, Washington
State University.)

retained placenta; and birth of dead, weak, incoordinated, or permanently blind calves caused by bone abnormalities in the optic foramen
that constricts the optic nerve (Miller, 1979). If born alive, weak calves
have trouble getting to their feet and lack the instinct to nurse. Vitamin
A-deficient newborn calves may have very severe diarrhea, which may
soon be followed by death. In young calves, signs of vitamin A deficiency also include watery eyes and nasal discharge, and sometimes muscular incoordination, staggering gait, and convulsive seizures. However, in
the calf, elevated cerebrospinal fluid pressure is the earliest change specific for vitamin A deficiency.

The classic sign of vitamin A deficiency in cattle is night blindness.
As vitamin A deficiency develops, the animal's adaptation to darkness is
reduced, and night blindness occurs; this condition is readily detected
when animals encounter obstacles in dim light. Blindness or night blindness may be the first noticeable sign of vitamin A deficiency in rapidly
growing cattle fed high-concentrate diets. In severe vitamin A deficiency, characteristic changes occur in the eye, including excessive watering,
keratitis, softening and cloudiness of the cornea, and development of
xerophthalmia characterized by drying of the conjunctiva. However, in
the eyes of cattle, copious lacrimation (rather than xerophthalmia) is the
most prominent clinical sign of vitamin A deficiency (Maynard et al.,

51

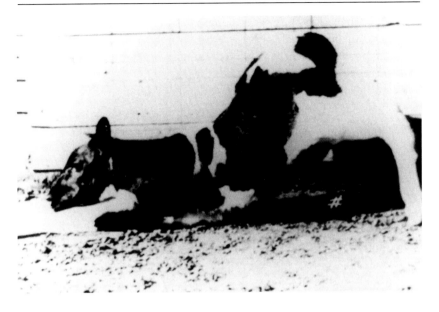

Fig. 2.11 Vitamin A-deficient calf shows incoordination and weakness. (Courtesy of J.W. Thomas, Michigan State University.)

1979). Blindness may follow eye infection caused by the deficiency.

Vitamin A is involved in normal bone development; when it is deficient, the bones are altered in shape during growth, and the teeth are affected. Failure of the spine and some other bones to develop normally results in pressure and degeneration of the nerves. For example, blindness in calves results from constriction of the optic nerve caused by a narrowing of the bone canal through which it passes (Maynard et al., 1979). Bone changes may also be responsible for muscular incoordination and other nervous signs shown by vitamin A-deficient cattle.

In finishing cattle, generalized edema may occur, with signs of lameness in the hock and knee joints and swelling in the brisket area (NRC, 1996). Booth et al. (1987) reported that feedlot cattle had low concentration of serum vitamin A; appeared blind; and had fixed dilated pupils, severe ataxia, and poor weight gains. Feedlot cattle with mild vitamin A deficiency reduce their feed intake and do not make satisfactory weight gains. Lowered feed intake may result in deficiencies of other nutrients when the diet is borderline in these nutrients.

As part of the major role of maintaining a healthy epithelium, vitamin A and β–carotene have been shown to have an important role in reducing the incidence and severity of mastitis in dairy cows (Oldham et al., 1986; Chew, 1987). A diet adequate in vitamin A and β–carotene are necessary for nutritional protection against this disease.

Vitamin A-deficient cattle have depressed activity of natural killer cells, decreased antibody production, decreased responsiveness of lymphocytes to mitogenic stimulation, and increased susceptibility to infection (Ross, 1992; Nonnecke et al., 1993; Michal et al., 1994; Rajaraman et al., 1998).

Vitamin A helps maintain normal immune resistance (immunostimulation), while the antioxidant activity of β–carotene increases the bactericidal activity of blood and milk polymorphonuclear neutrophils against *S. aureus* (Daniel et al., 1991). In addition, some studies have shown that β–carotene has a favorable effect on fertility of heifers and lactating cows (Bonsembiante et al., 1980). However, other studies (Akordor et al., 1986; Oldham et al., 1991) have shown no effect of β–carotene on reproductive performance or incidence of mastitis. Additional studies are needed to clarify the physiological role of β–carotene as differences in results may relate to different body stores of both β–carotene and vitamin A in experimental animals.

In the 1950s, it was discovered that cattle developed signs of vitamin A deficiency that was originally referred to as X disease (hyperkeratosis). This disease was due to feeds that contained highly chlorinated naphthalene found in lubricating oil. Because of the depressed vitamin A levels in blood plasma, it was concluded that the toxic substance interfered with the conversion of carotene to vitamin A (Maynard et al., 1979). Removal of naphthalenes from oils eliminated X disease.

Studies have shown that vitamin A-deficient cattle lack heat tolerance. Deficient cattle stood and panted considerably, and their daily feed consumption decreased (Perry, 1980), while vitamin A-supplemented cattle showed improved hot-weather tolerance and spent much of the time chewing their cud.

VITAMIN A DEFICIENCY IN SHEEP

Clinical signs of vitamin A deficiency in sheep (Fig. 2.12) are similar to those in cattle; night blindness is the common means of determining the deficiency (NRC, 1985). Vitamin A deficiency results in keratinization of the respiratory, alimentary, reproductive, and urinary tracts, and ocular epithelia. Keratinization causes lowered resistance to infections. The immune response is decreased in lambs with low vitamin A status (Bruns and Webb, 1990).

Additional clinical signs of vitamin A deficiency in sheep include growth retardation, bone malformation, degeneration of the reproduc-

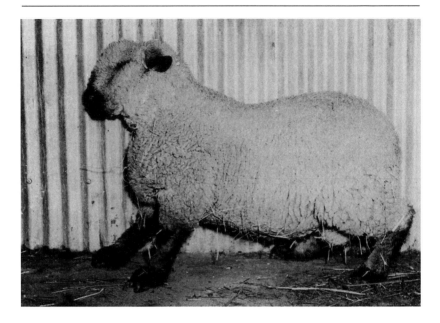

Fig. 2.12 Typical appearance of a vitamin A-deficient lamb. Note the extreme weakness and swayed back. This was followed by the inability to stand. (Courtesy of T.J. Cunha and Washington State University.)

tive organs, and elevated pressure in cerebrospinal fluid. Deficiency interferes with normal development of bone, which may relate to muscular incoordination and nervous signs. Vitamin A deficiency can also result in lambs born weak, malformed, or dead. In addition, retained placenta occurs in vitamin A-deficient ewes.

Vitamin A deficiency has resulted in low semen quality in rams (Lindley et al., 1949). Vitamin A deficiency has detrimental effects on wool production and characteristics, including shortened wool fibers and decreased fiber thickness, strength, and elongation (Farid and Ghanem, 1982).

VITAMIN A DEFICIENCY IN GOATS

In goats, vitamin A deficiency often appears first as a rough, dull hair coat condition. Goats deficient in vitamin A show keratinization of the epithelia of the respiratory, alimentary, reproductive, and urinary tracts, and of the eye (NRC, 1981). Signs include multiple infections, poor bone development, birth of abnormal offspring, and vision impairment. Night blindness is the classic sign of deficiency. Experimentally produced signs of vitamin A deficiency in goats include loss of appetite, loss of weight, unthrifty appearance, night blindness, and thick nasal discharge (Schmidt, 1941).

In India, limited work with vitamin A-deficient goats suggests that the deficiency may lead to urinary calculi (Majumdar and Gupta, 1960). Lack of vitamin A may produce temporarily impaired fertility or permanent infertility and, after kidding, metritis may be caused by damage to the integrity of the uterine mucosa (Guss, 1977). In fully grown goats, reduced fertility of the female and male is the more common clinical sign; the animals show poor conception rates during short or delayed heat periods, and reduced semen quality.

Swine

In pigs, the absence of vitamin A results principally in nervous signs such as unsteady gait, incoordination, trembling of the legs, spasms, and paralysis (Hentges et al., 1952) (Fig. 2.13). Eye lesions are less common. In pigs, the effect of vitamin A deficiency on appetite or rate of gain does not occur until eventual paralysis and weakness prohibit movement to the feeder (Cunha, 1977).

During reproduction and lactation, a vitamin A deficiency in the sow produces the following clinical signs: failure of estrus, resorption of young, wobbly gait, weaving and crossing of the hind legs while walking, dropping of the ears, curving with head down to one side, impaired vision, spasms, and loss of control of hindquarters and forequarters and thus inability to stand up (Cunha, 1977). Depending on degree of severity of vitamin A deficiency, fetuses were resorbed, born dead, or carried to term. Fetuses carried to term had a variety of defects, including various stages of arrested formation of the eyes as well as complete lack of eyeballs. Other defects included harelip, cleft palate, misplaced kidneys, accessory earlike growths, having only one eye, having one large and one small eye, and bilateral cryptorchidism (Cunha, 1977). Vitamin A appears to improve reproductive performance of gilts by decreasing embryonic mortality, resulting in more pigs per litter (Brief and Chew, 1985).

Field trials have indicated that litter size could be increased by 0.6 to 1.5 pigs per litter by injecting sows with vitamin A at weaning (Whaley et al., 1997). The correlation between size of the embryo and the retinol content in uterine flushings is high (r = 0.97) (Trout et al., 1992; Seijas, 1995). Retinol in the uterine secretions may function by protecting the conceptus against the oxidizing activity of uteroferrin (Vallet, 1995). Consequently, RBP may have several functions in the reproductive tract of pigs: (1) transfer of retinol to the fetus, (2) protec-

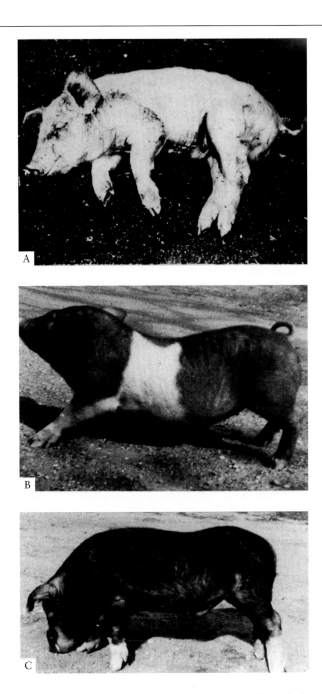

Fig. 2.13 Vitamin A deficiency in growing pigs: (A) partial paralysis and sebor-rhea, (B) initial stage of spasm, (C) lordosis and weakness of hind legs. (Courtesy of J.F. Hentges, R.H. Grummer, and the University of Wisconsin.)

tion of tissues against oxidative reactions, and (3) provision of a substrate to generate retinoic acid and other biologically active metabolites of retinol.

The effect of administering vitamin A on subsequent reproductive performance has had mixed responses (Pusateri et al., 1999). Coffey and Britt (1993) demonstrated that after the injection of 200 mg of provitamin A (β–carotene) at weaning, litter size was increased in multiparous but not in primiparous sows. In contrast, Tokach et al. (1994) conducted a study on a commercial swine farm with 956 sows and demonstrated that a single injection of β–carotene, vitamin A, or a combination of the two at weaning did not affect subsequent reproductive performance.

Poultry

Clinical signs of vitamin A deficiency are similar among chickens, turkeys, and other poultry species. On the same low vitamin A diet, turkeys and Japanese quail would exhibit clinical signs earlier than chickens due to their high requirement for the vitamin. In poultry, lack of vitamin A in the diet causes slower growth (Fig. 2.14), lowered resistance to disease, eye lesions, muscular incoordination (Fig. 2.15), and other signs (Scott et al., 1982). As deficiency progresses in adult poultry, the chickens become emaciated and weak, and their feathers are ruffled. A marked decrease in egg production occurs, and the length of time between clutches increases greatly. Hatchability is decreased, and embryonic mortality in eggs from affected birds increases. A watery discharge from the nostrils and eyes is noted, and eyelids are often stuck together. Average survival time of the progeny fed a diet with no vitamin A increased in a linear fashion with the increasing levels of vitamin A in the maternal turkey diet (Jensen, 1965).

Vitamin A level of the hen's diet is positively correlated with the growth of chicks and poults from that hen, and the level of vitamin A in the chick's and poult's diet is positively correlated with growth. Clearly, a deficiency of vitamin A will produce loss of appetite and reduction in growth. Severe deficiency will produce ataxia and death if not corrected (Hill, 1961).

When day-old chicks are given a diet with no vitamin A, clinical signs may appear at the end of the first week if the chicks are progeny of hens receiving a diet low in vitamin A. If chicks are progeny of hens receiving high levels of vitamin A, signs of deficiency may not appear until chicks are 6 or 7 weeks of age even though they are receiving a diet completely devoid of vitamin A (Scott et al., 1982). Gross signs of vitamin A deficiency in chicks are characterized by anorexia, cessation of

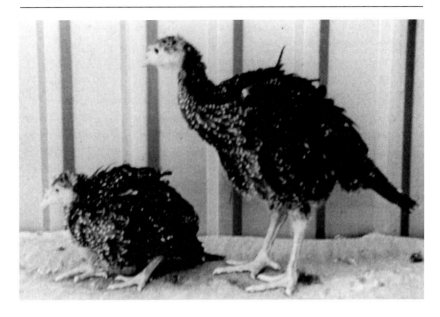

Fig. 2.14 Six-week-old turkeys: Left: fed a vitamin A-deficient diet; Right: fed a control diet. (Courtesy of L.M. Potter, Virginia Polytechnic Institute.)

growth, drowsiness, weakness, incoordination, emaciation, and ruffled plumage. The mucous epithelium is replaced by a stratified squamous, keratinizing epithelium. As a result of mucous membrane breakdown, bacteria and other pathogenic microorganisms may invade these tissues and enter the body, thereby producing infections that are secondary to original signs of vitamin A deficiency. The mucous membranes of the nasal passage, mouth, esophagus, and pharynx of poultry are affected and develop white pustules (Scott et al., 1982). The kidneys may be distended with uric acid deposits, and the epithelium of the eye is affected, producing exudates and eventually resulting in xerophthalmia. Clearly, there is a breakdown of the epithelium of many systems in the body due to vitamin A deficiency. Loss of membrane integrity, in turn, alters water retention (Lopen et al., 1973) and impairs the ability to withstand infection (Sijtsma et al., 1989). Inadequate vitamin A also reduces the immune system's response to challenge and further contributes to disease susceptibility (Davis and Sell, 1989). Viral infections have been found to impair the vitamin A status of chickens (West et al., 1992).

Vitamin A deficiency can cause alterations in bone growth, which create several areas of compression on the central nervous system, causing a loss in mobility (Howell and Thompson, 1967). Nockels (1988)

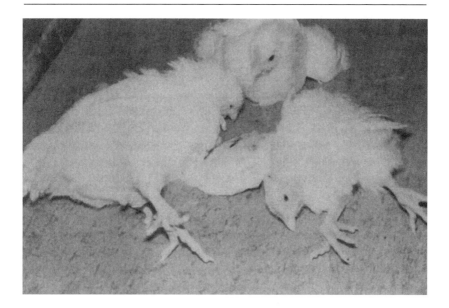

Fig. 2.15 Ataxia in chicks due to dietary deficiency of vitamin A. (Courtesy of M.L. Scott, Cornell University.)

reported that hypothyroidism is an early indication of vitamin A deficiency in chicks. Reductions in testes size, circulating testosterone, and fertility have been reported in vitamin A-deficient cockerels (Hall et al., 1980).

Horses

The importance of vitamin A to the overall health and well-being of horses has been well documented. Night blindness, lacrimation, keratinization of the cornea and respiratory system, reproductive difficulties, capricious appetite, progressive weakness, and death occur in horses deficient in vitamin A (NRC, 1989b).

During the winter, vitamin A depletion has been observed in grazing horses (Greiwe-Crandell et al., 1997) and in stabled horses fed conserved feeds (Mäenpää et al., 1988). Vitamin A depletion had adverse effects on growth and reproduction in horses (McDowell et al., 1995).

In a lengthy experiment with vitamin A-deficient horses, all horses developed night blindness that abated when dietary vitamin A was provided (Howell et al., 1941). Upon withdrawal of vitamin A supplements, night blindness again appeared in the animals.

Histological changes in the retinas of vitamin A-deficient horses have been shown (NRC, 1989b). Copious lacrimation is characteristically associated with vitamin A deficiency along with varying degrees of corneal keratinization.

Greiwe-Crandell et al. (1997) reported that vitamin A status in depleted mares was improved by supplementation with retinyl palmitate. However, in mares with no access to pasture, supplementation with twice the currently recommended amount of vitamin A barely matched the vitamin A status of unsupplemented mares on green pasture.

Other Animal Species

CATS

Vitamin A deficiency in cats is characterized by lack of growth, loss of weight, and poor appetite after 2 to 3 months of feeding a diet deficient in vitamin A. Muscle wasting is severe, while stored body fat may be nearly normal. Epithelial tissues and mucous glands forming the membrane lining of the alimentary, respiratory, urinary, and reproductive tracts as well as the membrane covering the eye and eyelids are markedly impaired by vitamin A deficiency (Gershoff et al., 1957).

Night blindness can be detected early in vitamin A-deficient kittens. As the deficiency progresses, the pupillary reflex to light is delayed from 1 to 2 seconds in the normal state to 5 to 10 seconds in the deficient state. Irreversible degeneration occurs in the rods and cones (visual cells) of the retina. Unfortunately, assessment of night blindness in cats has not been adequately distinguished from retinal degeneration due to taurine deficiency (Knopf et al., 1978), since all experimental A-deficient diets to date have used casein as the source of protein, a procedure which depletes taurine in cats.

With vitamin A deficiency, bones become thickened and constrict the central nervous system. Ataxia, stiff gait, and hydrocephalus in newborn kittens from deficient dams suggest increased cerebrospinal fluid pressure, whereas the description of cleft palate suggests deranged intrauterine mitosis and cell differentiation (Ralston Purina, 1987).

Male cats become sterile from testicular hypoplasia; females with severe vitamin A deficiency do not ovulate. With a lesser degree of deficiency, queens conceive and implantation occurs, but resorption or abortion of the fetus results at approximately the 49th day of pregnancy (Gershoff et al., 1957).

Bartsch et al. (1975) described ataxia, star gazing, blindness, and intermittent convulsions in African lion cubs presumed to be vitamin A-deficient. There was severe thickening of the cranium, compression of the brain, and partial herniation of the cerebellum.

DOGS

Vitamin A deficiency is usually confined to young animals, and advanced deficiency is always associated with cessation of growth or even weight loss and eye problems. Signs of xerophthalmia (excessive dryness of the eye), night blindness, conjunctivitis, corneal opacity and ulceration, and skin lesions are associated with rough hair coat, anorexia, growth depression, and muscle weakness (Singh et al., 1965). Respiratory infection in prolonged deficiency often results in death.

Deafness and facial paralysis occurred in puppies with severe chronic deficiency when bone growth of the skull was altered by inadequate remodeling and excessive periosteal growth to constrict cranial nerves. Blood and liver concentrations of vitamin A were negligible in these cases. Mellanby (1938) established that such damage to the cochlear and vestibular divisions of the eighth cranial nerve, plus serious labyrinthitis, may induce deafness. Similar damage may also affect function of the optic nerve, although this only has been observed after prolonged experimental deficiency (NRC, 1985a).

Vitamin A deficiency is generally a disease in growing pups, as adults seldom develop signs due to their extremely slow depletion of liver stores. In fact, several litters of pups have been produced while the dam was maintained on a vitamin A-deficient diet (Ralston Purina, 1987).

FISH

General signs of vitamin A deficiency in fish are impaired growth, exophthalmos, eye lens displacement, corneal thinning and expansion, degeneration of retina, edema, and depigmentation (NRC, 1993). Vitamin A deficiency in rainbow trout causes anemia, twisted gill opercula, and hemorrhages in the eyes and base of fins (Kitamura et al., 1967). Brook trout exhibit poor growth, high mortality, and eye lesions, such as edematous eyes, displaced lens, and degeneration of the retina when fed a vitamin A-deficient diet (Poston et al., 1977). Anorexia, pale body color, hemorrhagic skin and fins, exophthalmia, and twisted gill opercula occur in vitamin A-deficient common carp (Aoe et al., 1968). Rapidly growing yellowtail fingerlings fed a vitamin A-deficient diet develop deficiency signs in 20 days, including arrested growth of gill opercula, dark pigmentation, anemia, and hemorrhage in the eyes and liver, accompanied by high mortality (Hosokawa, 1989).

FOXES

Foxes fed a diet deficient in vitamin A develop a series of nervous derangements, usually manifested in this order: first, trembling or cocking of the head; next, unsteadiness (resulting from a disturbed sense of balance); then a tendency to run in circles (NRC, 1982a).

LABORATORY ANIMALS

Signs of vitamin A deficiency can be divided into six categories (Smith, 1990; NRC, 1995): (1) defect in vision, (2) bone defects, (3) increase in cerebral spinal fluid pressure, (4) reproductive failure (cessation of spermatogenesis in males and cornification of the reproductive tract in females), (5) epithelial metaplasia and keratinization and (6) growth failure. Insufficient vitamin A in rats leads to reduced efficiency of the urea synthesis pathway, thus accounting for the increased amino nitrogen excretion that is seen with the deficiency.

In mice, one of the early and significant consequences of vitamin A deficiency is impairment of the functional immune system. As the deficiency progresses, many epithelial tissues become keratinized, including those of the seminal vesicles, testes, bladder, kidney, trachea, esophagus, salivary glands, and lungs (Van Pelt and De Rooij, 1990; NRC, 1995). In the guinea pig, the first evidence of vitamin A deficiency is poor growth, then weight loss, followed by incrustations of eyelids and severe dermatitis resulting from bacterial infection (NRC, 1995). Often, animals develop pneumonia prior to death. Vitamin A-deficient hamsters develop abnormally and have coarse and sparse hair, xerophthalmia, and keratinized stratified tracheal lining (NRC, 1995).

NONHUMAN PRIMATES

In rhesus and cebus monkeys, the first manifestations of deficiency are weakness, diarrhea, loss of appetite, and an apparent increase in susceptibility to respiratory infection (NRC, 1978). With more severe deficiency, pathological changes in the eye become apparent. Two of four pregnancies carried to term by rhesus monkeys, which were maintained on marginal intakes of vitamin A, produced infants with congenital xerophthalmia, and a third infant developed xerophthalmia after receiving a vitamin A-deficient diet for 2 years (NRC, 1978).

RABBITS

Signs of vitamin A deficiency in rabbits are similar to those described for other animals and include retarded growth, neural lesions, ataxia, spastic paralysis, xerophthalmia, and impaired reproduction (NRC, 1977).

Humans

Throughout history, night blindness and xerophthalmia have been the major signs of vitamin A deficiency in humans. Xerophthalmia includes various stages of conjunctival xerosis, Bitot's spots, and corneal involvement and ulceration. Bitot's spots—foamy white accumulations of sloughed cells that usually appear on the temporal quadrant of the conjunctiva—are used as a clinical indicator of vitamin A deficiency in young children (Olson, 1991). Skin changes have also been observed, most specifically follicular hyperkeratosis (Olson, 1991).

Xerophthalmia is the most common cause of blindness in young children throughout the world (Fig. 2.16), with as many as 5 million Asian children developing xerophthalmia each year (Sommer et al., 1981). One-tenth of children with xerophthalmia have severe corneal involvement, and half of them become blind. Xerophthalmia is recog-

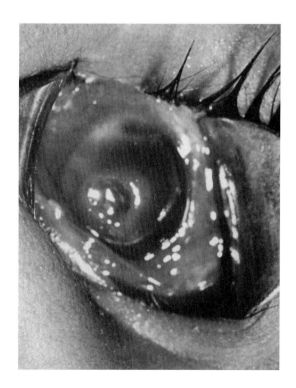

Fig. 2.16
Keratomalacia in a Jordanian infant with severe vitamin A deficiency. The central area of the cornea is undergoing typical colliquative necrosis. Sight is irrevocably lost at this advanced stage. (Courtesy of D.S. McLauren, Royal Infirmary, Edinburgh, Scotland.)

nized as endemic in many countries in southern and eastern Asia, parts of Latin America, and in many countries in Africa and the Middle East. Vitamin A deficiency remains the second major nutritional problem among children in many countries, including Bangladesh, India, Indonesia, Brazil, and other developing countries. An estimated 20 to 40 million children worldwide have at least mild vitamin A deficiency, nearly half of whom are said to reside in India (United Nations Administrative Committee, 1987).

Vitamin A deficiency affects about 100 million young children worldwide and has been long known to cause blindness. It has now become increasingly clear that even mild vitamin A deficiency also impairs the immune system, reducing children's resistance to diarrhea, which kills 2.2 million children a year, and measles, which kills nearly 1 million annually (UNICEF, 1998).

The group most vulnerable to vitamin A deficiency is children from birth to 6 years of age because of their low liver reserves; low protein, lipid, and vegetable intakes; and increased requirements due to rapid growth rate. Likewise, vitamin A deficiency for which night blindness is a marker is a problem for pregnant lactating women in rural Nepal, with health consequences for women and their infants (Katz et al., 1995). The mortality rate among children with mild xerophthalmia (night blindness and/or Bitot's spots) is on average four times the rate, and in some age groups, 8 to 12 times the rate, of children without xerophthalmia (Sommer et al., 1986). In Indonesia, a 34% difference in mortality was observed between preschool children who received vitamin A supplements for 1 year and those who received none (Sommer et al., 1986).

An early manifestation of vitamin A deficiency is premature growth (West et al., 1997) followed by infection of a wide variety of organs, overwhelming sepsis, and death. Death may frequently precede the onset of eye manifestations of deficiency. Many studies have shown that even mild vitamin A deficiency leads to patchy keratinization of the epithelial lining of the gastrointestinal tract, respiratory tract, urogenital tract, and skin. Five to six times more children in the developing world are likely to be subclinically than clinically deficient in vitamin A (Underwood, 1994).

Lack of vitamin A has been associated with an increased susceptibility to infections, especially of the respiratory and digestive tracts (Milton et al., 1987). Immune mechanisms become impaired and antibody synthesis is diminished. Large-dose vitamin A supplementation has improved vitamin A status and reduced childhood mortality (Rahmatullah et al., 1991; West et al., 1991; Fawzi et al., 1994). Regular intake of food rich in vitamin A is associated with reduced incidence of diarrhea and measles (Fawzi et al., 1995).

Vitamin A deficiency in humans occurs in endemic proportions in many developing countries and is seen only occasionally in technologically developed societies in patients with severe malabsorption, transport disorders, or liver disease (McLaren, 1984). It has been reported, however, that alcohol consumption results in significant hepatic vitamin A depletion, due perhaps to associated failure to consume an adequate diet. Also, drugs such as phenobarbital or food additives such as butylated hydroxytoluene (BHT), when combined with ethanol, result in a striking depletion of hepatic vitamin A concentrations in rats (Leo et al., 1987).

Vitamin A deficiency in humans under natural conditions is not wholly comparable to the human volunteers or experimental animals on an otherwise good diet lacking only vitamin A. Under field conditions, vitamin A deficiency is nearly always accompanied by protein-energy malnutrition, is exacerbated by parasitic infections, and is frequently complicated by intercurrent infections. Diarrheal diseases are a major cause of childhood morbidity and mortality in developing countries, causing approximately 4 million deaths per year in children younger than 5 years of age (Claeson and Merson, 1990). In areas where vitamin A status is suboptimal, children with even mild vitamin A deficiency appear to be at greater risk of developing diarrheal diseases than those with adequate vitamin A status (Bhandari et al., 1997). Chronic diarrhea is associated with reduced absorption of vitamin A (Liuzzi et al., 1998). It has been postulated that between 90 and 100 million children (predominantly in developing countries) who have some level of vitamin A deficiency are at risk of poor health and death (Underwood, 1994).

Deficiency Incidence and Relation to Vitamin A Body Stores

The circumstances most conducive to vitamin A deficiencies in livestock are (1) extended periods of drought, resulting in pastures becoming dry and bleached with no green color; (2) diets composed primarily of concentrates and no green pasture; (3) feeding mainly corn silage and a concentrate mixture low in vitamin A activity; (4) young animals fed milk from mothers on low intake of vitamin A or carotene, or poultry hatched where previous diets were low in vitamin A value; (5) young animals fed relatively little whole milk or colostrum; and (6) substituting yellow corn for grains containing no carotene. Mild vitamin A deficiency, especially in winter (or during the dry season) and early spring, is fairly common.

When grazing livestock receive a modest amount of fresh green pasture forage, there is little likelihood of deficiency. Likewise, with a substantial amount of good silage made from green forage, or with liberal feeding of fresh hay that has a good green color, deficiency will not occur. However, low-quality forages and weathered and leached hay may contain very little available carotene. Amounts of carotene in fresh green forages are very high relative to dietary requirements. Thus, a small quantity of fresh pasture forage will fully supply the need for vitamin A.

One of the most frequent stress conditions for grazing livestock in many parts of the world is low intake of carotene under conditions of winter feeding or protracted drought. When normal seasonal cycles prevail, and rainfall is sufficient to provide 4 months or more of green grazing, mature animals store sufficient vitamin A to carry them for many months on dry feed, including grain and roughage that is low in carotene. However, when severe and prolonged drought conditions prevail, especially during the normal green grazing period, signs of vitamin A deficiency may occur in adult animals. Geographical locations where vitamin A deficiency might be expected would therefore be in regions with long dry seasons. Many tropical regions in Africa, Asia, and Latin America routinely have dry seasons lasting 6 months or longer. In India, conditions reportedly permit fair grazing for only 3 months of the year (Ray, 1963). With the cessation of the monsoon rains, grasses mature rapidly, with a large drop in their carotene content. The value has been found to decrease from 100 to 200 mg per kilogram on a dry-matter basis in the middle of the rainy season to as low as 0.5 to 1 mg per kilogram during the dry season. As a result, clinical signs such as night blindness, blindness in newborn calves, and birth of weak calves have been reported in all parts of India.

In the various vitamin A supplementation trials to improve ruminant livestock production, contradictions on the benefits of supplementation have been reported. Overall, it has been shown beneficial to supplement grazing livestock with vitamin A, especially in middle to late dry season, and to feedlot cattle not receiving green forages. A general rule of thumb is that forages with a bright green color are always adequate in vitamin A value (carotene).

Deficiencies of other nutrients interfere with vitamin A metabolism and can result in vitamin A deficiency. Both protein and zinc have been shown to be required for mobilization of vitamin A from liver (see Deficiency, Ruminants). Vitamin A is required for intestinal absorption of zinc (Berzin and Bauman, 1987) in poultry, while zinc influences vitamin A by affecting RBP synthesis and release from the liver (Brown et al., 1976).

Liver is the main vitamin A storage site for humans as well as for farm species. Although most of the vitamin A reserves are in the liver, when carotene intake is high, some is stored in fat. During periods of low dietary carotene, this stored vitamin A can be mobilized and utilized without signs of vitamin A deficiency. At birth, the ruminant usually does not have sufficient vitamin A reserves to provide for its needs for any substantial time. Accordingly, it is important that young ruminants receive colostrum, which generally is rich in vitamin A, within a few days after birth. If the cow has received a diet low in vitamin A, the newborn calf is likely to be susceptible to a vitamin A deficiency because body reserves are low and colostrum will have a subnormal content (Miller et al., 1969). Likewise, if the hen received a diet deficient in vitamin A, chicks will develop the deficiency.

Grazing livestock with access to green, high-quality pastures can store sufficient vitamin A in the liver to be adequate for periods of low intake during the winter or dry season, perhaps as long as 4 to 6 months. Cattle grazing good pasture will have 30 to 80 ppm of liver vitamin A (Rumsey, 1975), and cattle entering the feedlot with 20 to 40 ppm will have adequate liver stores for 3 to 4 months (Perry et al., 1967). Intramuscular injection of 1 million IU of emulsified vitamin A apparently provides sufficient vitamin A to prevent deficiency signs for 2 to 4 months in growing or breeding beef cattle (NRC, 1996).

Because of vitamin A storage, sheep that graze on green forage during the normal growing season may be able to do reasonably well on a low-carotene diet of dry feed for periods of 4 to 6 months (NRC, 1985b). Goats that have had access to good-quality green feed can probably depend on vitamin A stores for a minimum of 3 months without detrimental effects (NRC, 1981). The tendency of goats to search out palatable green plant parts ensures it an advantage over other ruminant species. However, goats that are forced to consume more conventional cattle or sheep diets because of the unavailability of browse would not have such an advantage (NRC, 1981).

Florida beef cattle finished on Roselawn St. Augustine grass during summer did not require supplemental vitamin A for production; however, 25,000 IU per animal daily increased weight gains by approximately 10% when cattle were pastured during the winter (Chapman et al., 1964). In a study of nine cattle ranches from four regions in Florida, forage carotene and consequently liver vitamin A were lower during the winter than the summer (Kiatoko et al., 1982). In this study, cattle in the

67

northern-most region, with fewer total grazing days, had significantly lower liver vitamin A than cattle in the other three regions and approached critical levels.

Storage of vitamin A is considerable for humans and farm species that consume diets with high vitamin A value. If sows have built up stores of vitamin A until they are 8 to 9 months of age and are then placed on a diet practically devoid of carotene or vitamin A, they still can produce at least two normal litters (Selke et al., 1967). Well-nourished humans have at least several months' supply that the body can utilize (RDA, 1989).

Assessment of Status

A number of criteria are available to evaluate the status of livestock, including production response, liver vitamin A stores, plasma vitamin A, and cerebrospinal fluid pressure. Vitamin A level of blood may also reflect the nutritional status with respect to vitamin A (Green et al., 1987); however, blood vitamin A concentrations are governed by extent of liver stores as well as by current intake. In fact, in some species, blood level tends to be maintained until liver stores are exhausted when the diet is devoid of the vitamin. For this reason, a normal blood level cannot be interpreted to ensure that current intake is adequate, but a low level indicates a deficiency.

A plasma vitamin A level less than 20 µg/100 ml in Holstein calves suggests a deficiency (Eaton et al., 1970), and a plasma level of 10 µg/100 ml indicates an advanced deficiency. For beef cattle, Perry et al. (1967) suggested that plasma vitamin A is probably an accurate indicator of a borderline deficiency, with a level of less than 40 µg of vitamin A per 100 ml of blood serum indicating deficiency.

In dairy cattle, liver vitamin A values below 1 IU/kg were indicative of a critical deficiency (NRC, 1989a). Feedlot performance of beef cattle was good as long as liver vitamin A stores were above 2 IU/kg (Kohlmeier and Burroughs, 1970). In dairy calves, cerebrospinal fluid pressure rises at a rapid rate after liver concentrations of vitamin A fall below 1 to 2 ppm. Cattle showed a positive response to supplemental vitamin A when their liver concentrations were as low as 3 to 4 ppm (Perry et al., 1967).

One cannot determine the exact status of vitamin A storage in the pig by analyzing the blood for vitamin A. When vitamin A values drop below 10 µg/g in the liver and below 10 µg/100 ml in the plasma, the pig is quite deficient in vitamin A (Cunha, 1977). Liver biopsies for determination of liver vitamin A values would give the best indication of vitamin A storage or status in the pig as well as for most species.

The vitamin A content of liver of newly hatched chicks is an excellent measure of the vitamin A nutrition of breeding hens. Vitamin A deficiency will not occur in chickens having storage levels above 2 to 5 IU vitamin A per gram of liver. Thus, throughout the life of the chicken, vitamin A content of liver serves as a good measure for assessing vitamin A status (Scott et al., 1982). Liver vitamin A concentration of calves is associated with the carotene intake of their mothers (Flachowsky et al., 1993).

A simple test for night blindness evaluation in many animals (e.g., dogs and cats) can be made by darkening an unfamiliar room and observing the animals' movements in dim red light (Ralston Purina, 1987). More detailed analysis is possible with the electroretinogram in the anesthetized animal.

The overall methods that are used to determine vitamin A status in humans include dietary assessment, clinical evaluation, retinal function tests, and biochemical assessment. These methods of evaluation have been discussed in a review article (Underwood, 1990).

SUPPLEMENTATION

Supplemental vitamin A may be administered (1) as part of a concentrate or liquid supplement, (2) as included with a free-choice mineral mixture, (3) as an injectable product, and (4) in drinking water preparations. The most convenient and often most effective way to provide vitamin A to livestock is to include it with concentrate mixtures that will provide uniform consumption of the vitamin. For grazing livestock, however, providing vitamin A in concentrate mixtures generally is not economically feasible. Most vitamin A preparations used today in animal applications are administered orally as an ingredient to blend uniformly in dry feed. With the advent of low-cost synthetic vitamin A, fish oils are used only to a limited extent in various world regions.

In feed manufacturing, liquids such as oils are sprayed onto the feed in the batch or continuous blending operation, the amount being controlled volumetrically. In some cases the use of synthetic vitamin A with antioxidants in oil dilutions has continued; the oil addition plays a secondary role of reducing dustiness of feed and/or supplying an added source of calories (Bauernfeind and DeRitter, 1972).

Because of the lack of stability of vitamin A, particularly regarding exposure to oxygen, trace minerals, pelleting, feed storage, and other factors, the feed industry has readily accepted the dry stabilized forms of the vitamin. Stabilized and protectively coated (or beaded) forms of vitamin A slow destruction of the vitamin, but for highest potency, fresh supplies of the mixture should be available on a regular basis. Practical considerations that affect vitamin A stability are listed in Table 2.8. The gelatin beadlet in which the vitamin A ester (palmitate or acetate) is emulsified into a gelatin-plasticizer-antioxidant viscous liquid formulation and spray-dried into discrete dry particles results in products with good chemical stability, good physical stability, and excellent biological availability (Bauernfeind and DeRitter, 1972).

Supplemental vitamin A may be needed when (1) feed consists of poor-quality forage with little or no green color, (2) diets are composed primarily of concentrates and no green pasture, (3) feed consists mainly of corn silage and a concentrate mixture low in vitamin A activity, (4) young ruminants are receiving milk from cows fed a diet low in vitamin A or carotene, (5) calves are fed relatively little whole milk or colostrum, and (6) purchased cattle are of unknown background and in unthrifty condition, and body stores of vitamin A might be suboptimal (Perry, 1980).

Vitamin A assimilation was decreased, and its utilization was increased by infection (Nockels, 1988). Aflatoxin ingestion has also been reported to reduce vitamin A stores in the liver and induce its deficiency. Chickens showed decreased tissue accumulation of oxy-carotenoid pigments when fed aflatoxin. It is therefore important that animals that are sick or are receiving vitamin A antagonists receive diets that are fortified with the vitamin.

The use of concentrate feeds in place of forages is probably the largest single factor that has increased the need for vitamin A supplements in ruminant diets. Inefficient utilization of carotene from corn and the destruction of carotene and vitamin A in the rumen are reasons for adding supplemental vitamin A to high-concentrate diets, regardless of the vitamin A levels supplied by feedstuffs in these diets, to meet the total daily requirement (Rumsey, 1975). Weiss (1998) suggests that the requirement for vitamin A should be increased by approximately 50% for dairy cattle because of differences in bioavailability between β-carotene and retinyl esters.

Vitamin A is often included, along with vitamins D and E, in liquid feed supplements in addition to molasses, fat, urea, and selected minerals. Since the viscosity, pH, and solids content of liquid feed supplements vary considerably, the development of vitamin A forms that would blend

■ Table 2.8 Practical Factors That Affect the Stability of Vitamin A

Factors Detrimental to Stability
    Long storage of the vitamin product before mixing or of the feed product after mixing
    Vitamin premixes containing minerals
    High environmental temperature and humidity
    Pelleting, blocking, and extrusion
    Hot feed bins that sweat inside upon cooling
    Rancid fat in the feed
    Rain leaks in feed bins or storage facilities

Factors Promoting Stability
    Minimum time between manufacture of the vitamin product and consumption by
        the animal
    Storing vitamins in a cool, dark, dry area in closed containers
    Not mixing vitamins and minerals in the same premix until ready to mix the feed
    Not mixing deliquescent substances such as choline chloride with the vitamins
    Using good-quality feed ingredients and vitamins
    Good maintenance of storage bins and other equipment
    Coordination between production and purchasing to obtain a quality product that
        will not be stored an excessively long time before use

Source: Modified by personal communication (1985) with Dr. Charles H. McGinnis Jr., Manager of Nutritional Services, Rhône-Poulenc, Inc., Atlanta, Georgia.

uniformly and be stable in such a product of variable composition and characteristics represented a new challenge in the technology of vitamin A application. Products of choice are liquid emulsions of fat-soluble vitamins A, D, and E in a tested formulation of emulsifiers, antioxidants, synergists, preservatives, and carriers.

For grazing livestock, vitamin A can be provided as part of a free-choice mineral mixture as an alternative to mixing it with the feed. The greatest limitation of administering vitamin A with free-choice minerals is unknown consumption by individual animals and destruction of the vitamin with time. Vitamin A stability in a mineral mix is affected by abrasion, moisture, and prooxidant action of trace metals, particularly copper. Mitchell (1967) reported virtual destruction of gelatinized vitamin A when mixed with salt after 5 weeks. Apparently enough moisture was picked up from humid air, and perhaps saliva from cattle, to induce caking. This may have dissolved some of the gelatin coating, resulting in loss of vitamin A potency. Improved coatings of vitamin A are more insoluble in water and prevent exposure to air and the catalyzing effects of mineral contact.

Many livestock producers have followed the practice of intramuscular injection with a vitamin A concentrate. This has become a means of administering vitamin A either as a therapeutic measure or, more frequently, as a prophylactic approach when oral or dietary administration

71

is inconvenient or impossible. Feedlot cattle with an unknown history are often given an injection of vitamin A (e.g. 1,000,000 IU) as part of the adaptation or preconditioning process before the animal adjusts to the new environment and the high-energy fattening ration. Recommended high doses of vitamin A for ruminants are presented in Table 2.9.

Very high doses of vitamin A are also important under intensive housing conditions, where there are increased requirements in early life, or under conditions of stress. The practice has been found particularly valuable under the following circumstances (Hoffmann-La Roche, 1967): for day-old chicks before transport; for laying hens when, for reasons unknown, laying performance suddenly drops; for piglets and calves during weaning or changeover to milk substitutes; as an adjuvant in treatment of attacks by intestinal parasites, lungworms, and other parasites; and for newly arrived feedlot cattle.

Administration of vitamin A in very high levels in drinking water or by injection is recommended to support any specific measures used in treatment of diseased and convalescent animals. This is particularly true for animals in which vitamin A stores may have been depleted due to fever or in animals suffering from intestinal disorders when vitamin A absorption is seriously impaired. Also, very high levels of vitamin A may be beneficial in reducing the incidence of mastitis in dairy cows (Chew, 1987).

The level of vitamin A supplementation used should be based primarily on the degree of the deficiency that could potentially be problematic. As with most nutrients, a borderline deficiency is more likely than a severe deficiency. A marginal deficiency adversely affecting performance by a few percentage points is not easily detected (Miller, 1979). Based on the positive results that may be derived, and considering that vitamin A supplementation is inexpensive and (reportedly) nontoxic at recommended levels, it seems beneficial to administer supplemental vitamin A to livestock that are not grazing or receiving green pastures (roughages) and to those that are sick or under stress. Vitamin A injection is one good way to determine if a deficiency exists by injecting half the animals and using the others as controls. This can be done when it would be difficult to conduct complicated experiments.

Supplementation of pet foods would be particularly essential if organ meats rich in vitamin A (particularly liver and kidney) were not part of the diets. Some commercial foods for dogs and cats contain insufficient vitamin A. In 89 Australian brands, 8% of the dog foods and 14% of the cat foods had vitamin A concentrations below the minimum

■ Table 2.9   Recommendation for Periodic Administration of High Doses of Vitamin A
to Ruminants

Animal	IU per animal
Cattle	
Calves	200,000–500,000
Cattle (rearing)	1,000,000–1,500,000
Cattle (fattening)	1,000,000–2,000,000
Cattle (dairy)	2,000,000 (1 month before calving)
Breeding bulls	2,000,000–3,000,000 (2 months before and at the beginning of service)
Sheep	
Suckling and weaned lambs	100,000–500,000
Rams	1,000,000 (2 months before and at the beginning of service)
Ewes	1,000,000 (during service and a month before lambing)

Source: Adapted from Hoffmann-La Roche (1967).

recommended for dogs and pregnant or lactating cats (Heanes, 1990). In contrast, canned pet foods stated to contain liver or kidney showed favorable vitamin A concentrations.

The importance of synthetic retinoids in veterinary dermatology is now being explored. In dogs, the retinoids have been used primarily to treat skin diseases purported to be keratinization disorders. Various skin disorders, including sebaceous adenitis, canine ichthyosis, solar-induced precancerous lesions, and squamous cell carcinoma have all responded to retinoid therapy (Power and Ihrke, 1990; Power et al., 1992). In both dogs and cats with mycosis fungoides, isotretinoin seems to be a well-tolerated and relieving type of therapy. Cure is not always achieved, but the length and quality of life in treated animals are improved. The recommended dosage of isotretinoin in dogs and cats is between 1 and 3 mg per kilogram per day. Isotretinoin is available by prescription as Accutane in 10-, 20-, or 40-mg capsules and is sold prepackaged in 10-capsule units. The recommended dosage of etretinate used for keratinization disorders in dogs is 0.75 to 1 mg per kilogram per day. Initial response to retinoid therapy may not be apparent until 45 to 60 days of treatment (Power and Ihrke, 1990).

The major source of supplemental vitamin A used in diets is *trans*-retinyl acetate (McGinnis, 1988). The acetate, propionate and palmitate esters are chemically synthesized by vitamin A manufacturers. These are available in gelatin beadlet product forms for protection against oxidative destruction in premixes mash, and cubed and pelleted feeds. Carbohydrates, gelatin, and antioxidants are also generally included inside the beadlets to stabilize the vitamin A. These provide physical and chemical protection against factors normally present in feed that are destructive to vitamin A. The vitamin A acetate products most frequently used in feeds contain 650,000 IU or United States Pharmacopeia Units (USP) per gram of product.

Additional research is needed to establish whether supplemental β–carotene helps reduce mastitis incidence and improve reproductive performance. Experiments conducted so far to determine if β–carotene affects mastitis and/or reproduction are limited and conflicting. Likewise, the effect of supplemental β–carotene on reproduction function in mares is inconclusive (Peltier et al., 1997). One reason for the conflicting results is that the vitamin A and β–carotene status of livestock can vary greatly. Many feeds, especially green forages, contain large amounts of β–carotene, and animals can store vast quantities of vitamin A in the liver. Diets containing stored roughages such as wheat straw, corn silage, and dried beet pulp are low in β–carotene (Bonsembiante et al., 1980). According to Adams and Zimmerman (1984), analysis of various feedstuffs from different regions of the United States showed that in the absence of fresh pasture or good quality forage, diets may not provide sufficient β–carotene. Analysis also showed that samples of moldy corn averaged 98% less carotene than sound corn.

In industrialized countries, xerophthalmia due to primary vitamin A deficiency is rarely seen because of the availability of adequate fruits, vegetables, and animal food combined with fortified food such as margarine. Loss of animal products rich in vitamin A can quickly bring about deficiency of the vitamin where previously there was no problem. Many rural Sudanese have depended on milk from their livestock as their main source of vitamin A. Droughts, however, have caused animal losses, thus limiting vitamin A intake from milk products (Nestel et al., 1993).

The primary causes of hypovitaminosis A are ignorance, both natural and human-induced catastrophes, economic deprivation, and disease. Inexpensive foods that contain carotenoids and vitamin A are nonetheless available in most areas where vitamin A deficiency is prevalent, but, for a variety of reasons, they are not consumed in adequate amounts (Olson, 1994). Also, chronic alcohol consumption can reduce retinoic acid concentrations and diminish retinoid signaling (Wang, 1999).

Elimination of vitamin A deficiency is a global priority. Periodic supplementation using a large dose of vitamin A is the most widely used intervention in controlling deficiency. The current World Health Organization recommendation for universal prophylactic dosing in areas where vitamin A deficiency is a public health problem is 210 μmol every 3 to 6 months for children 1 to 6 years of age (Humphrey et al., 1994).

In developing countries, both marginal vitamin A status and intestinal helminths (e.g., *Ascaris lumbricoides*) are common among children (Tanumihardjo et al., 1996). The combination of deworming and vitamin A supplementation in a single program should be considered.

For humans, a number of reports have illustrated the benefits of supplemental vitamin A for conditions not associated with night blindness and xerophthalmia (see Functions and Deficiency sections). The results of a dozen field studies conducted in Brazil, Ghana, India, Indonesia, Nepal, and elsewhere indicate that supplementing the diets of children who are at risk of vitamin A deficiency can reduce deaths from diarrhea by 35 to 50%, and the vitamin can almost halve the number of deaths due to measles (UNICEF, 1998).

Supplemental retinoids have been successfully used as inhibitors of carcinogenesis and have important roles in optimizing immune response. Numerous clinical studies have demonstrated beneficial effects of retinoids on skin diseases such as acne, psoriasis, rosacea, ichthyoses, keratodermas, and skin cancers and their precursors, as well as a reversal of the effects of photoaging (Futoryan and Gilchrest, 1994). Retinoid-based creams applied to skin result in a younger appearance (e.g., reduced wrinkling). Retinoic acid has recently been shown as a therapy for emphysema because it regenerated lung alveoli in a rat study (Massaro and Massaro, 1997).

β-CAROTENE FUNCTION INDEPENDENT OF VITAMIN A

Carotenoids have been shown to have biological actions independent of vitamin A (Olson, 1989; Chew, 1995). Some animal studies indicate that certain carotenoids with antioxidant capacities, but without vitamin A activity, can enhance many aspects of immune functions, can act directly as antimutagens and anticarcinogens, can protect against radiation damage, and can block the damaging effects of photosensitizers. In animal models, β–carotene and canthaxanthin have protected against UV-induced skin cancer as well as some chemically induced tumors. In some of these models, enhancement of tumor immunity has been suggested as a possible mechanism of action of these carotenoids (Bendich, 1989). β–Carotene can function as a chain-breaking antioxidant; it deactivates reactive chemical species such as singlet oxygen, triplet photochemical sensitizers, and free radicals, which would otherwise induce potentially harmful processes (e.g., lipid peroxidation).

Cows supplemented with 300 mg of β–carotene per day had a lower incidence of intramammary infections than cows supplemented with preformed vitamin A or the unsupplemented control group. It was also demonstrated that dairy cows supplemented with 300 mg of β–carotene per day during the dry period maintained blood concentrations of β–carotene and had a lower incidence of mastitis than those supplemented with vitamin A alone (Chew and Johnston, 1985). β–Carotene enhances blastogenic responses of lymphocytes and increases cytotoxic activities of natural killer cells and cytokine production by macrophages (Chew, 1993).

Polymorphonuclear neutrophils (PMNs) are the major line of defense against bacteria in the mammary gland. β–Carotene supplementation seems to exert a stabilizing effect on PMN and lymphocyte function during the period around dry-off (Tjoelker et al., 1990). Daniel et al. (1991a,b) reported that β–carotene enhanced the bactericidal activity of blood and milk PMN against *S. aureus* but did not affect phagocytosis. Vitamin A either had no effect or suppressed bactericidal activity and phagocytosis. Control of free radicals is important for bactericidal activity but not for phagocytosis. The antioxidant activity of vitamin A is not important; it does not quench or remove free radicals. β–Carotene, on the other hand, has significant antioxidant properties and effectively quenches singlet oxygen free radicals (Di Mascio et al., 1991; Zamora et al., 1991).

A comprehensive review of the reproductive effects of carotene and/or vitamin A in ruminants has been reported (Hoffmann-La Roche, 1994). Since 1976, a number of studies have indicated that β–carotene has a function independent of vitamin A in dairy cattle. Dairy cattle receiving extra β–carotene have a higher intensity of estrus, increased conception rates, and reduced frequency of follicular cysts than controls. The corpus luteum of the cow has higher β–carotene concentrations than any other organ, and it has been suggested that β–carotene has a specific effect on reproduction in addition to its role as a precursor of vitamin A. Graves-Hoagland et al. (1988) suggest a positive relationship between β–carotene and luteal cell progesterone during the winter when plasma β–carotene and vitamin A are decreased. Other studies with cattle have been reported in which pregnancy rates were lower with low dietary β–carotene but were adequate in vitamin A (Cooke and Combden, 1978; Bonsembiante et al., 1980). However, other studies of cattle failed to detect differences between groups supplemented with β–carotene and control groups in the above-mentioned responses (Folman et al., 1979; Wang et al., 1988; Aréchiga et al., 1998b). Aréchiga et al. (1998a) reported that in cows fed β–carotene the pregnancy rate at 120 days postpartum was 14.3% higher, and milk yield was 6 to 11% higher than in controls.

Injectable β–carotene has increased conception rates in swine and improved live births and live weights in pigs (Chew, 1993). Contradictory results were obtained from studies that investigated the effect of supplemental β–carotene on reproductive function in mares. β–Carotene supplementation had a positive effect on the pregnancy rate of mares in some studies (Ahlswede and Konermann, 1980; Peltier et al., 1997).

There are significant new views on the health benefits of megavitamin doses, particularly the antioxidant vitamins (C, E, and β–carotene). Because damage to mammalian tissues induced by free radicals is believed to contribute to the aging process and to the development of some degenerative diseases (Canfield et al., 1992), it has been proposed that dietary carotenoids serve as antioxidants in tissues (Thurnham, 1994). This possibility is supported by numerous epidemiological studies that indicate an inverse association between the increased intake of carotenoid-rich fruits and vegetables and the incidence of disease.

There has been much research regarding the potential protective effects of carotenoids against chronic diseases (Cooper et al., 1999b). Studies have shown inverse relationships between serum levels of one or more carotenoids and a number of diseases, including cancer (Van Poppel and Goldbohn, 1995), cardiovascular disease (Gaziano and Hennekens, 1993; VERIS, 1996), eye diseases of age-related macular degeneration (Snodderly, 1995), and nuclear sclerotic and cortical cataracts (Mares-Perlman et al., 1995). In relation to cancer, in vitro studies have demonstrated that carotenoids can inhibit chemically induced neoplastic transformation (Bertram and Bortkiewicz, 1995), induce remission of oral leukoplakia (Garewal, 1995), quench free radicals such as singlet oxygen (Sies and Stahl, 1995), and modulate immune activity (Meydani et al., 1995). There is recent evidence that some of the carotenoid protection against cancer relates to gene regulation (Bertram, 1999).

Several hundred carotenoid research studies have been published since 1996, when two major intervention trials showed a lack of protective effect of β-carotene supplements against lung cancer. Recent epidemiologic studies, however, continue to show an association between high dietary intake of β-carotene and lower risk of lung cancer (Cooper, 1999a).

The predominant carotenoids in human tissues are β–carotene and lycopene. Compared with other carotenoids and other antioxidant compounds, including vitamin E, lycopene has been reported to be a more efficient quencher of singlet oxygen in vitro (Di Mascio et al., 1991). Lycopene disappearance precedes the disappearance of β–carotene when human low-density lipoprotein is oxidized in vitro (Esterbauer et al., 1989). When skin is subjected to UV light stress, more skin lycopene is destroyed compared with β–carotene, suggesting a role of lycopene in mitigating oxidative damage in tissues (Ribaya-Mercado et al., 1995). One study suggests that eating tomatoes, which are rich in lycopene, can significantly reduce the risk of heart attacks and prostate cancer.

TOXICITY

In general, the possibility of vitamin toxicities for livestock and poultry is remote. However, of all vitamins, vitamin A is most likely to be provided in toxic concentrations to both humans and livestock, and excess vitamin A has been demonstrated to have toxic effects in most species studied. Presumed upper safe levels are 4 to 10 times the nutritional requirements for nonruminant animals, including birds and fishes, and about 30 times the requirements for ruminants (NRC, 1987). A high tolerance for ruminants may be due in part to some microbial degradation of vitamin A in the rumen (Rode et al., 1990). Most of the harmful effects have been obtained by feeding over 100 times the daily requirements for a period of time. Thus, small excesses of vitamin A for short periods should not exert any harmful effects. Recommended upper safe levels of vitamin A for livestock and poultry are presented in Table 2.10 (NRC, 1987).

Large doses can be toxic, and many cases of overdoses have been reported in various species. The most characteristic signs of hypervitaminosis A are skeletal malformations, spontaneous fractures, and internal hemorrhage (NRC, 1987). Other signs include loss of appetite, slow growth, weight loss, skin thickening, suppressed keratinization, increased blood-clotting time, reduced erythrocyte count, enteritis, congenital abnormalities, and conjunctivitis. Degenerative atrophy, fatty infiltration, and reduced function of liver and kidney are also typical. A report on clinical signs of hypervitaminosis A in rainbow trout (*Salmo*

■ Table 2.10   Presumed Safe Upper Levels of Vitamin A (IU/kg Diet) for Livestock and Poultry

Animal	Presumed Safe Level[a]
Birds	
Chicken, growing	15,000
Chicken, laying	40,000
Duck	40,000
Goose	15,000
Quail	25,000
Turkey, growing	15,000
Turkey, breeding	24,000
Cat	100,000
Cattle, feedlot	66,000
Cattle, pregnant, lactating, or bulls	66,000
Dog	33,330
Fish	
Catfish	33,330
Salmon	25,000
Trout	25,000
Goat	45,000
Horse	16,000
Monkey	100,000
Rabbit	16,000
Sheep	45,000
Swine, growing	20,000
Swine, breeding	40,000

Source: Adapted from NRC (1987).
[a]For chronic dietary administration.

gairdneri) listed growth depression; increased mortality; abnormal and necrotic anal, caudal, pectoral, and pelvic fins; and pale yellow fragile livers (Hilton, 1983). Bone abnormalities may include extensive bone resorption and narrowing of the bone shaft, bone fragility, and short bones because of retarded growth. Abnormalities in bone modeling are the essential causes of fractures, and the cartilage matrix of bone may be destroyed. For example, high levels of vitamin A injected into rabbits may cause ears to curl because of the destruction of cartilage.

Pet foods or vitamin A medication can result in hypervitaminosis A. The use of vitamin A in dermatology therapy of dogs and the inclusion of livestock by-products high in vitamin A in canned dog foods have raised concerns about subclinical, long-term vitamin A toxicosis (Hoffmann-La Roche, 1998). Hypervitaminosis A in cats is most frequently associated with diets having a high liver or fish liver oil content (Goldman, 1992; Goldston and Hoskins, 1995). When a cat is found to be sick, and its diet consists wholly or partly of raw liver, vitamin A toxicity should be suspected. The feeding of raw liver should be stopped and a balanced feline diet instituted (Goldman, 1992). Cats consuming raw beef liver containing 20,000 to 40,000 µg per kilogram for 2 to 5 years produced the main clinical findings of cutaneous hyperesthesia of neck and forelegs, forelimb lameness, pain and skeletal immobility due to bony exostoses of the cervical vertebrae, and tendinous tuberosities of long bones (Seawright et al., 1965).

It is believed that release of lysosomal enzymes is responsible for degradative changes observed in tissues and intact animals suffering from hypervitaminosis A (Fell and Thomas, 1960). In hypervitaminosis A, retinol penetrates the lipid of the membrane and causes it to expand, and because the protein of the membrane is relatively inelastic, the membrane is therefore weakened. Thus, many phenomena in hypervitaminosis A can be explained in terms of damage to membranes either of cells or of organelles within cells.

Excess vitamin A affects metabolism of other fat-soluble vitamins with competition for absorption and transport demonstrated. Therefore, in diets containing barely adequate levels of vitamins D, E, and K, a marked increase in dietary vitamin A may cause decreases in growth or egg production due to a deficiency of one or more of the other fat-soluble vitamins rather than a toxic effect of vitamin A. Retinoid-induced hemorrhaging in rats fed diets deficient in vitamin K have been reported (McCarthy et al., 1989). The mechanisms of absorption and transport apparently are similar for the carotenoid pigments and the fat-soluble vitamins. A marked increase in dietary vitamin A has been shown to interfere with absorption of carotenoids, thereby resulting in decreased pigmentation for poultry.

High dietary levels of vitamin A have depressed vitamin E utilization in most animals studied (Schelling et al., 1995; Franklin et al., 1998). However, levels of vitamin A fed to dairy cattle were in excess by approximately tenfold to highest levels being fed commercially (Schelling et al., 1995). In swine, high levels of injectable vitamin A had little or no effect on serum and tissue vitamin E concentrations (Anderson et al., 1997).

The efficiency of carotene conversion to vitamin A declines progressively with increasing intakes (see Requirements). This appears to be a natural homeostatic control mechanism that protects grazing livestock from any harmful effects due to great abundance of carotene present in high-quality, fresh forages when they are the major feed for long periods (Miller, 1979). Likewise, comparatively rapid disposal of very high levels of stored vitamin A is a protective mechanism. On a practical basis, toxicity is more easily caused by vitamin A than by carotene. Even so, vitamin A toxicity is not a practical problem for livestock, except when unreasonably large amounts are given accidentally (Miller, 1979).

The symptomatology of hypervitaminosis A in humans varies considerably depending on the age of the subject and the duration of the excessive intake. The young child is especially susceptible, with toxicity occurring in children taking therapeutic doses prescribed for various skin problems. The onset of clinical vitamin A toxicity is insidious and usually follows consumption of doses of the order of 100,000 IU per day for periods ranging from weeks to months. The varied clinical signs and symptoms are well documented and include headache and other symptoms attributable to increased intracranial pressure, dermatological changes, pruritic skin rash, irritability, pain in arms and legs, and hydrocephalus in children. Plasma vitamin A is always elevated, usually well above 200 μg per deciliter.

Arctic and Antarctic explorers have suffered from acute toxicity after eating polar bear or seal liver. It has been calculated that consumption of 500 g of polar bear liver (13,000–18,000 IU of vitamin A/g) would result in a toxic dose (Sebrell and Harris, 1967). Symptoms of this acute polar bear liver poisoning, which may appear within 2 to 4 hours, are drowsiness, sluggishness, irritability or an irresistible desire to sleep, severe headache, and vomiting. The medical literature records death following intake of a single dose of 1,000,000 IU in adults and 500,000 IU in children.

Historically, it has been known for centuries among Eskimos and Arctic travelers that the ingestion of polar bear liver by men and dogs causes severe illness (Rodahl, 1949). There are stories of polar bear liver being given to dogs, which later became sick and eventually suffered from loss of hair. It is also said that the Eskimos threw the polar bear livers into the sea to keep the dogs from getting them. On the other hand, it is known that dogs are reluctant to eat polar bear liver, as is generally experienced by the European trappers in northeastern Greenland with their sledge dogs. On one occasion a liver was given to a very hungry dog, which ate a small portion of the liver and subsequently suffered from diarrhea (Rodahl, 1949).

It is interesting that gulls and ravens avoid polar bear liver. On one occasion ravens pecked a hole in the abdominal wall of a dead bear and ate all the entrails but left the liver untouched. From the footsteps in the snow around the carcass, it could be concluded that a large number of birds had been there (Rodahl, 1949).

Hypervitaminosis A in humans is becoming a clinical problem of increasing frequency as a result of self-medication and overprescription.

According to McLaren (1982), vitamin A accumulation in human liver with age signifies that hypervitaminosis A is also becoming a public health problem in Western countries. He points out that habitual intake of vitamin A in the United States and Europe is greater than the recommended daily allowance, the body content of vitamin A is in excess of that of other vitamins in relationship to requirements, and the rate of catabolism of retinol is exponential, regardless of stores. Excess retinol intake may explain the high incidence of osteoporosis in Northern Europe (Whiting and Lemke, 1999). Explicit warnings for both children and adults are provided by the RDA (1989) regarding excessive vitamin A intakes of more than 25,000 IU on a regular basis.

■ REFERENCES

Adams, C.R., and Zimmerman, C.R. (1984). *Feedstuffs 56*, 35.
Ahlswede, L, and Konermann, H. (1980). *Der praktische Tierarzt 61*, 47.
Ahmed, F., Jones, D.B., and Jackson, A.A. (1990). *Br. J. Nutr. 63*, 363.
Akordor, F.Y., Stone, J.B., Walton, J.S., Leslie, K.E., and Buchanan-Smith, J.B. (1986). *J. Dairy Sci. 69*, 2173.
Anderson, L.E., Myer, R.O., Brendemuhl, J.H., and McDowell, L.R. (1997). *Reprod. Nutr. Dev. 37*, 213.
Anonymous (1977). *Nutr. Rev. 35*, 305.
Anonymous (1991). *Nutr. Rev. 49*, 243.
Anonymous (1993). *Nutr. Rev. 51*, 81.
Aoe, H.I., Masuda, T., Mimura, T., Saito, T., and Komo, A. (1968). *Bull. Jpn. Soc. Sci. Fish. 34*, 959.
Aréchiga, C.F., Staples, C.R., McDowell, L.R., and Hansen, P.J. (1998a). *J. Dairy Sci. 81*, 390.
Aréchiga, C.F., Vázquez-Flores, S., Ortíz, O., Hernández-Cerón, J., Porras, A., McDowell, L.R., and Hansen, P.J. (1998b). *Theriogenology 50*, 65.
Arykroyd, W.R. (1958). *Fed. Proc. Fed. Am. Soc. Exp. Biol. 17*, 103.
Bardos, L. (1991). *Magyar-Allatorvosok-Lapja 46*, 167.
Bartsch, R.D., Imes Jr., G.D., and Smit, J.P.J. (1975). *Onderstepoort J. Vet. Res. 42*, 43.
Barua, A.B. (1997). *Nutr. Rev. 55*, 259.
Bauernfeind, J.C. (1972). *J. Agric. Food Chem. 20*, 456.
Bauernfeind, J.C., and DeRitter, E. (1972). *Feedstuffs 44* (36), 34.
Bebravicius, V., Medzevicius, A., and Medzevicius, A. (1987). *Acta Parasitologica Lituanica 22*, 102.
Beeson, W.M. (1965). *Fed. Proc. Fed. Am. Soc. Exp. Biol. 24*, 924.
Bendich, A. (1989). *J. Nutr. 119*, 135.
Bertram, J.S. (1999). *Nutr. Rev. 57*, 182.
Bertram, J.S., and Bortkiewicz, H. (1995). *Am J. Clin. Nutr. 62*, 1327S.
Berzin, N., and Bauman, V.K. (1987). *Br. J. Nutr. 57*, 255.

Bhandari, N., Bahl, R., Sazawal, S., and Bhan, M.K. (1997). *J. Nutr.* 127, 59.
Bierer, T.L., Merchen, N.R., and Erdman, J.W. (1995). *J. Nutr.* 125, 1569.
Blomhoff, R., Green, M.H., Green, J.B., Berg, T., and Norum, K.R. (1991). *Physiol. Rev.* 71, 951.
Bonsembiante, M., Bittante, G., and Andrighetto, I. (1980). *Zoot. Nutr. Anim.* 6, 47.
Booth, A., Reid, M., and Clark, T. (1987). *J. Am. Vet. Med. Assoc.* 190, 1305.
Braude, R., Foot, A.S., Henry, K.M., Kon, S.K., Thompson, S.Y., and Mead, T.H. (1941). *Biochem J.* 35, 693.
Brief, S., and Chew, B.P. (1985). *J. Anim. Sci.* 60, 998.
Brown, E.D., Chen, W., and Smith, J.C. (1976). *J. Nutr.* 106, 563.
Brubacher, G.B., and Weiser, H. (1985). *Int. J. Vitam. Nutr. Res.* 55, 5.
Bruns, N.J., and Webb, K.E. (1990). *J. Anim. Sci.* 68, 454.
Canfield, L.M., Foprage, J.W., and Valenzuela, J.G. (1992). *Proc. Soc. Exp. Biol. Med.* 200, 260.
Chapman, H.L, Shirley, R.L., Palmer, A.Z., Haines, C.E., Carpenter, J.W., and Cunha, T.J. (1964). *J. Anim. Sci.* 23, 669.
Chew, B.P. (1987). *J. Dairy Sci.* 70, 2732.
Chew, B.P. (1993). *J. Dairy Sci.* 76, 2804.
Chew, B.P. (1995). *J. Nutr.* 125, 1804S.
Chew, B.P., and Johnston, L.A. (1985). *J. Dairy Sci.* 68(Suppl. 1), 191(Abstr.).
Chew, B.P., Luedecke, L.O., and Holpuch, D.M. (1984). *J. Dairy Sci.* 67, 2566.
Chhabra, A., and Arora, S.P. (1987). *Indian J. Dairy Sci.* 40, 322.
Chhabra, A., Arora, S.P., and Kishan, J. (1980). *Indian J. Anim. Sci.* 50, 879.
Claeson, M., and Merson, M.H. (1990). *Pediatr. Infect. Dis. J.* 9, 345.
Clawitter, J.W., Trout, E., Burke, M.G., Areghi, S., and Roberts, R.M. (1990). *J.Biol. Chem.* 265, 3248.
Coelho, M.B. (1991). Vitamin Stability in Premixes and Feeds: A Practical Approach, p. 56. BASF Technical Symp., Bloomington, Minnesota.
Coffey, M.T., and Britt, J.H. (1993). *J. Anim. Sci.* 71, 1198.
Cooke, B.C., and Combden, N.A. (1978). *Anim. Prod.* 26, 356(Abstr.).
Cooper, D.A. (1999a). *Nutr. Rev.* 57, 133.
Cooper, D.A. (1999b). *Nutr. Rev.* 57, 201.
Cunha, T.J. (1977). Swine Feeding and Nutrition. Academic Press, New York.
Dahlquist, S.P., and Chew, B.P. (1985). *J. Dairy Sci.* 68(Suppl. 1), 191(Abstr.).
Daniel, L.R., Chew, B.P., Tanaka, T.S., and Tjoelker, L.W. (1991). *J. Dairy Sci.* 74, 124.
Dash, S.K., and Mitchell, D.J. (1976). *Anim. Nutr. Health* Oct. 16-17.
Davis, C.Y., and Sell, J.L. (1983). *J. Nutr.* 113, 1914.
Davis, C.Y., and Sell, J.L. (1989). *Poult. Sci.* 68, 136.
Di Mascio, P., Murphy, M.E., and Sies, H. (1991). *Am. J. Clin. Nutr.* 53, 194S.
Donoghue, S., Donawick, W.J., and Kronfeld, D.S. (1983). *J. Nutr.* 113, 2197.
Eaton, H.D., Lucas, J.J., Neilson, S.W., and Helmboldt, C.F. (1970). *J. Dairy Sci.* 53, 1775.
Ensminger, M.E., and Olentine, C.G. (1978). Feeds and Nutrition. Ensminger, Clovis, California.
Erdman, J.W., Thatcher, A.J., Hofmann, N.E., Lederman, J.D., Block, S.S., Lee, C.M., and Mokady, S. (1998). *J. Nutr.* 128, 2013.

Esterbauer, H., Striegl, G., Puhl, H., and Rotheneder, M. (1989). *Free Radic. Res. Commun. 6*, 67.

Farid, M.F.A., and Ghanem, Y.S. (1982). *World Rev. Anim. Prod. 18*, 75.

Fawzi, W.W., Herrera, M.G., Willett, W.C., Nestel, P., El Amin, A., Lipsitz, S., and Mohamed, K.A. (1994). *Am J. Clin. Nutr. 59*, 401.

Fawzi, W.W., Herrera, M.G., Willett, W.C., Nestel, P., El Amin, A., and Mohamed, K.A. (1995). *J. Nutr. 125*, 1211.

Fell, H.B., and Thomas, L. (1960). *J. Exp. Med. 111*, 719.

Fichter, S.A., and Mitchell, G.E. (1997). *J. Anim. Sci. 72*(Suppl. 1), 266(Abstr.).

Flachowsky, G., Heidemann, B., Schlenzig, M., Wilk, H., and Hennig, A. (1993). *Z. Ernährung Swiss 32*, 21.

Folman, Y., Ascarelli, F., Hertz, Z., Rosenberg, M., Davidson, M., and Halevi, A. (1979). *Br. J. Nutr. 41*, 353.

Franklin, S.T., Sorenson, C.E., and Hammell, D.C. (1998). *J. Dairy Sci. 81*, 2623.

Funk, C. (1922). The Vitamins. Williams and Wilkins Co., Baltimore.

Futoryan, T., and Gilchrest, B.A. (1994). *Nutr. Rev. 52*, 299.

Garewal, H. (1995). *Am J. Clin. Nutr. 62*, 1401S.

Gaziano, J.M., and Hennekens, C.H. (1993). *Ann. N.Y. Acad. Sci. 691*, 148.

Gershoff, S.N., Andrus, S.B., Hegsted, D.M., and Lentini, E.A. (1957). *Lab. Invest. 6*, 227.

Goldman, A.L. (1992). *J. Am. Vet. Med. Assoc. 200*(12), 1970.

Goldston, R.T., and Hoskins, J.D. (1995). *In* Geriatrics and Gerontology of the Dog and Cat, p. 310. W.B. Saunders Co., Phildelphia.

Goodman, D.S. (1980). *Fed. Proc. Fed. Am. Soc. Exp. Biol. 39*, 2716.

Grace, M.L., and Bernhard, R.A. (1984). *J. Dairy Sci. 67*, 1646.

Graves-Hoagland, R.L., Hoaglund, T.A., and Woody, C.O. (1988). *J. Dairy Sci. 71*, 1058.

Green, M.H., Green, J.B., and Lewis, K.C. (1987). *J. Nutr. 117*, 694.

Greiwe-Crandell, K.M., Kronfeld, D.S., Gay, L., Sklan, D., Tiegs, W., and Harris, P.A. (1997). *J. Anim. Sci. 75*, 2684.

Guerin, H.B. (1981). *J. Anim. Sci. 53*, 758.

Guss, S.B. (1977). Management and Diseases of Dairy Goats. Dairy Goat Journal Publ. Corp., Scottsdale, Arizona.

Halevy, O., Arazi, Y., Melamed, D., Friedman, A., and Sklan, D. (1994). *J. Nutr. 124*, 2139.

Hall, W.C., Damjanou, I., Nielsen, S.W., van der Heide, L., and Eaton, H.D. (1980). *Am. J. Vet. Res. 41*, 586.

Harmon, B.G., Miller, E.R., Hoefer, J.A., Ullrey, D.E., and Leucke, R.W. (1963). *J. Nutr. 79*, 263.

Harris Jr., B. (1975). *Feedstuffs 47*, 42.

Heanes, D.L. (1990). *Aust. Vet. J. 67*(8), 291.

Hentges, J.F., Grummer, R.H., Phillips, P.H., Bohstedt, G., and Sorensen, D.K. (1952). *J. Am. Vet. Med. Assoc. 120*, 213.

Herrick, J.B. (1972). *Vet. Med. 67*, 906.

Hidiroglou, N., McDowell, L.R., and Boning, A. (1986). *Int. J. Vitam. Nutr. Res. 56*, 339.

Hill, C.H. (1961). *Poult. Sci. 40*, 762.

Hilton, J.W. (1983). *J. Nutr. 113*, 1737.

Hoffmann-La Roche (1967). Vitamin A, the Key-stone of Animal Nutrition. Hoffmann-La Roche, Basel, Switzerland.

Hoffmann-La Roche (1994). *In* Vitamin Nutrition for Ruminants RCD8775/894. Hoffmann-La Roche Inc., Nutley, New Jersey.

Hoffmann-La Roche (1998). *In* Vitamin Nutrition for Dogs and Cats. Hoffmann-La Roche, Nutley, New Jersey (In Press).

Horst, R.L., Reinhardt, T.A., Goff, J.P., Nonnecke, B.J., Gambhir, V.K., Fiorella, P.D., and Napoli, J.L. (1995). *Biodhem. 34*, 1203.

Hosokawa, H. (1989). The vitamin requirements of fingerling yellowtail *Seriola quinqueradiata*. Ph.D. Dissertation, Kochi University, Japan.

Howell, C.E., Hart, G.H., and Ittner, N.R. (1941). *Am. J. Vet. Res. 2*, 60.

Howell, J., McC., and Thompson, J.N. (1967). *Br. J. Nutr. 21*, 741.

Humphrey, J.H., Natadisastra, G., Friedman, D.S., Tielsch, J.M., West, K.P., and Sommer, A. (1994). *J. Nutr. 124*, 1172.

Hussein, L., and El-Tohamy, M. (1990). *Int. J. Vitam. Nutr. Res. 60*, 229.

Jensen, L.S. (1965). *Poult. Sci. 44*, 1609.

Johnson, E.J., Qin, J., Krinsky, N.I., and Russell, R.M. (1997). *J. Nutr. 127*, 1833.

Kasner, P., Chambon, P., and Leid, M. (1994). *In* Vitamin A in Health and Disease, p. 189 (R. Blomhoff, ed.). Marcel Dekker, New York.

Katz, J. Khatry, S.K., West, K.P., Humphrey, J.H., LeClerq, S.C., Pradhan, E.K., Pohkrel, R.P., and Sommer, A. (1995). *J. Nutr. 125*, 2122.

Kelley, K., and Easter, R. (1987). *Feedstuffs 59*(22), 14.

Kiatoko, M., McDowell, L.R., Bertrand, J.E., Chapman, H.L., Pate, F.M., Martin, F.G., and Conrad. J.H. (1982). *J. Anim. Sci. 55*, 28.

Kitamura, S., Suwa, T., Ohara, S., and Nakagawa, K. (1967). *Bull. Jpn. Soc. Sci. Fish. 33*, 1126.

Kliewer, S.A., Umesono, K., Evans, R.M., and Mangelsdorf, D. (1994). *In* Vitamin A in Health and Diseases, p. 239 (R. Blomhoff, ed.). Marcel Dekker, New York.

Knopf, K., Sturman, J.A., Armstrong, M., and Hayes, K.C. (1978). *J. Nutr. 108*, 773.

Kohlmeier, R.H., and Burroughs, W. (1970). *J. Anim. Sci. 30*, 1012.

Krishnan, S., Bhuyan, U.N., Talwar, G.P., and Ramalingas Wami, R. (1974). *Immunology 27*, 383.

Larkin, P.J., and Yates, R.J. (1964). *E. Afr. Aric. For. J. 30*, 11.

Leo, M.A., Lowe, N., and Lieber, C.S. (1987). *J. Nutr. 117*, 70.

Lindley, C.E., Brugman, H.H., Cunha, T.J., and Warwick, E.J. (1949). *J. Anim. Sci. 8*, 590.

Liuzzi, J.P., Cioccia, A.M., and Hevia, P. (1998). *J. Nutr. 128*, 2467.

Loosli, J.K. (1991). *In* Animal Science Handbook (P.A. Putnam, ed). Academic Press, San Diego.

Lopen, G.A., Phillips, R.W., and Nockels, C.F. (1973). *Proc. Soc. Exp. Biol. Med. 144*, 54.

Mäenpää, P.H., Pirhonen, A., and Koskinen, E. (1988). *J. Anim. Sci. 66*, 1424.

Majumdar, B.N., and Gupta, B.N. (1960). *Ind. J. Med. Res. 48*, 388.

Mares-Perlman, J.A., Brady, W.E., Klein, B.E.K., Palta, M., Bowe, P., and

Stacewicz-Sapuntzakis, M. (1995). *Invest. Ophthalmol. Vis. Sci. 36*, 276.

Martin, F.J., Ullrey, D.E., Miller, E.R., Kemp, K.E., Geasler,M.R., and Henderson, H.E. (1971). *J. Anim. Sci. 32*, 1233.

Massaro, G.D., and Massaro, D. (1997). *Nat. Med. 3*, 675.

Maynard, L.A., Loosli, J.K., Hintz, H.F., and Warner, R.G. (1979). Animal Nutrition, p. 283, 7th Ed. McGraw-Hill, New York.

McCarthy, D.J., Lindamood, C., Gundberg, C.M., and Hill, D.L. (1989). *Toxicology and Applied Pharmacology 97*, 300.

McCollum, E.V. (1957). *In* A History of Nutrition, p. 217. Houghton Mifflin, Boston.

McDowell, K.J., Adams, M.H., Franklin, K.M., and Baker, C.B. (1995). *Biol. Reprod. 52*, 438.

McDowell, L.R. (1985). Nutrition of Grazing Ruminants in Warm Climates. Academic Press, San Diego.

McDowell, L.R. (1992). Minerals in Animals and Human Nutrition. Academic Press, San Diego.

McDowell, L.R. (1997). Minerals for Grazing Ruminants in Tropical Regions, 3rd Ed. University of Florida, Gainesville.

McGhee, J.R., Mestecky, J., Dertzbaugh, M.T., Eldridge, J.H., Hirasawa, M. and Kiyono, H. (1992). *Vaccine 10*, 75.

McGinnis Jr., C.H. (1988). *In* Proc. 1988 Georgia Nutrition Conference for the Feed Industry, Athens, Georgia.

McLaren, D.S. (1982). *Nutr. Rev. 40*, 303.

McLaren, D.S. (1984). *In* Nutrition Reviews, Present Knowledge in Nutrition, p. 192 (R.E. Olson, ed). Nutrition Foundation, Washington, D.C.

McLaren, D.S. (1986). *In* Vitamin A Deficiency and Its Control, p. 1 (J.C. Bauernfeind, ed). Academic Press, Orlando, Florida.

Mellanby, E. (1938). *J. Physiol. 94*, 316.

Meydani, S.N., Wu, D., Santos, M.S., and Hayek, M.G. (1995). *Am. J. Clin. Nutr, 62*, 1462S.

Michal, J.J., Heirman, L.R., Wong, T.S., and Chew, B.P. (1994). *J. Dairy Sci. 77*, 1408.

Miller, R.W., Hemken, R.W., Waldo, D.R., and Moore, L.A. (1969). *J. Dairy Sci. 52*, 1998.

Miller, W.J. (1979). Dairy Cattle Feeding and Nutrition. Academic Press, New York.

Milton, R.C. Reddy, V., and Naidu, A.N. (1987). *Am. J. Clin. Nutr. 46*, 827.

Mitchell, G.E. (1967). *J. Am. Vet. Med. Assoc. 151*, 430.

Moore, A.C., Gugger, E.T., and Erdman, J.W. (1996). *J. Nutr. 126*, 2904.

Morand-Fehr, P. (1981). *In* Goat Production, p. 193 (C. Gall, ed). Academic Press, New York.

Nestel, P., Herrera, M.G., El Amin, A., Fawzi, W.W., Mohammed, K.A., and Weld, L. (1993). *J. Nutr. 123*, 2115.

Nockels, C.F. (1988). *In* Proc. 1988 Georgia Nutrition Conference for the Feed Industry, Athens, Georgia.

Nonnecke, B.J., Reinhardt, T.A., and Franklin, S.T. (1993). *J. Dairy Sci. 76*, 2175.

NRC. Nutrient Requirements of Domestic Animals. National Academy of

Sciences-National Research Council, Washington, D.C. (1977). Nutrient Requirements of Rabbits, 2nd Ed. (1978). Nutrient Requirements of Nonhuman Primates. (1981). Nutrient Requirements of Goats. (1982a). Nutrient Requirements of Mink and Foxes. (1985a). Nutrient Requirements of Dogs, 2nd Ed. (1985b). Nutrient Requirements of Sheep, 5th Ed. (1986). Nutrient Requirements of Cats, 3rd Ed. (1989a). Nutrient Requirements of Dairy Cattle, 6th Ed. (1989b). Nutrient Requirements of Horses, 5th Ed. (1993). Nutrient Requirements of Fish. (1994). Nutrient Requirements of Poultry, 9th Ed. (1995). Nutrient Requirements of Laboratory Animals, 4th Ed. (1996). Nutrient Requirements of Beef Cattle, 7th Ed. (1998). Nutrient Requirements of Swine, 10th Ed.

NRC. (1982b). United States-Canadian Tables of Feed Composition, 3rd Ed. National Academy of Sciences-National Research Council, Washington, D.C.

NRC. (1987). Vitamin Tolerance of Animals. National Academy of Sciences-National Research Council, Washington, D.C.

Oldham, E.R., Eberhart, R.J., and Muller, L.D. (1986). *J. Dairy Sci.* 69(Suppl. 1), 103.

Oldham, E.R., Eberhart, R.J., and Muller, L.D. (1991). *J. Dairy Sci. 74,* 3775.

Olson, J.A. (1989). *J. Nutr. 119,* 94.

Olson, J.A. (1991). *In* Handbook of Vitamins (L.J. Machlin, ed). Marcel Dekker, Inc., New York.

Olson, J.A. (1994). *J. Nutr. 124,* 1461S.

Ong, D.E. (1993). *J. Nutr. 123,* 351.

Peltier, M.M., Peltier, M.R., Sharp, D.C., and Ott, E.A. (1997). *Theriogenology 48,* 893.

Perry, T.W. (1980). Beef Cattle Feeding and Nutrition, Academic Press, New York.

Perry, T.W., Beeson, W.M., Smith, W.H., and Mohler, M.T. (1967). *J. Anim. Sci. 26,* 115.

Pit, G.A.J. (1985). *In* Fat-Soluble Vitamins, p. 1. (A.T. Diplock, ed.). Technomic Publ., Lancaster, Pennsylvania.

Poor, C.L., Bierer, T.L., Merchen, N.R., Fahey, G.C., and Erdman, J.W. (1993). *J. Nutr. 123,* 1296.

Poston, H.A., Riis, R.C., Rumsey, G.L., and Ketola, H.G. (1977). *Cornell Vet. 67,* 472.

Power, H.T., and Ihrke, P.J. (1990). *Vet. Clin. North Am. Small Anim. Pract. 20*(6), 1525.

Power, H.T., Ihrke, P.J., Stannard, A.A., and Backus, K.Q. (1992). *J. Am. Vet. Med. Assoc. 201*(3), 419.

Pusateri, A.E., Diekman, M.A., and Singleton, W.L. (1998). *J. Anim. Sci.* 77, 1532.

Quackenbush, F.W. (1963). *Cereal Chem. 40,* 266.

Rahmatullah, L., Underwood, B.A., Thulasiraj, R.D., and Milton, R.C. (1991). *Am. J. Clin. Nutr. 54,* 568.

87

Raila, J., Eisenach, C., Buchholz, I., and Schweigert, F.J. (1997). *J. Anim. Sci.* 75(Suppl. 1), 226(Abstr.).

Rajaraman, V., Nonnecke, B.J., Franklin, S.T., Hammell, D.C., and Horst, R.L. (1998). *J. Dairy Sci.* 81, 3278.

Ralston Purina. (1987). Nutrition and Management of Dogs and Cats. Ralston Purina Co., St. Louis, Missouri.

Ray, S.M. (1963). *Proc. World Conf. Anim. Prod. 1st Rome 2,* 190(Abstr.).

RDA (1989). Recommended Dietary Allowances, 9th Ed. National Academy of Sciences-National Research Council, Washington, D.C.

Ribaya-Mercado, J.D., Garmyn, M., Gilchrest, B.A., and Russell, R.M. (1995). *J. Nutr. 125,* 1854.

Rodahl, K. (1949). *Norsk Polarinstitutt Bull. No. 92.* Oslo, Norway.

Rode, L.M., McAllister, T.A., and Cheng, K.J. (1990). *Can. J. Anim. Sci. 70,* 227.

Roels, O.A., Trout, M., and Dujacquier, R. (1958). *J. Nutr. 65,* 115.

Ross, A.C. (1992). *Proc. Soc. Exp. Biol. Med. 200,* 303.

Ross, A.C. (1993). *J. Nutr. 123,* 346.

Rumsey, T.S. (1975). *Feedstuffs 47,* 30.

Russell, W.C. (1929). *J. Biol. Chem. 85,* 289.

Safonova, I., Amri, E., and Ailhaud, G. (1994). *Mol. Cell. Endocrinol. 104,* 201.

Schelling, G.T., Roeder, R.A., Garber, M.J., and Pumfrey, W.M. (1995). *J. Nutr. 125,* 1799S.

Schmidt, H. (1941). *Am. J. Vet. Res. 2,* 373.

Schweigert, F.J., Vehlein-Harrell, S., and Zucker, H. (1990). *J. Vet. Med. 37,* 605.

Scott, M.L., Nesheim, M.C., and Young, R.J. (1982). Nutrition of the Chicken, p. 119. Scott, Ithaca, New York.

Seawright, A.A., English, P.B., and Gartner, R.J.W. (1965). *Nature 206,* 1171.

Sebrell Jr., W.H., and Harris, R.S. (1967). The Vitamins, p. 3. Academic Press, New York.

Seijas, H.C. (1995). *In* Ph.D. Dissertation, Ohio State University, Columbus.

Selke, M.R., Barnhart, C.E., and Chaney, C.H. (1967). *J. Anim. Sci. 26,* 759.

Semba, R.D. (1998). *Nutr. Rev. 56,* S38.

Serman, V., and Mazija, H. (1985). *Veterinarski Archiv 55(1),* 1.

Shields, R.G., Campbell, D.R., Hughes, D.M., and Dillingham, D.A. (1982). *Feedstuffs 22,* 27.

Shin, D., and McGrane, M.M. (1997). *J. Nutr. 127,* 1274.

Sies, H., and Stahl, W. (1995). *Am. J. Clin. Nutr. 62,* 1322S.

Sijtsma, S.R., West, C.E., Rombout, J.H.W.M., and van der Zijpp, A.J. (1989). *J. Nutr. 119,* 932.

Singh, M.M., Sinha, G.K., and Gupta, B.N. (1965). *Ind. Vet. J. 42,* 879.

Smith, J.E. (1990). *Methods Enzymol. 190,* 229.

Snodderly, D.M. (1995). *Am. J. Clin. Nutr. 62*(Suppl.), 1448S.

Sommer, A., Tarwotijo, I., Djunaedi, E., West, K.P., Loeden, A.A., Tilden, R., and Mele, L. (1986). *Lancet 1 (9481),* 1169.

Sommer, A., Tarwotijo, I., Hussani, G., Susanto, D., and Soegiharto, T. (1981). *Lancet 1 (8235),* 1407.

Stahl, W., Schwarz, W., Von Laar, J., and Sies, H. (1995). *J. Nutr. 125,* 2128.

Stephensen, C.B., Blount, S.R., Schoeb, T.R., and Park, J.Y. (1993). *J. Nutr. 823,* 833.

Stephensen, C.B., Moldoveanu, Z., and Gangopadhyay, N.N. (1996). *J. Nutr. 126,* 94.

Suryawan, A., and Hu, C.Y. (1997). *J. Anim. Sci. 75,* 112.

Takyi, E.E.K. (1999). *J. Nutr. 129,* 1549.

Tanumihardjo, S.A., Permaesih, D., Rustan, E., Rusmil, K., Fatah, A.C., Wilbur, S., Karyadi, D., and Olson, J.A. (1996). *J. Nutr. 126,* 451.

Thurnham, D.I. (1994). *Proc. Nutr. Soc. 53,* 77.

Tjoelker, L.W., Chew, B.P., Tanaka, T.S., and Daniel, L.R. (1990). *J. Dairy Sci. 73,* 1017.

Tokach, M.D., Goodband, R.D., and Nelssen, J.L. (1994). *In* Kansas State University Swine Day, Kansas State University, Manhattan, Kansas.

Trout, W.E., Hall, J.A., Stallings-Mann, M.L., Galvin, J.M., Anthony, R.V., and Roberts, R.M. (1992). *Endocrinology 130,* 2557.

Ullrey, D.E. (1972). *J. Anim. Sci. 35,* 648.

Underwood, B.A. (1990). *J. Nutr. 120,* 1459.

Underwood, B.A. (1994). *J. Nutr. 124,* 1467S.

UNICEF. (1988). *Nutr. Rev. 56,* 115.

United Nations Administrative Committee on Coordination-Subcommittee on Nutrition. (1987). *First Report on the World Nutrition Situation,* p. 36. United Nations, Geneva.

Vallet, J.L. (1994). *J. Anim. Sci. 72,* 2449.

Vallet, J.L. (1995). *Biol. Reprod. 53,* 1436.

Van den Berg, H. (1999). *Nutr. Rev. 57,* 1.

Van der Pol, F., Purnomo, S.U., and Van Rosmalen, H.A. (1988). *Nutr. Rep. Int. 37,* 785.

Van Pelt, A.M.M., and De Rooij, D.G. (1990). *Biol. Reprod. 43,* 363.

Van Poppel, G., and Goldbohn, R.A. (1995). *Am. J. Clin. Nutr. 62,* 1393S.

Van Vliet, T., Van Vlissingen, M.F., Van Schaik, F., and Van den Berg, H. (1996). *J. Nutr. 126,* 499.

VERIS. (1996). *In* VERIS Research Summary, November. VERIS Research Information Service, La Grange, Illinois.

Wald, G. (1968). *Science 162,* 230.

Wang, J.Y., Owen, F.G., and Larson, L.L. (1988). *J. Dairy Sci. 71,* 181.

Wang, X. (1999). *Nutr. Rev. 57,* 51.

Weiss, W.P. (1998). *J. Dairy Sci. 81,* 2493.

West, C.E., Sijtsma, S.R., Kouwenhoven, B., Rombout, J.H.W.M., and van der Zijpp, A.J. (1992). *J. Nutr. 122,* 333.

West, K.P., LeClerq, S.C., Shrestha, S.R., Wu, L.S., Pradhan, E.K., Khatry, S.K., Katz, J., Adhikari, R., and Sommer, A. (1997). *J. Nutr. 127,* 1957.

West, K.P., Pokhrel, R.P., Katz, J., LeClerq, S.C., Khatry, S.K., Shrestha, S.R., Pradhan, E.K., Tielsch, J.M., Pandey, M.R., and Sommer, A. (1991). *Lancet 338 (8759),* 67.

Whaley, S.L., Hedgpeth, V.S., and Britt, J.H. (1997). *J. Anim. Sci. 75,* 1071.

White, W.S., Peck, K.M., Ulman, E.A., and Erdman, J.W. (1993). *J. Nutr. 123,* 1129.

Whiting, S.J., and Lemke, B. (1999). *Nutr. Rev. 57,* 192.

Wiedermann, U., Hanson, L.A., Holmgren, J., Kahu, H., and Dahlgren, U.I. (1993). *Infect. Immun. 61,* 3952.

Wing, J.M. (1969). *J. Dairy Sci. 52,* 479.

Wolf, G. (1991). *Nutr. Rev. 49*(1), 1.

Wolf, G. (1992). *Nutr. Rev. 50,* 292.

Wolf, G. (1995). *Nutr. Rev. 53*(5), 134.

Wolf, G. (1998). *Nutr. Rev. 56,* 156.

Zamora, R., Hidalgo, F.J., and Tappel, A.L. (1991). *J. Nutr. 121,* 30.

Zhao, Z., and Ross, C. (1995). *J. Nutr. 125,* 2064.

VITAMIN D

INTRODUCTION

Vitamin D is thought of as the "sunshine vitamin" because it is synthesized by various materials when they are exposed to sufficient sunlight. The two major natural sources of vitamin D are cholecalciferol (vitamin D_3, which occurs in animals) and ergocalciferol (vitamin D_2, which occurs predominantly in plants). In this chapter, the term vitamin D in the absence of a subscript will imply either vitamin D_2 or vitamin D_3. Under modern farming conditions, many animals, particularly swine and poultry, are raised in total confinement with little or no exposure to natural sunlight. Even though with adequate sunlight exposure, vitamin D is not needed in the diet, it still fits the definition of a vitamin in all respects for animals and humans who are confined indoors away from the sun. In recent years vitamin D receptors have been found in tissues not associated with the traditional role of calcium (Ca) metabolism. The additional roles of vitamin D await further elucidation.

HISTORY

Historical aspects of vitamin D have been reviewed by DeLuca (1979), Holick (1987), Loosli (1991), and Collins and Norman (1991). Vitamin D-deficiency rickets is a disease known since antiquity. There is evidence that rickets occurred in Neanderthal man about 50,000 B.C. In 525 B.C., there was a battle between Persia and Egypt, and 100 years later, the battlefield was visited by the Greek historian Herodotus. Herodotus noted that Persian skulls were so fragile they broke when struck by a pebble, while Egyptian skulls were strong. The difference related to sunlight and vitamin D activity; Egyptians went bareheaded from childhood while Persians covered their heads with turbans. Hippocrates described conditions that resembled rickets, and Soranus Ephesius (born A.D. 130) provided a classic description referring to "the backbone bending" and "legs twisted at the thighs" in a disease noted to be more common in smoky cities than in the country (Arneil, 1975).

Since the Middle Ages, it was observed that sunlight seemed to have health-giving effects. During the early stages of the Industrial Revolution in the late eighteenth and early nineteenth centuries, there was a mass migration of population from the rural countryside into the industrial centers of Great Britain and Europe. Young children of the working class who lived in the densely populated cities were affected by a severe bone-deforming disease. The combination of industrial pollution and narrow, shaded alleyways prevented children who were reared in this environment from being exposed to sunlight. When necropsy studies were performed on children who died of various causes, it was found in Leyden, The Netherlands, that 85 to 90% of these children suffered from rickets (Holick, 1987).

In 1822 Sniadecki suggested that rickets was caused by lack of exposure to sunlight. He observed that children who lived in inner cities of Warsaw, Poland, had a very high incidence of rickets, whereas children living on the farms on the outskirts of the city essentially were free of this disease. Almost 70 years later Palm concluded from an epidemiological survey that the common denominator in rickets in children was lack of exposure to sunlight. He encouraged systematic sunbathing as a means of preventing and curing rickets. The majority of scientists and physicians at the time did not believe that simple exposure to sunlight could cure or prevent this bone-deforming disease.

In the early twentieth century, Sir Edward Mellanby began his work on rickets, which was in epidemic proportions in the human population in his native England. Mellanby attempted to produce rickets by nutritional means, and in 1922 he succeeded in producing the disease in dogs maintained on a diet of oatmeal and, unplanned by him, in absence of sunlight. However, we now know sunlight would not have been a factor since vitamin D is not produced in the skin of this species (How et al., 1994a). Although Mellanby incorrectly concluded that the healing of rickets was a property of the fat-soluble vitamin A, he placed the study of rickets on an experimental basis.

McCollum, who had discovered the fat-soluble vitamin A, realized that the antirachitic activity discovered by Mellanby was distinct from the antixerophthalmia activity in cod liver oil. McCollum bubbled oxygen through cod liver oil and heated it to destroy the vitamin A activity, but the properties of cod liver oil in prevention and cure of rickets remained. Therefore, in 1922 he concluded that this unknown substance represented a new fat-soluble vitamin, which he called vitamin D.

Although it was known that ultraviolet (UV) light and vitamin D from cod liver oil were both equally effective in preventing and curing rickets, the close interdependence of these two factors was not immediately realized. Goldblatt and Soames (1923) conducted experiments in which they irradiated rachitic rats with UV light, removed their livers, and demonstrated that they contained the antirachitic substance, whereas if they were not irradiated, no antirachitic substance could be detected. Steenbock and Black (1924) then realized that UV irradiation was causing the alteration of some substance in animals and proceeded to demonstrate that UV irradiation of not only the animals but of their food could heal or prevent rickets.

These important discoveries led to the use of UV light irradiation of foods such as milk and butter to fortify them with vitamin D and thus eliminate rickets as a major medical problem. In addition, the demonstration that irradiation of food resulted in the production of an antirachitic factor provided the key for the isolation and chemical characterization of vitamin D_2 from the provitamin ergosterol, and that irradiation of skin produced vitamin D_3 from the provitamin 7-dehydrocholesterol. In 1932, the structure of vitamin D_2 was simultaneously determined by Windaus in Germany, who named it vitamin D_2, and by Askew in England, who named it ergocalciferol. In 1936, Windaus succeeded in identifying the structure of vitamin D_3. Vitamin D_1 had been isolated earlier by Windaus and his colleagues but was later shown to be a combination of vitamin D_2 and an irradiation side product, lumisterol.

A new phase of vitamin D research began in the late 1960s and has resulted in a complete change in attitude regarding the problems associated with this substance. It is now recognized that vitamin D is simply the precursor of a steroid hormone, 1,25-dihydroxyvitamin D [1,25-$(OH)_2D$], sometimes referred to as calcitrol. In 1966, DeLuca (1979) demonstrated the disappearance of vitamin D_3 following administration and the appearance of several metabolites that possessed more potent antirachitic activity. The first of these metabolites, 25-hydroxyvitamin D(25-OHD), was found to be produced in the liver. The 25-OHD form of vitamin D was chemically synthesized by Blunt and coworkers in 1968. Using the radioactively labeled chemical, 25-OHD was shown to be metabolically altered to at least three dihydroxy compounds, the most important thought to be 1,25-$(OH)_2D$. In the early 1970s, it was determined that the kidney was the principal site of 1,25-$(OH)_2D$ production. From the discoveries that this biologically active vitamin D metabolite is produced exclusively in kidney and is found in the nuclei of intestinal cells came the concept that, in terms of its structure and mode of action, vitamin D is similar to steroid hormones. The discovery that the biological actions of vitamin D can be explained by a hormone-like mechanism of action marked the beginning of the modern era of vitamin D research.

CHEMICAL STRUCTURE, PROPERTIES, AND ANTAGONISTS

Vitamin D designates a group of closely related compounds that possess antirachitic activity. It may be supplied through the diet or by irradiation of the body. There are about 10 provitamins that, after irradiation, form compounds having variable antirachitic activity. The two most prominent members of this group are ergocalciferol (vitamin D_2) and cholecalciferol (vitamin D_3). Chemical structures of ergocalciferol and cholecalciferol and their precursors, ergosterol and 7-dehydrocholesterol, are shown in Fig. 3.1. All sterols possessing vitamin D activity have the same steroid nucleus; they differ only in the nature of the side chain attached to carbon 17.

Ergocalciferol is derived from a common plant steroid, ergosterol, and is the usual dietary source of vitamin D. Cholecalciferol is produced exclusively from animal products. 7-Dehydrocholesterol is derived from cholesterol or squalene, which is synthesized in the body and present in large amounts in skin, intestinal wall, and other tissues. Vitamin D precursors have no antirachitic activity until the B-ring is opened between the 9 and 10 positions by irradiation and a double bond is formed between carbons 10 and 19 to form vitamin D.

Vitamin D in the pure form occurs as colorless crystals that are insoluble in water but readily soluble in alcohol and other organic solvents. It is less soluble in vegetable oils. Cholecalciferol crystallizes as fine white needles from diluted acetone and has a melting point between 84 and 85°C. Vitamin D can be destroyed by overtreatment with UV light and by peroxidation in the presence of rancidifying polyunsaturated fatty acids. Like vitamins A and E, unless vitamin D_3 is stabilized it is destroyed by oxidation. Its oxidative destruction is increased by heat, moisture, and trace minerals. There is less destruction of vitamin D_3 in freeze-dried fish meals during drying, possibly because of decreased atmospheric oxygen (Scott and Latshaw, 1994). There is negligible loss of crystalline cholecalciferol over 1 year of storage in amber evacuated

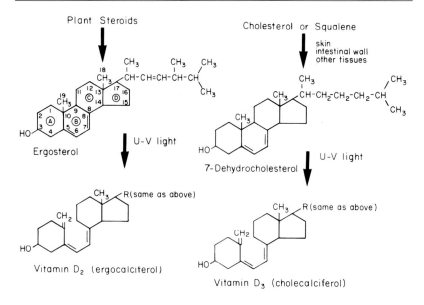

Fig. 3.1 Vitamin D_2 (ergocalciferol), vitamin D_3 (cholecalciferol), and their precursors in animal (7-dehydrocholesterol) and plant (ergosterol) tissues.

capsules at refrigerator temperatures or of ergocalciferol for 9 months. Solutions in corn oil stored in amber bottles have shown no loss of activity during 30 months of storage. Overirradiation of ergocalciferol or cholecalciferol produces numerous irradiation products such as tachysterols, supra-sterol$_1$, supra-sterol$_2$, and others. Some of these compounds have partial vitamin D activity, some are toxic, and some may be potent antagonists of vitamin D (Scott et al., 1982).

ANALYTICAL PROCEDURES

Vitamin D activity can be expressed in units based on a bioassay in vitamin D-deficient rats or chicks. When assayed in the rachitic rat, ergocalciferol and cholecalciferol are equally active with a potency of 40,000 units/mg of pure steroid. However, in chicks and other birds, ergocalciferol has only about one-tenth the activity of cholecalciferol (Chen and Bosmann, 1964). One international or USP unit of vitamin D activity is defined as the activity of 0.025 μg of vitamin D_3 contained in the USP vitamin D reference standard. For poultry, the term *international chick unit* (ICU) is employed with reference to use of D_3 versus D_2.

95

Methods of analysis for vitamin D are complex and somewhat difficult because there are so many isomers, and not all are biologically active. The standard method for assay of vitamin D supplements for feeds is a biological assay. Vitamin D is the only vitamin in which a biological method has not been largely replaced by a chemical, physical, or microbiological assay. The rat is often used to assay products for human and animal use, but the chick is the assay animal of choice in assessing supplements intended for poultry feeding because of unequal activity of vitamin D_2 and D_3 for this species compared with most mammals. Vitamin D_3 biological assay using young chicks has been standardized by the Association of Analytical Official Chemists. It involves feeding a standard rachitogenic ration to young chicks for a 21-day period and determining the ash content of dry fat-free tibia, either from chicks that have received the supplements containing unknown quantities of vitamin D or from those receiving standard quantities of a vitamin D reference standard (Scott et al., 1982).

A curative method involves developing rickets in young rats and chicks; then graded increments of unknown samples and standard vitamin D are added to diets for 7 days, followed by a "line test." This test entails staining a section of the metaphysis of the proximal end of the tibia with silver nitrate ($AgNO_3$) to show deposition of Ca salts. The silver precipitates the PO_4 and, on exposure to light, Ag_3PO_4 is reduced to Ag, which deposits in a black line. Bones are then graded numerically according to degree of calcification. Also, x-rays may be taken instead of using the line test. Chemical and physical methods to analyze vitamin D generally lack sensitivity of biological assays. Thus, they are not adequate for measuring samples that contain low concentrations of vitamin D. However, these physical and chemical means of vitamin D determination have the advantage of being less time-consuming than biological assays and are frequently used on samples known to contain high levels of vitamin D (Collins and Norman, 1991).

Physical and chemical methods of vitamin D analysis include UV absorption, colorimetric procedures, fluorescence spectroscopy, gas chromatography/mass spectroscopy, competitive binding assays, and high-pressure liquid chromatography (HPLC). The HPLC procedure is very promising, with the separation process resulting in an exceedingly high resolving capability and increased sensitivity (Collins and Norman, 1991; Matilla et al., 1995). A major advantage of HPLC is that compounds are not altered by the heat of gas-liquid chromatography, so they may be detected as the actual known compounds. Other benefits of using HPLC are the reduced labor and time required to separate vitamin

D and its metabolites. Compounds may be identified by the retention time of either an internal or external standard and a new technique of stop flow in which the UV spectrum of the molecule separated may be examined.

METABOLISM

Absorption and Conversion from Precursors

Vitamin D obtained from the diet is absorbed from the intestinal tract, with conflicting reports as to which portion of the small intestine serves as the primary absorption site. It has also been suggested that the largest amount of dietary vitamin D is more likely to be absorbed in the ileum because of longer retention time of food in the distal portion of the intestine (Norman and DeLuca, 1963).

Vitamin D is absorbed from the intestinal tract in association with fats, as are all the fat-soluble vitamins. Like the others, it requires the presence of bile salts for absorption. Because it is fat soluble, vitamin D is absorbed with other neutral lipids via chylomicra into the lymphatic system of mammals or the portal circulation of birds and fishes. It has been reported that only 50% of a dose of vitamin D is absorbed. However, considering that sufficient vitamin D is usually produced by daily exposure to sunlight, it is not surprising that the body has not evolved a more efficient mechanism for dietary vitamin D absorption (Collins and Norman, 1991).

Cholecalciferol is produced by irradiation of 7-dehydrocholesterol with UV light either from the sun or from an artificial source. Cholecalciferol is synthesized in the outer skin layers. Presence of the provitamin 7-dehydrocholesterol in the epidermis of the skin and sebaceous secretions is well recognized. In poultry, Tian et al. (1994) reported that in the chicken, the skin of legs and feet contains about 30 times as much 7-dehydrocholesterol (provitamin D_3) as the body skin.

Vitamin D is synthesized in the skin of many herbivores and omnivores, including humans, rats, pigs, horses, poultry, sheep, and cattle. However, little 7-dehydrocholesterol is found in the skin of cats and dogs (and likely other carnivores), and therefore little vitamin D is produced in the skin (How et al., 1995).

During exposure to sunlight, the high-energy UV photons (290–315 nm) penetrate the epidermis and photolyze 7-dehydrocholesterol (provitamin D_3) to previtamin D_3. Once formed, previtamin D_3 undergoes a thermally induced isomerization to vitamin D_3 that takes 2 to 3 days to reach completion. In poultry, the time course revealed a fourfold increase in the circulating concentration of vitamin D_3, with a peak about 30 hours postradiation (Tian et al., 1994). Approximately 15% of provitamin D_3 in human skin exposed to 10 minutes of simulated sunlight is converted in the stratum basale to vitamin D_3 (Holick et al., 1981). Longer exposure times do not significantly increase D_3 concentrations in the epidermis. Heuser and Norris (1929) showed that 11 to 45 minutes of sunshine daily were sufficient to prevent rickets in growing chicks, and that no further improvements in growth were obtained under these conditions by adding cod liver oil. During initial exposure to sunlight, provitamin D_3 in the human epidermis is efficiently converted to previtamin D_3. However, because previtamin D_3 is also labile to sunlight, once it is formed, it begins to photolyze to additional photoproducts, principally luminsterol and tachysterol. The net result is that prolonged exposure to sunlight does not significantly increase the previtamin D_3 concentration above about 15% of the initial provitamin D_3 concentrations (Holick, 1987).

More than 90% of previtamin D_3 synthesis in skin occurs in the epidermis. The cholecalciferol formed by irradiation of the 7-dehydrocholesterol in the skin is absorbed through the skin and transported by the blood to the lipids throughout the body. Clearly, absorption can take place, because rickets can be successfully treated by rubbing cod liver oil on the skin. Once vitamin D_3 is formed, it is transported in the blood. Some of the vitamin D_3 formed in and on the skin ends up in the digestive tract as many animals consume the vitamin as they lick their skin and hair.

Conversion to Metabolically Active Forms

Prior to 1968, it was almost universally thought that cholecalciferol and ergocalciferol (D_3 and D_2) were the circulating antirachitic agents in the living animal system. Starting in 1968, DeLuca and a number of other researchers demonstrated that vitamin D undergoes a multiple series of transformations and multi-site interactions in the living system (DeLuca, 1979). Whether the vitamin is ingested orally or produced photochemically in the skin, these chemical changes occur before any significant biological response is registered in the intestine or bone. Production and metabolism of the vitamin D necessary to activate the target organs are illustrated in Fig. 3.2.

Once vitamin D (D_2, D_3, or both) enters the blood, it circulates at relatively low concentrations. This phenomenon is probably a result of its rapid accumulation in the liver. Once in the liver, the first transfor-

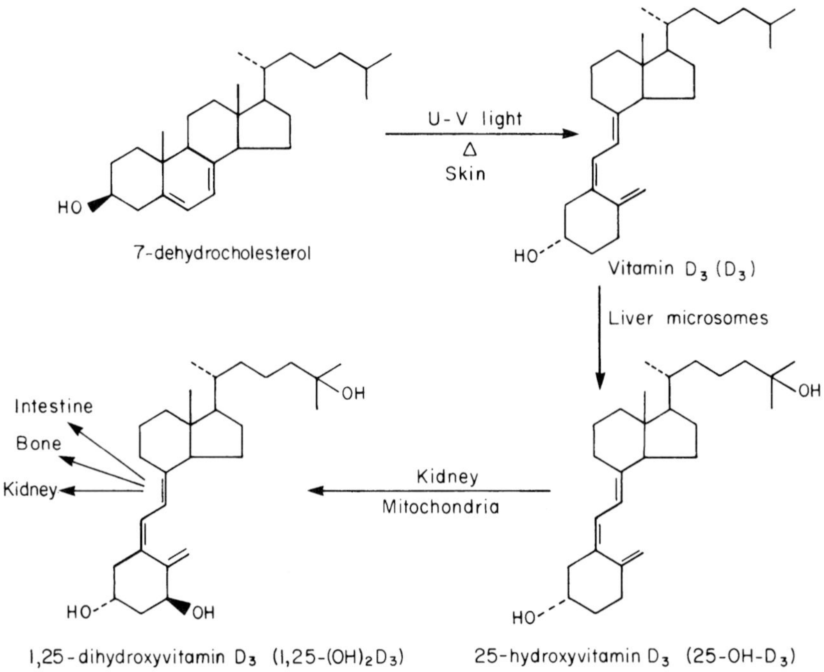

Fig. 3.2 The functional metabolism of vitamin D_3 necessary to activate the target organs of intestine, bone, and kidney.

mation occurs, in which a microsomal system hydroxylates the 25-carbon in the side chain to produce 25-OH vitamin D. This metabolite is the major circulating form of vitamin D under normal conditions and during vitamin D excess (Littledike and Horst, 1982).

Conversion to 25-OHD takes place predominantly in the microsomes but also in the mitochondria. The mitochondrial enzyme is a high-capacity, low-affinity enzyme and is thought to hydroxylate vitamin D under conditions of high substrate concentrations, such as vitamin D toxicity. Liver is the major site of 25-hydroxylation of vitamin D; however, the intestine and kidney can also produce 25-OHD, although the amount of 25-hydroxylation taking place in these organs is small (Tucker et al., 1973). In the chicken, the D-25-hydroxylase enzyme exists in the extrahepatic tissues, including the intestine and kidney, but in mammals, the liver is the predominant site.

The 25-OHD is then transported to the kidney on the vitamin D transport globulin, where it can be converted to a variety of compounds, of which the most important appears to be $1,25\text{-}(OH)_2D_3$ (also called calcitrol) (DeLuca, 1990). This reaction occurs in the mitochondrial fraction and is catalyzed by a three-component, mixed-function monoxygenase involving NADPH, molecular oxygen, a flavoprotein, an iron-sulfur protein, and cytochrome P-450 (Ghazarian et al., 1974). The 1,25-$(OH)_2$D that is formed in the kidney is then transported to the intestine, bones, or elsewhere in the kidney, where it is involved in the metabolism of Ca and phosphorus (P). The hormonal form is the metabolically active form of the vitamin that functions in intestine and bone, whereas 25-OHD and vitamin D do not function at these specific sites under physiological conditions (DeLuca, 1990).

Production of 1,25-$(OH)_2$D is very carefully regulated by parathyroid hormone in response to serum Ca and phosphate concentrations. Removal of parathyroid glands results in an animal's inability to adapt to varying Ca demands by increasing intestinal Ca absorption. It is now known that the most important point of regulation of the vitamin D endocrine system occurs through the stringent control of the activity of the renal 1-hydroxylase. In this way, the production of the hormone 1,25-$(OH)_2$D can be modulated according to the Ca needs of the organism (Collins and Norman, 1991). Factors known to affect the activity of the 1-hydroxylase include Ca, parathyroid hormone, and vitamin D status. Both intestinal and serum 1,25-$(OH)_2$D concentrations and activity of 1-hydroxylase are inversely related to dietary and serum Ca concentrations.

Later, it was found that the hormone 1,25-$(OH)_2$D is produced by its endocrine gland, the kidney, and a paracrine system (Norman, 1995). The 1-hydroxylase activities have been confirmed in placenta and in cultured cell lines (skin, bone, embryonic intestine).

Epidermal cells (keratinocytes) produce vitamin D; metabolize it to its most biologically active form, 1,25-$(OH)_2$D; and in response to the 1,25-$(OH)_2$D, there is a decrease in proliferation and an increase in differentiation (Bikle, 1995). 1,25-$(OH)_2$D production by keratinocytes is tightly controlled and changes as the cells differentiate, increasing during the early stages of differentiation and then decreasing again as terminal differentiation ensues.

Besides 1,25-$(OH)_2$D, the kidney also converts 25-OHD to other known compounds, including 24,25-$(OH)_2$D, 25-26-$(OH)_2$D, and 1,24,25-$(OH)_2$D. The role of these compounds in function or inactivation of vitamin D has not been fully evaluated, and significant physiological roles are yet to be discovered. Although controversy exists, it has been suggested that 24,25-$(OH)_2$D is responsible for the mineralization of bone and for the suppression of parathyroid hormone secretion.

Bordier et al. (1978) showed that 24,25-$(OH)_2D_3$ is required with 1,25-$(OH)_2D_3$ for normal healing of osteomalacia in humans. Dogs with impaired renal function had depressed serum concentration of 24,25-$(OH)_2D_3$, but no clinical benefit was observed when this form of vitamin D was administered (Dzanis et al., 1992). The hormonal role of 24,25-$(OH)_2D$ is very tentative. Although it has been shown that 24-hydroxylation appears to have a role in bone mineralization, it is also believed to be involved in the elimination pathway for 25-hydroxy and 1,25-dihydroxy vitamin D.

Henry and Norman (1978) have shown that hatchability of eggs from hens is severely depressed in vitamin D-deficient hens even when they are fed 1,25-$(OH)_2D_3$. Evidently, 1,25-$(OH)_2D_3$ is effective in maintaining blood Ca levels so that egg production and egg shell thickness remain normal. However, without vitamin D, the upper mandible of the chicks fails to develop, and consequently, the chicks cannot crack the shell, resulting in mortality. The suggestion was made that chick mortality resulted from lack of 24,25-$(OH)_2D$. However, the reason for the chick deaths related to failure of 1,25-$(OH)_2D_3$ being passed from the hen to the egg, as D_3 and 25-OHD_3 are readily passed to the egg.

Transport

Vitamin D in plasma, coming from either diet or the skin, is picked up for transport to the liver by a plasma protein called vitamin D-binding protein (DBP; also called transcalciferin), which is synthesized in the liver. In mammals, vitamin D, 25-OHD, and possibly 24,25-$(OH)_2D$ and 1,25-$(OH)_2D$, are all transported by DBP. This protein has a molecular weight of 50,000 to 60,000 and in humans appears to be a single-chain polypeptide. The DBP binds 25-OHD (the major circulating metabolite) with a higher affinity than it binds vitamin D or 1,25-$(OH)_2D_3$ (Haddad and Walgate, 1976). With radioactively labeled metabolites, Hay and Watson (1976) observed in 65 of the 72 species of mammals studied that the vitamin D metabolites associated with a protein of α-globulin mobility as determined by disk gel electrophoresis. This was also observed in bony fish, reptiles, and some species of birds. However, for several mammalian species and in four species of birds, 25-OHD was carried on albumin or on a protein with albumin-like electrophoretic mobility.

Storage and Placental Transfer

In contrast to aquatic species, which store significant amounts of vitamin D in liver, land animals and humans do not store appreciable amounts of the vitamin. The body has some ability to store the vitamin, although to a much lesser extent than is the case for vitamin A. Principal stores of vitamin D occur in blood and liver, but it is also found in lungs, kidneys, and elsewhere. Since it was known that liver serves as a storage site for vitamin A, another fat-soluble vitamin, it was thought that the liver also functioned as a storage site for vitamin D. However, it has since been shown that blood has the highest concentration of vitamin D compared with other tissues; in pigs, the amount of vitamin D in blood is several times higher than that in liver (Quaterman et al., 1964).

The persistence of vitamin D in animals during periods of vitamin D deficiency may be explained by slow turnover rate of vitamin D in certain tissues, such as skin and adipose tissue. During times of deprivation, vitamin D in these tissues is released slowly, thus meeting vitamin D needs of the animal over a longer period (Collins and Norman, 1991).

Transplacental movement of Ca increases dramatically during the last trimester of gestation in all species observed. It is well established that in most mammalian species, fetal plasma Ca levels are higher than maternal levels at term. In sheep, passive diffusion accounts for a minor component of placental Ca movement, with active transport mechanisms responsible for more than 90% (Braithwaite et al., 1972). In the pregnant rat (and perhaps humans), $1,25\text{-}(OH)_2D$ is a critical factor in the maintenance of sufficient maternal Ca for transport to the fetus and may play a role in normal skeletal development of the neonate (Lester, 1986). Although there is no large transfer to the fetus, liberal intake during gestation provides a sufficient store in newborns to help prevent early rickets. For example, newborn lambs can be provided enough in this way to meet their needs for 6 weeks. Parenteral cholecalciferol treatment of sows before parturition proved an effective means of supplementing young piglets with cholecalciferol (via the sow's milk) and its more polar metabolites via placental transport (Goff et al., 1984).

Excretion

Excretion of absorbed vitamin D and its metabolites occurs primarily in feces with the aid of bile salts. Very little vitamin D appears in urine. Ohnuma et al. (1980) suggested that the metabolite $1,25\text{-}(OH)_2D_3\text{-}26,23\text{-}lactone$ may represent one of the first steps in the catabolism of $1,25\text{-}(OH)_2D_3$. Because the half-life of $25,26\text{-}(OH)_2D$ in serum is only 10 days, this metabolite might have an excretory role.

FUNCTIONS

The general function of vitamin D is to elevate plasma Ca and P to a level that will support normal mineralization of bone as well as other body functions. The active form of vitamin D, 1,25-$(OH)_2$D, functions as a steroid hormone. The hormone is produced by an endocrine gland, circulated in blood bound to a carrier protein (DBP), and transported to target tissues.

In the target tissue, the hormone enters the cell and binds to a cytosolic receptor or a nuclear receptor. 1,25-$(OH)_2$D regulates gene expression through its binding to tissue-specific receptors and subsequent interaction between the bound receptor and the DNA (Collins and Norman, 1991; DeLuca and Zierold, 1998). The receptor-hormone complex moves to the nucleus, where it binds to the chromatin and stimulates the transcription of particular genes to produce specific mRNAs, which code for the synthesis of specific proteins. Evidence for transcription regulation of a specific gene typically includes 1,25-$(OH)_2$D–induced modulation in mRNA levels. Additionally, evidence may include measurements of transcription and/or the presence of a vitamin D-responsive element within the promoter region of the gene (Hannah and Norman, 1994). Recent research provides evidence that a membrane-bound receptor, in addition to nuclear receptors, exists (Fleet, 1999).

The 1,25-$(OH)_2D_3$ receptor has been extensively characterized, and the cDNA for the human receptor has been cloned (Baker et al., 1988). The 1,25-$(OH)_2D_3$ receptor is a protein with a molecular weight of about 67,000 daltons. The nucleotide sequence of the bovine vitamin D_3 receptor has been reported (Neibergs et al., 1996).

Common vitamin D receptor gene alleles have been shown to contribute to the genetic variability in bone mass and bone turnover; however, the physiological mechanisms involved are unknown. The vitamin D receptor alleles are associated with differences in the vitamin D endocrine system and may have important implications in relation to the pathophysiology of osteoporosis (Howard et al., 1995; Eisman, 1998).

Recent studies have identified a heterodimer of the vitamin D receptor (VDR) and a vitamin A receptor (RXR) within the nucleus of the cell as the active complex for mediating positive transcriptional effects of 1,25-$(OH)_2$D. The two receptors (vitamins D and A) selectively interact with specific hormone response elements composed of direct repeats of specific nucleotides located in the promoter of regulated genes. The complex that binds to these elements actually consists of three distinct elements: the 1,25-$(OH)_2D_3$ hormonal ligand, the vitamin D receptor (VDR), and one of the vitamin A (retinoid) X receptors (RXR) (Kliewer et al., 1992; Whitfield et al., 1995).

Since the late 1980s, it has become apparent that 1,25-$(OH)_2D_3$ also has the potential to generate biological actions through mechanisms not dependent on regulation of gene transcription (Norman, 1995). Research suggests that 1,25-$(OH)_2D_3$ may also generate biological responses via signal transduction mechanisms that are independent of the nuclear VDRs, which are termed nongenomic pathways. Nongenomic responses can include stimulation of membrane lipid turnover, activation of Ca^{2+} channels, and elevation of intracellular Ca^{2+} concentrations, all of which have been shown to occur within seconds after addition of 1,25-$(OH)_2D_3$. Progress has been made in identifying and purifying an integral protein of the basal lateral membrane that may be a receptor for 1,25-$(OH)_2D_3$ (Nemere, 1995). These studies have provided definite correlations between binding to the solubilized membrane receptor and the ability to initiate transcaltachia (the rapid hormonal stimulation of Ca transport). The involvement in genomic and nongenomic signal transduction pathways is not unique to the steroid hormone 1,25-$(OH)_2D_3$; these same pathways are also utilized by virtually all steroid hormones (Nemere et al., 1993).

Relationship to Calcium and Phosphorus Homeostasis

Tetany in humans and animals results if plasma Ca levels are appreciably below normal. Two hormones—thyrocalcitonin (calcitonin) and parathyroid hormone (PTH)—function in a delicate relationship with 1,25-$(OH)_2D$ to control blood Ca and P levels. Production rate of 1,25-$(OH)_2D$ is under physiological control as well as dietary control (see Metabolism, Conversion to Metabolically Active Forms). Calcitonin, contrary to the other two, regulates high serum Ca levels by (1) depressing gut absorption, (2) halting bone demineralization, and (3) reabsorption in the kidney. Vitamin D brings about an elevation of plasma Ca and P by stimulating specific pump mechanisms in the intestine, bone, and kidney. These three sources of Ca and P thus provide reservoirs that enable vitamin D to elevate the levels of Ca and P in blood to levels that are necessary for normal bone mineralization and for other functions ascribed to Ca.

Intestinal Effects

It is well known that vitamin D stimulates active transport of Ca and P across intestinal epithelium. This stimulation involves the parathyroid hormone directly and the active form of vitamin D. Parathyroid hormone indirectly stimulates intestinal Ca absorption by stimulating production of $1,25\text{-}(OH)_2D$ under conditions of hypocalcemia. As the human body becomes vitamin D insufficient, the efficiency of intestinal Ca absorption decreases from approximately 30 to 50% to no more than 15%.

The mechanism whereby vitamin D stimulates Ca and P absorption is still not completely understood. Evidence (Wasserman, 1981) indicates that $1,25\text{-}(OH)_2D$ is transferred to the nucleus of the intestinal cell, where it interacts with the chromatin material. In response to the $1,25\text{-}(OH)_2D$, specific RNAs are elaborated by the nucleus, and when these are translated into specific proteins by ribosomes, the events leading to enhancement of Ca and P absorption occur (Scott et al., 1982).

In the intestine, $1,25\text{-}(OH)_2D$ promotes synthesis of Ca-binding protein (calbindin) and other proteins and stimulates Ca and P absorption. Vitamin D has also been reported to influence magnesium (Mg) absorption as well as Ca and P balance (Miller et al., 1965). Administration of $1,25\text{-}(OH)_2D_3$ to rachitic animals has been shown to stimulate the incorporation of [^{3}H] leucine into several proteins of the intestinal mucosa. This apparent increase in protein synthesis was accounted for at least in part by the discovery that $1,25\text{-}(OH)_2D$ induces synthesis of a specific intestinal protein that has been identified as calbindin. Calbindin is not present in the intestine of rachitic chicks but appears after vitamin D treatment.

Intestinal Ca transport relies on the integrated effects of both genomic and nongenomic mechanisms of hormone action. Two kinds of mucosal proteins are dependent on vitamin D: (1) calbindin and (2) intestinal membrane Ca-binding protein (IMCal). IMCal is a membrane component of the translocation mechanism rather than a cytosol constituent (Schachter and Kowarski, 1982). It is proposed that the primary nongenomic mechanism by which $1,25\text{-}(OH)_2D$ regulates Ca transport across the luminal membrane of the enterocyte involves inducing a specific alteration in membrane phosphatidylcholine content and structure, which leads to an increase in membrane fluidity and thereby to an increase in Ca transport rate. The size of the villus and the microvilli increases upon $1,25\text{-}(OH)_2D_3$ treatment. The brush border undergoes noticeable alterations in structure and composition of cell surface proteins and lipids, in a time frame corresponding to the increase in Ca^{2+} transport mediated by $1,25\text{-}(OH)_2D_3$ (Collins and Norman, 1991). In addition to inducing calbindin and IMCal, $1,25\text{-}(OH)_2D_3$ has been shown to increase levels of several other proteins in the intestinal mucosa. These include alkaline phosphatase, Ca-stimulated ATPase, and phytase enzyme activities (Collins and Norman, 1991). Once Ca is transported to the basolateral membrane, it is extruded from the cell against a 1,000-fold concentration gradient by Mg-dependent Ca-ATPase, which is also increased by 1,25-$(OH)_2D_3$ (Bronner, 1987).

Originally, it was believed that vitamin D did not regulate P absorption and transport, but in 1963, it was demonstrated, through the use of an in vitro inverted sac technique, that vitamin D does in fact play such a role (Harrison and Harrison, 1963). Little is known about the actual mechanism of phosphate transport, but phosphate is transported against an electrochemical potential gradient involving sodium in response to 1,25-$(OH)_2D_3$.

Bone Effects

Vitamin D plays roles both in the mineralization of bone as well as demineralization or mobilization of bone mineral. 1,25-$(OH)_2D$ is one of the factors controlling the balance between bone formation and resorption. In young animals during bone formation, minerals are deposited on the matrix. This is accompanied by an invasion of blood vessels that gives rise to trabecular bone. This process causes bones to elongate. During vitamin D deficiency, this organic matrix fails to mineralize, causing rickets in the young and osteomalacia in adults. 1,25-$(OH)_2D_3$ brings about mineralization of the bone matrix, and Weber et al. (1971) provided evidence that 1,25-$(OH)_2D_3$ is localized in the nuclei of bone cells. Also, there is some indication that 24,25-$(OH)_2D_3$ and possibly 25-OHD_3 may have unique actions on bone.

Vitamin D also plays a role in the mobilization of Ca from bone to the extracellular fluid compartment. This function is shared by PTH (Garabedian et al., 1974). However, little is known about the mechanism of bone reabsorption in response to these factors, although it may be similar or identical to the intestinal transport system. It is an active process requiring metabolic energy, and presumably it transports Ca and phosphate across the bone membrane by acting on osteocytes and osteoclasts.

Rapid, acute plasma Ca regulation is due to the interaction of plasma Ca with Ca-binding sites in bone mineral since blood is in contact with bone. Changes in plasma Ca are brought about by a change in the proportion of high- and low-affinity Ca-binding sites, access to which is regulated by osteoclasts and osteoblasts, respectively (Bronner and Stein, 1995). These cells, in turn, respond to hormonal signals by shape changes. Contraction of osteoclasts and corresponding expansion of osteoblasts make more high-affinity sites available, whereas osteoblast contraction and osteoclast expansion, make more low-affinity sites available, leading to a decrease or an increase in the blood Ca level, respectively.

Another role of vitamin D has been proposed in addition to its involvement in bone; namely, in the biosynthesis of collagen in preparation for mineralization (Gonnerman et al., 1976). A vitamin D deficiency causes inadequate cross-linking of collagen as a result of low lysyl oxidase activity, which is involved in a condensation reaction for the collagen cross-linking. This may be a direct effect of vitamin D or a result of mineral changes in blood; it is not considered a major function of vitamin D.

Kidney Effects

There is evidence that vitamin D functions in the distal renal tubules to improve Ca reabsorption and is mediated by calbindin (Bronner and Stein, 1995). It is known that 99% of the filtered load of Ca is reabsorbed in the absence of vitamin D and the parathyroid hormone. The remaining 1% is under control of these two hormonal agents, although it is not known whether they work in concert. It has been shown that $1,25\text{-}(OH)_2D_3$ functions in improving renal reabsorption of Ca (Sutton and Dirks, 1978). With intact parathyroids and without vitamin D, renal tubular resorption of inorganic phosphate decreases, thereby increasing phosphate clearance and resulting in hypophosphatemia, although the parathyroids maintain a normal plasma Ca level. With adequate vitamin D, greater reabsorption of P by the renal tubules occurs. Without intact parathyroids, vitamin D actually increases renal loss of P.

Calcium and Phosphorus Absorption by Ruminants

Calcium

There is clear evidence that sheep and cattle absorb Ca from their gut according to need and that they can alter the efficiency of absorption to meet a change in requirement. For example, Braithwaite and Riazuddin (1971) showed that young sheep with a high Ca requirement absorb Ca at a higher rate and with greater efficiency than mature animals with a low requirement. An increase in both absorption and efficiency of absorption also occurs in mature sheep when their requirement for Ca is increased through pregnancy or lactation or after a period of Ca deficiency (Braithwaite, 1974).

Studies in cattle have given similar results. Thus, the efficiency of absorption of Ca in the small intestine of the dairy cow has been shown to rise in response to a reduction in dietary Ca intake and to the onset of lactation (Scott and McLean, 1981). Calcium absorption has also been shown to be directly related to milk production, though in early lactation, when the demand for Ca is greatest, the increase in absorption falls short of the requirement, with the deficit being met by increased bone resorption (Braithwaite et al., 1969).

The mechanism by which Ca is adjusted in response to requirement has received much attention. In this sequence, a fall in plasma Ca concentration resulting from an increase in demand leads in turn to an increase in parathyroid hormone release. This then stimulates the increased production by the kidney of $1,25\text{-}(OH)_2D$, which acts on the gut to increase the production of calbindin and so accelerates Ca absorption. In a reverse manner, an increase in plasma Ca concentration causes suppression of parathyroid hormone release, a reduction in $1,25\text{-}(OH)_2D$ production, and reduced Ca absorption. Although all aspects of this system have not yet been fully examined in ruminants, it appears that the same mechanism operates, in that an increase in circulatory $1,25\text{-}(OH)_2D$ level has been found to precede the increase in Ca absorption that occurs in cattle soon after parturition (Horst et al., 1978).

Phosphorus Absorption

Sheep fed on roughage diets usually excrete little P in their urine (Scott and McLean, 1981), so control of P balance must therefore be achieved within the gut through control of either absorption or secretion or both. Saliva is the main contributor of P in the gut. Little or no net absorption of P appears to occur from either the forestomach or the large intestine, and it is generally accepted that the upper small intestine is the major absorptive site. Using sheep fitted with reentrant cannulas, several workers have shown that the secretion of P before the pylorus (salivary) is closely matched by net absorption in the small intestine. Ability to balance absorption against secretion has been shown to be unaffected by wide variations in dietary Ca:P values (Scott and McLean, 1981).

Until recently, secretion of P in saliva has usually been viewed in the context of its role as a buffer against the volatile fatty acids produced in the rumen. However, studies by Australian workers (Tomas, 1974) have suggested that salivary glands, apart from their role as a source of buffer, may also play an important role in P homeostasis by controlling the amount of P secreted into the gut. Evidence for this function was provided by sheep studies in which both parotid salivary ducts were ligated, a procedure that led to a small increase in urinary P excretion and a proportional reduction in fecal P excretion (Tomas and Somers, 1974). Similar changes in the pathway of P excretion were also seen in sheep in which part of the parotid salivary flow was collected and returned directly to the circulation.

Ruminants have a higher renal threshold for P excretion than do monogastric species, and it is important to consider what advantage this confers. Poor-quality roughage diets, apart from their low digestibility, also tend to contain little P (McDowell, 1997). Therefore, the ratio between the amount of P required for saliva production and dietary intake is wide. If the renal threshold for P excretion in ruminants were as low as in monogastric species, then at times when the concentration of inorganic P in the plasma rises in response to reabsorption, P would be excreted in the urine. This P would not, however, in any real sense be surplus to requirement, and its loss would have to be met from a diet low in available P. Under such conditions, there is clearly an advantage to the ruminant in maintaining the high renal threshold for P excretion.

Concentrate diets, especially those that include fish meal, contain much larger quantities of P than do roughage diets, to the point where intake may equal or exceed the amount secreted in the saliva. Under these conditions, need to control P absorption is clearly less critical and, as a result, a different level of control may operate. Increasing dietary P intake leads to increased absorption and increased urinary P excretion.

Administration of large amounts of parathyroid hormone over several days has been shown to reduce fecal P excretion in cattle (Mayer et al., 1968), though whether this was due to reduced secretion or increased absorption is not clear. In sheep, parathyroidectomy has been shown to result in a negative balance for both Ca and P, and it has been suggested that the effect on P balance was the result of a reduction in the amount of salivary P reabsorbed (McIntosh and Tomas, 1978). 1,25-$(OH)_2D$ has also been suggested as a possible regulator of intestinal P absorption in ruminants (Scott and McLean, 1981), though whether this was a primary effect or secondary to its effects on Ca absorption and deposition in bone is not clear.

Other Vitamin D Functions

The well-known effects of vitamin D relate to biochemical changes occurring in the intestine, bone, and kidney. Vitamin D has also been shown to be required for chick embryonic development. Vitamin D treatment stimulated yolk Ca mobilization, and the vitamin D-dependent Ca-binding protein, calbindin, is present in the yolk sac (Tuan and

Suyama, 1996). These findings strongly suggest that the hormonal action of 1,25-(OH)$_2$D on yolk sac Ca transport is mediated by the regulated expression and activity of calbindin, analogous to the response of the adult intestine. 1,25-(OH)$_2$D is also essential for the transport of eggshell Ca to the embryo across the chorioallantoic membrane (Elaroussi et al., 1994).

Vitamin D is important for more than just its traditional role in Ca metabolism. A receptor for the active metabolite 1,25-(OH)$_2$D has been isolated in the pancreas, parathyroid glands, bone marrow, certain cells of the ovary and brain, endocrine cells of the stomach, breast epithelial cells, skin fibroblasts, and keratinocytes, suggesting that 1,25-(OH)$_2$D has additional functions in a wide variety of cells, glands, and organs (Machlin and Sauberlich, 1994). In the pancreas, 1,25-(OH)$_2$D is essential for normal insulin secretion. Experiments with rats have shown that vitamin D increases insulin release from isolated perfused pancreas, both in the presence or absence of normal serum Ca levels (Cade and Norman, 1986). More than 50 genes have been reported to be transcriptionally regulated by 1,25-(OH)$_2$D (Hannah and Norman, 1994).

The actions of 1,25-(OH)$_2$D$_3$ are recognized as being involved in regulation of the growth and differentiation of a variety of cell types, including those of hematopoietic and immune systems (Lemire, 1992). Studies have suggested 1,25-(OH)$_2$D$_3$ as an immunoregulatory hormone. Elevated 1,25-(OH)$_2$D also has been associated with a significant 70% enhancement of lymphocyte proliferation in cells treated with pokeweed mitogen (Hustmeyer et al., 1994). 1,25-(OH)$_2$D$_3$ also inhibits growth of certain malignant cell types and promotes their differentiation (Colston et al., 1981; DeLuca, 1992). 1,25-(OH)$_2$D has been reported to inhibit proliferation of leukemic cells (Pakkala et al., 1995), breast cancer cells (Vink van Wijngaarden et al., 1995), and colorectal cancer cells (Cross et al., 1995). A deficiency of vitamin D may promote prostate cancer (Skowronski et al., 1995). Also, 1,25-(OH)$_2$D and its analogs may be effective in treating some forms of psoriasis (Kragballe et al., 1991). The therapeutic value of vitamin D and its analogs has been under rigorous evaluation in numerous laboratories around the world.

Thus, the concept has emerged that 1,25-(OH)$_2$D, and possibly other vitamin D metabolites, have functions that extend beyond those of regulating bone mineralization and intestinal Ca transport. The skin is one such tissue in which this broader role is being intensively explored. Besides producing vitamin D, epidermal cells (keratinocytes) make 1,25-(OH)$_2$D and respond to the 1,25-(OH)$_2$D they produce with a decrease in proliferation and an increase in differentiation (Bikle et al., 1995). 1,25-(OH)$_2$D production by keratinocytes is tightly controlled and changes as the cells differentiate, increasing during the early stages of differentiation and then decreasing again as terminal differentiation ensues. The 1,25-(OH)$_2$D produced endogenously or supplied exogenously acts in concert with Ca and products of phosphoinositide metabolism to stimulate the transition from a proliferating basal cell to a terminally differentiated corneocyte. The mechanisms involved include changes in gene transcription and messenger RNA stability.

REQUIREMENTS

Most animals and humans do not have a nutritional requirement for vitamin D when sufficient sunlight is available, since vitamin D$_3$ is produced in skin through action of UV light on 7-dehydrocholesterol.

Unlike humans, rats, common poultry, and livestock, dogs and cats (and perhaps other carnivores) have a nutritional requirement for vitamin D even when sufficient sunlight is available, since vitamin D$_3$ is not produced in skin through action of UV irradiation on 7-dehydrocholesterol in sufficient quantities to prevent rickets (How et al., 1994a,b, 1995). Hazewinkel et al. (1987) found that rickets in dogs could not be prevented or treated by UV radiation; treated dogs developed clinical, biochemical, and histological signs of rickets. In the skin of the dog and cat, the concentrations of the precursor 7-dehydrocholesterol are low, and the precursor is inadequately converted to vitamin D. It is suggested that carnivores do not need to provide their own vitamin D, since fat, liver, and blood of their prey will fulfill this need (How et al., 1995). In addition to sunlight, other factors influencing dietary vitamin D requirements include (1) amount and ratio of dietary Ca and P, (2) availability of P and Ca, (3) species, and (4) physiological factors.

Vitamin D becomes a nutritionally important factor in the absence of sufficient sunlight. Sunlight that comes through ordinary window glass is ineffective in producing vitamin D in skin, since glass does not allow penetration of UV rays, and its effectiveness is dependent on length and intensity of UV rays that reach the body. The radiation that reaches the earth contains only a small part of the UV range that has an antirachitic effect. Sunlight is more potent in the tropics than in the temperate or arctic zones, more potent in summer than in winter, more potent at noon than in the morning or evening, and more potent at high altitudes. Sunlight provides most of its antirachitic powers during the 4 hours around noon.

Season and latitude greatly influence skin synthesis of vitamin D_3. In Boston (42.2°N), previtamin D_3 was produced in the irradiated skin samples exposed to sunlight from March through October, but not at all from November through February (Webb et al., 1988). In Edmonton, Alberta, Canada (52° N), the effective period for the synthesis of previtamin D_3 commenced at the beginning of April and ceased after October. In Los Angeles (34° N) and Puerto Rico (18°N), sunlight effectively photoconverted 7-dehydrocholesterol to previtamin D_3 even in the middle of winter. These data confirm that the conversion of 7-dehydrocholesterol to previtamin D_3 is dependent on the intensity of UV radiation as affected by the zenith angle of the sun at various latitudes and by seasons of the year.

Besides geographical and seasonal considerations, sunlight may be blocked by many means. Potency of UV light varies greatly with differences in atmospheric conditions and because of clouds, mist, or smoke. Air pollution screens out many UV rays as does the use of sunscreens. Air pollution became prevalent during the Industrial Revolution and, at the same time, the incidence of rickets became widespread in industrial cities. It is now known that this epidemic of rickets was partly due to the lack of sunlight because of the presence of air pollution. Thus, rickets has been called the first air-pollution disease. Animals housed for much of the year must depend on their feed for the vitamin D they need; in a modern agricultural economy, this applies particularly to intensive swine and poultry production.

The colors of the coat and skin are important in determining response to irradiation. UV irradiation is more effective on exposed skin than through a heavy coat of hair. Irradiation is less effective on dark-pigmented skin. This has been shown to be true for white and black breeds of hogs as well as for people. White pigs have taken about twice as long as colored pigs to show signs of vitamin D deficiency (Cunha, 1977).

In white humans, 20 to 30% of the UV radiation is transmitted through the epidermis, while in black people, less than 5% of the UV radiation penetrates the epidermis (Holick, 1987). When specimens of surgically obtained white and black skin were exposed to simulated sunlight under the same conditions, longer exposure times were needed to maximize vitamin D_3 formation in the samples of black skin. As skin pigmentation increased, the time required to maximize vitamin D_3 formation increased from 30 minutes to 3 hours.

Aging has an effect on the cutaneous production of vitamin D_3. In humans older than about 20 years, skin thickness decreases linearly with time. A comparison of amounts of previtamin D_3 generated in the skin of young and elderly subjects showed that aging can decrease more than twofold the capacity of the skin to produce previtamin D_3 (Holick, 1986).

Amounts of dietary Ca and P, and the physical and chemical forms in which they are presented, must be considered when determining vitamin D requirements. High dietary Ca concentrations can precipitate phosphates as insoluble Ca phosphate. If Ca is given in the form of a relatively insoluble compound, or even a Ca compound that is normally easily soluble but is too coarsely ground, it may be comparatively unavailable, for example, coarse limestone (Ca carbonate) (Franklin and Johnstone, 1948). Soluble Ca salts are more readily absorbed, and oxalates tend to interfere with absorption, but some of this interference can be overcome by dietary vitamin D or irradiation.

Correspondingly, while the P of inorganic orthophosphate tends to be well absorbed, other factors being favorable, that of phytic acid (see Chapter 17), which is the predominant P compound of unprocessed cereal grains and oilseeds, seems to be poorly available except to species (such as ruminants) with massive populations of microorganisms in the gut that synthesize phytase enzymes. Phosphorus absorption is mostly independent of vitamin D intake, with the inefficient absorption and the improvement upon vitamin administration being a result of improving Ca absorption.

The need for vitamin D depends to a large extent on the Ca-P ratio. As this ratio becomes either wider or narrower than the optimum, the vitamin D requirement increases, but no amount will compensate for severe deficiencies of either Ca or P. The dietary dry matter of rapidly growing young stock should contain approximately 0.6 to 1.2% Ca, with a Ca-P ratio in the range of about 1.2:1 to 1.5:1. For adult maintenance, lower Ca levels and wider Ca-P ratios are possible. In these situations, vitamin D requirements seem to be at a minimum, and risks of vitamin D deficiency are less probable. The young rat needs very little vitamin D. Indeed, to make the species suitably responsive in the biological assay of the vitamin, the dietary P content has to be kept low and the Ca-P ratio high (Abrams, 1978).

Intestinal pH as well as other dietary nutrients influence Ca and P requirements, and thus vitamin D requirements. Fermentation of excess carbohydrates makes intestinal contents more acid, which favors both Ca and P absorption, probably by converting less soluble alkaline salts to the more soluble acid salts. High intakes of fats containing higher fatty acids increase highly insoluble Ca soaps. Potassium may increase P absorption, but cations that form insoluble phosphates such as iron and aluminum interfere.

Vitamin D requirements of various species (Table 3.1) are sufficiently high to produce normal growth, calcification, production, and reproduction in the absence of sunlight, provided that diets contain recommended levels of Ca and available P. Species differences can be illustrated by the fact that adequate intakes of Ca and P in a diet that contains only enough vitamin D to produce normal bone in rats or pigs will quickly cause the development of rickets in chicks. Turkeys and pheasants have higher requirements than chicks. Surprisingly, human babies

■ Table 3.1   Vitamin D Requirements for Various Animals and Humans

Animal	Purpose or Class	Requirement[a]	Reference
Beef cattle	Adult	275 IU/kg	NRC (1996)
Dairy cattle	Milk replacer	300 IU/kg	NRC (1989a)
	Growing bulls	300 IU/kg	NRC (1989a)
	Lactating	1,000 IU/kg	NRC (1989a)
Goat	All classes	1,400 IU/kg	Morand-Fehr (1981)
Chicken	Leghorn, 0–18 weeks	200 ICU/kg	NRC (1994)
	Leghorn, laying (100-g intake)	300 ICU/kg	NRC (1994)
	Broilers, 0–8 weeks	200 ICU/kg	NRC (1994)
Duck (Peking)	0–7 weeks	400 ICU/kg	NRC (1994)
Geese	All classes	200 IU/kg	NRC (1994)
Japanese quail	Growing	750 ICU/kg	NRC (1994)
Turkey	All classes	1,100 ICU/kg	NRC (1994)
Sheep	Adult	555 IU/100 kg body weight	NRC (1985b)
Swine	Growing-finishing, 3–10 kg	220 IU/kg	NRC (1998)
	Growing-finishing, 20–120 kg	150 IU/kg	NRC (1998)
	Adult	200 IU/kg	NRC (1998)
Horse	Maintenance and working	300 IU/kg	NRC (1989b)
	Growing	800 IU/kg	NRC (1989b)
	Pregnancy and lactation	600 IU/kg	NRC (1989b)
Cat	Growing	500 IU/kg	NRC (1986)
Dog	Growing	22 IU/kg body weight	NRC (1985a)
Fish	Catfish	250–1,000 mg/kg	NRC (1993)
	Rainbow trout	1,600–2,400 IU/kg	NRC (1993)
Rat	Growing-reproductive	1,000 IU/kg	NRC (1995)
Mouse	Growing	1,000 IU/kg	NRC (1995)
Guinea pig	Growing	1,000 IU/kg	NRC (1995)
Human	Children	400 IU/day	RDA (1989)
	Adults	200–400 IU/day	RDA (1989)
	Lactating	400 IU/day	RDA (1989)

[a]Expressed as per unit of animal feed on either as-fed (approximately 90% dry matter) or dry basis (see Appendix, Tables A1a,b). Human data are expressed as IU/day (1 IU = 0.025 μg vitamin D).

are more like birds in this respect than like the other mammals mentioned. Greater absorption of Ca and greater growth rates occurred in full-term infants given 400 IU per day compared to those given 100 IU per day, although 100 IU is enough to prevent rickets (Collins and Norman, 1991). In addition to the RDA (1989) suggested requirements for humans, it is recognized that without casual exposure to sunlight, the dietary intake for vitamin D should be at least two to three times more than the recommended intake (Holick, 1995).

NATURAL SOURCES

Ergocalciferol and cholecalciferol contents of natural materials are shown in Table 3.2. Sources of vitamin D are natural foods, irradiated sebaceous material licked from skin or hair, and directly absorbed products or irradiation formed on or in the skin.

In dogs and cats (and presumably other carnivores), vitamin D must be obtained from dietary sources due to the inability of these species to synthesize and utilize vitamin D from precursors in the skin (How et al., 1995). The distribution of vitamin D is very limited in nature, although provitamins D occur widely. Of feeds for livestock, grains, roots, and oilseeds, as well as their numerous by-products, contain insignificant amounts of vitamin D. With a few notable exceptions, vitamin D_3 is not found in plants. Those exceptions include the species *Solanum malacoxylon*, *Cestrum diurnum*, and *Trisetum flavescens* (see Toxicity), in which vitamin D occurs as water-soluble β–glycosides of vitamin D_3, 25-OHD_3 and 1,25-$(OH)_2D_3$.

Typical green forages are extremely poor in vitamin D. However, when plants—especially pasture species—begin to die and the fading leaves are favorably exposed to UV light, some vitamin D_2 is formed. So arises the vitamin D of hay, the potency of which depends on local climatic conditions, for if it is made very quickly in the absence of direct sunlight and is baled when still quite green, its potency will be low. The principal source of the antirachitic factor in the diets of farm animals is thus provided by the action of radiant energy upon ergosterol in forages. Legume hay that is cured to preserve most of its leaves and green color contains considerable amounts. Alfalfa, for example, will range from 650 to 2,200 IU/kg (Maynard et al., 1979); timothy and other grass hays contain less. Stemmy hay that is lacking in leaves and color and has been exposed to a minimum of sunlight may contain none, whether legume or nonlegume. The antirachitic value of the alfalfa crop increases with state of maturity because of the increase in dead leaves.

■ Table 3.2   Vitamin D Concentrations in Various Foods and Feedstuffs

Food or Feedstuff	IU/100 g[a] Ergocalciferol (D$_2$)
Alfalfa pasture	4.6
Alfalfa hay, sun cured	142
Alfalfa silage	12
Alfalfa wilted silage	60
Birdsfoot trefoil hay, sun cured	142
Barley straw	60
Cocoa shell meal, sun dried	3,500
Corn grain	0
Corn silage	13
Molasses, sugar beet	58
Red clover, fresh	4.7
Red clover, sun cured	192
Sorghum grain	2.6
Sorghum silage	66

Food or Feedstuff	IU/100 g Cholecalciferol (D$_3$)
Blue fin tuna liver oil	4,000,000
Cod liver oil meal	4,000
Cod liver oil	10,000
Eggs	100
Halibut liver oil	120,000
Herring, entire body oil	10,000
Menhaden, entire body oil	5,000
Milk, cow's whole (summer)	4
Milk, cow's whole (winter)	1
Sardine, entire body oil	8,000
Sturgeon liver oil	0
Swordfish liver oil	1,000,000

Sources: Adapted from NRC (1982b) and Scott et al. (1982).
[a]Concentrations are on as fed-basis.

Artificially dried and barn-cured hay contains less vitamin D than hay that is properly sun cured. Even hay dried in the dark immediately after cutting contains some of the vitamin, because the dead or injured leaves on the growing plant respond to irradiation even though the living tissues do not. This fact is also largely responsible for the vitamin D found in corn silage (Maynard et al., 1979). Under normal conditions, even wilted legume silage furnishes ample vitamin D for dairy calves.

For non–forage-consuming species, the vitamin D that occurs naturally in unfortified food is generally derived from animal products. Saltwater fish, such as herring, salmon, and sardines, contains substantial amounts of vitamin D, and fish liver oils are extremely rich sources. The probable origin of vitamin D in fish liver is a result of food chains from plankton (Takeuchi et al., 1991). Veal, beef, unfortified milk, and butter supply only small quantities. Among animal products, eggs, especially the yolks, are a good source if the hen's diet is rich in the vitamin. Milk contains a variable amount in its fat fraction (5 to 40 IU in cow's milk per quart), but neither cow's milk nor human milk contains enough to protect the baby against rickets. Cow's milk is reportedly higher in vitamin D when produced during the summer rather than winter.

It has generally been assumed that for all but a few species, vitamin D_2 and vitamin D_3 are equally potent. In poultry, other birds, and a few of the rarer mammals, including some New World monkeys, vitamin D_3 has been found to be many times more potent than D_2 on a weight basis. Vitamin D_3 may be 30 times more effective than D_2 for poultry; therefore, plant sources (vitamin D_2) of the vitamin should not be provided to these species. The dogma that mammals (other than the New World monkey) do not discriminate between the two sources has been proven incorrect. Data for pigs (Horst and Napoli, 1981) and ruminants (Sommerfeldt et al., 1981) have suggested that these species discriminate in the metabolism of vitamin D_2 and D_3, with vitamin D_3 being the preferred substrate. Pigs given oral doses of a mixture of vitamin D_2 and D_3 (1:w/w) had significantly higher concentrations of plasma vitamin D_3, 25-OHD_3, 24,25-$(OH)_2D_3$, and 1,25-$(OH)_2D_3$ than those of corresponding counterparts given vitamin D_2. Sommerfeldt et al. (1983) reported that the amount of 1,25-$(OH)_2D$ in the plasma of ergocalciferol-treated dairy calves was one-half to one-fourth the amount in the plasma of cholecalciferol-treated calves. Discrimination against vitamin D_2 by ruminants may be in part a result of its preferred degradation by rumen microbes or its less efficient absorption by the intestine. Similarly, Harrington and Page (1983) found vitamin D_3 to be more hypercalcemic and overtly toxic to horses than vitamin D_2, likewise suggesting preference for D_3. Vitamin D_3 has been reported to be at least three times as effective as vitamin D_2 in satisfying the vitamin D requirement in trout (NRC, 1993). Although the more recent data suggest a preference for D_2 by a number of animals, in practice D_2 is still relatively comparable to D_3 in antirachitic function except for poultry and certain monkeys.

DEFICIENCY

Effects of Deficiency

The outstanding disease of vitamin D deficiency is rickets, generally characterized by a decreased concentration of Ca and P in the organic matrices of cartilage and bone. The signs and symptoms are similar to those of a lack of Ca or P or both, as all three are concerned with proper bone formation. In the adult, osteomalacia is the counterpart of rickets and, since cartilage growth has ceased, is characterized by a decreased concentration of Ca and P in the bone matrix. Osteoporosis is defined as a decrease in the amount of bone, leading to fractures after minimal trauma. In osteoporosis, bone mineral and protein matrix are lost, resulting in less overall bone but normal composition. Osteomalacia is also characterized by inadequate bone mineralization; however, in contrast to osteoporosis, persons with osteomalacia have normal protein matrix that is not fully mineralized. When bone mass becomes too low, mechanical support and skeletal integrity cannot be maintained, and fractures can occur with minimal trauma.

Clinical signs of vitamin D deficiency are seen mainly in the young. General consequences of deficiency can appear as inhibited growth, weight loss, and reduced or lost appetite before characteristic signs that relate primarily to the bone system become apparent. The role of vitamin D in the adult appears to be much less important except during reproduction and lactation. Congenital malformations in newborns result from extreme deficiencies in the diet of the mother during gestation, and the mother's skeleton is injured as well.

The same disruption of the orderly processes of bone formation with vitamin D deficiency occurs in animals as it does in humans and includes the following characteristics (Kramer and Gribetz, 1971):

1. Failure of Ca salt deposition in the cartilage matrix.
2. Failure of cartilage cells to mature, leading to their accumulation rather than destruction.
3. Compression of the proliferating cartilage cells.
4. Elongation, swelling, and degeneration of proliferative cartilage.
5. Abnormal pattern of invasion of cartilage by capillaries.

Outward signs of rickets include the following skeletal changes, varying somewhat with species depending on anatomy and severity:

1. Weak bones, causing curving and bending of bones.
2. Enlarged hock and knee joints.
3. Tendency to drag hind legs.
4. Beaded ribs and deformed thorax.

Although there appear to be differences between species in the susceptibility of different bones to such degenerative changes, differences that probably reflect bodily conformation (e.g., pigs compared with sheep) and stance (e.g., humans compared with the common quadrupeds), there is nevertheless an apparent common pattern (Abrams, 1978). Spongy parts of individual bones, and bones relatively rich in spongy tissue, are first and worst affected. As in simple Ca deficiency, the vertebrae and the bones of the head suffer the greatest degree of resorption. Next come the scapula, sternum, and ribs. The most resistant bones are the metatarsals and the shafts of long bones.

Ruminants

Clinical signs of vitamin D deficiency in ruminants are decreased appetite and growth rate, digestive disturbances, rickets (Figs. 3.3 and 3.4), stiffness in gait, labored breathing, irritability, weakness, and occasionally tetany and convulsions. There is enlargement of joints, slight arching of the back, and bowing of legs, with erosion of joint surfaces

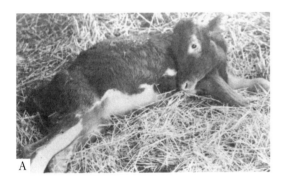

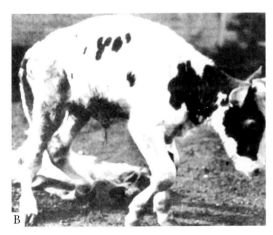

Fig. 3.3 Calves developed severe rickets while receiving ration deficient in vitamin D, and kept away from sunlight. (A: Courtesy of W. Krauss, Ohio Agriculture Experiment Station. B: Courtesy of Michigan Agriculture Experiment Station, NRC, 1958.)

119

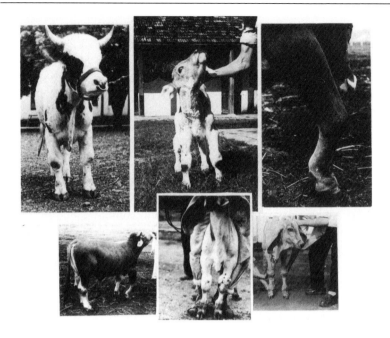

Fig. 3.4 Calves and young bulls with rickets. (Courtesy of the late Francisco Megale, Universidade Federal de Minas Gerais, Escola de Veterinaria, Belo Horizante, MG, Brazil.)

causing difficulty in locomotion (NRC, 1996). Young ruminants may be born dead, weak, or deformed.

Clinical signs involving bones begin with thickening and swelling of the metacarpal or metatarsal bones. As the disease progresses, the forelegs bend forward or sideways. In severe or prolonged vitamin D deficiency, tension of the muscles will cause bending and twisting of long bones to give the characteristic deformity of bone. There is enlargement at ends of bones from deposition of excess cartilage, giving the characteristic "beading" effect along the sternum where ribs attach (NRC, 1989a, 1996). The lower jaw bone (mandible) becomes thick and soft; in severe cases, eating is then difficult. Calves may experience slobbering, inability to close the mouth, and protrusion of the tongue (Craig and Davis, 1943). Joints (particularly the knee and hock) become swollen and stiff, the pastern straight, and the back humped. In more severe cases, synovial fluid accumulates in the joints (NRC, 1989a). Posterior paralysis may also occur as the result of fractured vertebrae. The structural weakness of the bones appears to be related to poor mineralization. The advanced stages of the disease are marked by stiffness of gait, dragging of the hind feet, irritability, tetany, labored and fast breathing, weakness, anorexia, and retardation of growth. Calves may be born dead, weak, or deformed (Rupel et al., 1933).

Clinical signs of vitamin D deficiency in sheep and goats are similar to those in cattle, including rickets in young animals and osteomalacia in adults (NRC, 1981, 1985b). An early report of rickets in Scotland referred to the condition as "bent leg," which occurred in ram lambs 7 to 12 months of age (Elliot and Crichton, 1926). The condition was prevented by administration of small doses of vitamin D in the form of cod liver oil. Newborn lambs can receive enough vitamin D from their dams to prevent early rickets if the dams have adequate storage (Church and Pond, 1974). Newborn kids had rickets if the dam was deficient in vitamin D during pregnancy (NRC, 1981).

In older animals with vitamin D deficiency (osteomalacia), bones become weak and fracture easily, and posterior paralysis may accompany vertebral fractures. In dairy cattle, milk production may be decreased and estrus inhibited by inadequate vitamin D (NRC, 1989a). Cows fed a diet deficient in vitamin D and kept out of direct sunlight showed definite signs of vitamin D deficiency within 6 to 10 months (Wallis, 1944). Functions that deplete vitamin D are high milk production and advancing pregnancy, especially during the last few months before calving. The visible signs of vitamin D deficiency in dairy cows are similar to those of rickets in calves. The animal begins to show stiffness in limbs and joints, which makes it difficult to walk, lie down, and get up. The knees, hocks, and other joints become swollen, tender, and stiff. The knees often spring forward, the posterior joints straighten, and the animal is tilted on its toes. The hair becomes coarse and rough, and the animal has an overall appearance of unthriftiness (Wallis, 1944). As the deficiency advances, the back often becomes stiff, humped, bent, and flexed. In vitamin D-deficient herds, calving rates are lower and calves have been born dead or weak.

Milk fever (parturient paresis) is a paralyzing metabolic disease caused by hypocalcemia near parturition and initiation of lactation in high milk-producing dairy cows. Milk fever is an impaired metabolic condition that is related to Ca status, previous Ca intake, and malfunction of the hormone form of vitamin D [1,25-$(OH)_2$D] and PTH. Animals that develop milk fever are unable to meet the sudden demand for Ca that is brought about by the initiation of lactation. Milk fever usually occurs within 72 hours after parturition and is manifested by circulatory collapse, generalized paresis, and depression of consciousness. The most obvious and consistent abnormality is acute hypocalcemia, in which serum Ca decreases from a normal 8 to 10 mg/dL to 3 to 7 mg/dL (average, 5 mg/dL). Early in the onset, the cow may exhibit some unsteadiness as she walks. More frequently, the cow is found lying on her sternum with her head displaced to one side, causing a kink in the neck, or turned into the flank. The eyes are dull and staring and the pupils dilated. If treatment is delayed many hours, the dullness gives way to coma, which becomes progressively deeper, leading to death.

Aged cows are at the greatest risk of developing milk fever. Heifers almost never develop milk fever. Older animals have a decreased response to dietary Ca stress due to both decreased production of 1,25-$(OH)_2D$ and decreased response to the 1,25-$(OH)_2D$. Target tissues of cows with milk fever may have defective hormone receptors, and the number of receptors declines with age. In older animals, fewer osteoclasts exist to respond to hormone stimulation, which delays the ability of bone to contribute Ca to the plasma Ca pool (Goff et al., 1989). The aging process is also associated with reduced renal 1α-hydroxylase response to Ca stress, therefore reducing the amount of 1,25-$(OH)_2D$ produced from 25-OHD (Goff et al., 1991b).

Parturient paresis also occurs in ewes. It is a disturbance of metabolism in pregnant and lactating ewes characterized by acute hypocalcemia and the rapid development of hyperexcitability, ataxia, paresis, coma, and death. The disease occurs any time from 5 weeks before to 10 weeks after lambing, principally in highly conditioned older ewes at pasture. The onset can be associated with an abrupt changing of feed, a sudden change in weather, or short periods of fasting imposed by circumstances such as shearing or transportation. The degree of involvement of vitamin D with Ca metabolism in parturient paresis with sheep is unclear.

Vitamin D should be supplied to growing animals that are denied sunlight over extended periods because of cloud cover or confinement housing. In northern latitudes during winter, photochemical conversion of provitamin D to its active compound in the skin of ruminants is limited because of insufficient UV radiation. Hidiroglou et al. (1979) reported that 25-OHD was higher in plasma of cattle in summer than in winter. Richter et al. (1990) found that 25-OHD concentrations of blood plasma were higher if bulls were kept outdoors versus indoors (21.1 versus 14.3 ng per milliliter, respectively). Vitamin D deficiency may be observed in young ruminants that are closely confined and do not consume sun-cured roughage. Hidiroglou et al. (1978) reported the clinical history of a flock of sheep kept under total confinement that showed a high incidence (8%) of an osteodystrophic condition (a vitamin D-responsive disease). A form of osteodystrophia has also been produced experimentally in goats (NRC, 1981).

When grazing ruminants have normal exposure to direct sunlight or are fed normal amounts of sun-cured forage, little chance for vitamin D deficiency exists. However, seasons of minimum sunlight, artificially cured forages, sheep with full fleece, feedlot animals without access to sunlight or sun-cured forages, and high-producing dairy cows with limited access to sunlight or sun-cured forage may lead to the need for dietary supplementation.

Swine

In swine, vitamin D deficiency causes poor growth, stiffness, lameness (Fig. 3.5), stilted gait, a general tendency to "go down," or lose the use of the limbs (posterior paralysis), frequent cases of fractures, softness of bones, bone deformities, beading of the ribs, enlargement and erosion of joints, and unthriftiness (Cunha, 1977). Bones may also be deformed by the weight of the animal and the pull of body muscles.

Pigs with severe vitamin D deficiency may exhibit signs of Ca and

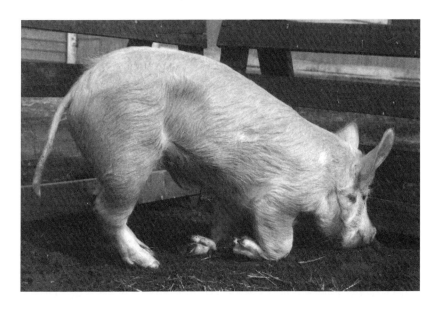

Fig. 3.5 Pig with advanced rickets caused by lack of vitamin D. The pig was not exposed to sunlight. It shows leg abnormalities and was unable to walk; it later responded to supplementary vitamin D. (Courtesy of J.M. Bell, University of Saskatchewan, Canada.)

magnesium deficiency, including tetany (NRC, 1998). It takes 4 to 6 months for pigs fed a vitamin D-deficient diet to develop signs of a deficiency (Johnson and Palmer, 1939; Quarterman et al., 1964).

The trend toward confinement of swine in completely enclosed houses through the life cycle increases the importance of adequate dietary vitamin D fortification. Goff et al. (1984) concluded that subclinical rickets may become more of a problem as swine producers convert to swine-confinement operations, which deprive sows and piglets of the UV irradiation needed for endogenous production of cholecalciferol. Research has shown that sunshine cannot always be depended on to meet vitamin D requirements of growing or finishing pigs during winter months in northern latitudes.

Of all the vitamins provided in swine feeds, vitamin D is one of two (the other is vitamin B_{12}) that is most likely to be deficient. Typical grain- and soybean-based diets contain virtually none of the vitamin. Also, the trend toward complete confinement will eliminate UV light as a source of the vitamin; therefore, supplemental vitamin D must be provided for all swine operations in which growing and breeding animals remain in confinement.

Poultry

Little difference exists among poultry species in relation to clinical signs of deficiency. Clinical signs in all poultry species include rickets and lowered growth rate, egg production, and hatchability.

In addition to retarded growth, the first sign of vitamin D deficiency in chicks is rickets, which is characterized by severe weakness of the legs. During vitamin D deficiency, growing birds develop hypocalcemia, which in turn stunts skeletal development through widened cartilage at epiphyses of long bones and weakened shafts (NRC, 1994). Young, growing chickens and turkeys tend to rest frequently in a squatting position, are disinclined to walk, and have a lame, stiff-legged gait. These are distinguished from the clinical signs of vitamin A deficiency in that vitamin D-deficient birds are alert rather than droopy, and walk with a lame rather than a staggering gait (ataxia). The beaks and claws become soft and pliable (Fig. 3.6), usually between 2 and 3 weeks of age. The most characteristic internal sign of vitamin D deficiency in chicks is a beading of the ribs at their juncture with the spinal column (Scott et al., 1982).

In chronic vitamin D deficiency, marked skeletal distortions become apparent (Scott et al., 1982), in which the spinal column may bend downward in the sacral and coccygeal region. The sternum usually

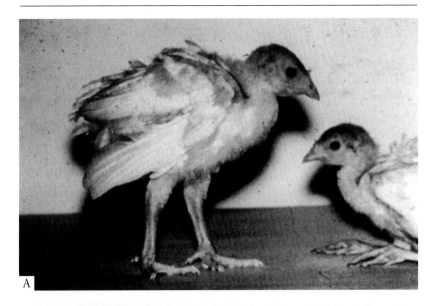

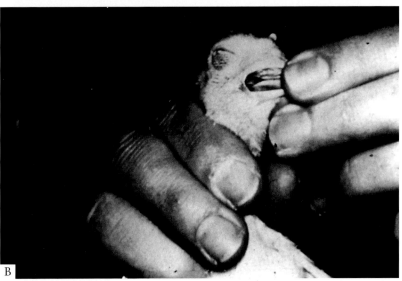

Fig. 3.6 Vitamin D-deficient and normal poult: (A) Note rubbery beak from vitamin D deficiency; (B) (Courtesy of L.S. Jensen and Washington State University.)

shows both a lateral bend and an acute dent near the middle of the breast. These changes reduce the size of the thorax, with consequent crowding of the vital organs.

A disease condition known as endochondral ossification defects (EOD) produces bone deformations, fractures, and lameness in broiler chickens throughout the world within the first few weeks after hatching. Flocks with a high incidence of EOD have significantly lower bone ash and $1,25\text{-}(OH)_2D_3$ than do mildly affected flocks, and it seems probable that higher systemic concentrations of $1,25\text{-}(OH)_2D_3$ between 7 and 14 days of age will enhance the ability of broiler chickens to effectively mineralize the cartilaginous growth plates in the appendicular skeleton during early bone maturation (Vaiano et al., 1994).

As in many other nutritional diseases of poultry, the feathers soon become ruffled. In red or buff-colored breeds of chickens, vitamin D deficiency causes an abnormal black pigmentation of some of the feathers, especially those of the wings. If the deficiency is very marked, the blackening becomes pronounced, and nearly all the feathers may be affected (NRC, 1994). When vitamin D is supplied in adequate quantity, the new feathers and newer parts of older feathers are normal in color, although the discolored portion remains black.

Signs of vitamin D deficiency begin to occur in laying hens in confinement about 1 to 2 months after they are deprived of vitamin D. When laying chickens are fed a diet deficient in vitamin D, the first sign of the deficiency is a thinning of the shells of their eggs. Commercial layers will continue to lay eggs with reduced shell quantity for weeks. If the diet is also completely devoid of vitamin D_3, egg production may decrease rapidly, and eggs with a very thin shell or no shell will be produced. In laying hens, eggshell strength tends to decrease as the hens age. The decline in shell strength may be due to a decrease in the hen's ability to synthesize $1,25\text{-}(OH)_2D$. A study of the effect of dietary $1,25\text{-}(OH)_2D_3$ on eggshell strength in older hens found that within 3 weeks, the percentage of cracked or broken eggs was lower for hens supplemented with $1,25\text{-}(OH)_2D$ (Tsang, 1992).

Vitamin D nutriture of the hen also influences its content in egg yolk and the subsequent need for this vitamin by the chick (Stevens and Blair, 1985). Hatchability is markedly reduced, with embryos frequently dying at 18 to 19 days of age. These embryos show a short upper mandible or incomplete formation at the base of the beak. Eventually, breast bones become noticeably less rigid, and there may be beading at the ends of the ribs. Individual hens may show temporary loss of use of the legs, with recovery after laying an egg (usually shell-less) (Scott et al., 1982). During periods of extreme leg weakness, hens show a characteristic posture that has been described as a penguin-like squat.

Of all vitamins provided in poultry feeds, vitamin D is one of two (the other is vitamin B_{12}) that is most likely to be deficient. Typical grain- and soybean-based diets contain virtually none of these vitamins. Also (as mentioned for swine above), the trend to complete confinement will eliminate UV light as a source of the vitamin; therefore, supplemental vitamin D must be provided for all poultry operations in which birds remain in confinement.

Horses

Deficiency of Ca, P, or vitamin D can cause bone deformities in the horse caused by the weight of the animal and the pull of the muscles on weak, porous bones. Vitamin D deficiency is characterized by reduced bone calcification, stiff and swollen joints, stiffness of gait, bone deformities, frequent fractures, and reduction in serum Ca and P (NRC, 1989b). El Shorafa et al. (1979) observed that early stages of rickets in ponies included decreased bone ash, decreased cortical area and bone density, and delayed epiphyseal closure.

Young Shetland ponies kept outdoors in Florida clearly do not need dietary vitamin D (El Shorafa et al., 1979). However, when they were deprived of sunlight and no vitamin D was included in the diet, ponies lost their appetite and had difficulty standing.

Grazing horses or horses that exercise regularly in sunlight and consume sun-cured hay will get the amount of vitamin D they require. However, if exposure to sunlight is restricted by confinement, hay may not always supply the requirement. Sunlight provides most of its antirachitic powers during the 4 hours around noon. This should be considered by those who exercise race horses briefly in the early morning before housing them for the rest of the day (Abrams, 1978).

Other Animal Species

DOGS AND CATS

The dog was one of the first animals in which rickets was produced experimentally. In 1922, Mellanby produced rickets in dogs by feeding them oatmeal (NRC, 1985a). Rickets in dogs is radiographically, histopathologically, and biochemically similar to the disorder as manifested in other animals or in human beings. Rickets with typical bone lesions is readily produced in dogs, but clinical signs are frequently confounded by simultaneous deficiency or imbalance of Ca and P (NRC, 1985a), both of which result in initial hypocalcemia.

Campbell and Douglas (1965) fed a diet of 0.5% Ca and 0.3% P, with no supplemental vitamin D, to puppies for 15 weeks without signs of rickets or osteoporosis. However, when the diet contained 0.08 to 0.10% Ca and 0.13 to 0.15% P and no supplemental vitamin D, rickets complicated by osteoporosis was observed.

A diagnosis of rickets in a 12-week-old female St. Bernard was attributed to an inborn error in vitamin D metabolism (Johnson et al., 1988). Physical examination revealed enlargement of the costochondral junctions and the distal metaphyses of the radius, ulna, femur, and tibia. When the dog was standing, its elbows were slightly abducted, and there was mild valgus deviation of the front paws. The dog showed no lameness but was lethargic and inactive. Radiographically, the physes were enlarged radially and axially, and metaphyseal bone adjacent to the physes was widened and cup-shaped. Serum biochemical abnormalities were hypocalcemia, hypomagnesemia, and hyperparathyroidism.

Severe rickets in kittens resulted in enlarged costochondral junctions ("rachitic rosary"), with disorganization in new bone formation and excessive osteoid (NRC, 1986). Classic signs of rickets are rare in kittens but can arise from queens fed vitamin D-deficient diets.

Severe rickets in kittens was produced using vitamin D-deficient diets containing either 1% Ca and 1% P or 2% Ca and 0.65% P (Gershoff et al., 1957). Weight gain was less with the latter diet, and rickets was less severe. Rickets that developed in about 4 to 5 months was characterized by radiographic and morphological changes that were similar to bone lesions observed in other species with the disease. The cats that died during acute rickets had a lower percent of femur ash than cats supplemented with vitamin D.

FISH

Channel catfish raised in aquaria and fed a vitamin D-deficient diet for 16 weeks showed reduced weight gain, lower body ash, lower body P, and lower body Ca than controls (NRC, 1993). Reduced growth with vitamin D deficiency has also been reported with juvenile lobsters, juvenile grass shrimp, blue tilapia, and trout (NRC, 1993; O'Connell and Gatlin, 1994; Shiau and Hwang, 1994). Although effects of vitamin D_3 on mineralization of hard tissues were negligible in blue tilapia, weight gains were reduced with deficiency (O'Connell and Gatlin, 1994).

Signs of vitamin D deficiency in trout include slow growth, impaired

Ca homeostasis manifested by clinical signs of tetany of the white skeletal muscles, and ultrastructural changes in the white muscle fibers of the musculature (Barnett et al., 1982; NRC, 1993). No changes in bone ash have been detected in this species of fish. A lordosis-like droopy tail syndrome observed in vitamin D-deficient trout (Barnett et al., 1982) was suggested to be related to muscle weakness.

FOXES AND MINK

Rickets can be produced in both foxes and mink by feeding diets having low vitamin D content and abnormal Ca-P ratios (NRC, 1982a). Signs of rickets in growing kits are generally seen between 2 and 4 months of age.

LABORATORY ANIMALS

Rickets is classically brought about in rats by a diet lacking vitamin D, adequate in Ca, and low in P. Bones of rachitic rats show decreased or absent calcification, with wide areas of uncalcified cartilage at the junction of diaphysis and epiphysis. Bone ash may be less than half normal (NRC, 1995).

Guinea pigs housed without access to UV light and fed a purified diet low in vitamin D, with 0.028% Ca and 0.2% P, did not grow normally and developed rickets. Typical lesions occurred in the zone of cartilage proliferation at the epiphyseal plate of long bones and ribs. Also, incisors exhibited a high degree of enamel hypoplasia, while enamel and dentin were disorganized and irregular, with poor calcification (NRC, 1995). Hamsters do not require dietary vitamin D for prevention of rickets when the dietary Ca-P ratio is about 2:1 and Ca is at 0.6% (NRC, 1995). However, Sergeev et al. (1990) reported changes in vitamin D status of guinea pigs fed a vitamin D-deficient diet containing 6 g Ca/kg diet and 6 g P/kg diet. Serum Ca and P concentrations were reduced, serum alkaline phosphatase was increased, serum 25-OHD concentrations were extremely low, kidney 1-α-hydroxylase activity was more than twice the normal concentration, and bone Ca content was about four-fifths of the control concentration. Rickets may be induced in hamsters in the absence of vitamin D and when dietary Ca is 4 g/kg and P is 0.2 g/kg (NRC, 1995).

NONHUMAN PRIMATES

Softening, demineralization, and fibrous dysplasia of bone, which are compatible with a diagnosis of rickets and responsive to vitamin D treatment, have been observed in many species of nonhuman primates

129

(NRC, 1978). Rickets also has been induced unintentionally in New World primates kept under laboratory conditions when it was incorrectly assumed that they could utilize vitamin D_2 as efficiently as D_3 (see Natural Sources).

Humans

Vitamin D deficiency in children leads to the pathological bone condition called rickets, which is characterized by disordered cartilage cell growth and enlargement of the epiphyseal growth plates in the long bones (Fraser, 1984). There is also a prominent accumulation of unmineralized bone matrix (osteoid) on trabecular bone surfaces. Classic bone symptoms associated with rickets, such as bowlegs (Fig. 3.7), knock-knees, curvature of the spine, and pelvic and thoracic deformities, result from the application of normal mechanical stress to demineralized bone (Collins and Norman, 1991). Beading of the ribs, referred to as the "ricketic rosary," is almost a constant sign after the age of 6 months, and is caused by the swollen cartilaginous ends of the ribs. The chest may be narrow and rather funnel-shaped, and described as a "pigeon" chest. In severe cases, this may interfere with breathing. Enlargement of bones, especially in the knees, wrists, and ankles, and changes in the costochondral junctions also occur. With these defects, the bones become structurally weak, bend under the weight of the child, and are liable to fracture. Rickets also results in inadequate mineralization of tooth enamel and dentin. If the disease occurs during the first 6 months of life, convulsions and tetany can develop.

When humans changed from a hunting and gathering culture to an agricultural one, they also moved from tropical and subtropical climates to temperate zones, where houses and clothes were necessary for protection from the cold for a considerable part of the year (Harrison, 1978). This limited the production of vitamin D in skin, particularly of infants during those months when exposure of large areas of skin to sunshine was not possible. When a further change to urban living occurred, children in crowded city slums had little opportunity for exposure to sunshine. As noted earlier, this was accentuated by the Industrial Revolution, during which the use of fossil fuels contaminated the atmosphere and thus blocked out UV radiation.

Rickets resulting from vitamin D deficiency became widespread in northern cities, particularly in the British Isles, Europe, the United States, and Canada. The disease usually appeared in the first year of life and was characterized by muscle weakness; deformities of long bones, including bowed legs; knuckle-like projections along the rib cage,

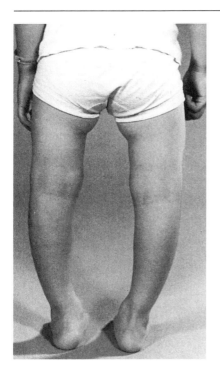 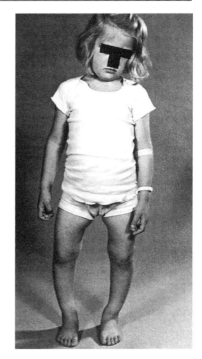

Fig. 3.7 Child with rickets exhibits marked bowlegs. Note the angle of the feet. (Courtesy of Alan T. Forrester, *Scope Manual on Nutrition*, The Upjohn Company, Kalamazoo, Michigan.)

known as the rachitic rosary; and deformities of the pelvis, which were often permanent. Consequences of this disease were quite profound, especially for young women, in whom a deformed pelvis would cause difficulty with childbirth and result in a high incidence of infant and maternal morbidity and mortality (Holick, 1987).

Osteomalacia occurs after skeletal development is complete. As in rickets, even though bone mineralization has ceased, collagen formation continues, resulting in formation of uncalcified bone matrix. In adults, the bones stop growing in length but are constantly remodeled. The main symptoms of osteomalacia are muscular weakness and bone pain. As the disease progresses, bone fractures occur.

Season and latitude greatly affect the ability of sunlight to promote synthesis of vitamin D_3 in skin; therefore, individuals from more temperate regions in the winter are more susceptible to vitamin D deficiency. Studies have indicated less vitamin D activity in northern climates

131

(see Natural Sources). In Manitoba, Canada, 43% of children and 76% of mothers had serum 25-OHD levels below the normal range (Lebrun et al., 1993). In a study of infant growth in two northern and two southern cities in China, infants from the more southern latitudes had the greatest body length (Feliciano et al., 1994). Rickets is not limited to northern climates; the disease was established in 41 Sudanese children (El-Hag and Karrar, 1995). Possible causes in the Sudan were poor socioeconomic background, inadequate dietary intake in both mothers and children, prolonged breast feeding, limited sun exposure, and type of residence.

Although it is accepted that vitamin D is absolutely essential for growing children, it is not well appreciated that it is also essential for maintenance of a healthy mineralized skeleton in adults. One reason for vitamin D deficiency in older populations is that individuals do not get enough exposure to sunlight. Older persons require more sunlight to get the same vitamin effect as do young individuals (see Requirements). A high incidence (73%) of vitamin D deficiency as evidenced by low blood 25-OHD was reported for elderly women in a nursing home in Holland (Lowik et al., 1992). The low 25-OHD concentrations were associated with limited exposure to UV radiation and nonusage of vitamin D supplements.

Holick (1987) observed that one of the primary causes of poor vitamin D nutrition in the elderly in the United States is a decrease in or complete abstinence from consumption of milk, which is the principal food source that is fortified with vitamin D. Also, milk and milk products are the principal sources of Ca and P in many diets. In Great Britain, where dairy products were not routinely fortified with vitamin D, it was found that 30% of women and 40% of men who incurred a hip fracture were deficient in vitamin D (Doppelt et al., 1983).

In relation to diet, alcoholics have a high risk of vitamin D deficiency. Low plasma 25-OHD was highly related to alcohol consumption (Guilland et al., 1994). Many studies have shown the indigenous elderly population and Asian immigrants to be groups at particular risk of vitamin D deficiency and osteomalacia. In one study, blood 25-OHD was significantly lower in elderly Asians (21/37) and young Asians (7/17) compared with white controls (Solanki et al., 1995).

Vitamin D is involved not only in the regulation of Ca homeostasis and bone metabolism, but in the regulation of cell proliferation, differentiation, and immune response. The extent of non–bone-related vitamin D deficiency is unknown. Vitamin D treatment to prevent various types of cancer and other conditions, such as psoriasis, may be based on the pharmacological effects of the vitamin versus a function of vitamin D. Vitamin D has a role in heart function as evidenced by abnormal electrocardiograms (Sood et al., 1995), with congestive heart failure reported as a result of the deficiency (Brunvand et al., 1995).

Assessment of Status

Several methods have been used to assess vitamin D nutritional status of individuals. Poor production rates in livestock as well as bone abnormalities in both animals and humans are the chief indications that vitamin D deficiency is substantially advanced. The incomplete calcification of the skeleton is easily detectable with x-rays, but, like other production-related signs, would not be specific for vitamin D deficiency versus other nutrient inadequacies.

Low serum Ca levels in the range of 5 to 7 mg/100 ml and high serum alkaline phosphatase activity can be used to diagnose rickets and osteomalacia. Also, a marked reduction in circulating $1,25$-$(OH)_2D$ levels in individuals with osteomalacia has been reported. The plasma concentration of 25-OHD is related to and therefore is an index of the vitamin D supply for both animals and humans. The concentration of 25-OHD in plasma, which is the principal form of vitamin D in plasma, is about 10 times and 500 to 1,000 times higher than those of $24,25$-$(OH)_2D$ and $1,25$-$(OH)_2D$, respectively (Fraser, 1984).

The circulating concentration of 25-OHD is a good index for determining the cumulative effect of sunlight on synthesis of vitamin D_3 in skin, and dietary sources of the vitamin. In plasma of the vitamin D-deficient child, a low concentration of 25-OHD (less than 5 ng/ml) has been found (Fraser, 1984). Oldham et al. (1980) fed a vitamin D-deficient diet to dogs. This diet required at least 3 months to depress the serum Ca approximately 2 mg/dL while lowering the serum 25-$(OH)_2D_3$ level to less than 0.4 ng/ml (30 to 60 ng/ml is the normal value for humans).

Toxicity caused by excess vitamin D administration is also associated with plasma 25-OHD; concentrations of more than 400 ng/ml have been reported (Hughes et al., 1976). Patients suffering from hypervitaminosis D have been shown to exhibit a 15-fold increase in plasma 25-OHD concentration compared with normal individuals.

Osteocalcin can also be used to evaluate bone mineralization. Carter et al. (1996) have suggested that serum osteocalcin and $1,25$-$(OH)_2D$ are better predictors of bone mineralization and/or turnover in pigs than is serum alkaline phosphatase.

SUPPLEMENTATION

For animals that are kept indoors or live in climates where the sunlight is not adequate for vitamin D production, the vitamin D content of the diet becomes important. In modern poultry, swine, and dairy operations, animals are often entirely without sunlight. Under these intensive conditions, supplemental vitamin D must be provided. It seems that supplementation is important for dogs and cats since studies have shown conclusively that neither dogs nor cats receive a significant benefit from synthesis of vitamin D in the skin through exposure to UV irradiation (How et al., 1994a,b, 1995).

Animals on pasture during the summer never suffer from the lack of the antirachitic factor even though their diet may be practically devoid of it. In winter, however, animals are outside only a part of the time, there are generally fewer sunny days, and the sunlight that reaches the animal is much less effective than in summer. In winter at far southern and northern latitudes, it is unsafe to rely on exposure to sunlight to provide the antirachitic factor as no significant production of vitamin D_3 in skin occurs (Webb et al., 1988). Milk is not especially rich in vitamin D, but young animals can obtain adequate amounts by skin irradiation if exposed to the sunlight for 1 to 2 hours per day. Sun-cured forage is the best natural source of vitamin D. Even silages generally have dead (thus sun-cured) leaves that will provide some vitamin D to growing animals housed indoors. However, it is probably prudent to provide a vitamin D supplement to young calves in their milk replacer and starter diets until they are turned out or are consuming adequate forage (e.g., 6 to 8 weeks).

Special Ca and P supplementation is required for high-producing dairy cows to prevent parturient paresis (milk fever). Parturient paresis can be prevented effectively by feeding a prepartum diet low in Ca and adequate in P. Prepartal low-Ca diets are associated with increased plasma PTH and $1,25\text{-}(OH)_2D_2$ and $1,25\text{-}(OH)_2D_3$ concentrations during the prepartal period. Green et al. (1981) suggested that these increased PTH and $1,25\text{-}(OH)_2D$ concentrations resulted in "prepared" and effective intestinal and bone Ca homeostatic mechanisms at parturition that prevented parturient paresis.

Supplemental vitamin D has been used to prevent parturient paresis in dairy cows for a number of years. Treatment with high levels of vitamin D has been successful, but toxicity problems have sometimes resulted, and for some animals, the disease has been induced by the treatment. Because of the extreme toxicity of vitamin D_3 in pregnant cows, and the low margin of safety between doses of vitamin D_3 that prevent milk fever and doses that induce milk fever, Littledike and Horst (1982) concluded that vitamin D_3 cannot be used practically to prevent milk fever when injected several weeks prepartum. However, a later report from the same laboratory provided data suggesting that injection of 24-F-1,25-$(OH)_2D_3$ (fluoridation at the 24R position) delivered at 7-day intervals prior to parturition can effectively reduce incidence of parturient paresis (Goff et al., 1988). This compound, however, never advanced beyond the experimental stage. An analogue that has been marketed in Israel and used with varying degrees of success was 1α-hydroxycholecalciferol [$1\alpha(OH)D_3$] (Sachs et al., 1977).

This analogue was developed as a precursor in the chemical synthesis of 1,25-$(OH)_2D_3$ and, fortunately, can be activated by the body following 25-hydroxylation in the liver to form 1,25-$(OH)_2D_3$. Use of this analogue, however, shared the disadvantages of earlier compounds: hypercalcemia was induced, and the endogenous synthesis of 1,25-$(OH)_2D_3$ was inhibited. Hodnett et al. (1992) used a combination of 25-OHD_3 plus 1α-hydroxycholecalciferol to reduce parturient paresis in dairy cows fed high dietary Ca. The incidence of the disease was reduced from 33 to 8%. Supplementation of 1α-hydroxycholecalciferol, which is less costly to produce than 1,25-$(OH)_2D_3$, has improved phytate P utilization in poultry but not swine (Biehl and Baker, 1997a,b).

Anion-cation balance of prepartum diets (sometimes referred to as acidity or alkalinity of a diet) also can influence the incidence of milk fever (Oetzel et al., 1988; Gaynor et al., 1989). Diets high in cations, especially sodium and potassium, tend to induce milk fever, but those high in anions, primarily chlorine and sulfur, can prevent milk fever. The incidence of milk fever depends on the abundance of the cations Na+ and K+ relative to the anions Cl- and SO_4^{2-}. This concept is now generally referred to as the cation-anion difference (CAD). Because most legumes and grasses are high in potassium, many of the commonly used prepartum diets are alkaline. Addition of anions to a prepartal diet is thought to induce metabolic acidosis in the cow, which facilitates bone Ca resorption and intestinal Ca absorption (Lomba et al., 1978; Fredeen et al., 1988; Horst et al., 1997). Diets higher in anions increase osteoclastic bone resorption and synthesis of 1,25-$(OH)_2D_3$ in cows (Goff et al., 1991a). Both of these physiological processes are controlled by PTH. Workers at the Rowett Research Institute (Abu Damir et al., 1994) have also reported that 1,25-$(OH)_2D_3$ production is enhanced in cows fed acidifying diets. Commercial preparations of HCL mixed into common feed ingredients as a premix could offer an inexpensive and palatable alternative to anionic salts as a means of controlling the incidence of milk fever in dairy cows (Goff and Horst, 1998).

Collectively, these data suggest that a major underlying cause of milk fever is metabolic alkalosis, which causes an inability of cow tissues to respond adequately to PTH (Horst et al., 1997). This lack of response in turn reduces the ability of the cow to draw on bone Ca stores, and reduces production of the second Ca-regulating hormone, 1,25-$(OH)_2D$, which is needed for active transport of Ca within the intestine. The presumption is that metabolic alkalosis somehow disrupts the integrity of PTH receptors on target tissues. Low CAD diets prevent metabolic alkalosis, increasing target tissue responsiveness to PTH, which controls renal 1α-hydroxylase and resorption of bone Ca.

Several options exist regarding methods for the control of milk fever (Horst et al., 1997). The current understanding of the CAD concept suggests that milk fever could be managed more effectively if dietary K were reduced (Goff and Horst, 1997). Calcium chloride has been used to reduce blood pH. This reduction is beneficial, but excessive oral Ca chloride can induce metabolic acidosis (Goff and Horst, 1994), which can cause inappetence at a time when feed intake is already compromised. Calcium propionate treatment has been beneficial in reducing subclinical hypocalcemia in all trials and reduced the incidence of milk fever in a herd having a problem with milk fever (Goff et al., 1996).

Due to lack of vitamin D in feeds and management systems without direct sunlight, modern livestock operations must provide a supplemental source of the vitamin. Vitamin D is available in two forms: vitamin D_3 of animal origin and vitamin D_2 of plant origin. Vitamin D_3 has been the primary source of supplemental vitamin D for domestic animals, whereas vitamin D_2 has been the chief source of supplemental vitamin D in foods and pharmaceuticals. Vitamin D_3 is commercially available as a resin, usually containing 24 to 26 million IU per gram, for use as the vitamin D source in various vitamin products. Vitamin D_3 products for feed include gelatin beadlets (with vitamin A), oil dilutions, oil absorbates, emulsions, and spray- and drum-dried powders. Test results have shown that the gelatin beadlet offers optimum vitamin D_3 stability. A commercially available vitamin product containing stabilized, high-purity vitamin D for feed or drinking water use should be used to ensure the vitamin D levels needed to prevent deficiency and allow optimum performance. Continued irradiation eventually destroys the vitamin D produced, but the chief cause of loss from foods is doubtless oxidation, as was recognized long ago (Fritz et al., 1942). Higher vitamin D levels in freeze-dried fish meals suggest less destruction during drying, possibly because of decreased atmospheric oxygen (Scott and Latshaw, 1994).

Stabilization of the vitamin can be achieved by (1) rapid compression of the mixed feed, for example, into cubes, so that air is excluded, (2) storing feed under cool, dry, dark conditions, (3) preventing close contact between the vitamin and potent metallic oxidation catalysts, for example, manganese, and (4) including natural or synthetic antioxidants in the mix. The vitamin can also be protected by enclosing it in tough, gelatin beadlets. But all stability is relative; warmth and moisture will soften gelatin, while temperatures below about 10°C cause it to become hard, brittle, and friable (Abrams, 1978).

Pure vitamin D_3 crystals or vitamin D_3 resin is very susceptible to degradation upon exposure to heat or contact with mineral elements. In fact, the resin is stored under refrigeration with nitrogen gas. Dry, stabilized supplements retain potency much longer and can be used in high-mineral supplements. It has been shown that vitamin D_3 is much more stable than D_2 in feeds containing minerals. When the unprotected vitamin is thinly spread over the surface of free-flowing powders, as in some of the mineral components of compound animal feeds, its life in storage may be no more than 1 month. In complete feeds and mineral-vitamin premixes, Schneider (1986) reported activity losses of 10 to 30% after either 4 or 6 months of storage at 22°C.

Stability of dry vitamin D supplements is affected most by high temperature, high moisture content, and contact with trace minerals such as ferrous sulfate, manganese oxide, and others. Hirsh (1982) reports the results of a "conventional" or nonstabilized vitamin D_3 product being mixed into a trace mineral premix or into animal feed and stored at ambient room temperature (20 to 25°C) for up to 12 weeks. The mash feed had lost 31% of its vitamin D activity after 12 weeks, and the trace mineral premix had lost 66% of its activity after only 6 weeks in storage.

In addition to providing supplemental vitamin D in feed and water, injectable sources are available. Parenteral vitamin D_3 treatment of sows before parturition provided an effective means of supplementing piglets with vitamin D_3 (via the sow's milk) and its dehydroxymetabolites by placental transport (Goff et al., 1984).

Naturally occurring sources of vitamin D in feeds must likewise be protected from loss. Poor handling of hay, which can otherwise be an important source of vitamin D and various other nutrients for forage-consuming animals, can lead to extensive fragmentation and loss of the leaf, which is much richer in vitamin D than the stem. Animals fed on grain, silage, or hay that is poorly produced or stored are extremely liable to have dietary deficiency of the vitamin (Abrams, 1978).

Cost of vitamin D supplementation to livestock diets is nominal (Rowland, 1982). In contrast, the cost of not adding enough vitamin D to prevent deficiencies is very high. Supplemental levels of vitamin D administered to livestock through the feed should be adjusted to provide the margin of safety needed to offset the factors influencing vitamin D needs. This is important to prevent deficiency and allow optimum performance.

Rowland (1982) notes that diets for young, rapidly growing chickens must contain liberal amounts of vitamin D to prevent field problems. He further observed that the NRC level (200 IU/kg of feed) for young chickens is extremely unrealistic for broilers. Even under low-stress research conditions, three to five times the NRC level is required to support maximum weight gain of broilers, and under commercial conditions, 10 times the NRC level is prudent for broilers fed under field conditions. The NRC vitamin D levels for laying hens and turkeys are somewhat more realistic, with a factor of five times the NRC level generally supporting optimum performance and providing some margin of safety (Rowland, 1982). The most logical approach is to adjust supplemental vitamin D levels to expected production conditions.

Besides inadequate quantities of dietary vitamin D, deficiencies may result from (1) errors in vitamin addition to diets, (2) inadequate mixing and distribution in feed, (3) separation of vitamin D particles after mixing, (4) instability of the vitamin content of the supplement, or (5) excessive length of storage of diets under environmental conditions causing vitamin D loss (Hirsch, 1982).

Supplementation considerations are dependent on other dietary ingredients. The requirements for vitamin D_3 are increased several-fold by inadequate levels of Ca and/or P or by improper ratios of these two elements in the diet (see Requirements). Vitamin D treatment considerably enhances Ca and P utilization in pigs fed on a phytate-P diet but does not completely overcome the negative effects of phytate feeding on mineral metabolism (Pointillart et al., 1986). A number of reports have indicated that molds in feeds interfere with vitamin D (Cunha, 1977); for example, when corn contains the mold *Fusarium roseum,* a metabolite of this mold prevents vitamin D_3 in the intestinal tract from being absorbed by the chick. Other molds may also be involved, and they result in a large percentage of birds with bone disorders. A number of flocks have been successfully treated by adding water-dispersible forms of vitamin D to drinking water at three to five times the normally recommended vitamin D levels.

Other factors that influence vitamin D status are diseases of the endocrine system, intestinal disorders, liver malfunction, kidney disorders, and drugs. Liver malfunction limits production of the active forms of the vitamin, while intestinal disorders reduce absorption. Persons with kidney failure are unable to synthesize 1,25-$(OH)_2$D, and for patients in renal dialysis who are waiting for a compatible kidney transplant donor, 1,25-$(OH)_2$D has been found to alleviate the painful and serious bone disease associated with chronic renal failure. The prolonged use of anticonvulsant drugs can result in an impaired response to vitamin D (Collins and Norman, 1991), and Cunha (personal communication, 1987) suggested the possibility that livestock with certain diseases or heavy infestation of internal parasites might be unable to synthesize the metabolically active forms of vitamin D as a result of liver or kidney damage. Unknown factors in feeds may increase vitamin D requirements. For example, there is evidence of a factor in rye and in soybean fractions that can produce malabsorption of this vitamin in the intestine (Mac-Auliff and McGinnis, 1976).

Widespread fortification of human diets with vitamin D and provision of oral supplements over the past 60 years have greatly reduced the incidence of rickets in children. However, most of the world's population still depends on exposure to sunlight for their vitamin D nutritional needs because very few natural foods contain sufficient quantities to meet the daily requirement. It has been assumed that in countries where food is fortified with vitamin D, such as the United States, exposure to sunlight is no longer necessary for vitamin D nutrition. Although this may be true for young children who drink milk fortified with vitamin D, many elderly persons who do not drink milk or take a vitamin D supplement are prone to vitamin D deficiency when they are not exposed to sufficient sunlight. Among the fortified foods are milk (both fresh and evaporated), margarine and butter, cereals, and chocolate mixes. Milk is fortified to supply 400 IU of vitamin D per quart, and margarine usually contains 4,400 or more IU per kilogram (Collins and Norman, 1991).

The major source of vitamin D for most humans is casual exposure to sunlight. It is estimated that more than 80 to 90% of the body's requirement for vitamin D comes from this source (Holick, 1994). Several factors can affect the cutaneous synthesis of vitamin D_3 (see Requirements). Anything that limits the amount of solar ultraviolet B (UVB) photons to reach the skin's surface and penetrate the viable epidermis can significantly affect this vital photosynthetic process. Skin pigment, clothing, and topically applied sunscreens absorb UVB photons and, therefore, can significantly diminish the synthesis of vitamin D_3 (Holick, 1994). The topical application of a sunscreen with a sun protection factor of 8 can almost completely eliminate the cutaneous production of vitamin D_3 and cause vitamin D deficiency (Matsuoka et al., 1988). This is probably not a logical concern as sufficient summer sunlight is received, probably through both the sunscreen itself and the lack of total skin cover at all times, to allow adequate vitamin D production in people who are advised to use sunscreens regularly (Marks et al., 1995). Season, latitude, and time of day can significantly affect the cutaneous production of vitamin D_3.

Many bone problems in humans are the result of Ca and/or vitamin D deficiencies. These problems are most severe in young children, adolescents, and elderly persons (manifested as hip fracture and fractures of the vertebrae). Bone problems are generally preventable by adequate dietary or supplementary Ca and vitamin D and exercise at a young age, with the goal of developing peak bone mass prior to advancing age. Optimal intake of both Ca and vitamin D may be an easily implemented strategy to maintain existing bone mass and reduce the risk of fracture in older men and women (O'Brien, 1998).

Epidemiological studies have suggested that sunlight deprivation, and the associated reduction in the circulating levels of vitamin D_3 derivatives, may lead to an increased incidence of carcinomas of the breast, colon, and prostate (Studzinski and Moore, 1995). Likewise, sunlight (vitamin D) may be a protective factor in ovarian cancer mortality (Lefkowitz and Garland, 1994).

The Food and Drug Administration does not permit $1,25\text{-}(OH)_2D$ to be added to feeds. However, this hormone or its analogs have proven effective in human medicine in treating psoriasis (Bikle, 1995), colorectal carcinoma (Cross et al., 1995), leukemia (Jung et al., 1994), breast cancer (James et al., 1994), and prostate cancer (Skowronski et al., 1995). This function relates to $1,25\text{-}(OH)_2D$ modulating cell growth and differentiation, including that of malignant cells.

TOXICITY

Excess consumption of vitamin A results in toxicity. After vitamin A, vitamin D is the vitamin most likely to be consumed in concentrations toxic to both humans and livestock. Excessive intake of vitamin D produces a variety of effects, all associated with abnormal elevation of blood Ca. Elevated blood Ca is caused by greatly stimulated bone resorption, as well as increased intestinal Ca absorption.

The main pathological effect of ingestion of massive doses of vitamin D is widespread calcification of soft tissues. Pathological changes in these tissues are observed to be inflammation, cellular degeneration, and calcification. Diffuse calcification affects the joints, synovial membranes, kidney, myocardium, pulmonary alveoli, parathyroids, pancreas, lymph glands, arteries, conjunctivae, and cornea. More advanced cases interfere with cartilage growth. The abnormal calcification is grossly observed as a whitish chalky material, and kidney insufficiency is the most critical development of these processes. Initial kidney damage is due to Ca deposition in distal tubules, causing inflammation and later obstruction, which in turn causes hypertension and related pathology. As would be expected, the skeletal system undergoes a simultaneous demineralization that results in the thinning of bones.

Other common observations of vitamin D toxicity are anorexia (loss of appetite), extensive weight loss, elevated blood Ca, and lowered blood phosphate. Many investigators have described the clinical signs of hypervitaminosis D in mammals (NRC, 1987). Cows receiving 30 million IU of vitamin D_2 orally for 11 days developed anorexia, reduced rumination, depression, premature ventricular systoles, and bradycardia. Toxicosis in monkeys resulted in weight loss, anorexia, elevated blood urea nitrogen, diarrhea, anemia, and upper respiratory infections. In pigs, signs of toxicity were anorexia, stiffness, lameness, arching of the back, polyuria, and aphonia. Dogs receiving toxic concentrations of vitamin D exhibited anorexia, polyuria, bloody diarrhea, polydipsia, prostration, and excessive calcification of the lungs (Morgan, 1947), while cats receiving excess vitamin D exhibited heavy calcification of arteries and the adrenals (Suter, 1957). Symptoms of vitamin D intoxication for humans include hypercalcemia, hypercalciuria, anorexia, nausea, vomiting, thirst, polyuria, muscular weakness, joint pains, diffuse demineralization of bones, and disorientation (Collins and Norman, 1991).

In poultry, excess vitamin D elevates $1,25-(OH)_2D$ with hypercalcemia and soft tissue mineralization (NRC, 1994). Leg problems may arise with growing birds because of bone Ca loss (Cruickshank and Sim, 1987), but few obvious changes occur with hens other than a general depression in performance (Ameenuddin et al., 1986). Toxic levels of vitamin D may be transferred into the egg to create similar problems for the embryo; however, the hypercalcemia occurs from shell resorption, and bone mineralization is enhanced (Narbaitz and Fragiskos, 1984).

141

Harrington and Page (1983) compared toxicity of D_2 to D_3 in horses. Signs of toxicity included weight loss, hypercalcemia, hyperphosphatemia, and cardiovascular calcinosis. However, the signs of illness, deviations of blood chemistry from normal, and severity of tissue pathology, were much more pronounced for vitamin D_3.

Severity of the effects and pathogenic lesions in vitamin D intoxication depend on such factors as the type of vitamin D (D_2 versus D_3), the dose, the functional state of the kidneys, and the composition of the diet (NRC, 1987). Studies indicate that vitamin D_3 is 10 to 20 times more toxic than vitamin D_2. When equal amounts of vitamin D_3 and vitamin D_2 are provided together in diets of mammals, the predominant circulating form of the vitamin is usually $25\text{-}OHD_3$ rather than $25\text{-}OHD_2$. Similarly, in toxicity experiments in which vitamin D_2 was less toxic than vitamin D_3, the metabolite $25\text{-}OHD_2$ was found to be present at lower plasma concentrations than $25\text{-}OHD_3$ (Harrington and Page, 1983).

Vitamin D toxicity is enhanced by elevated supplies of dietary Ca and P and is reduced when the diet is low in Ca. Toxicity is also reduced when the vitamin is accompanied by intakes of vitamin A or by thyroxin injections (Payne and Manston, 1967). Route of administration also influences toxicity. Parenteral administration of 15 million IU of vitamin D_3 in a single dose caused toxicity and death in many pregnant dairy cows (Littledike and Horst, 1982). On the other hand, oral administration of 20 to 30 million IU of vitamin D_2 daily for 7 days resulted in little or no toxicity in pregnant dairy cows (Hibbs and Pounden, 1955). Rumen microbes are capable of metabolizing vitamin D to an inactive compound, which may partially explain the difference in toxicity between oral and parenteral vitamin D. The toxic dose of vitamin D is quite variable, with an important factor being duration of intake, as this is a cumulative toxicity. However, there is marked variation among individuals in tolerance to excessive doses of vitamin D, the mechanism of which is unknown. Some species are less affected by toxicity due to vitamin D metabolism differences. For example, in the hooded seal, there is increased conversion of 25-OHD to $24,25\text{-}(OH)_2D$ and a high capacity for vitamin D storage in its large blubber mass, which provides resistance for this species to toxicity (Keiver et al., 1988).

Although it is usually assumed that living plants do not contain vitamin D_2, some plants contain compounds that have vitamin D activity (Mello and Habermehl, 1995). Grazing animals in several parts of the world develop calcinosis, a disease characterized by the deposition of Ca salts in soft tissues (Carrillo, 1973; Morris, 1982). The ingestion of the leaves of the shrub *Solanum malacoxylon* by grazing animals causes enzootic calcinosis in Argentina and Brazil, where the disease is referred to as *enteque seco* and *espichamento*, respectively. As few as 50 fresh leaves per day (200 g of fresh leaves per week) over a period of 8 to 20 weeks are enough for the disease to develop in cows (Fig. 3.8) (Okada et al., 1977).

Another solanaceous plant, *Cestrium diurnum* (a large ornamental plant), causes calcinosis in grazing animals in Florida, while the grass *Trisetum flavescens* is the causative agent in the Alpine regions in Europe. *Solanum torvum* is suspected of causing calcinosis in cattle in Papua, New Guinea. A condition known as "humpy-back," in which clinical symptoms reminiscent of calcinosis occur, may be caused by sheep grazing the fruits of *S. esuriale* in Australia. In Jamaica, "Manchester wasting disease" and in Hawaii, "Naalehu disease" are conditions seen in cattle that are virtually identical to *enteque seco* in relation to clinical and pathological signs (Wasserman, 1975; Arnold and Fincham, 1997).

The calcinogenic factor in *S. malacoxylon* and *C. diurnum* is a water-soluble glycoside of $1,25\text{-}(OH)_2D_3$ (Wasserman, 1975). The digestive system of the animal releases the sterol, which promotes a massive increase in the absorption of dietary Ca and P such that accommodation of these elements by the normal physiological processes is ineffective, and soft tissue calcification results. Vitamin D_3 has been identified in *T. flavescens* but at concentrations that would not be calcinogenic. Evidence is emerging that the grass may also contain $1,25\text{-}(OH)_2D_3$ or a substance able to mimic its actions as well as an aqueous-soluble factor that promotes phosphate absorption.

During development of plant-induced calcinosis diseases, destruction of connective tissues occurs, and this precedes mineralization in which magnesium is involved as well as Ca and phosphate. Clinical signs of the disease are stiffened and painful gait, with progressive weight loss. If the animals are removed in the early stages from the affected areas, they recover quickly, but they may die if they are not removed. In advanced cases, joints cannot be extended completely, and animals tend to walk with an arched back, carrying the weight on the forepart of the hooves.

Animals with calcinosis may also show signs of acute cardiac and pulmonary insufficiency. Postmortem examination shows widespread metastatic calcification of the vascular system and soft tissues. The heart and aorta exhibit the most marked effects, and calcification in the lung develops later than in the vascular system. Cartilage of the appendicular

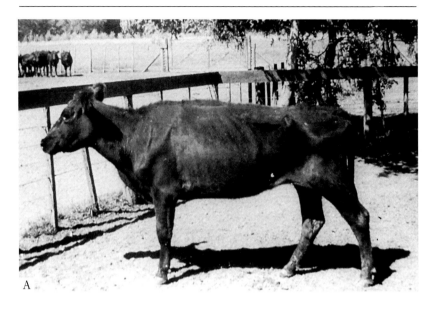

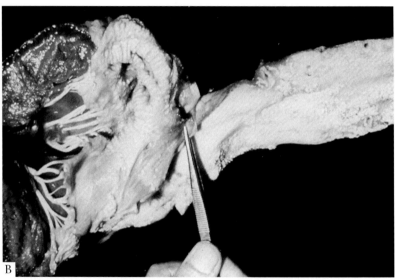

Fig. 3.8 Vitamin D toxicity (*enteque seco*) in Argentina: (A) Cow that had consumed the shrub *Solanum malacoxylon;* (B) Calcium deposits in soft tissue. (Courtesy of Bernardo Jorge Carrillo, CICV, INTA, Castelar, Argentina.)

144

skeleton is eroded in advanced cases, with the joints almost denuded of cartilage. The kidney may also show some calcification. Animals grazing in areas where the disease occurs show high serum levels of Ca and inorganic P. All clinical signs are similar to those found in vitamin D intoxication (Wolker and Carrillo, 1967).

It is clear that the calcinogenic plants are economically important, particularly because of their toxic effects. which result in enormous losses in meat and milk production (Morris, 1982). In some fields in Argentina, between 10 and 30% of cattle show signs of *enteque seco*, and *S. malacoxylon* is now regarded as one of the most important poisonous plants of that country. A survey conducted in Bavarian slaughterhouses revealed mineral deposits in soft tissues in 22 to 52% of cattle from the south of Bavaria that had been grazing at an altitude above 500 m. *Trisetum flavescens* is also an important toxic plant in these alpine pastures. In 1977, it was estimated that the annual loss in revenue resulting from *S. malacoxylon*-induced calcinosis in Argentina was of the order of $10 million. No assessment of the economic losses arising from plant-induced calcinosis is available for any other country.

With the exception of grazing animals consuming certain plants containing $1,25\text{-}(OH)_2D_3$ in several parts of the world, excessive amounts of vitamin D are not available from natural sources. Although certain fish liver and body oils are good sources of vitamin D, concentrations are not so high that toxic amounts of vitamin D would likely be ingested. Therefore, danger of vitamin D toxicosis is from dietary supplementation. Extensive whole-body irradiation with UV light will not result in vitamin D toxicity. Vitamin D toxicosis from dietary sources can result in 400 ng/ml of plasma 25-OHD, while extensive UV light exposure can result in only 40 to 80 ng of this transport form of vitamin D (Davie and Lawson, 1980). Therefore, supplying vitamin D by mouth bypasses protective mechanisms that prevent excessive 25-OHD formation.

For most species the presumed maximum safe level of vitamin D_3 for long-term feeding conditions (more than 60 days) is 4 to 10 times the recognized dietary requirement (NRC, 1987). Catfish and rainbow trout, on the other hand, can tolerate as much as 50 and 500 times their requirements, respectively. Under short-term feeding conditions (less than 60 days), most species can tolerate as much as 100 times their apparent dietary requirements. Table 3.3 provides recommendations for safe upper dietary levels of vitamin D_3 for animals.

Rodents are sensitive to vitamin D toxicity and have an LD_{50} of 43.6 mg/kg body weight for cholecalciferol compared to 88 and 200

■ Table 3.3   Estimation of Safe Upper Dietary Levels of Vitamin D₃ (IU/kg in Diet) for Animals

Animal	Dietary Requirement	Exposure Time	
		< 60 days	> 60 days
Birds			
Chicken	200	40,000	2,800
Japanese quail	1,200	120,000	4,700
Turkey	900	90,000	3,500
Cow	300	25,000	2,200
Fish			
Catfish	1,000		20,000
Rainbow trout	1,800		1,000,000
Horse	400		2,200
Sheep	275	25,000	2,200
Swine	220	33,000	2,200

Source: Modified from NRC (1987).

mg/kg in dogs and humans, respectively (Tindall, 1985). Cholecalciferol is marketed as an effective rodenticide, with low oral toxicity to nonrodent species. However, cholecalciferol rodenticides have caused significant toxicity in dogs at a fraction of the manufacturer's reported LD_{50} for dogs, 88 mg pure cholecalciferol per kilogram of body weight (Garlock et al., 1991). These researchers described a dog that consumed pure cholecalciferol in an estimated amount of 1.5 to 3.0 mg/kg body weight. Clinical signs most commonly associated with the resultant hypercalcemia were polyuria, polydipsia, depression, anorexia, weakness, and vomiting.

In the early stages of vitamin D intoxication, the effects are usually reversible. Treatment consists merely of withdrawing vitamin D and perhaps reducing dietary Ca intake until serum Ca levels fall. However, it is usually not immediately successful because of the long plasma half-life of vitamin D (5 to 7 days) and 25-OHD (20 to 30 days). This is in contrast to the short plasma half-life of 1α-OHD₃ (1 to 2 days) and 1,25-$(OH)_2D_3$ (4 to 8 hours). Sodium phytate, an agent that reduces intestinal Ca absorption, has also been used successfully in vitamin D toxicity management in monogastrics. This treatment would be of little benefit to ruminants because of the presence of rumen microbial phytases. There have also been reports that calcitonin, glucagon, and glucocorticoid therapy reduces serum Ca levels resulting from vitamin D intoxication (NRC, 1987).

■ REFERENCES

Abrams, J.T. (1978). *In* Handbook Series in Nutrition and Food, Section E: Nutritional Disorders (M. Rechcigl Jr., ed.), Vol. 2, p. 179. CRC Press, Boca Raton, Florida.

Abu Damir, H., Phillippo, M., Thorp, B.H., Milne, J.S., Dick, L., and Nevison, I.M. (1994). *Res. Vet. Sci. 56*, 310.

Ameenuddin, S., Sunde, M.L., DeLuca, H.F., and Cool, M.E. (1986). *Brit. Poult. Sci. 27*, 671.

Arneil, G.C. (1975). *Proc. Nutr. Sci. 34*, 101.

Arnold, R.M., and Fincham, I.H. (1997). *Trop. Anim. Health Prod. 29*, 174.

Baker, A.R., McDonnell, D.P., Hughes, M., Crisp, R.M., Manglesdorf, D.J., Haussler, M.R., Pike, J.W., Shine, J., and O'Malley, B.W. (1988). *Proc. Natl. Acad. Sci. 85*, 3294.

Barnett, B.J., Young, Cho, C., and Slinger, S.J. (1982). *J. Nutr. 112*, 2011.

Biehl, R.R., and Baker, D.H. (1997a). *J. Nutr. 127*, 2054.

Biehl, R.R., and Baker, D.H. (1997b). *J. Anim. Sci. 75*, 2986.

Bikle, D.D. (1995). *J. Nutr. 125*, 1709S.

Blunt, J.W., DeLuca, H.F., and Schnoes, H.K. (1968). *Biochemistry 7*, 3317.

Bordier, P., Rasmussen, H., Marie, P., Miravet, L., Gueris, J., and Ryckwaert, A. (1978). *J. Clin. Endocrinol. Metab. 46*, 284.

Braithwaite, G.D. (1974). *Br. J. Nutr. 31*, 319.

Braithwaite, G.D., and Riazuddin, S.H. (1971). *Br. J. Nutr. 26*, 215.

Braithwaite, G.D., Glascock, R.F., and Riazuddin, S.H. (1969). *Br. J. Nutr. 23*, 827.

Braithwaite, G.D., Glascock, R.F., and Riazuddin, S.H. (1972). *Br. J. Nutr. 27*, 417.

Bronner, F. (1987). *J. Nutr. 117*, 1347.

Bronner, F., and Stein, W.D. (1995). *J. Nutr. 125*, 1987S.

Brunvand, L., Haga, P., Tangsrud, S.E., and Haug, E. (1995). *Acta Paediatrica 84*, 106.

Cade, C., and Norman, A.W. (1986). *Endocrinology 119*, 84.

Campbell, J.R., and Douglas, T.A. (1965). *Br. J. Nutr. 19*, 339.

Carrillo, B.J. (1973). *Rev. Invest. Agropecu. Serv. 4, Patol. Anim. 10*, 65.

Carter, S.D., Cromwell, G.L., Combs, T.R., Colombo, G., and Fanti, P. (1996). *J. Anim. Sci. 74*, 2719.

Chen, Jr., P.S., and Bosmann, H.B. (1964). *Science 150*, 19.

Church, D.C., and Pond, W.G. (1974). Basic Animal Nutrition and Feeding. Albany Printing, Albany, New York.

Collins, E.D., and Norman, A.W. (1991). *In* Handbook of Vitamins (L. Machlin, ed.) p. 59. Marcel Dekker, New York.

Colston, K., Colston, M.J., and Feldman, D. (1981). *Endocrinology 108*, 1083.

Craig, J.F., and Davis, G.O. (1943). *J. Comp. Pathol. Ther. 53*, 196.

Cross, H.S., Hulla, W., Tong, W., and Peterlik, M. (1995). *J. Nutr. 125*, 2004S.

Cruickshank, J.J., and Sim, J.S. (1987). *Avian Dis. 31*, 332.

Cunha, T.J. (1977). Swine Feeding and Nutrition. Academic Press, New York.

Davie, M., and Lawson, D.E.M. (1980). *Clin. Sci. 58*, 235.

DeLuca, H.F. (1979). *Nutr. Rev. 37*, 161.

DeLuca, H.F. (1990). *In* Proc. 1990 National Feed Ingredients Association Nutrition Institute: Developments in Vitamin Nutrition and Health Applications, Kansas City, Missouri. National Feed Ingredients Association (NFIA), Des Moines, Iowa.

DeLuca, H.F. (1992). *Ann. N.Y. Acad. Sci. 669*, 59.

DeLuca, H.F., and Zierold, C. (1998). *Nutr. Rev. 56*, S 4.

Doppelt, S.H., Neer, R.M., Daly, M., Bourvet, L., Schiller, A., and Holick, M.F. (1983). *Orthop. Trans. 7*, 512.

Duncan, C.W. (1944). *J. Dairy Sci. 27*, 636.

Dzanis, D.A., Corbellini, C.N., Krook, L., and Kallfelz, F.A. (1992). *J. Nutr. 121*, 11S.

Eisman, J.A. (1998). *Nutr. Rev. 56*, S 22.

Elaroussi, M.A., Uhland-Smith, A., Hellwig, W., and DeLuca, H.F. (1994). *Biochem. Biophys. Acta 1192*, 1.

El-Hag, A.I., and Karrar, Z.A. (1995). *Annals Trop. Pediat. 15*, 69.

Elliot, W., and Crichton, A. (1926). *J. Agar. Sci. 16*, 65.

El Shorafa, W.M., Feaster, J.P., Ott, E.A., and Asquith, R.L. (1979). *J. Anim. Sci. 48*, 882.

Feliciano, E.S., Ho, M., Specker, B.L., Falciglia, G., Shui, Q.M., Yin, T.A., and Chen, X.C. (1994). *J. Trop. Pediat.* y40, 162.

Fleet, J.C. (1999). *Nutr. Rev. 57*, 60.

Franklin, M.C., and Johnstone, I.L. (1948). Maintenance of Serum Calcium Level by Calcium Supplements to the Diet, p. 63. C.S.I.R.O., Melbourne, Florida.

Fraser, D.R. (1984). *In* Nutrition Reviews, Present Knowledge in Nutrition (R.E. Olson, ed.), p. 209. Nutrition Foundation, Washington, D.C.

Fredeen, A.H., DePeters, E.J., and Baldwin, R.L. (1988). *J. Anim. Sci. 66*, 159.

Fritz, J.C., Archer, W.F., and Barker, D.K. (1942). *Poult. Sci. 21*, 361.

Garabedian, M., Tanaka, Y., Holick, M.F., and DeLuca, H.F. (1974). *Endocrinology 94*, 1022.

Garlock, S.M., Matz, M.E., and Shell, L.G. (1991). *J. An. Anim. Hosp. Assoc. 27*, 356.

Gaynor, P.J., Mueller, F.J., Miller, J.K., Ramsey, N., Goff, J.P., and Horst, R.L. (1989). *J. Dairy Sci. 72*, 2525.

Gershoff, S.N., Legg, M.A., O'Connor, F.J., and Hegsted, D.M. (1957). *J. Nutr. 63*, 79.

Ghazarian, J.G., Jefcoate, C.R., Knutson, J.C., Orme-Hohnson, W.H., and DeLuca, H.F. (1974). *J. Biol.Chem. 249*, 3026.

Goff, J.P., and Horst, R.L. (1994). *J. Dairy Sci. 77*, 1451.

Goff, J.P., and Horst, R.L. (1997). *J. Dairy Sci. 80*, 176.

Goff, J.P., and Horst, R.L. (1998). *J. Dairy Sci. 81*, 2874.

Goff, J.P., Horst, R.L., and Littledike, E.T. (1984). *J. Nutr. 114*, 163.

Goff, J.P., Horst, R.L., Beitz, D.E., and Littledike, E.T. (1988). *J. Dairy Sci. 71*, 1211.

Goff, J.P., Horst, R.L., Jardon, P.W., Borelli, C., and Wedam, J. (1996). *J. Dairy Sci. 79*, 378.

Goff, J.P., Horst, R.L., Mueller, F.J., Miller, J.K, Kiess, G.A., and Dowlen, H.H.

(1991a). *J. Dairy Sci. 74*, 3863.

Goff, J.P., Reinhardt, T.A., and Horst, R.L. (1989). *Endocrinology 125*, 49.

Goff, J.P., Reinhardt, T.A., and Horst, R.L. (1991b). *J. Dairy Sci. 74*, 4022.

Goldblatt, H., and Soames, K.M. (1923). *Blochem J. 17*, 446.

Gonnerman, W.A., Toverud, S.V., Ramp, W.K., and Mechanic, G.L. (1976). *Proc. Soc. Exp. Biol. Med. 151*, 453.

Green, H.B., Horst, R.L., Beitz, D.C., and Littledike, E.T. (1981). *J. Dairy Sci. 64*, 217.

Guilland, J.C., de Carvalho, M.J.C., Moreau, D., Boggio, V., Lhuissier, M., and Fuchs, F. (1994). *Nutr. Res. 14*, 1317.

Haddad, J.G., and Walgate, J. (1976). *J.Biol. Chem. 251*, 4803.

Hannah, S.S., and Norman, A.W. (1994). *Nutr. Rev. 52*, 376.

Harrington, D.D., and Page, E.H. (1983). *J. Am. Vet. Med. Assoc. 182*, 1358.

Harrison, H.C., and Harrison, H.E. (1963). *Am. J. Physiol. 205*, 107.

Harrison, H.E. (1978). *In* Handbook Series in Nutrition and Food, Section E: Nutritional Disorders (M. Rechcigl Jr., ed.), Vol. 3, p. 117. CRC Press, Boca Raton, Florida.

Hay, A.W.M., and Watson, G. (1976). *Comp. Biochem. Physiol. 56*, 167.

Hazewinkel, H.A.W., How, K.L., Bosch, R., Goedegebuure, S.A., and Voorhout, G. (1987). *In* Ernahrung, Fehlernäbrung und Diätetik Bei Hund und Katze (H. Meyer and E. KIenzle, eds.) p. 125. Hanover, Germany.

Henry, H.L., and Norman, A.W. (1978). *Science 201*, 853.

Heuser, G.F., and Norris, L.C. (1929). *Poult. Sci. 8*, 89.

Hibbs, J.W., and Pounden, W.D. (1955). *J. Dairy Sci. 38*, 65.

Hidiroglou, M., Prouix, J.G., and Roubos, D. (1979). *J. Dairy Sci. 62*, 1076.

Hidiroglou, M., Williams, C.J., and Ho, S.K. (1978). *Can. J. Anim. Sci. 58*, 621.

Hirsch, A. (1982). Vitamins—The Life Essentials, p. 1. National Feed Ingredients Association, Des Moines, Iowa.

Hodnett, D.W., Jorgensen, N.A., and DeLuca, H.F. (1992). *J. Dairy Sci. 75*, 485.

Holick, M.F. (1986). *Curr. Top. Nutr. Dis. 5*, 241.

Holick, M.F. (1987). *Fed. Proc. Fed. Am. Soc. Exp. Biol, 46*, 1876.

Holick, M.F. (1994). *Am. J. Clin. Nutr. 60*, 619.

Holick, M.F. (1995). *Am. J. Clin. Nutr. 61*, 638.

Holick, M.F., MacLaughlin, J.A., and Doppelt, S.H. (1981). *Science 211*, 590.

Horst, R.L., and Napoli, J.L. (1981). *Fed. Prod. Fed. Am. Soc. Exp. Biol. 40*, 898(Abstr.).

Horst, R.L., DeLuca, H.F., and Jorgensen, N.A. (1978). *Metab. Bone Dis. Relat. Res. 1*, 29.

Horst, R.L., Goff, J.P., Reinhardt, T.A., and Buxton, D.R. (1997). *J. Dairy Sci. 80*, 1269.

How, K.L., Hazewinkel, H.A.W., and Mol, J.A. (1994a). *Endocrinology 96*, 12.

How, K.L., Hazewinkel, H.A.W., and Mol, J.A. (1994b). *Vet. Rec. 134*, 384.

How, K.L., Hazewinkel, H.A.W., and Mol, J.A. (1995). Proc. Voorjaarsdagen Congress (H.P. Meyer and H.A.W. Hazewinkel, eds.) p. 1, Amsterdam.

Howard, G., Nguyen, T., Morrison, N., Watanabe, T., Sambrook, P, Eisman, J., and Kelly, P.J. (1995). *J. Clin. Endocrinol. Metab. 80*, 2800.

Hughes, M.R., Baylink, D.J., Jones, P.G., and Haussler, M.R. (1976). *J. Clin. Invest. 58*, 61.

Hustmeyer, F.G., Beitz, D.C., Goff, J.P., Nonnecke, B.J., Horst, R.L., and Reinhardt, T.A. (1994). *J. Dairy Sci.* 77, 3324.

James, S.Y., Mackay, A.G., Binderup, L., and Colston, K.W. (1994). *J. Endocrin.* 14, 555.

Johnson, D.W., and Palmer, L.S. (1939). *J. Agr. Res.* 58, 929.

Johnson, K.A., Church, D.B., Barton, R.J., and Wood, A.K.W. (1988). *J. Small Anim. Pract.* 29, 657.

Jung, S.J., Lee, Y.Y., Pakkala, S., DeVos, S., Elstner, E., Norman, A.W., Uskokovic, J.G.M., and Koeffler, H.P. (1994). *Leukemia Res.* 18, 453.

Keiver, K.M., Draper, H.H., and Ronald, K. (1988). *J. Nutr.* 118, 332.

Kliewer, S.A., Umesono, K., Mangelsdorf, D.J., and Evans, R.M. (1992). *Nature, 355,* 446.

Kragballe, K., Gjertsen, B.T., and DeHoop, D. (1991). *Lancet 337,* 193.

Kramer, B., and Gribetz, D. (1971). *In* The Vitamins (W.H. Sebrell Jr. and R.S. Harris, eds.), p. 259. Academic Press, New York.

Lebrun, J.B., Moffatt, M.E.K., Mundy, R.J.T., Sangster, R.K., Postl, B.D., Dooley, J.P., Dilling, L.A., Godel, J.C., and Haworth, J.C. (1993). *Can. J. Public Health 84,* 394.

Lefkowitz, E.S. and Garland, C.F. (1994). *Int. J. Epidemiol. 23,* 1133.

Lemire, J.M. (1992). *Cell Biochem. 49,* 26.

Lester, G.E. (1986). *Fed. Proc. Fed. Am. Soc. Exp. Biol. 45,* 2524.

Littledike, E.T., and Horst, R.L. (1982). *J. Dairy Sci. 65,* 749.

Lomba, F.G., Chauvaux, G., Teller, E., Lengele, L., and Beinfet, V. (1978). *Br. J. Nutr. 39,* 425.

Loosli, J.K. (1991). *In* Handbook of Animal Science (P.A. Putnam, ed.) Academic Press, San Diego.

Lowik, M.R.H., Van Den Berg, H., Schrijver J., Odink, J., Wedel, M., and Van Houten, P. (1992). *J. Am. Coll. Nutr. 11,* 673.

Mac-Auliff, T., and McGinnis, J. (1976). *Poult. Sci. 55,* 2059(Abstr.).

Machlin, L.J., and Sauberlich, H.E. (1994). *Nutr. Today Jan/Feb.,* 25.

Marks, R., Foley, P.A., Jolley, D., Knight, K.R., Harrison, J., and Thompson, S.C. (1995). *Arch. Dermatol. 13,* 415.

Matsuoka, L.Y., Wortsman, J., Hanifan, N., and Holick, M.F. (1988). *Arch. Dermatol. 124,* 1802.

Mattila, P.H., Piironen, V.I., Uusi-Rauva, E.J., and Koivistoinen, P.E. (1995). *J. Agri. Food Chem. 43,* 2394.

Mayer, G.P., Ramberg, C.F., and Kronfeld, D.S. (1968). *J. Nutr. 95,* 202.

Maynard, L.A., Loosli, J.K., Hintz, H.F., and Warner, R.G. (1979). Animal Nutrition, 7th Ed., p. 283. McGraw-Hill, New York.

McDowell, L.R. (1997). Minerals for Grazing Ruminants in Tropical Regions. University of Florida, Gainesville.

McIntosh, G.H., and Tomas, F.M. (1978). *Q. J. Exp. Physiol. 63,* 119.

Mello, J.R., and Habermehl, G. (1995). *Pesquisa Vet. Brasileria 15,* 73.

Miller, E.R., Ullrey, D.E., Zutaut, C.L., Hoeffer, J.A., and Luecke, R.W. (1965). *J. Nutr. 85,* 255.

Morand-Fehr, P. (1981). *In* Goat Production (G. Gall, ed.), p. 193. Academic Press, New York.

Morgan, A.F., Axelrod, H.E., and Groody, M. (1947). *Am. J. Physiol. 149*, 333.

Morris, K.M.L. (1982). *Vet. Hum. Toxicol. 24*, 34.

Narbaitz, R., and Fragiskos, B. (1984). *Calcif. Tissue Res. 36*, 392.

Neibergs, H.L., Bosworth, B.T., and Reinhardt, T.A. (1996). *J. Dairy Sci. 79*, 1313.

Nemere, I. (1995). *J. Nutr. 125*, 1695S.

Nemere, I., Zhou, I.X., and Norman, A.W. (1993). *Receptor 3*, 277.

Norman, A.W. (1995). *J. Nutr. 125*, 1687S.

Norman, A.W., and DeLuca, H.F. (1963). *Biochemistry 2*, 1160.

NRC. Nutrient Requirements of Domestic Animals. National Academy of Sciences-National Research Council, Washington, D.C.

(1978). Nutrient Requirements of Nonhuman Primates.

(1981). Nutrient Requirements of Goats.

(1982a). Nutrient Requirements of Mink and Foxes.

(1985a). Nutrient Requirements of Dogs, 2nd Ed.

(1985b). Nutrient Requirements of Sheep, 5th Ed.

(1986). Nutrient Requirements of Cats, 3rd Ed.

(1989a). Nutrient Requirements of Dairy Cattle, 6th Ed.

(1989b). Nutrient Requirements of Horses, 5th Ed.

(1993). Nutrient Requirements of Fish.

(1994). Nutrient Requirements of Poultry, 9th Ed.

(1995). Nutrient Requirements of Laboratory Animals, 4th Ed.

(1996). Nutrient Requirements of Beef Cattle, 7th Ed.

(1998). Nutrient Requirements of Swine, 10th Ed.

NRC. (1982b). United States-Canadian Tables of Feed Composition, 3rd Ed. National Academy of Sciences-National Research Council, Washington, D.C.

NRC. (1987). Vitamin Tolerance of Animals. National Academy of Sciences-National Research Council, Washington, D.C.

O'Brien, K.O. (1998). *Nutr. Rev. 56*, 148

O'Connell, J.P., and Gatlin, D.M. (1994). *Aquaculture 125*, 107.

Oetzel, G.R., Olson, J.D., Curtis, C.R., and Fettman, M.J. (1988). *J. Dairy Sci. 71*, 3302.

Ohnuma, N., Bannai, K., Yamagauchi, H., Hashimoto, Y., and Norman, A.W. (1980). *Arch. Biochem. Biophys. 204*, 387.

Okada, K.A., Carrillo, B.J., and Tilley, M. (1977). *Econ. Bot. 31*, 225.

Oldham, S.B., Mitnick, S.A., and Coburn, J.W. (1980). *J. Biol. Chem. 255*, 5789.

Pakkala, S., DeVos, S., Elstner, E., Rude, R.K., Uskokovic, M., Binderup, L., and Koeffler, H.P. (1995). *Leukemia Res. 18*, 65.

Payne, J.M., and Manston, R. (1967). *Vet. Rec. 81*, 214.

Pointillart, A., Fontaine, N., and Thomasset, M. (1986). *Brit. J. Nutr. 56*, 661.

Quaterman, J., Dalgarno, A.C., Adam, A., Fell, B.F., and Boyne, R. (1964). *Br. J. Nutr. 18*, 65.

RDA. (1989). Recommended Dietary Allowances, 9th Ed. National Academy of Sciences-National Research Council, Washington, D.C.

Richter, V.G.H., Flachowsky, F., Matthey, M., Ochrimenko, W.I., Wolfram, D., and Schade, T. (1990). *Vet. Med. 45*, 227.

Rowland, R. (1982). Vitamins—The Life Essentials, p. 1. National Feed Ingredients Association, Des Moines, Iowa.
Rupel, I.W., Bohstedt, G., and Hart, E.B. (1933). *Wisc. Agric. Exp. Stn. Res. Bull. 115.*
Sachs, M., Bar, A., Cohen, R., Mazur, Y., Mayer, E., and Horwitz, S. (1977). *Am. J. Vet. Res. 38,* 2039.
Schachter, D., and Kowarski, S. (1982). *Fed. Proc. Fed. Am. Soc. Exp. Biol. 41,* 84.
Schneider, J. (1986). In Proc. of the NFIA Nutrition Institute, p. 1, Ames, Iowa.
Scott, D., and McLean, A.F. (1981). *Proc. Nutr. Soc. 40,* 257.
Scott, K.C., and Latshaw, J.D. (1994). *Anim. Feed Sci. Tech. 47.* 99.
Scott, M.L., Nesheim, M.C., and Young, R.J. (1982). Nutrition of the Chicken, p. 119. Scott, Ithaca, New York.
Sergeev, I.N., Arkhapchev, Y.P., and Spirichev, V.B. (1990). *J. Nutr. 120,* 1185.
Shiau, S., and Hwang, J. (1994). *J. Nutr. 124,* 2445.
Skowronski, R.J., Peehl, D.M., and Feldman, D. (1995). *Endocrinology 136,* 20.
Solanki, T., Hyatt, R.H., Kemm, J.R., Hughes, E.A., and Cowan, R.A. (1995). *Age and Aging 24,* 103.
Sommerfeldt, J.L., Horst, R.L., Littledike, E.T., Beitz, D.C., and Napoli, J.L. (1981). *J. Dairy Sci. 64,* 157.
Sommerfeldt, J.L, Napoli, J.L., Littledike, E.T., Beitz, D.C., and Horst, R.L. (1983). *J. Nutr. 114,* 2595.
Sood, S., Reghunandanan, R., and Reghunandanan, V. (1995). *Indian J. Exp. Biol. 33,* 61.
Steenbock, H., and Black, A. (1924). *J. Biol. Chem. 61,* 405.
Stevens, V.I., and Blair, R. (1985). *Poult. Sci. 64,* 510.
Studzinski, G.P., and Moore, D.C. (1995). *Cancer Res. 55,* 4014.
Suter, P. (1957). *Schweiz. Arch. Tierheilkd. 99,* 421.
Sutton, R.A.L., and Dirks, J.H. (1978). *Fed. Proc. Fed. Am. Soc. Exp. Biol. 37,* 2112.
Takeuchi, A., Okano, T., Tanda, M., and Kobayashi, T. (1991). *Comp Biochem. Physiol. 100A,* 483.
Tian, X.Q., Chen, T.C., Liu, Z., Shao, Q., and Holick, M.F. (1994). *Endocrinology 135,* 655.
Tindall, B. (1985). *Anim. Health Nutr. 40,* 26.
Tomas, F.M. (1974). *Aust. J. Agric. 25,* 495.
Tomas, F.M., and Somers, M. (1974). *Aust. J. Agric. Res. 25,* 475.
Tsang, C.P.W. (1992) *Poult. Sci. 71,* 215.
Tuan, R.S., and Suyama, E. (1996). *J. Nutr. 126,* 1309S.
Tucker, G., Gagnon, R.E., and Hassler, M.R. (1973). *Arch. Biochem. Biophys. 155,* 47.
Vaiano, S.A., Azuolas, J.K., and Parkinson, G.B. (1994). *Poult. Sci. 73,* 1296.
Vink van Wijngaarden, T., Birkenhager, J.C., Kleinekoort, W.M., Van Den Bend, G.J., Pols, H.A., and Van Leeuwen, J.P. (1995). *Endocrinology 136,* 812.
Wallis, G.C. (1944). *S.D. Agric. Exp. Stn. Bull. No. 372.* South Dakota State University, Brookings.
Wasserman, R.H. (1975). *Nutr. Rev. 33,* 1.

Wasserman, R.H. (1981). *Fed. Proc Fed. Am. Soc. Exp. Biol. 40*, 68.
Webb, A.R., Kline, L., and Holick, M.F. (1988). *J. Clin. Endocrinol. Metab. 67*, 373.
Weber, J.C., Pons, V., and Kodicek, E. (1971). *Biochem J.. 125*, 147.
Whitfield, G.K., Hsieh, J., Jurutha, P.W., Selznick, S.H., Haussler, C.A., MacDonald, P.N., and Haussler, M.R. (1995). *J. Nutr. 125*, 1690S.
Wolker, N.A., and Carrillo, B.J. (1967). *Nature (London) 215*, 72.

VITAMIN E

INTRODUCTION

Vitamin E is recognized as an essential nutrient for all species of animals, including humans. However, opinions differ among research workers as well as practical livestock producers regarding conditions under which vitamin E supplementation is required and at what levels it should be fed. For years, vitamin E in human nutrition was described as "a vitamin looking for a disease." Some vitamin E-deficiency conditions that occurred in animals were not seen in humans; however, a number of medical claims for physiological benefits from the vitamin have been made. In more recent years, vitamin E has been shown to be important against free-radical injury; enhancing the immune response; and playing a role in prevention of cancer, heart disease, cataracts, Parkinson's disease, and a number of other disease conditions.

4

HISTORY

Excellent reviews of the history of vitamin E have been provided by Scott (1980) and Ullrey (1982). By the early 1920s, existence of vitamins A, B (thiamin), and C was established, and that of vitamin D was virtually assured.

As a result of the stimulus to experiment with purified diets that followed the discovery of the first vitamins, it was frequently observed that on certain diets, which were satisfactory for growth and health, rats failed to reproduce. Vitamin E was discovered in 1922 by Evans and Bishop (University of California, Berkeley) as an unidentified factor in vegetable oils required for reproduction in female rats. In their experiments, estrus, mating, and all detectable phases of the beginning of pregnancy were normal, but fetuses soon died and were resorbed unless the diet was supplemented with small amounts of wheat germ, dried alfalfa leaves, or fresh lettuce.

At first this substance was known as factor X, but Sure (1924) and Evans (1925) soon proposed the name vitamin E, since this was the next serial alphabetical designation. Vitamin E was isolated as α-tocopherol. The name tocopherol is derived from the Greek *tokos* meaning childbirth or offspring, the Greek *pherein* meaning to bring forth, and *ol* to designate an alcohol. The structure of α-tocopherol was determined by E. Fernholz in 1938, and the substance was first synthesized by P. Karrer, also in 1938. δ-Tocopherol was reported in 1947, and tocotrienols were described in about 1959.

It also became apparent that male rats were affected by a deficiency of this nutrient that resulted in testicular degeneration. Throughout the 1920s, vitamin E was recognized only as a factor required for reproduction in rats. Many clinical studies were undertaken to determine the effects of vitamin E on various reproductive problems in humans, though in most cases it was found to have little or no effect.

In 1931, Pappenheimer and Goettsch conducted a series of what became classic experiments showing that vitamin E is also required for prevention of encephalomalacia in chicks and of nutritional muscular dystrophy in rabbits and guinea pigs. By 1944, it was found that a multiplicity of clinical signs occur in animals suffering from vitamin E deficiency. In a single species, the chick, three distinct vitamin E deficiency diseases were documented: exudative diathesis, encephalomalacia, and muscular dystrophy. Also, embryonic failure in poultry was found to be caused by damage to the circulatory system.

The first controlled study of vitamin E deficiency in swine was that of Adamstone et al. (1949). These workers reported a decline in reproductive efficiency and signs of locomotor incoordination and muscular necrosis. Obel (1953) described a naturally occurring dietary disease in vitamin E-deficient swine that was characterized by hepatic necrosis, fibrinoid degeneration of blood vessel walls, and muscular dystrophy. In 1957, Klaus Schwarz and associates, studying dietary liver necrosis of rats receiving a diet low in vitamin E, showed that dried brewer's yeast, which contains no vitamin E, was as effective as vitamin E in preventing liver necrosis. Shortly after this discovery, selenium (Se) was found to be the active ingredient in brewer's yeast and able to replace vitamin E for prevention of exudative diathesis in poultry, tissue degeneration in swine, and muscular degeneration in young ruminants. Much confusion existed because earlier discoveries had shown that synthetic antioxidants as well as sulfur amino acids were as effective as vitamin E for prevention of some vitamin E deficiency diseases. Considerable effort has been made to clarify the mechanisms of vitamin E, Se, sulfur amino acids, and antioxidants in relation to diseases that are vitamin E responsive. Likewise, considerable research in the last 10 years has confirmed the beneficial aspects of vitamin E supplementation for both livestock and humans.

CHEMICAL STRUCTURE AND PROPERTIES

Vitamin E activity in food derives from a series of compounds of plant origin, the tocopherols and tocotrienols. Eight forms of vitamin E are found in nature: four tocopherols (α, β, γ, and δ) and four tocotrienols (α, β, γ, and δ). All have a 6-chromanol ring structure and a side chain. The structures of α-tocopherol and the commercially available α-tocopheryl acetate are presented in Fig. 4.1, while different active forms of vitamin E are shown in Fig. 4.2. Differences among α, β, γ, and δ are due to the placement of methyl groups on the ring. The difference between tocopherols and tocotrienols is due to unsaturation of the side chain in the latter.

The *dl*-α-tocopheryl acetate (also called all-rac-α-tocopheryl acetate) is accepted as the International Standard (1 mg = 1 international unit). Synthetic-free tocopherol, *dl*-α-tocopherol, has a potency of 1.1 IU/mg. Activity of naturally occurring α-tocopherol, *d*-α-tocopherol

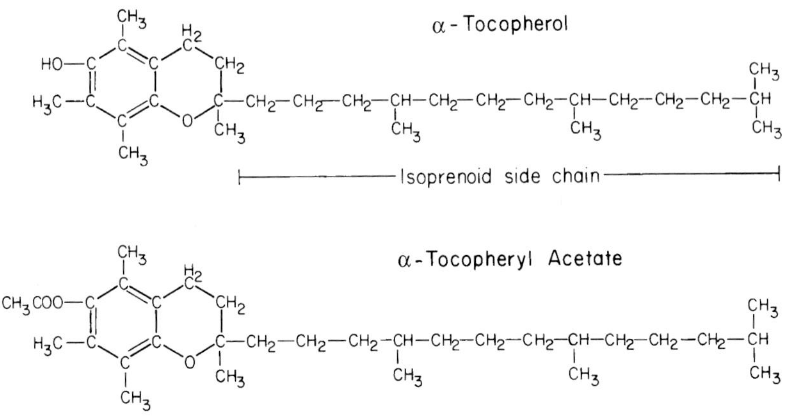

Fig. 4.1 Structure of α-tocopherol and α-tocopheryl acetate.

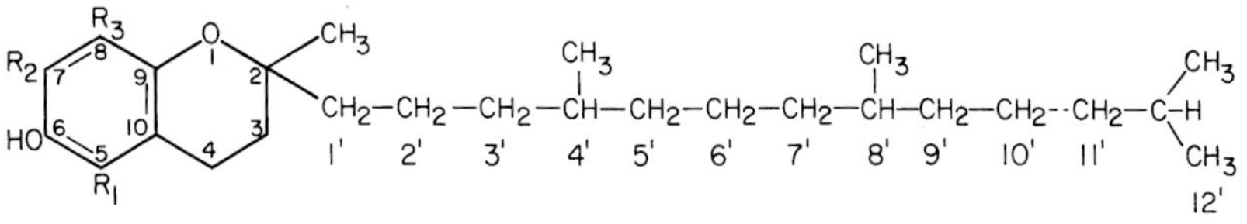

Tocopherol	$R_1(5)$	$R_2(7)$	$R_3(8)$	Side chain double bonds (3', 7', 11', positions)
α	CH_3	CH_3	CH_3	
β	CH_3	H	CH_3	
γ	H	CH_3	CH_3	
δ	H	H	CH_3	
α – tocotrienol	CH_3	CH_3	CH_3	+
β – tocotrienol	CH_3	H	CH_3	+
γ – tocotrienol	H	CH_3	CH_3	+
δ – tocotrienol	H	H	CH_3	+

Fig. 4.2 Structural differences among vitamin E forms.

(also called RRR-tocopherol, see below), is 1.49 IU/mg, and of its acetate, 1.36 IU/mg.

The *dl*-α-tocopheryl acetate is made by the extraction of natural tocopherols from vegetable oil. Extracted tocopherols undergo distillation to obtain the alpha form, and are then acetylated to produce the acetate ester. α-Tocopherol, the most active compound, is fully methylated, with methyl groups at positions 5, 7, and 8 (2 R, 4′R, 8′R-α-tocopherol, abbreviated RRR). The loss of one or both of the methyl groups at position 5 or 7 on the ring sharply reduces vitamin E activity of the structures. The position of the methyl groups influences the vitamin E activity of the molecule.

dl-α-Tocopheryl acetate is the most widely available source of vitamin E for supplementation. The acetate ester is very stable to in vitro oxidation and has no activity as an in vitro antioxidant. However, it is readily hydrolyzed in the intestine to nonesterified or free tocopherol, which is the potent in vivo antioxidant.

A number of vitamin E products are available that are highly effective in preventing or curing conditions associated with inadequate dietary vitamin E. Ochoa et al. (1992) compared six vitamin E sources that differed in relation to carrier used, emulsification, liquid or dry

158

product, and a micellized form. All tissues tested resulted in relatively similar tissue vitamin E concentrations. The naturally derived (d) and synthetic (dl) chemical forms of vitamin E are not used equally and because of this have different biopotencies. Technically, the d form should not be referred to as "natural" as it is derived from natural sources but then undergoes chemical processing (e.g., methylation and hydrogenation). Free d- and dl-α-tocopherol as alcohol forms and their respective ester forms have the highest biopotency. Since the free form is easily oxidized, more stable forms such as acetate and succinate esters have been synthesized with reduced biopotencies.

Serum and certain tissue vitamin E concentrations are influenced by method of supplementation, dosage levels, chemical formulation, and carrier of vitamin E supplements (Charmley et al., 1992; Hidiroglou et al., 1990; Hidiroglou and Charmley, 1991; Njeru et al., 1992, 1994b). Some studies with sheep and cattle have indicated that the d form resulted in higher serum and selected tissue α-tocopherol concentrations than the dl when administered on an equal IU basis (Hidiroglou and McDowell, 1987; Hidiroglou et al., 1988a,b). On the contrary, although higher serum α-tocopherol was found in preruminant calves (Roquet et al., 1992) and sheep (Hidiroglou et al., 1992a), and in selected tissues for sheep (Hidiroglou et al., 1994) for d versus dl forms of vitamin E, the relative IU biopotencies were similar. The ratios of d to dl-α-tocopherol were in close agreement with the established U.S. Pharmacopeia biopotency of 1.36 for d- to dl-α-tocopheryl acetate. It is not just natural versus synthetic that is important for vitamin E biopotency but also the ester and carrier used. In sheep, Hidiroglou and Singh (1991) reported that with equivalent IU dosage, the natural form of d-α-tocopheryl succinate had only one-third the biopotency of the synthetic dl-α-tocopheryl acetate, indicating that the ester succinate has less value than the acetate. Jensen et al. (1999) also found the acetate to be a better form of vitamin E than succinate.

Although less stable, alcohol forms of vitamin E resulted in higher concentrations of α-tocopherol in serum and tissues compared to ester forms (e.g., acetate) (Hidiroglou et al., 1988a, 1989; Ochoa et al., 1992). From a practical viewpoint, this may be important as there is a suggestion that a young ruminant may not utilize ester forms (e.g., acetate) as well as the alcohol forms of vitamin E for the first few weeks of life.

More research is needed to evaluate the different forms of vitamin E and the carriers of these products. Until more research is conducted, opinion will remain divided on biopotencies of various vitamin E forms, particularly *d* versus *dl*. Studies are needed to compare forms with dietary levels closer to ruminant vitamin E requirements since, for a number of nutrients, homeostasis mechanisms discriminate less between chemical forms when administered at the physiologically required concentration.

α-Tocopherol is a yellow oil that is insoluble in water but soluble in organic solvents. Tocopherols are extremely resistant to heat but are readily oxidized. Natural vitamin E is subject to destruction by oxidation, which is accelerated by heat, moisture, rancid fat, light, alkali, and certain trace minerals (e.g., copper and iron). α-Tocopherol is an excellent natural antioxidant that protects carotene and other oxidizable materials in feed and in the body. However, in the process of acting as an antioxidant, it is destroyed. Since esterification of the vitamin improves its stability, commercial supplements usually contain *d*-α-tocopheryl acetate or *dl*-α-tocopheryl acetate.

ANALYTICAL PROCEDURES

Many methods for the determination of tocopherols in feedstuffs and animal tissues have been introduced, most of them based on separation of the tocopherols by column, paper, or thin-layer chromatography, followed by a colorimetric reaction. Separation steps, however, are usually laborious and time consuming, and colorimetric reactions such as that of Emmerie and Engel are often subject to interference from other compounds (McMurray and Blanchflower, 1979). High-pressure liquid chromatography (HPLC) offers the possibility of combining rapid analysis with separation of tocopherols from interfering substances. The method consists of three main steps via extraction, saponification, and chromatography (McMurray and Blanchflower, 1979; Cohen and Lapointe, 1980). Either reverse-phase or normal-phase procedures are used, coupled with either fluorometric or ultraviolet detectors. The procedures are specific, rapid, simple, and very sensitive. With fluorometric detection, nanogram quantities can be detected; HPLC procedures permit separation and quantitation of the α, β, and γ isomers of tocopherol.

Biological assay methods for vitamin E determine the ability of an unknown to prevent or reverse specific vitamin E deficiency signs of animals in vivo (e.g., fetal resorption, encephalomalacia, muscular degeneration, erythrocyte hemolysis) or indications of vitamin E status (e.g., liver and serum concentrations). The biological assay developed by Herbert Evans was the rat fetal resorption test. International units have been established on the basis of the resorption test. This is the ultimate measure of vitamin E activity and is based on development of live fetuses in rats. Litter efficiency is calculated as the number of females with living young divided by total number of pregnancies.

Biological variations are inherent in bioassays, considerably more so than in chemical assays as a rule. They involve variations in response between individuals, families, strains, and species of animals, as well as management skill, stability of the test material, diet standardization and purity, and control of other environmental factors. Dietary history (particularly previous vitamin E intakes) of parent stock can have an influence. Table 4.1 illustrates a comparison among vitamin E forms related to biological assays.

METABOLISM

Absorption and Transport

Vitamin E absorption is related to fat digestion and is facilitated by bile and pancreatic lipase (Sitrin et al., 1987). The primary site of absorption appears to be the medial small intestine. Whether presented as free alcohol or as esters, most vitamin E is absorbed as the alcohol. Esters are largely hydrolyzed in the gut wall, and the free alcohol enters the intestinal lacteals and is transported via lymph to the general circulation. Medium-chain triglycerides particularly enhance absorption, whereas polyunsaturated fatty acids (PUFAs) are inhibitory. Balance

■ Table 4.1   Relative Biopotency of Vitamin E Forms

	Rat Antisterility	Rat Weight Gain	Rabbit Cure of Muscular Dystrophy	Hemolysis of Erythrocytes in vivo	Hemolysis of Erythrocytes in vitro
Tocopherols					
d-α	135	—	100	130	100
dl-α	100	100	90	100	100
d-β	54	—	30	30	40
dl-β	27	25	—	25	54
d-γ	1	—	20	4–22	30
dl-γ	1–11	19	6	18	67
d-δ	1	—	—	3	20
Tocotrienols					
d-β	5	—	—	1–5	133
d-α	29	—	—	23	106
d-γ	3	—	—	—	88

studies indicate that much less vitamin E is absorbed, or at least retained, in the body than vitamin A. Vitamin E recovered in feces from a test dose was found to range from 65 to 80% in the human, rabbit, and hen, although in chicks, it was reported at about 25%. It is not known how much fecal vitamin E represents unabsorbed tocopherol and how much may come via secretion in the bile. As the intake increases, the percentage of tocopherol absorbed decreases, suggesting a saturation process.

The tocopherol form, which is the naturally occurring one, is subject to destruction in the digestive tract to some extent, whereas the acetate ester is not. Much of the acetate is readily split off in the intestinal wall, and the alcohol is reformed and absorbed, thereby permitting the vitamin to function as a biological antioxidant. Any acetate form absorbed or injected into the body evidently is converted there to the alcohol form.

Vitamin E in plasma is attached mainly to lipoproteins in the globulin fraction within cells and occurs mainly in mitochondria and microsomes. The vitamin is taken up by the liver and is released in combination with low-density lipoprotein (LDL) cholesterol. Rates and amounts of absorption of the various tocopherols and tocotrienols are in the same general order of magnitude as their biological potencies. α-Tocopherol is absorbed best, with γ-tocopherol absorption 85% that of α-forms but with a more rapid excretion. One can generally assume that most of the vitamin E activity within plasma and other animal tissues is α-tocopherol (Ullrey, 1981). In humans, whose natural diet contains a high percentage of non-alpha forms, blood serum tocopherols identified consisted of about 87% α-, 11% γ-, and 2% β-tocopherol (Hoffmann-La Roche, 1972).

Placental and Mammary Transfer

Vitamin E does not cross the placenta in any appreciable amounts; however, it is concentrated in colostrum (Van Saun et al., 1989). With respect to neonatal ruminants (Hidiroglou et al., 1969; Van Saun et al., 1989) and baby pigs (Mahan, 1991), several investigators have reported limited placental transport of α-tocopherol, making neonates highly susceptible to vitamin E deficiency. This may be related to a decrease in efficiency of placental vitamin E transfer as gestation proceeds, a dilution effect as a result of rapid fetal growth, or a decrease in available maternal vitamin E. With limited placental transfer of vitamin E, newborns must rely heavily on ingestion of colostrum as a source of vitamin E. Van Saun et al. (1989) reported decreased fetal serum vitamin E concentrations with increasing fetal age. Additionally, these authors reported less decline in fetal serum vitamin E concentration during gestation in fetuses from vitamin E adequate dams.

There is inefficient placental transfer of vitamin E, but high levels of the vitamin have been shown in calves (Nockels, 1991) and lambs (Njeru et al., 1994a) after consumption of colostrum. Nockels (1991) reported α-tocopherol levels in plasma from beef calves prior to colostrum consumption and for several days thereafter. Precolostral plasma vitamin E levels averaged 0.2 μg/ml and increased to 3.3 μg/ml at 5 to 8 days of age. Njeru et al. (1994a) fed ewes dl-α-tocopheryl acetate at graded levels (0, 15, 30, and 60 IU per head daily) to study placental and mammary gland transfer. Supplemental vitamin E had no effect on serum α-tocopherol of lambs prior to nursing, averaging 0.35 μg/ml. By day 3, lamb serum tocopherol increased to 1.41, 1.84, 2.43, and 4.46 μg/ ml, respectively, for the four supplemental dietary levels of vitamin E (Table 4.2). Vitamin E at the given levels of supplementation increased colostral α-tocopherol at a linear rate of 3.3, 6.8, 8.0, and 9.6 μg/ml, respectively. The importance of providing colostrum rich in vitamin E is quite apparent, as both calves and lambs are born with low levels of the vitamin (Nockels, 1991; Njeru et al., 1994a). Low blood vitamin E may lead to diminished disease resistance and immune response in the neonate (Nockels, 1991).

Storage and Excretion

Vitamin E is stored throughout all body tissues; major deposits are in adipose tissue, liver, and muscle, with highest storage in the liver. However, liver contains only a small fraction of total body stores, in

■ Table 4.2 Effect of Supplemental Vitamin E to Prepartum Ewes on α-Tocopherol Concentration in Serum and Colostrum (μg/ml)

	Ewes		Lambs	
Supplemental Vitamin E (IU per day)	Serum at Parturition	Colostrum Day 1	Serum Prior to Nursing	Serum Day 3
0	0.94	3.3	0.40	1.41
15	1.94	6.8	0.40	1.84
30	2.53	8.0	0.38	2.43
60	4.07	9.6	0.23	4.46

Source: Njeru et al. (1994b).
Note: Treatments administered as dl-α-tocopheryl acetate 28 days prepartum through 28 days postpartum.
   Linear ($P < 0.05$) treatment effects for α-tocopherol in ewe serum and colostrum and lamb serum at day 3.

163

contrast to vitamin A, for which about 95% of the body reserves are in the liver. The extent of storage is shown by the fact that females born of mothers whose diets contained a liberal supply frequently have enough in their bodies at birth to carry them through a first pregnancy. Rats reared on natural foods rich in the vitamin and then placed on a deficient diet may produce three or four litters before exhausting their reserves (Maynard et al., 1979). However, Gallo-Torres (1980) reports that unlike vitamin A, lower body stores of vitamin E are available for periods of low dietary intake.

Tocopherol entering the circulatory system becomes distributed throughout the body, with most of it localizing in the fatty tissues. Subcellular fractions from different tissues vary considerably in their tocopherol content; the highest levels are found in membranous organelles, such as microsomes and mitochondria, which contain highly active redox systems (McCay et al., 1981; Taylor et al., 1976).

Small amounts of vitamin E will persist tenaciously in the body for a long time. However, stores are exhausted rapidly by PUFAs in the tissues; the rate of disappearance is proportional to the intake of PUFAs. A major excretion route of absorbed vitamin E is bile, in which tocopherol appears mostly in the free form. Usually less than 1% of orally ingested vitamin E is excreted in the urine.

FUNCTIONS

Vitamin E has been shown to be essential for integrity and optimum function of the reproductive, muscular, circulatory, nervous, and immune systems (Hoekstra, 1975; Sheffy and Schultz, 1979; Bendich, 1987; McDowell et al., 1996). It is well established that some functions of vitamin E, however, can be fulfilled in part or entirely by traces of Se or by certain synthetic antioxidants. Even the sulfur-bearing amino acids, cystine and methionine, affect certain vitamin E functions. Much evidence points to undiscovered metabolic roles for vitamin E that may be paralleled biologically by roles of Se and possible other substances. The most widely accepted functions of vitamin E are discussed in this section.

Vitamin E as a Biological Antioxidant

Vitamin E has a number of different but related functions. One of the most important functions is its role as an intercellular and intracellular antioxidant. Vitamin E is part of the body's intracellular defense against the adverse effects of reactive oxygen and free radicals that initiate oxidation of unsaturated phospholipids (Chow, 1979) and critical sulfhydryl groups (Brownlee et al., 1977). Vitamin E functions as a quenching agent for free radical molecules with single, highly reactive electrons in their outer shells. Free radicals attract a hydrogen atom, along with its electron, away from the chain structure of a PUFA, satisfying the electron needs of the original free radical but leaving the PUFA short one electron. Thus, a fatty acid free radical is formed that joins with molecular oxygen to form a peroxyl radical that steals a hydrogen-electron unit from yet another PUFA. This reaction can continue in a chain, resulting in the destruction of thousands of PUFA molecules (Gardner, 1989; Herdt and Stowe, 1991). Free radicals can be extremely damaging to biological systems (Padh, 1991). Free radicals, including hydroxy, hypochlorite, peroxy, alkoxy, superoxide, hydrogen peroxide, and singlet oxygen, are generated by autoxidation or radiation, or from activities of some oxidases, dehydrogenases, and peroxidases.

Highly reactive oxygen species, such as superoxide anion radical (O_2), hydroxyl radical (HO), hydrogen peroxide (H_2O_2), and singlet oxygen (O_2), are continuously produced in the course of normal aerobic cellular metabolism. Also, phagocytic granulocytes undergo respiratory burst to produce oxygen radicals to destroy the intracellular pathogens. However, these oxidative products can, in turn, damage healthy cells if they are not eliminated. Antioxidants serve to stabilize these highly reactive free radicals, thereby maintaining the structural and functional integrity of cells (Chew, 1995). Therefore, antioxidants are very important to the immune defense and health of humans and animals.

The antioxidant function of vitamin E is closely related to and synergistic with the role of Se. Selenium has been shown to act in aqueous cell media (cytosol and mitochondrial matrix) by destroying hydrogen peroxide and hydroperoxides via the enzyme glutathione peroxidase (GSH_{px}) of which it is a co-factor. In this capacity, it prevents oxidation of unsaturated lipid materials within cells, thus protecting fats within the cell membrane from breaking down. It is the oxidation of vitamin E that prevents oxidation of other lipid materials to free radicals and peroxides within cells, thus protecting the cell membrane from damage (Drouchner, 1976). If lipid hydroperoxides are allowed to form in the absence of adequate tocopherols, direct cellular tissue damage can result, in which peroxidation of lipids destroys structural integrity of the cell and causes metabolic derangements.

Vitamin E reacts or functions as a chain-breaking antioxidant, thereby neutralizing free radicals and preventing oxidation of lipids within membranes. Free radicals may not only damage their cell of origin but migrate and damage adjacent cells in which more free radicals are produced in a chain reaction leading to tissue destruction (Nockels, 1991). At least one important function of vitamin E is to interrupt production of free radicals at the initial stage. Myodystrophic tissue is common in cases of vitamin E-Se deficiency with leakage of cellular compounds such as creatinine and various transaminases through affected membranes into plasma. The more active the cell (e.g., the cells of skeletal and involuntary muscles), the greater the inflow of lipids for energy supply and the greater the risk of tissue damage if vitamin E is limiting. This antioxidant property also ensures erythrocyte stability and maintenance of capillary blood vessel integrity.

Interruption of fat peroxidation by tocopherol explains the well-established observation that dietary tocopherols protect or spare body supplies of such oxidizable materials as vitamin A, vitamin C, and the carotenes. Certain deficiency signs of vitamin E (e.g., muscular dystrophy) can be prevented by diet supplementation with other antioxidants, thus lending support to the antioxidant role of tocopherols. Semen quality of boars was improved with Se and vitamin E supplementation, with vitamin E playing a role in maintaining sperm integrity in combination with Se (Marin-Guzman et al., 1989). Chemical antioxidants are stored only at very low levels, thus they are not as effective as tocopherol. It is clear that highly unsaturated fatty acids in the diet increase vitamin E requirements. When acting as an antioxidant, vitamin E supplies become depleted, thus furnishing an explanation for the often observed fact that the presence of dietary unsaturated fats (susceptible to peroxidation) augments or precipitates vitamin E deficiency.

Membrane Structure and Prostaglandin Synthesis

α-Tocopherol may be involved in the formation of structural components of biological membranes, thus exerting a unique influence on architecture of membrane phospholipids (Ullrey, 1981). It is reported that α-tocopherol stimulated the incorporation of ^{14}C from linoleic acid into arachidonic acid in fibroblast phospholipids. Also, it was found that α-tocopherol exerted a pronounced stimulatory influence on formation of prostaglandin E from arachidonic acid, while a chemical antioxidant had no effect.

Blood Clotting

Vitamin E is an inhibitor of platelet aggregation in pigs (McIntosh et al., 1985), and may play a role by inhibiting peroxidation of arachidonic acid, which is required for formation of prostaglandins involved in platelet aggregation (Panganamala and Cornwell, 1982; Machlin, 1991).

Disease Resistance

In addition to the relationship of vitamin E and Se, vitamin E, vitamin C, and β-carotene as antioxidant vitamins together have important tissue defense mechanisms against free-radical damage. The dietary and tissue balance of all these nutrients are important in protecting tissues against free-radical damage. Both in vitro and in vivo studies showed that the antioxidant vitamins generally enhance different aspects of cellular and noncellular (humoral) immunity. The antioxidant function of these vitamins could, at least in part, enhance immunity by maintaining the functional and structural integrity of important immune cells. A compromised immune system will affect animal health and result in reduced animal production efficiency through increased susceptibility to diseases, thereby leading to increased animal morbidity and mortality.

One function of vitamin C is that this vitamin can regenerate the reduced form of α-tocopherol, perhaps accounting for observed sparing effects of these vitamins (Jacob, 1995; Tanaka et al., 1997). In the process of sparing fatty acid oxidation, tocopherol is oxidized to the tocopheryl free radical. Ascorbic acid can donate an electron to the tocopheryl free radical, regenerating the reduced antioxidant form of tocopherol.

Considerable attention is being directed to the role vitamin E and Se play in protecting leukocytes and macrophages during phagocytosis, the mechanism whereby animals immunologically kill invading bacteria. Both vitamin E and Se may help these cells to survive the toxic products that are produced in order to effectively kill ingested bacteria (Badwey and Karnovsky, 1980). Macrophages and neutrophils from vitamin E-deficient animals have decreased phagocytic activity (Burkholder and Swecker, 1990).

Since vitamin E acts as a tissue antioxidant and aids in quenching free-radicals produced in the body, any infection or other stress factors may exacerbate depletion of the limited vitamin E stores from various tissues. With respect to immunocompetency, dietary requirements may be adequate for normal growth and production; however, higher levels have been shown to positively influence both cellular and humoral immune status of ruminant species. The former two responses are generally used as criteria for determining the requirement of a nutrient. During stress and disease, there is an increase in production of glucocorticoids, epinephrine, eicosanoids, and phagocytic activity. Eicosanoid and corticoid synthesis and phagocytic respiratory bursts are prominent producers of free radicals that challenge the animal's antioxidant systems. Vitamin E has been implicated in stimulation of serum antibody synthesis, particularly IgG antibodies (Tengerdy, 1980). The protective effects of vitamin E on animal health may be involved with its role in reduction of glucocorticoids, which are known to be immunosuppressive (Golub and Gershwin, 1985). In rats, an in vivo inflammatory challenge decreased vitamin E blood and liver concentrations (Fritsche and McGuire, 1996). Vitamin E also most likely has an immuno-enhancing effect by virtue of altering arachidonic acid metabolism and subsequent synthesis of prostaglandin, thromboxanes, and leukotrienes. Under stress conditions, increased levels of these compounds by endogenous synthesis or exogenous entry may adversely affect immune cell function (Hadden, 1987).

The effects of vitamin E and Se supplementation on protection against infection by several types of pathogenic organisms, as well as antibody titers and phagocytosis of the pathogens, have been reported for calves (Cipriano et al., 1982; Reddy et al., 1987a; Rajaraman et al., 1998) and lambs (Reffett et al., 1988; Finch and Turner, 1989; Turner and Finch, 1990). As an example, calves receiving 125 IU of vitamin E daily were able to maximize their immune responses compared with calves receiving low dietary vitamin E (Reddy et al., 1987b). In sows, vitamin E restriction depressed lymphocytes and polymorphonuclear cells for immune function (Wuryastuti et al., 1993). Dogs with vitamin E deficiency had a depressed proliferative lymphocyte responsiveness (Langweiler et al., 1983).

Antioxidants, including vitamin E, play a role in resistance to viral infection. Vitamin E deficiency allows a normally benign virus to cause disease (Beck et al., 1994). In mice, enhanced virulence of a virus resulted in myocardial injury that was prevented with vitamin E adequacy. Selenium or vitamin E deficiency leads to a change in viral phenotype, such that an avirulent strain of a virus becomes virulent and a virulent strain becomes more virulent (Beck, 1997).

Electron Transport and Deoxyribonucleic Acid (DNA)

There is limited evidence that vitamin E is involved in biological oxidation-reduction reactions (Hoffmann-La Roche, 1972). Vitamin E also appears to regulate the biosynthesis of DNA within cells.

Relationship to Toxic Elements or Substances

Both vitamin E and Se provide protection against toxicity with three classes of heavy metals (Whanger, 1981). In one class, which includes metals like cadmium and mercury, Se is highly effective in altering toxicities, but vitamin E has little influence. In the second class, which includes silver and arsenic, vitamin E is highly effective; Se is also effective but only at relatively high levels. The third class, which includes lead, is counteracted by vitamin E, but Se has little effect.

Vitamin E can be effective against other toxic substances. For example, treatment with vitamin E gave protection to weanling pigs against monensin-induced skeletal muscle damage (Van Vleet et al., 1987).

Relationship with Selenium in Tissue Protection

There is a close working relationship between vitamin E and Se within tissues. Selenium has a sparing effect on vitamin E and delays onset of deficiency signs. Likewise, vitamin E and sulfur amino acids partially protect against or delay onset of several forms of Se deficiency syndromes. Tissue breakdown occurs in most species receiving diets deficient in both vitamin E and Se, mainly through peroxidation. Peroxides and hydroperoxides are highly destructive to tissue integrity and lead to disease development. It appears that vitamin E in cellular and subcellular membranes is the first line of defense against peroxidation of vital phospholipids, but even with adequate vitamin E, some peroxides are formed. Selenium, as part of the enzyme glutathione peroxidase, is a second line of defense that destroys these peroxides before they have an opportunity to cause damage to membranes. Therefore, Se, vitamin E, and sulfur-containing amino acids, through different biochemical mechanisms, are capable of preventing some of the same nutritional diseases. Vitamin E prevents fatty acid hydroperoxide formation, sulfur amino acids are precursors of glutathione peroxidase, and Se is a component of glutathione peroxidase (Smith et al., 1974).

To some extent, vitamin E and Se are mutually replaceable, but there are lower limits below which substitution is ineffective. In diets severely deficient in Se, vitamin E does not prevent or cure exudative diathesis, whereas addition of as little as 0.05 ppm Se completely prevents this disease (Scott, 1980).

Other Functions

Scott et al. (1982) reported additional functions of vitamin E, including (1) normal phosphorylation reactions, especially of high-energy phosphate compounds, such as creatine phosphate and adenosine triphosphate; (2) a role in synthesis of vitamin C; (3) a role in synthesis of ubiquinone; and (4) a role in sulfur amino acid metabolism. Pappu et al. (1978) reported on the role of vitamin E in vitamin B_{12} metabolism. A deficiency of vitamin E interferes with conversion of vitamin B_{12} to its coenzyme 5'-deoxyadenosylcobalamin and concomitantly metabolism of methylmalonyl-CoA to succinyl-CoA. Turley and Brewster (1993) suggested that in humans, cellular deficiency of adenosylcobalamin may be one mechanism by which vitamin E deficiency leads to neurologic injury. In rats, vitamin E deficiency has been reported to inhibit vitamin D metabolism in the liver and kidneys with the formation of active metabolites and decreases in the concentration of the hormone-receptor complexes in the target tissue. Liver vitamin D hydroxylase activity decreased by 39%, 25-OHD_3 1-hydroxylase activity in the kidneys by 22%, and 24-hydroxylase activity by 52% (Sergeev et al., 1990).

REQUIREMENTS

Estimated vitamin E requirements for selected animals and humans are presented in Table 4.3. Scott (1980), after reviewing the literature, concluded that the minimum vitamin E requirement of normal animals and humans is approximately 30 ppm of diet. Vitamin E requirements are exceedingly difficult to determine because of the interrelationships with other dietary factors (see Functions and Deficiency sections). The requirement may be increased with increasing levels of PUFA, oxidizing agents, vitamin A, carotenoids, gossypol, or trace minerals and decreased with increasing levels of fat-soluble antioxidants, sulfur amino acids, or Se (Dove and Ewan, 1990; Nockels, 1990; Hidiroglou et al., 1992b; McDowell et al., 1996; Franklin et al., 1998). On otherwise adequate diets containing sufficient cystine and methionine and containing a minimum of PUFA, vitamin E requirements appear to be low. This is evidenced by difficulties in producing deficiency signs on such diets under optimum environmental conditions.

The levels of PUFA found in unsaturated oils such as cod liver oil, corn oil, soybean oil, sunflower seed oil, and linseed oil increase vitamin E requirements. This is especially true if these oils are allowed to undergo oxidative rancidity in the diet or are in the process of peroxidation

■ Table 4.3   Vitamin E Requirements for Various Animals and Humans

Animal	Purpose or Class	Requirement[a]	Reference
Beef cattle	Growing	15–60 IU/kg	NRC (1996)
Dairy cattle	Milk replacer	40 IU/kg	NRC (1989a)
	Growing	25 IU/kg	NRC (1989a)
	Lactating cows and bulls	15 IU/kg	NRC (1989a)
Goat	All classes	100 IU/kg	Morand-Fehr (1981)
Chicken	Leghorn, 0–6 weeks	10 IU/kg	NRC (1994)
	Leghorn, 6–18 weeks	5 IU/kg	NRC (1994)
	Laying (100 g intake)	5 IU/kg	NRC (1994)
	Broilers, 0–8 weeks	10 IU/kg	NRC (1994)
Duck	Growing, 0–7 weeks	10 IU/kg	NRC (1994)
Turkey	All classes	10–12 IU/kg	NRC (1994)
Sheep	All classes	15–20 IU/kg	NRC (1985b)
Horse	Growing, pregnant, lactating, and working	80 IU/kg	NRC (1989b)
	Maintenance	50 IU/kg	NRC (1989b)
Swine	All classes	11–44 IU/kg	NRC (1998)
Mink	Growing	25 IU/kg	NRC (1982a)
Cat	All classes	30 IU/kg	NRC (1986)
Dog	Growing	22 IU/kg	NRC (1985a)
Rabbit	All classes	40 IU/kg	NRC (1977)
Fish	Catfish	25–50 IU/kg	NRC (1993)
	Pacific salmon	30–50 IU/kg	NRC (1993)
	Rainbow trout	15–100 IU/kg	NRC (1993)
Rat	All classes	18 IU/kg	NRC (1995)
Mouse	All classes	22 IU/kg	NRC (1995)
Human	Infants	3–4 mg/day	RDA (1989)
	Children	6–7 mg/day	RDA (1989)
	Adults	8–12 mg/day	RDA (1989)

[a]Expressed as per unit of animal feed on either as-fed (approximately 90% dry matter) or dry basis (see Appendix, Tables A1a,b). Human data are expressed as mg α-tocopherol equivalents/day.

when consumed by the animal. If they become completely rancid before ingestion, the only damage is the destruction of the vitamin E present in the oil and in the feed containing the rancidifying oil. But if they are undergoing active oxidative rancidity at the time of consumption, they apparently cause destruction of body stores of vitamin E as well (Scott et al., 1982). The vitamin E requirement for dogs is five times higher under conditions of high PUFA intake (NRC, 1985a). The amount of vitamin E required per gram of PUFA is dependent on experimental conditions, species differences, levels and kinds of PUFA, and test used (Lopez-Bote et al., 1997; McGuire et al., 1997). Nevertheless, for a number of species, 0.6 IU of vitamin E per gram of PUFA is inadequate, and 1 IU is a realistic minimum (Hoffmann-La Roche, 1972). A combination of stress of infection and presence of oxidized fats in swine diets was reported to exaggerate vitamin E needs still further (Tiege et al., 1978). These researchers reported that supplements of 100 IU of vitamin E per kilogram of diet and 0.1 ppm Se did not entirely prevent deficiency lesions in weanling pigs afflicted with dysentery and fed 3% cod liver oil.

Of all factors, the most important determinant of vitamin E requirements is the dietary concentrations of unsaturated fatty acids. A diet that contains high levels of fish oil may cause a threefold to fourfold increase in a cat's daily requirement for α-tocopherol. Early cases of steatitis (yellow fat disease) occurred almost exclusively in cats that were fed a canned, commercial fish-based cat food, of which red tuna was the principal type of fish.

Since the PUFA content of membranes can be altered by dietary fats, it is not surprising that the dietary requirement for vitamin E is closely related to the dietary concentration of PUFAs. When a large amount of polyunsaturated fat is fed after it has been stripped of tocopherols, as much as 100 mg of α-tocopherol per kilogram of diet may be insufficient to protect against lipofuscin formation (Hayes et al., 1969).

Harris and Embree (1963) proposed a dietary α-tocopherol:PUFA ratio (mg/g) of 0.6:1 as a minimum to protect against PUFA peroxidation. This is a step in being more accurate for determining vitamin E requirements for animals; however, it should be realized that some PUFAs require much more vitamin E to counteract detrimental effects than others. Fish-oil PUFAs, which contain arachidonic acid (20:4), docosapentaenoic acid (22:5), and docosahexaenoic acid (22:6), require much more vitamin E for stabilization than typical plant PUFAs, such as linoleic acid (18:2) and linolenic acid (18:3). The longer the carbon chain of a fatty acid and the more double bonds, the greater the vitamin E requirement. As an example, when 5% tuna oil (long carbon chain and greater unsaturation) was substituted for 5% of the lard (shorter carbon chain and less unsaturation), steatitis was severe in cats unsupplemented with vitamin E. The severity of steatitis was diminished by supplemental vitamin E, but was not entirely prevented by 34 IU/kg of diet. When 136 IU/kg of diet were provided, no lesions were seen (Gershoff and Norkin, 1962). By-product organs (e.g., liver) in the diet would also have more of the longer-chained, more unsaturated fatty acids.

The amount of vitamin E needed to maintain adequate growth and reproduction would not necessarily be enough to ensure optimal immune function as noted previously (Weiss, 1998). For example, in the

172

rat, Bendich et al. (1986) reported that 15 IU/kg vitamin E of diet prevented muscle abnormalities and 50 IU/kg of diet was necessary to prevent red blood cell breakdown, but for maximum lymphocyte stimulation, 200 IU of vitamin E per kilogram of diet was required. In pigs, 150 IU/kg of supplemental vitamin E resulted in a higher activity of lysozyme and a higher rate of yeast lysis (Riedel-Caspari et al., 1986). Reduced mortality and increased humoral immune titers were reported when chicks infected with *Escherichia coli* were supplemented with 150 or 300 mg of *dl*-α-tocopherol/kg (Heinzerling et al., 1974).

Stress, exercise, infection, and tissue trauma all increase vitamin E requirements (Nockels, 1991). Handling and bleeding heifers periodically in a 10-day period resulted in a large decrease in the vitamin E content of red blood cells and a 62% decrease in neutrophil vitamin E levels (Nockels, 1991). Vitamin E supplementation to stressed calves increased immune response (Golub and Gershwin, 1985). Nockels et al. (1996) noted that for most sampled tissues, stress did not affect α-tocopherol concentration, although other indicators confirmed a deficiency.

Requirements of both vitamin E and Se are greatly dependent on the dietary concentrations of each other (see Functions and Deficiency sections). As noted earlier, they are mutually replaceable above certain limits. Chicks consuming a diet containing 100 IU/kg vitamin E required 0.01 ppm Se, while those receiving no added vitamin E required 0.05 ppm Se (Thompson and Scott, 1969).

Vitamin E is known to reduce the Se requirement in at least two ways: (1) by maintaining body Se in an active form, or preventing body loss; and (2) by preventing destruction of membrane lipids within the membrane, thereby inhibiting the production of hydroperoxides and reducing the amount of glutathione peroxidase needed to destroy peroxides formed in the cell. Selenium is known to spare vitamin E in at least three ways: (1) it is required to preserve the integrity of the pancreas, which allows normal fat digestion and thus normal vitamin E absorption; (2) it reduces the amount of vitamin E required to maintain the integrity of lipid membranes via glutathione peroxidase; and (3) it aids in some unknown way in retention of vitamin E in the blood plasma.

Determination of vitamin E requirements is further complicated because the body has a fairly large ability to store both vitamin E and Se. Sows maintained on a diet deficient in vitamin E and Se produced normal piglets during the first reproductive cycle of the deficiency, and clinical deficiency signs occurred only after five such cycles (Glienke and Ewan, 1974). A number of studies to establish requirements for both nutrients have underestimated the requirements by failing to account for their augmentation from both body stores as well as experimental dietary concentrations.

It has been concluded that in humans, a daily intake of 3 to 15 mg of tocopherol is required from natural diets (RDA, 1989). However, the allowances will not be adequate in individuals who, for a variety of reasons, do not absorb fat efficiently or who have medical conditions that result in an abnormal vitamin E status in the blood and tissues. As in other species, the human requirement for vitamin E is related to dietary intake of PUFA. However, in normal diets in the United States, this relationship is probably of little significance, inasmuch as primary dietary sources of PUFA—vegetable oils, margarine, and shortening—are also rich sources of vitamin E. This situation is not true when foods consumed contain the longer-chained fatty acids (e.g., fish oils).

NATURAL SOURCES

Many vitamin E analyses of foods and feedstuffs have been reported using a variety of analytical techniques; however, there is a lack of characterization of individual tocopherols in the majority of analyses. Total tocopherol analysis of a food or feedstuff is of limited value in providing a reliable estimate of the biological vitamin E value. The occurrence of tocopherols (and tocotrienols) other than alpha (Table 4.4), as well as the prevalence of non–tocopherol-reducing substances in natural products, has led to analytical examination of these materials by techniques capable of precise quantitation of individual species.

Because α-tocopherol is the most active form of vitamin E, many

■ Table 4.4   Tocopherols in Selected Feedstuffs (ppm)

Feedstuff	α	β	γ	δ
Barley	4	3	0.5	0.1
Corn	6	—[a]	38	Trace
Oats	7	2	3	—
Rye	8	4	6	—
Wheat	10	9	—	0.8
Corn oil	112	50	602	18
Cottonseed oil	389	—	387	—
Palm oil	256	—	316	70
Safflower oil	387	—	174	240
Soybean oil	101	—	593	264
Wheat germ oil	1,330	710	260	271

Source: Modified from Ullrey (1981).
[a]No value reported.

nutritionists prefer listing this form in feeds versus the unreliable total tocopherol values. Some of the less active tocopherols, particularly γ-tocopherol, are present in mixed diets in amounts two to four times greater than that of α-tocopherol. Cort et al. (1983), utilizing HPLC assay procedures, which allow separation of alpha and non-alpha forms of both tocopherol and tocotrienols, determined that corn, corn gluten meal, oats, barley, and wheat contained significant amounts of γ-tocotrienol, which has minimal biological activity. For purposes of calculating total vitamin E activity of mixed diets, milligrams of β-tocopherol should be multiplied by 0.5, those of γ-tocopherol by 0.1, and those of δ-tocopherol by 0.3 (RDA, 1989). These three forms, in addition to α-tocopherol, provide the only significant vitamin E activity in typical diets. If only α-tocopherol in a mixed diet is reported, the value in milligrams should be increased by 20% (multiply by 1.2) to account for other tocopherols that are present, thus giving an approximation of total vitamin E activity as milligrams of α-tocopherol equivalents. The α-tocopherol concentrations of various foods and feedstuffs are listed in Table 4.5.

Vitamin E is widespread in nature, with the richest sources being vegetable oils, cereal products containing oils, eggs, and liver. In nature, the synthesis of vitamin E is a function of plants, and thus, their products are by far the principal sources. It is abundant in whole cereal grains, particularly in germ, and thus in by-products containing the germ. There is wide variation in vitamin content of particular feeds, with many feeds having a threefold to tenfold range in reported α-tocopherol values.

Milk is highly variable in vitamin E content. As a source of vitamin E, there can be a fivefold seasonal difference in the α-tocopherol content of cow's milk. The vitamin E content of colostrum is of special importance for the newborn, because at birth, many species have very small amounts of vitamin E in their tissues. Hidiroglou (1989) reported that colostrum from dairy cows has a mean value of 1.9 µg α-tocopherol per milliliter and declines at 30 days to 0.3 µg α-tocopherol per milliliter. In this study, milk tocopherol was raised from 0.3 µg/ml to 1.6 µg/ml 12 hours after an intraperitoneal injection of dl-α-tocopheryl acetate. Supplemental vitamin E administered to ewes at graded levels of 0, 15, 30, and 60 IU (as dl-α-tocopheryl acetate) increased colostral α-tocopherol at a linear rate of 3.3, 6.8, 8.1, and 9.6 µg/ml, respectively (Njeru et al., 1994a). In sows, colostrum α-tocopherol concentration can be elevated by increasing the gestation dietary level of vitamin E or via injection during the last 14 days of pregnancy (Chung and Mahan, 1995).

■ Table 4.5   α-Tocopherol Content of Feeds (ppm)

Source	Mean	Range
Alfalfa meal, dehydrated 17% protein	73	28–121
Alfalfa meal, sun cured 13% protein	41	18–61
Alfalfa hay	53	23–102
Barley, whole	36	22–43
Beef, meat	6	5–8
Brewer's grains, dried	27	17–48
Butter	24	10–33
Chicken, meat	3	2–4
Corn, whole	20	11–35
Cottonseed meal	9	2–16
Distiller's grains, dehydrated	30	17–40
Eggs	11	8–12
Fat, animal	8	2–16
Fish, halibut	9	4–13
Fish (seafood product), shrimp	9	6–19
Fish meal, herring	17	8–31
Fish meal, Peruvian	2	1–3
Lard	12	2–30
Linseed meal	8	3–10
Meat and bonemeal	1	1–2
Milo	12	10–16
Molasses, cane	5	3–9
Oats, whole	20	18–24
Pork, meat	5	4–6
Poultry by-products meal	2	1–4
Rice, brown	13.5	13–14
Rice, bran	61	34–87
Sorghum, grain	12	10–16
Soybean meal, solvent process	3	1–5
Wheat, whole	11	3–15
Wheat, bran	17	15–19

Source: Adapted from Bauernfeind (1980) and Ullrey (1981).
Note: When only α-tocopherol in a mixed diet is available, multiply value by 1.2 to account for the other tocopherols present.

Colostrum α-tocopherol concentration was approximately five times higher than later milks (Mahan and Vallet, 1997).

Animal by-products supply only small amounts of vitamin E, and milk and dairy products are often poor sources. Eggs, particularly the yolks, make a significant contribution depending on the diet of the hen. Wheat germ oil is the most concentrated natural source, and various other oils, such as soybean and peanut, and particularly cottonseed, are also rich sources of vitamin E. Unfortunately, most of the oilseed meals that are part of pet-food diets are almost devoid of these oils because of their removal by solvent extraction (Maynard et al., 1979). Green forage and other leafy materials, including good-quality hay, are very good sources; alfalfa is especially rich. Concentration of tocopherols per unit dry matter in fresh herbage is between 5 and 10 times as great as that in some cereals or their by-products (Hardy and Frape, 1983). Variability in forage vitamin E content is so great, both between and within farms, that one must have current results or representative samples to ensure proper vitamin E fortification programs (Harvey and Bieber-Wlaschny, 1988). These authors indicated that previously published values on vitamin E content of forages are unacceptable for use in feed formulation.

Stability of all naturally occurring tocopherols is poor, and substantial losses of vitamin E activity occur in feedstuffs when processed and stored, as well as in manufacturing and storage of finished feeds (Coelho, 1991; Dove and Ewan, 1991; McDowell et al., 1996). Vitamin E sources in these ingredients are unstable under conditions that promote oxidation of feedstuffs—heat, oxygen, moisture, oxidizing fats, and trace minerals. Vegetable oils that normally are excellent sources of vitamin E can contain extremely little if oxidation has been promoted. Not only does oxidized oil have little or no vitamin E, but it will destroy the vitamin of other feed ingredients and deplete animal tissue stores of vitamin E. Rats fed a diet containing 15% oxidized frying oil had significantly lower α-tocopherol in plasma and tissues (Liu and Huang, 1995, 1996).

For concentrates, oxidation increases following grinding, mixing with minerals, addition of fat, and pelleting. When feeds are pelleted, destruction of both vitamins E and A may occur if the diet does not contain sufficient antioxidants to prevent their accelerated oxidation under conditions of moisture and high temperature. Iron salts (e.g., ferric chloride) can completely destroy vitamin E. Dove and Ewan (1991) observed that the rate of oxidation of natural tocopherols is increased in swine diets containing increased levels of copper, iron, zinc, and manganese. High dietary copper in swine diets decreased serum tocopherols (Dove and Ewan, 1990). Both nitrogen trichloride and chlorine dioxide, at concentrations usually used to bleach flour, will destroy much of the vitamin E activity in flour. According to Moore et al. (1957), baking destroyed 47% of remaining tocopherols in treated flour.

Artificial dehydration or processing of forages and grains will reduce availability of tocopherol as well as that of Se. For example, King et al. (1967) reported that 80% of the vitamin E is lost in hay making, whereas ensiling or rapid dehydration of forages retains most of the vitamin. Vitamin E content in forage is affected by stage of maturity at the time of forage cutting and the period between cutting and dehydration. Storage losses can reach 50% in 1 month, and losses during drying in the swath can amount to as much as 50% within 4 days. Vitamin E losses of 54 to 73% have been observed in alfalfa stored at 33°C for 12 weeks, and 5 to 33% losses have been obtained with commercial dehydration of alfalfa.

In a study testing vitamin E stability, Orstadius et al. (1963) reported that vitamin E content of corn was reduced from 30 to 50 mg/kg to about 5 mg/kg dry weight as a result of artificial drying at 100°C for 24 hours under a continuous flow of air. Similarly, Adams (1973) reported that artificial drying of corn for 40 minutes at 74°C produced an average 19% loss of α-tocopherol and 12% loss of other tocopherols. When corn was dried for 54 minutes at 93°C, the α-tocopherol loss averaged 41%. Young et al. (1975) reported a concentration of 9.3 and 20 mg/kg α-tocopherol in artificially dried corn versus undried, respectively. Preservation of moist grains by ensiling caused almost complete loss of vitamin E activity. Corn stored as acid-treated (propionic or acetic-propionic mixture), high-moisture corn contained approximately 1 mg/kg dry matter of α-tocopherol, whereas similar corn artificially dried contained approximately 5.7 mg/kg (Young et al., 1978). Apparently, damage is not due to moisture alone but to the combined propionic acid-moisture effect (McMurray et al., 1980). Further decomposition of α-tocopherol occurs over a more extended period, until the grain eventually has α-tocopherol levels of less than 1 mg/kg, which is commonly found in propionic acid-treated barley.

DEFICIENCY

Vitamin E displays the greatest versatility of all vitamins in the range of deficiency signs. Deficiency signs differ among species and even within the same species. The amount of vitamin E required in diets can vary depending on such factors as levels of PUFAs, Se, antioxidants, and sulfur amino acids in feed. Deficiency diseases and compounds preventing them are shown in Table 4.6.

Blaxter (1962) reported that muscular dystrophy seemed to be the one syndrome commonly encountered in vitamin E deficiency in all species. He cited references indicating that muscular degeneration that can be prevented with vitamin E occurs in all laboratory and farm animals, including camels, buffalos, kangaroos, and quokkas. In some 20 different animal species, tocopherol deficiency leads to muscular dystrophy. Fundamentally, this is Zenker's degeneration of both skeletal and cardiac muscle fibers. Connective tissue replacement that follows is observed grossly as white striations in the muscle bundles (Smith, 1970).

Occurrence of muscular dystrophy is worldwide, but its incidence,

■ Table 4.6 Vitamin E Deficiency Diseases As Influenced by Other Factors

Disease	Experimental Animal	Tissue Affected	PUFA Influence	Prevented by — Vitamin E	Prevented by — Se	Prevented by — Antioxidant	Prevented by — Sulfur Amino Acids
Reproductive failure							
Embryonic degeneration							
Type A	Rat, hamster, mouse, hen, turkey	Vascular system of embryo	X	X		X	
Type B	Cow, ewe			—[a]	X[b]		
Sterility (male)	Rat, guinea pig, hamster, dog, cock, rabbit, monkey	Male gonads		X			
Neuropathy	Chick, human	Brain	X	X		X	
Liver, blood, brain, capillaries, pancreas							
Necrosis	Rat, pig	Liver		X	X		
Fibrosis	Chick, mouse	Pancreas			X		X
Erythrocyte hemolysis	Rat, chick, human (premature infant), calf, dog, monkey	Erythrocytes	X	X		X	
Plasma protein loss	Chick, turkey	Serum albumin		X	X		
Anemia	Monkey	Bone marrow		X		X	
Encephalomalacia	Chick	Cerebellum	X	X		X	
Exudative diathesis	Chick, turkey	Vascular system	X	X	X		
Kidney degeneration	Rat, mouse, monkey, mink	Kidney tubular	X	X	X		
Steatitis (ceroid)	Mink, pig, chick	Adipose tissue	X	X		X	
Depigmentation	Rat	Incisors	X	X		X	

■ Table 4.6 *Continued*

Disease	Experimental Animal	Tissue Affected	PUFA Influence	Prevented by Vitamin E	Prevented by Se	Prevented by Antioxidant	Sulfur Amino Acids
Nutritional myopathies							
Type A (nutritional muscular dystrophy)	Rabbit, guinea pig, monkey, duck, mouse, mink, dog	Skeletal muscle		X		?	
Type B (white muscle disease)	Lamb, calf, kid, foal	Skeletal and heart muscles		—[a]	X[b]		
Type C	Turkey	Gizzard, heart		—[a]	X		
Type D	Chicken	Skeletal muscle	—[c]	X			
Retinopathy	Dog, monkey, rat	Retinal pigment epithelium (photoreceptor cells)	X	X			X
Dermatosis	Dog	Skin					
Immunodeficiency	Dog, chick, mouse, sheep, pig	Reticuloendothelial	X	X	X		

Sources: Modified from Scott (1980) and Sheffy and Williams (1981).
[a]Not effective in diets severely deficient in selenium.
[b]When added to diets containing low levels of vitamin E.
[c]A low level (0.5%) of linoleic acid is necessary to produce dystrophy; higher levels did not increase vitamin E required for prevention.

180

or at least diagnosis, particularly in a mild or subclinical form, varies widely in different countries and regions within countries (McDowell, 1997). Considerable research has revealed the positive relationship between Se content in soil and geographical occurrence of muscular dystrophy that responds to vitamin E and Se.

Effects of Deficiency

Ruminants

White muscle disease (WMD; also known as nutritional muscular dystrophy), a serious muscle degeneration disease in young ruminants, is caused by Se deficiency but is influenced by vitamin E status. White muscle disease occurs with two clinical patterns; the first is a congenital type of muscular dystrophy in which young ruminants are stillborn or die within a few days of birth after sudden physical exertion, such as nursing or running. The second pattern (delayed WMD) develops after birth; it is observed most frequently in lambs within 3 to 6 weeks of birth but may occur as late as 4 months after birth. The condition in calves is generally manifested at 1 to 4 months of age.

Typically, WMD is characterized by generalized weakness, stiffness, and deterioration of muscles; affected animals have difficulty standing (Figs. 4.3 and 4.4). Affected animals have difficulty standing and exhibit crossover walking and impaired suckling ability because the tongue musculature is affected (Muth, 1955). Calves with WMD have chalky white striations, degeneration, and necrosis in the skeletal muscles and heart (Fig. 4.3). Often, death occurs suddenly from heart failure as a result of severe damage to the heart muscle. In calves with milder cases, in which the chief clinical signs are stiffness and difficulty standing, dramatic, rapid improvement can result with vitamin E-Se injections.

An acute and chronic as well as a peracute form of the disease can be distinguished in older calves, usually already in the finishing period. In particular, stress situations such as transport, regrouping, or abrupt changes in feed composition are generally considered precipitating factors. Sudden death without previous unmistakable signs of disease is the main feature of the peracute condition (Bostedt, 1980). The cause is usually found in advanced degeneration of the myocardium, and motor disturbances such as an unsteady gait or stiff-calf disease; hard lumbar, neck, and forelimb muscles; muscle tremor; and perspiration are encountered in the acute form.

In Florida, the condition is most common in "buckling" calves that

181

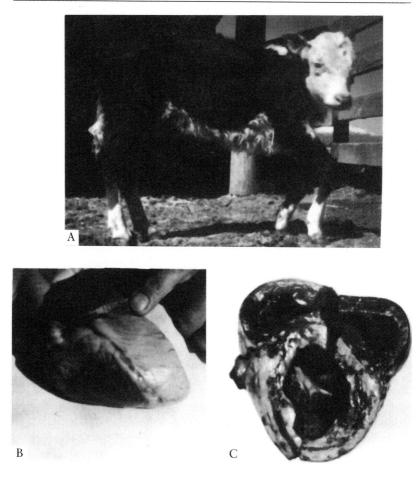

Fig. 4.3 White muscle disease in a calf about 3 months old. (A) Lameness and generalized weakness of muscles can be seen. (B and C) Abnormal white areas in the heart muscle. (Courtesy of O.H. Muth, College of Veterinary Medicine, Oregon State University.)

come off the truck or out of the processing chute with weakness of rear legs, buckling of fetlocks, and frequently a generalized shaking or quivering of muscles (Figs. 4.5 and 4.6). Many calves become progressively worse until they are unable to rise and may appear to be paralyzed. Many animals will be down or continue to buckle for extended periods, and death loss is high in severe cases. Calves with excitable temperaments appear to be most affected. Postmortem examination of affected calves reveals pale chalky streaks in the muscles of the hamstring and

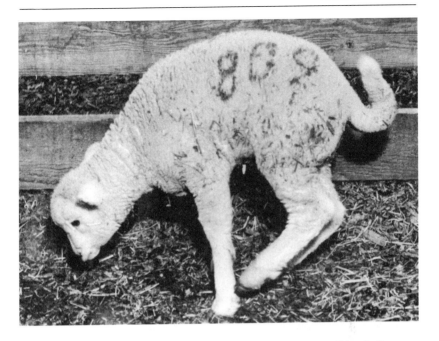

Fig. 4.4 Vitamin E-selenium deficiency in sheep is known as stiff-lamb disease or white muscle disease. This lamb is unable to stand as a result of tissue degeneration. (Courtesy of O.H. Muth, College of Veterinary Medicine, Oregon State University.)

back, and the heart, rib muscles, and diaphragm may also be affected (McDowell, 1985).

In lambs, WMD (also known as stiff-lamb disease) takes a course similar to that found in calves. There are motor disturbances such as unsteady gait (Fig. 4.4); stiffness in rear quarters, neck, and forelimb muscles; and arched back. Muscle tremor and perspiration are encountered in the acute form. On necropsy, the disease is manifested as white striations in cardiac muscles and is characterized by bilateral lesions in skeletal muscles. A gradual swelling of the muscles, particularly in the lumbar and rear thigh regions, gives the erroneous impression of an especially muscular young animal. In addition to the peracute form encountered in calves (changes primarily in the myocardium), chronic cardiac muscle degeneration is also found in the lamb. Despite good initial development, affected lambs quickly lose weight after the third week of life and are unthrifty. They try to avoid any strain and usually stand apart from the herd. Cardiac arrhythmia and increased heart rate can

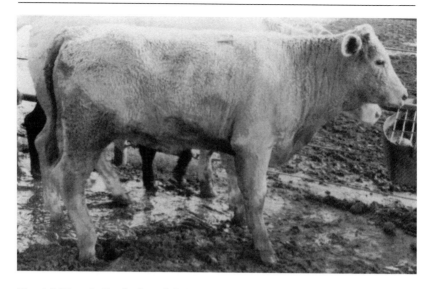

Fig. 4.5 Vitamin E-selenium deficiency is seen as flexion of the hock and fetlock joints as a result of decreased support by the gastrocnemius muscle, which is severely affected by myodegeneration. (Courtesy of Bob Mason and University of Florida.)

result even after slight exercise. In the advanced stage, animals eat little feed and rapidly waste away.

Other conditions responsive to vitamin E-Se are not restricted to young animals and relate to unthriftiness ("illthrift"), occurring in lambs and hoggets at pasture (Underwood, 1981). Yearling sheep can also be affected by WMD. In sheep of 9 to 12 months of age, the disease is frequently observed following driving, with the rapid onset of listlessness, stiffness, inability to stand, prostration, and, in the most acute cases, death within 24 hours (Andrews et al., 1968). Hartley and Grant (1961) reported that the incidence of barren ewes was reduced from over 30 to 5% with Se administration. Farms in New Zealand have had lamb losses as high as 40 to 50%. Vitamin E reduced losses by only 60%; Se, by 96%.

The immune response in sheep has been improved with supplemental vitamin E. Vitamin E improved disease resistance in lambs challenged with chlamydia (Stephens et al., 1979). Reffett et al. (1988) reported that vitamin E and Se independently increased the immune response of lambs challenged with a viral pathogen. Myopathic lambs exhibited low lymphocyte responses when deficient in vitamin E and Se (Finch and Turner, 1989; Turner and Finch, 1990). The poor lymphocyte responses

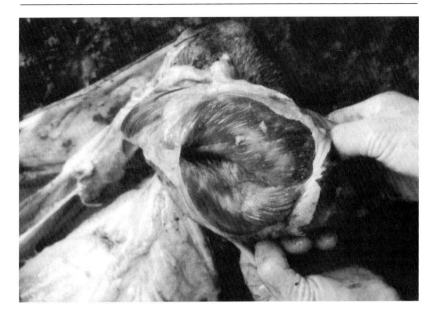

Fig. 4.6 Vitamin E-selenium deficiency in cattle is manifested as white muscle disease or necrosis of the gastrocnemius muscle; chalky white streaks are evident in the belly of the muscle. (Courtesy of Bob Mason and University of Florida.)

of the lambs with nutritional myopathy was rapidly reversed by intramuscular administration of these nutrients, with the prophylaxis most effective during the first 5 weeks of life (Finch and Turner, 1989).

Deficiency of vitamin E and/or Se in the goat, as in other ruminants, results mainly in WMD. Kids especially suffer from this disturbance of muscle metabolism, as they are born with little or no reserves of the fat-soluble vitamins A, D, and E. Sudden death of young kids under 2 weeks of age may reveal postmortem evidence of muscle disease and degeneration in the heart or diaphragm. In older kids and mature animals, the disease may occur after sudden exercise, and the animals show bilateral stiffness, usually in their hind legs.

In preruminant calves, WMD has been easily induced by feeding polyunsaturated oils; however, it was thought unlikely that unsaturated fats were responsible for the disease in ruminating calves because of the apparent near 100% hydrogenation of all unsaturated fatty acids by the rumen microflora (Noble et al., 1974). However, one study indicated that unsaturated fatty acids from lipids in grasses can act as substitutes for the peroxidative challenge in nutritional muscular dystrophy in

185

calves (McMurray and Rice, 1984). Nutritional degenerative myopathy in older calves occured most frequently at turnout to spring pasture (Anderson et al., 1976). McMurray et al. (1980) showed that PUFAs were capable of escaping ruminal hydrogenation at turnout, resulting in a threefold increase of plasma linolenic acid within 3 days of turnout. Rice et al. (1981) showed that linolenic acid, if protected from ruminal hydrogenation, rapidly reaches high levels in blood and is associated with a rise in plasma creatine phosphokinase, indicating muscular degenerative myopathy.

Most nutritional myopathy cases have involved young ruminants, with effects less fully described for adult animals. However, degenerative myopathy in adult cattle has been reported (Van Vleet et al., 1977; Gitter and Bradley, 1978; Hutchinson et al., 1982), and a group of yearling Chianina heifers experienced abortion, stillbirth, and periparturient recumbency (Hutchinson et al., 1982). Necropsy and tissue analyses revealed myodegeneration and a combined deficiency of vitamin E and Se. Rapid growth in these heifers, coupled with stresses of late pregnancy and parturition, may have contributed to this vitamin E deficiency. A myopathic condition affecting yearling cattle was reported by Barton and Allen (1973) and was associated with animals fed grains treated with propionic acid, which is known to destroy vitamin E.

Attempts to establish a practical role for vitamin E in ruminant reproductive deficiencies of both males and females have been limited. The relationship to reproduction is of special interest since early rat research demonstrated that reproductive failure was a key feature of vitamin E deficiency. In one experiment, four generations of female and male dairy cattle were fed diets low in vitamin E (Gullickson et al., 1949). Although growth, reproduction, and milk production were normal, several cattle died suddenly of apparent heart failure between 21 months and 5 years of age. Large doses of vitamins A, D, E, and C were reported to favorably affect some characteristics of semen and sperm (Kozicki et al., 1981).

Recent research has shown that vitamin E supplementation is beneficial for male reproduction in bulls fed high concentrations of gossypol. Velásquez-Pereira et al. (1998) reported that bulls receiving 14 mg of free gossypol per kilogram of body weight had a lower ($P < 0.05$) percentage of normal sperm than those that also received supplemental vitamin E (31 and 55%, respectively; Table 4.7). Likewise, sperm production per gram of parenchyma and total daily sperm production were higher ($P < 0.05$) when gossypol-treated animals also received vitamin

E. Bulls receiving gossypol exhibited more sexual inactivity ($P < 0.05$) than bulls receiving other treatment (Table 4.8). Vitamin E supplementation in bulls receiving gossypol improved number of mounts in the first test and time of first service in the second test. The final conclusion based on these data is that vitamin E is effective in reducing or eliminating important gossypol toxicity effects for male cattle (Velasquez-Pereira et al., 1998, 1999).

From a different aspect of reproduction in dairy cattle, Harrison et al. (1984) reported that supplemental vitamin E was required in addition to Se for prevention of retained placenta. Groups administered vitamin E alone, Se alone, and controls had a retained-placenta incidence of 17.5% compared to 0% for animals receiving both vitamin E and Se. Other research found that the incidence of retained placenta (22.1%) was not reduced by a combination of vitamin E and Se or by Se alone (Hidiroglou et al., 1987). In high-producing dairy goats, deficiency manifested itself in poor involution of the uterus, with accompanying retained placenta and metritis following kidding (Guss, 1977).

Adequate amounts of vitamin E in the diet are needed to prevent oxidative flavors in milk. However, the cost is high, with efficiency of transfer into milk less than 2% (NRC, 1989a).

■ Table 4.7 Relationship of Gossypol and Vitamin E on Semen Characteristics of Dairy Bulls

	Treatment		
Item	Control[a]	+ Gossypol[b]	+ Gossypol + Vitamin E[c]
Normal, %	64.7 ± 6.4[g]	31.4 ± 7.4[h]	54.6 ± 6.4[g]
Abnormal (DIC)[d], %	4.4 ± 1.3[g]	13.4 ± 1.5[h]	4.8 ± 1.2[g]
DSPG[e] (x10^6/g)	14.6 ± 1.0[g]	10.2 ± 1.0[h]	17.6 ± 1.0[g]
DSP[f] (x10^9)	3.2 ± 3.0[g]	2.2 ± 3.0[h]	4.1 ± 3.0[g]

Source: From Velásquez-Pereira et al. (1998).
Note: Least square means ± SEM.
[a]Diet based on soybean meal, corn, and 30 IU vitamin E/kg of supplement.
[b]Diet containing 14 mg free gossypol/kg body weight per day and 30 IU vitamin E/kg of supplement.
[c]Diet containing 14 mg free gossypol/kg body weight per day and 4,000 IU vitamin E per bull per day.
[d]Midpiece abnormalities evaluated in isotonic formal saline using differential-phase microscopy.
[e]Daily sperm production per gram of parenchyma.
[f]Daily sperm production total.
[g,h]Means in a row with different superscripts differ when $P < 0.05$.

187

■ Table 4.8   Effects of Gossypol and Vitamin E on Sex Drive of Holstein Bulls

Item	Month	Control[b]	+ Gossypol[c]	+ Gossypol + Vitamin E[d]
Libido score	16	10.4 ± 0.7	8.9 ± 0.5	$10.0 \pm .6$
No. of mounts	12	$5.7^a \pm 1.2$	$3.2^b \pm 1.1$	$6.3^a \pm 1.2$
	16	9.4 ± 1.3	9.5 ± 0.9	7.9 ± 1.1
No. of services	16	2.4 ± 0.5	1.7 ± 0.4	2.3 ± 0.4
Time of mounts (sec)	16	$38^a \pm 7$	$29^{a,b} \pm 5$	$21^b \pm 5$
Time of first service (sec)	12	223 ± 94	232 ± 69	206 ± 69
	16	$154^{a,b} \pm 71$	$213^a \pm 52$	$69^b \pm 60$
Sexual inactivity (min)	12	$1.2^d \pm 0.8$	$3.9^c \pm 0.7$	$1.7^d \pm 0.8$
	16	0.1 ± 0.2	0.1 ± 0.1	0.2 ± 0.2

Source: From Velásquez-Pereira et al. (1998).
Notes: Each treatment represented eight animals.
     Animals received 14 mg free gossypol per kg body weight (except controls).
     Vitamin E–treated animals received 4,000 IU vitamin E per day as dl-α-tocopheryl acetate.
     [a,b]Means with different superscripts in the same row differ ($P < 0.01$).
     [c,d]Means with different superscripts in the same row differ ($P < 0.05$).

Swine

In pigs, most signs of vitamin E deficiency have been associated with Se deficiency, and scientists usually refer to vitamin E and/or Se deficiency since it is not clear which is involved, and generally, dietary levels of both must be low to bring about deficiency signs and lesions. Since the early 1950s, reports in the European literature have revealed tissue-degeneration signs in swine under field conditions associated with vitamin E deficiency; the significance of Se deficiency was not realized until 1957.

Muscular dystrophy and hepatosis dietetica (toxic liver dystrophy) were particularly widespread in the swine industry in Sweden. Obel (1953) reported that records from the State Veterinary Medical Institute of Stockholm from 1947 to 1952 revealed that of 4,382 pigs autopsied, over 10% suffered from hepatosis dietetica.

Vitamin E-Se deficiencies have been readily produced in swine diets through use of both highly unsaturated fats (e.g., cod liver oil) and rancid fats. However, naturally occurring vitamin E-Se deficiencies were not reported in the United States until the late 1960s (Michel et al., 1969), and in the 1970s, they became widespread. High incidence of vitamin E-Se deficiencies in swine was believed to be due to a number of factors (Trapp et al., 1970), including (1) swine raised in complete confinement without access to pasture, (2) low Se content in midwestern U.S. feeds, (3) solvent-extracted protein supplements low in vitamin E, (4) limited feeding programs for sows, (5) loss of vitamin E and Se from corn due to oxidation as a result of air and heat drying or storing high-moisture grains, and (6) selection of meatier-type pigs that require more Se. Evidence also suggests that moldy feed in bulk-holding bins may produce mycotoxins that either inhibit the uptake of vitamin E in the small intestine or affect the antioxidant balance of cells.

An increase in confinement rearing of swine on concrete floors or slats has been accompanied by a decrease in the utilization of pasture and forages. Such crops not only are excellent sources of vitamin E but also provide the more highly available form of the vitamin, α- versus γ-tocopherol.

Vitamin E-Se deficiency in swine is often associated with sudden death. In most cases, clinical signs of the condition were not observed prior to death (Michel et al., 1969; Trapp et al., 1970), although occasionally, pigs were observed with clinical signs of icterus, difficult locomotion, reluctance to move, and weakness. Clinical signs also include peripheral cyanosis (particularly of the ears), dyspnea (abdominal respiration), and weak pulse, all occurring shortly before death. In many cases, the faster-growing, more thrifty-appearing pigs died suddenly.

The most common pathological lesions include massive hepatic necrosis (hepatosis dietetica) (Figs. 4.7 through 4.9), degenerative myopathy of cardiac and skeletal muscles (Figs. 4.10 and 4.11), edema, esophagogastric ulceration, icterus, nephrosis, hemoglobinuria, acute congestion, hemorrhaging (Fig. 4.12) in various tissues (Trapp et al., 1970; Piper et al., 1975), and yellowish discoloration of adipose tissue (yellow fat).

Many pathology reports of vitamin E-Se deficiency have noted that the most striking lesion was liver necrosis (Trapp et al., 1970); however, bilateral paleness of skeletal muscles was the gross lesion most commonly found. In some pigs, microscopic lesions in liver were either absent or minimal, whereas changes in skeletal muscles were extensive. In other cases, the reverse was true.

Other conditions reported in swine herds with vitamin E-Se deficiency include mastitis-metritis-agalactia syndrome (MMA) in sows, spraddled rear legs in newborn pigs, gastric ulcers, infertility, and poor skin condition. These conditions were believed initially to be unrelated to pig deaths due to vitamin E-Se deficiency. However, after supplementation with dietary vitamin E or injections of Se and vitamin E, a noticeable reduction in these conditions occurred (Trapp et al., 1970).

189

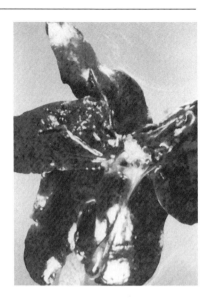

Fig. 4.7 Lesions in growing pig fed diet low in vitamin E (7.0 IU α-tocopherol/kg diet and selenium (0.061 ppm). Liver with severe acute lesions is characteristic of hepatosis dietetica, consisting of a mosaic pattern of deep red and yellow lobules of massive coagulation necrosis. (Courtesy of L.R. McDowell, R.C. Piper, and Washington State University.)

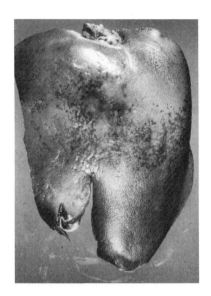

Fig. 4.8 Lesions in growing pig fed diet low in vitamin E (7.0 IU α-tocopherol/kg diet) and selenium (0.061 ppm). In subacute dietary massive hepatic necrosis, the lesions are more chronic than those seen in the liver of pig in Fig. 4.7, in that many hepatic lobules are atrophic and collapsed, causing a pitted appearance on the surface of the liver. (Courtesy of L.R. McDowell, R.C. Piper, and Washington State University.)

Whitehair et al. (1983) provided evidence that the MMA syndrome may be ameliorated by supplementation of the gestation-lactation diet with vitamin E and Se. In one experiment, vitamin E was shown to help reduce the incidence of MMA from 50 to 14% (Ullrey, 1969). Occurrence of MMA was reduced from 39 to 24% in two studies involving 191 farrowings (Ullrey et al., 1971). Diets low in Vitamin E-

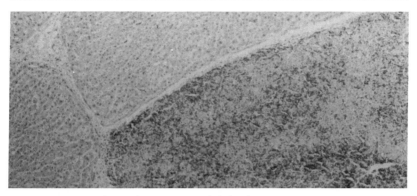

Fig. 4.9 Lesions in liver of growing pig fed diet low in vitamin E (7.0 IU α-tocopherol/kg diet) and selenium (0.061 ppm). Individual hepatic lobule has undergone acute massive coagulation necrosis, and the necrosis cells are being replaced by blood. Note the normal adjacent lobule. (Courtesy of L.R. McDowell, R.C. Piper, and Washington State University.)

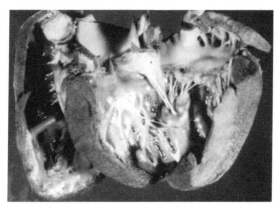

Fig. 4.10 Lesions in heart of growing pig fed diet low in vitamin E (7.0 IU α-tocopherol/kg diet) and selenium (0.061 ppm). Note the degenerative nutritional cardiac myopathy and the large pale areas due to degeneration and necrosis of myocardial fibers that are most severe along the inner border of the left ventricle. (Courtesy of L.R. McDowell, R.C. Piper, and Washington State University.)

Se for long periods will affect reproductive efficiency of boars (Marin-Guzman et al., 1997). Sperm motility was found to decline, and the percentage of abnormal sperm increased.

Studies by Tiege et al. (1978) have shown that susceptibility of pigs to dysentery resulting from exposure to the spirochete *Treponema hyodysenteriae* was greatly increased by the combined dietary deficiencies of

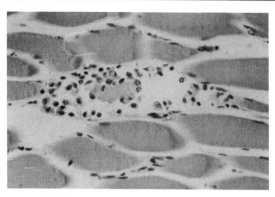

Fig. 4.11 Lesions in skeletal muscle of pig fed diet low in vitamin E (7.0 IU α-tocopherol/kg diet) and selenium (0.061 ppm). A muscle fiber (low power) of the biceps fermoris is undergoing degeneration, surrounded by normal fibers. Cytoplasm is breaking up into granules from enzymatic digestion as the fiber is invaded by macrophages. (Courtesy of L.R. McDowell, R.C. Piper, and Washington State University.)

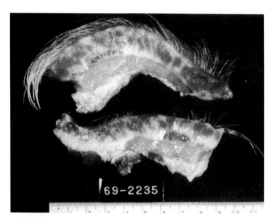

Fig. 4.12 Skin lesion in growing pig fed diet low in vitamin E (7.0 IU α-tocopherol/kg diet) and selenium (0.061 ppm). The skin is from a pig with severe congestion and hemorrhage. The hemorrhage extended throughout the epidermis, dermis, and subcutaneous fat and down to the cutaneous musculature. (Courtesy of L.R. McDowell, R.C. Piper, and Washington State University.)

vitamin E and Se. In studies with young pigs, supplemental vitamin E has been beneficial in increasing the humoral response against sheep red blood cells (Peplowski et al., 1981; Morrow et al., 1987). Depressed peripheral blood lymphocytes and polymorphonuclear cell immune functions were found in vitamin E-restricted sows (Wuryastuti et al., 1993).

The vitamin E-Se deficiency syndromes (nutrition-related microangiopathy; nutritional hepatic dystrophy; muscle degeneration in the back, pelvis, and upper thigh) can, however, also be found in the fattening and reproductive stages of pig production (Bostedt, 1980). At an early age, it is particularly myocardial damage, also known as nutritional microangiopathy or mulberry heart disease, that may cause substantial losses within a litter. This is the most serious of disorders, since when heart muscle tissue is damaged, the result is usually sudden death. There may be hemorrhagic lesions within the heart that give the characteristic mulberry appearance of mulberry heart disease.

There is a low tolerance of vitamin E- and Se-deficient baby pigs to intramuscular injections of iron dextrose for prevention of anemia. At 2 or 3 days, piglets die from iron shock if given routine treatment with iron, with death resulting from an iron-induced lipid peroxidation in tissues. Pretreatment with vitamin E, Se, or ethoxyquin was protective against toxic effects of injectable iron (Tollerz and Lannek, 1964; Hill et al., 1999).

Maximum incidence of death due to vitamin E-Se deficiency generally occurs at 6 to 8 weeks of age, with the incidence declining up to the sixteenth week of life; however, conceptuses can be adversely affected prior to parturition, resulting in stillborn pigs (Putnam, 1984). Vitamin E deficiency can also occur in fattening and reproductive stages of swine production (Bostedt, 1980). Clinical conditions characterized by cellular damage most often occur after a period of stress, such as change of feed or housing, transportation, or weaning. A Michigan survey diagnosed vitamin E-Se deficiencies in swine herds, with mortality ranging from 3 to 10% (Michel et al., 1969; Trapp et al., 1970). One producer, however, lost approximately 300 of 800 pigs weaned.

It has been realized for many years that vitamin E-deficient animals are more subject to the effects of stress than normal animals. The concept of stress is difficult to define, but experience has shown that dietary and environmental abnormalities of various kinds can lead to clinical signs of disease and death in animals deprived of vitamin E. Death is often associated with unaccustomed muscular activity. Incidence of death in baby pigs is greatly increased because of fighting when animals are weaned and mixed with different litters. Castration, an additional cause of stress, has been implicated as a cause of early death in pigs deficient in vitamin E and Se (Piper et al., 1975).

Poultry

Vitamin E deficiency in poultry can result in at least three conditions: exudative diathesis (Fig. 4.13), with signs of subcutaneous edema

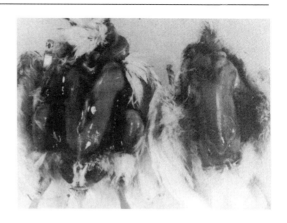

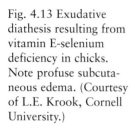

Fig. 4.13 Exudative
diathesis resulting from
vitamin E-selenium
deficiency in chicks.
Note profuse subcuta-
neous edema. (Courtesy
of L.E. Krook, Cornell
University.)

and, in severe cases, blackening of the affected parts, apathy, and inappetence; encephalomalacia ("crazy chick disease") (Fig. 4.14), characterized by ataxia, head retraction, and "cycling" with legs; and muscular dystrophy (Fig. 4.15) (Scott et al., 1982).

CHICKENS

Exudative diathesis in chicks is a severe edema produced by a
marked increase in capillary permeability. The subcutaneous edema
soon progresses to a hemorrhagic stage, producing a blue-green discoloration of the skin. Affected chicks show reduced spontaneous activity
and food intake; if not treated with vitamin E or Se, they survive usually no more than 2 to 6 days. Both vitamin E and Se are involved in prevention of exudative diathesis and nutritional muscular dystrophy. In
diets severely deficient in Se, however, vitamin E does not prevent or
cure exudative diathesis, whereas addition of as little as 0.05 ppm of
dietary Se completely prevents this disease.

Encephalomalacia generally affects chicks from 2 to 6 weeks of age
and results from hemorrhages and edema within the cerebellum.
Degeneration of the Purkinje layer of cells in the cerebellum results in
nervous signs typified as sudden prostration, with toes and legs outstretched, toes flexed, and head outstretched (NRC, 1994). At least one
important function of vitamin E is to interrupt the production of free
radicals at the initial stage of encephalomalacia. The quantitative need
for vitamin E for this function depends on the amount of linoleic acid in
the diet. Selenium is ineffective in preventing encephalomalacia, while
synthetic antioxidants are partially effective. The fact that low concentrations of antioxidants are capable of preventing encephalomalacia in

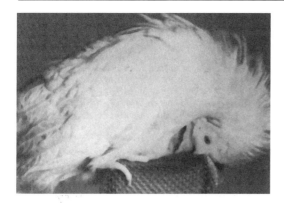

Fig. 4.14 Encephalomalacia in a chick fed a vitamin E-deficient diet. This disease is caused by deficiency of vitamin E or antioxidants. Selenium supplementation of the diet will not prevent it. (Courtesy of M.L. Scott, Cornell University.)

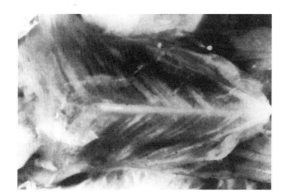

Fig. 4.15 Nutritional muscular dystrophy in chick fed a vitamin E-deficient diet low in sulfur amino acids. The diet contained an antioxidant and 0.1 ppm of selenium to prevent encephalomalacia and exudative diathesis. Note the white degenerated muscle fibers in the breast and thigh. (Courtesy of M.L. Scott, Cornell University.)

chicks but fail to prevent exudative diathesis or muscular dystrophy in the same chicks strongly suggests that in preventing encephalomalacia vitamin E acts as an antioxidant.

When vitamin E deficiency is accompanied by sulfur amino acid deficiency, chicks show severe nutritional muscular dystrophy, especially of breast muscle, at about 4 weeks of age. Cystine is likewise effective in preventing nutritional muscular dystrophy in vitamin E-deficient chicks. Cystine, however, is apparently ineffective in preventing the dystrophic condition in other animals. Although vitamin E and Se are generally both highly effective in preventing exudative diathesis, Se is only partially effective in protecting against muscular dystrophy in chicks when added in the presence of a low level of dietary vitamin E. Much larger quantities of Se are required to reduce the incidence of dystrophy in chicks receiving a vitamin E-deficient diet low in methionine and cystine (Scott et al., 1982).

Prolonged vitamin E deficiency can result in permanent sterility. Hatchability of eggs from vitamin E-deficient hens is reduced (NRC, 1994), and embryonic mortality may be high during the first 4 days of incubation and during later stages as a result of circulatory failure. Males become infertile because sperm become incompetent (Friedrichsen et al., 1980).

TURKEYS AND OTHER POULTRY SPECIES

The combined deficiency of vitamin E and Se in poults was found to produce a mild type of exudative diathesis (Creech et al., 1957). This condition was characterized by hemorrhaging on the inner margins of the thighs and caudal breast muscles; in contrast to the exudative diathesis of the vitamin E- and Se-deficient chick, it involved only a mild edema. In ducklings, exudative diathesis would appear to be more similar to that of the chick, i.e., green edema of the subcutaneous tissues can be seen most frequently on the thigh, with associated petechial hemorrhages of the thigh musculature (Combs and Combs, 1986). The appearance of exudative diathesis is infrequent and occurs in association with only the more severe cases of nutritional muscular dystrophy in deficient ducklings (Jager, 1977). In Japanese quail, the combined deficiency of vitamin E and Se has only produced exudative diathesis in some animals.

Degeneration of the smooth muscle of the gizzard is the most characteristic sign of Se deficiency in the young turkey poult. In marked contrast to the skeletal myopathy of the vitamin E-deficient chick, gizzard myopathy in vitamin E- and Se-deficient poults is not prevented by dietary sulfur containing amino acids but is completely prevented by supplements of Se (Walter and Jensen, 1963). However, the dietary level of vitamin E affects the amount of Se required for the prevention of the disorder. It was necessary to use a basal diet low in methionine and vitamin E, as well as Se, in order to produce gizzard myopathy experimentally. Muscular dystrophy in ducklings is characterized by degeneration of the sarcoplasmic reticulum and mitochondria of the smooth muscle of the duodenum and gizzard, and are prevented with either vitamin E or Se.

Vitamin E deficiency is also known to reduce hatchability in turkey eggs (Jensen and McGinnis, 1957). Turkey embryos deficient in vitamin E may have eyes that protrude with a bulging of the cornea. In Japanese quail, embryonic survival (i.e., egg hatchability) was markedly depressed among females reared to maturity with vitamin E- and Se-deficient diets.

Many of the surviving progeny of vitamin E- and Se-deficient females showed extreme generalized muscular weakness and prostration after hatching (Jensen, 1968).

Horses

The newborn foal that is born with nutritional muscular dystrophy usually exhibits various clinical signs in this acute phase of vitamin E-Se deficiency. Animals can hardly stand up and give the impression of general weakness. After laborious attempts to struggle to its feet, the foal stands rather awkwardly and stiffly. If neck muscles are affected, suckling is substantially impaired, and the foal is unable to raise its head to the mother's udder, although it gives the impression of wishing to suckle (Bostedt, 1980). Changes affect predominantly pectoral, intercostal, and diaphragm muscles and result in accelerated, intermittent, primarily abdominal respiration that can be incorrectly diagnosed as bronchial pneumonia or dry pleurisy. Movement of the thorax appears to cause pain. Dysphagia is a common finding (Dill and Rebhun, 1985), perhaps because pain is especially prominent during extension and rotation of the head and neck (Moore and Kohn, 1991). The dysphagia might also be due to the weakening of the lingual and pharyngeal muscles and even the masticatory muscles. Cardiac arrhythmia is another clinical sign that occurs as a result of muscle changes in the heart.

As with calves, the musculature of the tongue may be affected. In spite of their obvious appetite, the animals are unable to swallow milk, and the slightly opened mouth allows milk to leak out or trickle from their nostrils. The stomach is empty and the belly drawn up, so that the person in charge of the mare frequently consults a veterinarian for what is believed to be a lack of milk. Foals affected in this manner usually die during the first few days of life; the animal's death is accelerated by hypostatic or deglutition pneumonia or by neonate infections arising from immunological disorders caused by an inadequate intake of colostrum or from cardiovascular insufficiency (Bostedt, 1980).

In older foals (6 to 12 weeks), the progressive degeneration of motor muscles rather than changes in the head and thoracic muscles are the first indications of the disease. Typical signs are an increasingly clumsy gait and unsteady movements of the hindquarters. These foals also lie down a great deal and can hardly be made to stand (Bostedt, 1980). The urine may be coffee-colored because of myoglobin released from damaged muscle cells. As the condition worsens, the foal remains permanently in the lying position.

Combinations of vitamin E and Se have been used in the treatment of the "tying-up" syndrome in horses (Hintz, 1996), which is characterized by lameness and rigidity of the loin muscles. However, no experimental evidence to confirm the value of vitamin E in the condition has been provided. Likewise, published studies concerning the influence of vitamin E on reproduction have been contradictory.

It has been suggested that vitamin E alone or with Se is essential for the development of resistance to diseases such as influenza and tetanus in horses (Hintz, 1996). Horses fed a diet containing 80 IU of vitamin E per kilogram had greater immune responses than when fed diets containing 18 IU per kilogram (Baalsrud and Overnes, 1986).

Vitamin E supplementation has been claimed to enhance performance in horses, but few controlled studies have been conducted. Putnam (1986) concluded, apparently from field observations, that performance could be enhanced by a daily intake of 2,000 mg of vitamin E. Dewes (1981) reported that the performance of horses might be improved by vitamin E-Se supplementation due to relief from pain in the musculature of the neck.

It is hypothesized that vitamin E plays an oxidative role in equine motor neuron disease (EMND) and equine degenerative myeloencephalopathy (EDM). Both are neurodegenerative diseases that result in a loss of motor neurons and, subsequently, muscle mass. The absence of pasture, the feeding of marginal-quality hay, and high concentrates without additional vitamin E supplementation in part help to explain vitamin E-deficiency states in horses with EMND and EDM. Thus far, definitive causes for both EMND and EDM remain elusive. However, pathological evidence for each disorder presents a strong case for vitamin E involvement (NRC, 1989b; Hintz, 1996).

Other Animal Species

DOGS

Definite clinical cases of vitamin E deficiency have been well documented in dogs. Particularly prominent indications of vitamin E deficiency were degeneration of skeletal muscle associated with muscle weakness, degeneration of testicular germinal epithelium and failure of spermatogenesis, failure of gestation, weak and dead pups, and brown pigmentation (lipofuscinosis) of intestinal smooth muscle (NRC, 1985a).

Van Kruiningen (1967) reported a brown bowel in malabsorbing boxer dogs with granulomatous colitis, and the condition was eventually reproduced experimentally by Hayes et al. (1969), who fed varying levels of polyunsaturated fat to vitamin E-deficient weanling puppies over a 16-week period. The puppies developed an increased susceptibility to hemolysis of red blood cells as well as brown bowel, mild muscle degeneration, and neural-axonal dystrophy.

Retinal degeneration was described by Hayes and Rousseau (1970) and reproduced experimentally (Riis et al., 1981) in puppies fed a diet containing stripped corn oil. In as few as 3 months, ophthalmoscopic lesions were visible, which represented lipid peroxidation and disruption of photoreceptors, with accumulation of lipofuscin pigment.

The effect of vitamin E deficiency on reproduction has been reported by Anderson et al. (1939; 1940) and Elvehjem et al. (1944), who described a nutritional deficiency syndrome in puppies from bitches fed evaporated or pasteurized milk diets for extended periods. Lactating dams and puppies developed festering skin lesions, and the puppies developed muscle weakness and hemorrhages of body cavities and brain. Other pups were stillborn or died shortly after birth. The syndrome was alleviated by weekly feeding of 40 mg of vitamin E to the bitch during pregnancy.

A combined vitamin E-Se deficiency described by Van Vleet (1975) included muscle weakness, subcutaneous edema, anorexia, depression, dyspnea, and coma. Pathological examination revealed extensive skeletal muscle degeneration and regeneration, focal subendocardial necrosis, lipofuscinosis, and renal mineralization.

Deficiency of vitamin E has been implicated in the development of certain dermatological disorders in dogs (Anderson et al., 1939; Worden, 1958; Sheffy, 1979; Scott and Walton, 1985; Scott and Sheffy, 1987; Miller, 1989; Codner and Thatcher, 1993). The occurrence of these skin disorders has been associated with decreased blood levels of vitamin E. It has been postulated that subclinical vitamin E deficiency causes suppression of the immune system, which in turn increases a dog's susceptibility to Demodex (skin lesions caused by the demodectic mange mite, Demodex canis). When a group of dogs with demodicosis was treated with supplemental vitamin E, significant levels of improvement were reported. However, other researchers have been unable to reproduce these results.

Scott and Sheffy (1987) experimentally produced vitamin E deficiency skin disorders. They were characterized clinically by an early keratinization defect (seborrhea sicca), a later inflammatory stage (erythroderma), and a tendency to develop secondary pyoderma. The vitamin E anti-inflammatory effect may be related to stabilization of cell and lysosomal membranes against damage induced by free radicals and peroxides. By reducing oxidative damage to cells, vitamin E may inhibit immune-mediated or neoplastic skin diseases associated with ultraviolet irradiation.

Vitamin E therapy has been reported to be effective in dogs with discoid lupus erythematosus (Scott et al., 1983) and has been suggested as therapy for dogs with dermatomyositis (Hargis et al., 1985; Muller et al., 1989). Vitamin E supplementation has also been evaluated in dogs with acanthosis nigricans. Eight dachshunds with primary acanthosis nigricans showed improvement after 60 days of vitamin E therapy (200 mg twice daily) (Scott and Walton, 1985). All dogs responded with gradual elimination of pruritus, inflammation, lichenification, greasiness, and odor.

CATS

Steatitis (yellow fat disease) results when sources of highly unsaturated fatty acids (e.g., tuna fish oil, cod liver oil, and unrefined herring oil) have been fed in the absence of adequate supplemental vitamin E. The condition was known as yellow fat after the peroxidized ceroid in adipose tissue. It was characterized by extreme hyperesthesia, fever, and a marked rise in leucocytes, primarily as neutrophils and eosinophils. Anorexia, weight loss, listlessness or overt neurological dysfunction and muscle spasms, harsh hair coat, and palpable lumps in the subcutaneous fat were characteristic. Additional signs were focal interstitial myocarditis and, rarely, muscle fiber degeneration, focal myositis of the skeletal muscle, and periportal mononuclear infiltration in the liver (Gershoff and Norkin, 1962). Affected cats are often lethargic and febrile and exhibit pain on gentle palpation. Subcutaneous and abdominal fat may feel firm or lumpy, and draining tracts may develop. Microscopically, the fat shows focal neutrophilic infiltration with some mononuclear cells. Acid-fast ceroid pigment is present as globules and as peripheral rings in the fat-cell vacuoles (NRC, 1986). The white blood cell count is usually elevated (24,000 to 70,000 µg/ml), primarily as a result of neutrophilia, and reflects the degree of fat necrosis.

Vitamin E deficiency in cats became a significant clinical problem when fish products were first used in commercial cat foods that contained inadequate levels of tocopherol (Cordy, 1954; Munson et al., 1958). Later cases of the disease occurred in cats that were fed diets consisting wholly or largely of canned red tuna or fish scraps. Red tuna packed in oil contains high levels of PUFA and low levels of vitamin E. The addition of large amounts of fish products to a cat's diet appears to be the primary cause of this disease.

Stephan and Hayes (1978) induced severe vitamin E deficiency with hemolytic anemia and steatitis by feeding a diet containing 15% stripped safflower oil without α-tocopherol. Clinical signs of deficiency were prevented by supplementing with α-tocopheryl acetate at 100 IU per kg.

FISH

Channel catfish fed a vitamin E-deficient diet containing oxidized menhaden oil exhibited reduced growth, muscular dystrophy, fatty livers, anemia, exudative diathesis, and depigmentation in 16 weeks. Sekoke disease is a condition in common carp characterized by a marked loss of flesh. The disease in carp results from feeding oxidized silk worm pupae and is completely prevented with supplemental vitamin E.

Vitamin E deficiency signs have been described for chinook salmon, Atlantic salmon, channel catfish, common carp, rainbow trout, and yellowtail (NRC, 1993). The signs of vitamin E deficiency in various fishes are similar and include muscular dystrophy, involving atrophy and necrosis of white muscle fibers; edema of heart, muscle, and other tissues due to increased capillary permeability, which allows exudates to escape and accumulate (these are often green as a result of hemoglobin breakdown); anemia and impaired erythropoiesis; depigmentation; and ceroid pigment in the liver. The incidence and severity of these deficiency signs were shown to be enhanced when diets deficient in both vitamin E and Se were fed to Atlantic salmon (Poston et al., 1976), rainbow trout (Bell et al., 1985), and channel catfish (Gatlin et al., 1986).

FOXES AND MINK

Diets containing rancid fats or high in unsaturated fat cause "yellow fat" disease (steatitis) in foxes and mink as well as in cats. The most frequent clinical sign in animals with uncomplicated vitamin E deficiency was sudden death due to minor stress (NRC, 1982a). Selenium had some, but not complete, vitamin E-sparing effect.

Signs of steatitis in both foxes and mink are most evident among fast-growing male pups. Acute and subacute cases frequently occur. In fur-bearing animals, anemia is often found in chronic cases of yellow fat disease. A pronounced fragility of the red blood cells and an increased number of leukocytes and thrombocytes are frequent. In the postmortem examination, the musculature often appears light and musty, and fatty degeneration is usually discovered in the parenchymatous organs and in the musculature. The skin is of poor quality and loses hair easily, both during and after tanning (Helgebostad and Ender, 1973).

201

LABORATORY ANIMALS

Intrauterine death and resorption of fetuses in rats was the first evidence that led to the discovery of vitamin E. Other signs of vitamin E deficiency in rats are increased red blood cell hemolysis, skeletal muscle degeneration, accumulation of yellow pigment in smooth muscles; irreversible degeneration of the seminiferous epithelium of the testis in the male, which occurs by age 40 to 50 days; humped-back condition; rough coat, skin ulcers; neural lesions; and impaired learning ability (Sarter and Van Der Linde, 1987; NRC, 1995).

Pappenheimer (1942) reported muscular dystrophy and hyaline degeneration in vitamin E-deficient mice but at a lower incidence than was observed in rats. Spermatogenesis remained active in vitamin E-deficient mice for up to 439 days (Pappenheimer, 1942). Feeding a vitamin E-deficient diet increased pathology in hearts of mice infected with a virus (Beck et al., 1994), indicating an immune response for vitamin E in mice.

Diet-induced muscular dystrophy was produced in the guinea pig when 5 to 20 g of cod liver oil per kilogram was included in the diet. The research of Shimotori et al. (1940) related vitamin E deficiency to muscular dystrophy. Vitamin E-deficient guinea pigs lost weight with degeneration of skeletal muscle. In males, testes atrophied and developed degenerative changes in the seminiferous tubules, with clumping or complete disappearance of spermatozoa and spermatids. Fetal malformations, resorption, and death occurred in pregnant females (NRC, 1995).

NONHUMAN PRIMATES

When deprived of vitamin E for prolonged periods, usually a year or more, rhesus and cebus monkeys developed a characteristic anemia and muscular dystrophy (NRC, 1978). Anemia resulted in the production of defective erythrocytes, with muscular dystrophy closely resembling vitamin E deficiency in other species.

RABBITS

Muscular dystrophy in rabbits is caused primarily by vitamin E deficiency. The rabbit appears to be unusual in that Se has neither a protective nor sparing effect on muscular dystrophy that is preventable by vitamin E (Hove et al., 1958). Signs of this syndrome include degeneration of the skeletal and cardiac muscles, paralysis, and fatty liver (Bragdon and Levine, 1949). Ringer and Abrams (1970) encountered widespread signs of vitamin E deficiency in a commercial herd of rabbits fed a natural diet that provided 16.7 ppm of vitamin E. Tissues from rabbits fed ω-3 fatty acids rather than ω-6 and ω-9 were more susceptible to oxidation, with α-tocopherol lowering lipid oxidation (Lopez-Bote et al., 1997).

EXOTIC ANIMALS

Numerous cases of vitamin E deficiency have been diagnosed in zoo and wildlife species (Dierenfeld and Traber, 1992). Increased longevity of species in zoos, possibly limited genetic variability, and various stress factors contribute to the increasing number of clinical reports; however, dietary deficiency of vitamin E is likely the single most important determinant underlying current observations (Dierenfeld, 1994). Cervids (deer) and bovids (antelope) with vitamin E deficiency display cardiac and skeletal muscle dystrophy (Liu et al., 1985; Dierenfeld, 1989). Zebras suffer deterioration of the myelin sheath and spinal cord with vitamin E deficiency, clinically displayed as asymmetric weakness and ataxia (Liu et al., 1983). Both the elephant and rhinoceros appear to have limited absorption of dietary vitamin E, perhaps due to minimal dietary lipid levels in zoo feeds. Elephants with deficiency have heart lesions similar to those of swine with microangiopathy (Dierenfeld and Dolensek, 1988), whereas rhinos display skeletal and cardiac muscle myopathies. Among all exotic birds examined, species with carnivorous or granivorous feeding habits are most severely affected by vitamin E deficiency. Deficiency signs include decreased hatchability through pipping and cardiac muscle degeneration (Liu et al., 1985; Dierenfeld, 1989).

Humans

At one time, it was believed that in the United States and other developed countries, vitamin E intake of most adult human populations was considered adequate for maintenance, growth, and reproduction in normal individuals. This view is radically changing as supplemental vitamin E has shown benefits for improving the immune system; for prevention of cancer, thrombosis and cardiovascular diseases, cataracts, arthritis, and Parkinson's disease; and as an antidote to toxic substances and other pathological processes and diseases (Tengerdy, 1989; Padh, 1991; Consumer Report on Health, 1993; Langseth, 1995a,b; Chew, 1995). The various signs of vitamin E deficiency in humans often are believed to be manifestations of membrane dysfunction resulting from the oxidative degradation of polyunsaturated membrane phospholipids and/or the disruption of other critical cellular processes. Free radicals can be extremely damaging to biological systems (Padh, 1991). Antioxidants stabilize these highly reactive free radicals, thereby maintaining the structural and functional integrity of cells (Chew, 1995). Therefore, antioxidants are very important to immune defense and health of both humans and animals. Tissue defense mechanisms against free-radical damage include vitamin E, vitamin C, and β-carotene as the major vitamin antioxidant sources.

New findings on vitamin E and cardiovascular diseases were summarized by Langseth (1995a) as follows:

1. The use of vitamin supplements—especially vitamin E—was associated with a significantly reduced risk of coronary disease in Canadian men.

2. Low vitamin E intake was associated with elevated coronary mortality in Finnish men and women.

3. Vitamin E enhanced the benefits of aspirin in reducing the incidence of stroke in high-risk patients.

4. Vitamin E supplements slowed progression of coronary artery lesions, both in men taking cholesterol-lowering drugs and in those taking inactive placebos.

5. Vitamin E supplements lowered the risk of recurrence of coronary blockage in patients who had been treated for previous blockages.

6. Two studies of diabetics (a group at high risk for cardiovascular disease) showed beneficial changes in lipid peroxidation and other biochemical factors after vitamin E supplementation.

Jialal and Grundy (1993) reported that combined supplementation with vitamin C, β-carotene, and α-tocopherol is not superior to high-dose α-tocopherol alone in inhibiting low-density lipoprotein oxidation. Hence, α-tocopherol therapy should be favored in future coronary prevention trials involving antioxidants.

Cancer-prevention findings related to vitamin E have been summarized (Consumer Report on Health, 1993; Langseth, 1995a). In addition to possibly helping prevent cancer by keeping cells from becoming oxidized and turning cancerous, vitamin E might fight the disease indirectly by boosting the immune system. People who had taken vitamin E supplements for at least 6 months were half as likely to develop cancers of the mouth and throat. The evidence suggests that people who consume the most vitamin E may have a slightly lower risk of cancers of the colon, rectum, esophagus, and lung. One study reported a 34% decrease in prostate cancer and a 16% decrease in colorectal cancer. Preliminary research has hinted that certain forms of vitamin E applied to the skin might help protect against skin cancer caused by sun exposure.

In animal species, there is considerable evidence of beneficial effects of vitamin E on the immune response. In humans, however, there are only limited data on the relation between vitamin E status and the immune system. In a French study of healthy elderly subjects, the level of plasma vitamin E was inversely correlated with the number of infections the subjects experienced in the 3 years previous to the study (Chavance et al., 1989). In a double-blind, placebo-controlled trial, healthy older adults (60 years or older) improved some in vivo and in vitro parameters of immune function as a result of receiving supplemental vitamin E (Meydani, 1995).

A myriad of neurological abnormalities can be found in the presence of vitamin E deficiency. Cavalier and Gambetti (1981) reported dystrophic axons in the nucleus gracilis and demyelination of the fasciculus gracilis in patients with cystic fibrosis. In a review, Sokol (1989) reported that vitamin E deficiency in humans results in loss of deep tendon reflexes, truncal and limb ataxia, reduced perception of vibration and position, ophthalmoplegia, muscle weakness, dysarthria, and scoliosis.

Additional human diseases that are alleviated by vitamin E include thrombophlebitis and intermittent claudication, both of which involve blood flow, particularly in the extremities of elderly persons (Haeger, 1974). Low levels of vitamin E also have been found in the plasma of many persons with absorptive defects (Sitrin et al., 1987). Patients suffering from sprue, cystic fibrosis of the pancreas with accompanying steatorrhea, or any other disease that causes malabsorption of fat also show a marked decrease in plasma tocopherol levels.

Plasma vitamin E concentration in the newborn infant is about one-third that of adults, with that in the low-birth-weight (LBW) infant even lower. This is primarily a reflection of lower concentration of blood lipids in newborn infants that is due to inefficient placental transfer of the vitamin. Serum vitamin E levels increase during pregnancy, while fetal levels remain low, at about 25% of the maternal level. In the United States, edema and anemia attributed to vitamin E deficiency have been reported in LBW infants fed low-vitamin E commercial formulas made with polyunsaturated fat (Oski and Barness, 1967). Premature infants fed these formulas with inadequate vitamin E develop hemolytic anemia, resulting in shortened life span of red blood cells.

Numerous researchers have reviewed the effects of vitamin E on human diseases and presented two extreme points of view: (1) One group claims that vitamin E is a cure for almost every known disease;

the other group holds that vitamin E has not been proved scientifically to have any of the effects attributed to it. (2) The second viewpoint—that vitamin E is of little value—is no longer valid, as many studies have shown the positive benefits of vitamin E supplementation for the prevention and cure of many disease conditions.

Assessment of Status

Confirmation of a low vitamin E and/or Se status in animals is obtained when specific deficiency diseases associated with lack of these nutrients are present. Likewise, gross lesions and histopathological examinations provide definite evidence of vitamin E and/or Se deficiency.

Muscular damage as a result of vitamin E and/or Se deficiency causes leakage of intercellular contents into the blood. Thus, elevated levels of selected enzymes (above the normal concentrations for particular species) serve as diagnostic aids in detecting tissue degeneration. Serum enzyme concentrations used to follow incidence of nutritional muscular dystrophy include serum glutamic-oxaloacetic-transaminase (SGOT), aspartate amino transferase (ASPAT), lactic dehydrogenase (LDH), creatine phosphokinase (CPK), and malate dehydrogenase (MDH). A distinction regarding type of tissue degeneration can sometimes be made. For example, in swine, SGOT and ornithine carbamyl transferase (OCT) are useful indicators of muscular dystrophy and liver necrosis, respectively (Wretlind et al., 1959). Enzyme tests are very sensitive, and an elevation of enzyme activity in serum is usually discovered before any pathological changes or clinical signs appear (Tollersrud, 1973).

In addition to serum enzyme determinations, other laboratory tests devised to assist in diagnosis of vitamin E and Se deficiency include (1) vitamin E and Se analyses of feeds, blood, and tissues and (2) electrocardiogram changes that reflect heart muscle injury. Low tissue concentrations of glutathione peroxidase, an enzyme that contains Se, is a relatively good status indicator of this element. However, an in vitro hemolysis test is an indicator of vitamin E but not Se status.

Nutritional status with respect to vitamin E is commonly estimated from plasma (or serum) concentration. There is a relatively high correlation between plasma and liver levels of α-tocopherol (also between amount of dietary α-tocopherol administered and plasma levels). This has been observed in rats, chicks, pigs, lambs, and calves within rather wide ranges of intake. There is a much higher correlation between blood and liver concentrations for vitamin E than for vitamin A. Plasma tocopherol concentrations of 0.5 to 1 μg/ml are considered low in most animal species, with less than 0.5 µg/ml generally considered a vitamin E deficiency. Thus, plasma α-tocopherol concentrations can be used for assay purposes without the necessity of liver biopsy or animal slaughter (Ullrey, 1981; Njeru et al., 1994b).

In normal adult human populations of the United States, the range of total plasma tocopherols is 0.5 to 1.2 µg/ml, with values for α-tocopherol 10 to 15% lower (Bieri and Prival, 1965). It is generally accepted that a plasma level of total tocopherols below 0.5 µg/ml is undesirable, although it has not been shown that lower concentrations in adults, unless they continue a year or longer, are associated with inadequate tissue concentrations. Plasma tocopherol concentrations are highly correlated with total lipid, with less than 0.6 to 0.8 µg/g lipid considered deficient in humans (Machlin, 1991).

For a number of disease conditions, it is important to know the status of Se as well as vitamin E. For many species, Se concentrations in liver, renal cortex, and blood (as well as other tissues) each adequately portray Se status. For example, swine hepatic, renal cortex, and blood Se concentrations of 0.25, 2.5, and 0.1 ppm (dry basis), respectively, were determined to be critical levels below which clinical illness, death, or lesions of vitamin E-Se deficiency could be expected (McDowell et al., 1977). Serum or plasma Se is considered a good status indicator, with less than 0.03 ppm being critical for cattle (McDowell, 1985).

SUPPLEMENTATION

Methods of providing supplemental vitamin E are (1) as part of a concentrate or liquid supplement, (2) included with a free-choice mineral mixture, (3) as an injectable product, and (4) in drinking water preparations.

To offset losses of vitamin E activity in feedstuffs, diets should be adequately fortified with vitamin E. The principal commercially available forms of vitamin E used in food, feed, and pharmaceutical industries are acetate and hydrogen succinate esters of RRR α-tocopherol and the acetate ester of all-rac-α-tocopherol (Table 4.9). During commercial synthesis of dl-α-tocopherol, it is esterified to acetate to stabilize it, with the ester extremely resistant to oxidation. Thus, dl-α-tocopherol acetate does not act as an antioxidant in the feed and has antioxidant activity only after it is hydrolyzed in the intestine and free dl-α-tocopherol is released and absorbed.

The acetate forms of α-tocopherol are commercially available from two basic sources (Hoffmann-La Roche, 1972): (1) d-α-tocopheryl

■ Table 4.9   Forms of α-Tocopherol Commercially Available

Form	IU/mg
dl-α-Tocopheryl acetate (all-rac)	1.00
dl-α-Tocopherol (all-rac)	1.10
d-α-Tocopheryl acetate (RRR)	1.36
d-α-Tocopherol (RRR)	1.49
dl-α-Tocopheryl acid succinate (all-rac)	0.89
d-α-Tocopheryl acid succinate (RRR)	1.21

acetate is made by extraction of natural tocopherols from by-products of vegetable oil refining, molecular distillation to obtain the alpha form, and then acetylation to form the acetate ester, and (2) *dl*-α-tocopheryl acetate is made by complete chemical synthesis, producing a racemic mixture of equal parts of *d* and *l* isomers. The *d* and *l* forms differ only in spatial placement of the isoprenoid side chain.

Commercially, the *dl*- and *d*-α-tocopheryl acetates are available in purified form or in various dilutions, including (Hoffmann-La Roche, 1972) (1) a highly concentrated oily form for further processing; (2) emulsions incorporated in powders for use in dry premixes or water-dispersible preparations; (3) beadlets or powders consisting of the tocopheryl acetate incorporated in oil, or in emulsifiable form mixed with gelatin and sugar, gum acacia, soy grits, or dextrin as carriers (such beadlets or powders may be further diluted to lower potencies in a feed ingredient or water-soluble material and are primarily for use in feed); and (4) adsorbates of the oily tocopheryl acetate on selected carriers, in free-flowing "dry" powder, meal, or granules. This type is for use in feeds only. Vitamin E as the acetate form is highly stable in vitamin premixes, with 98% retention after 6 months, but in the alcohol form is completely destroyed during that time (Coelho, 1991).

Even though the ester is more stable than the natural free or alcohol form, it is desirable to further stabilize it by a gelatin coating or adsorption technique that reduces it to a beadlet, granule, or powder form to be added more easily and uniformly to animal feeds (Bauernfeind, 1969). Both types of products are quite stable. Stabilized *dl*-α-tocopheryl acetate gelatin beadlets have been blended in mash feed that also has been pelleted and stored with satisfactory stability results.

Injectable vitamin E preparations are also available, which contain free *d*- or *dl*-α-tocopherol or their esters. Liquid emulsions of appropriate types are used in drinking water and liquid feeds, in regular feed, and for injection. In this form, α-tocopherol is more efficiently absorbed from intramuscular injection sites than a water-miscible preparation containing α-tocopheryl acetate or either form dissolved in an oily base (Machlin, 1991). Products containing vitamin E and Se are often given intramuscularly to animals exhibiting clinical signs of muscular degeneration. Response to treatment of this condition is extremely variable depending on degree of muscular degeneration. However, intramuscular injection of α-tocopherol and Se to young ruminants usually provides a rapid means of alleviating deficiencies of these nutrients (McDowell, 1992). For cattle, animals that are down are unlikely to survive, while animals showing moderate weakness of the rear limbs or slight buckling of fetlocks may respond. Total recovery may require several days to 1 month (Mason et al., 1985). However, affected animals are particularly responsive to treatment, generally gaining ability to walk unassisted 3 to 5 days following vitamin E-Se therapy.

Some cattle ranchers make it a practice to inject newborn calves intramuscularly with a combination of vitamin E and Se. For dystrophic lambs, an oral therapeutic dose of 500 mg of dl-α-tocopherol followed by 100 mg on alternate days until recovery was successful (Rumsey, 1975). Reddy et al. (1987a) concluded that supplementation of conventional dairy calf diets with 125 to 250 IU vitamin E per animal daily increases performance compared to controls. Stuart (1987) recommended that weaned calves with transit shrink receive 400 IU of vitamin E daily during arrival to a feedlot finishing program, while those with minimal shrink receive 100 to 200 IU. The recommended amount for yearling cattle was 200 to 400 IU vitamin E, depending on previous dietary history in relation to vitamin E and Se. Most preventive preparations for WMD in ruminants contain a combination of both vitamin E and Se. As a preventive measure, they should be administered to pregnant cows during the second trimester and again 30 days prior to calving.

Supplementing vitamin E in well-balanced diets has been shown to increase humoral immunity for ruminants (Hoffmann-La Roche, 1994) and monogastric species (Langweiler et al., 1983; Wuryastuti et al., 1993). These results suggest that the criteria for establishing requirements based on overt deficiencies or growth do not consider optimal health (Hoffmann-La Roche, 1991). The effects of oral vitamin E supplementation in young calves was evaluated by Cipriano et al. (1982). Calves were fed skimmed colostrum and supplemented with either 0 or 1,000 mg dl-α-tocopheryl acetate for 6 weeks in a vitamin E-deficient diet. Conventionally managed calves were included as positive controls. Vitamin E-supplemented calves had greater plasma α-tocopherol concentrations as well as mean lymphocyte blastogenesis response to phytohemagglutinin (PTH) expressed as mean lymphocyte stimulation indices (LSIs) at 6 weeks. These authors suggested that the enhancing effect of vitamin E on immune response of cattle could have been partially masked in this study by feeding of diets high in emulsified fats.

Vitamin E administration to calves enhanced immune response and weight gain, while enzymes of muscle origin (e.g., creatine kinase and serum glutamic oxaloacetic transaminase) and plasma cortisol concentration were decreased (Reddy et al., 1987b). Vitamin E also positively influenced neutrophil-mediated antibody-dependent cellular cytotoxicity and phagocytosis as well as lymphocyte stimulation in calves fed milk replacer (Pruiett et al., 1989).

In a series of 28-day feedlot receiving trials, Lee et al. (1985) observed an improvement in early performance of newly arrived growing cattle supplemented with 450 IU vitamin E (as dl-α-tocopheryl acetate) per head per day that were stressed by long-distance shipment and changes from green forages to high-grain feedlot diets. Depression of circulating cortisol concentrations may explain the improved gain and feed efficiency in this trial.

Gill et al. (1986) supplemented newly received feedlot cattle with 1,600 IU of vitamin E (as dl-α-tocopheryl acetate) per head per day for the first 21 days and 800 IU for the remaining 7 days of a 28-day trial. Average daily gain and gain-feed ratios were improved by 23.2 and 28.6%, respectively, for vitamin E-supplemented stressed cattle (Table 4.10). The number of sick pen days per head was reduced by 15.6%, and morbidity was reduced by 13.4% with vitamin E supplementation. The growth response to vitamin E could be related to the fact that young, rapidly growing animals are in a metabolically demanding state resulting from overall tissue growth, which has a high energy demand. Vitamin E is an integral part of this response via its ability to quench free radicals, which are generated during the course of metabolism.

Supplemental levels of vitamin E higher than those recommended for dairy cattle by the NRC (1989a) have been beneficial in the control of mastitis. Smith and Conrad (1987) reported that intramammary infection was reduced 42.2% in vitamin E- and Se-supplemented versus unsupplemented controls. The duration of all intramammary infections in lactation was reduced 40 to 50% in supplemented heifers. Weiss et al. (1990) reported that clinical mastitis was negatively related to plasma Se concentration and concentration of vitamin E in the diet.

Many new intramammary infections (IMIs) occur in the 2 weeks before and after calving. Deficiencies of either vitamin E or Se have been associated with increased incidence and severity of IMI, increased clini-

■ Table 4.10 Effects of Vitamin E Supplementation on Performance, Morbidity, and Mortality of Stressed Cattle

Item	Control	Vitamin E[a]
No. of head	252	250
Average daily gain (kg)	0.43[b]	0.53[c]
Feed conversion	18.56	15.06
No. of sick days	3.2	2.7
Morbidity (%)	43.2	37.5
Mortality (%)	1.8	l.6

Source: From Gill et al. (1986).
[a]1,600 IU of vitamin E per head per day for first 21 days and 800 IU for the last 7 days.
[b,c]Means with different superscripts differ ($P < 0.01$).

cal mastitis cases, and higher somatic cell counts in individual cows and bulk tank milk. Somatic cell counts are a primary indicator of mastitis and milk quality in dairy herds. The polymorphonuclear neutrophil (PMN) is a major defense mechanism against infection in the bovine mammary gland. A known consequence of vitamin E and Se deficiency is impaired PMN activity, and postpartum vitamin E deficiency is frequently observed in dairy cows. Dietary supplementation with vitamin E and Se results in a more rapid PMN influx into milk following intramammary bacterial challenge and increased intracellular kill of ingested bacteria by PMN. In one study, subcutaneous injections of vitamin E approximately 10 and 5 days before calving successfully elevated PMN α-tocopherol concentrations during the periparturient period and negated the suppressed intracellular kill of bacteria by PMN that commonly is observed around calving (Smith et al., 1997).

Diets of multiparous dairy cows were supplemented with either 0 or 1,000 IU of vitamin E (as dl-α-tocopheryl acetate) during the dry period (Smith et al., 1984). Cows were additionally administered Se at the rate of 0 or 0.1 mg/kg body weight via intramuscular injection 21 days prepartum. No vitamin E or Se was supplemented during lactation. Incidence of new clinical cases of mastitis was reduced by 37% in both groups receiving vitamin E compared to controls. The reduction in clinical mastitis was only 12% when cows were injected with Se but not supplemented with dietary vitamin E. These authors also reported that clinical cases in the vitamin E-supplemented, Se-injected cows were consistently of shorter duration than those occurring in all other groups. Erskine et al. (1989) investigated specific effects of Se status of dairy cat-

211

tle on the induction of mastitis by *E. coli*. Bacterial concentrations were significantly higher in Se-deficient than in Se-adequate cows, and Se supplementation reduced both severity and duration of clinical mastitis.

Plasma concentrations of α-tocopherol decreased at calving for cows fed dietary treatments with low or intermediate concentrations of vitamin E, but not for cows fed the high vitamin E treatment (Weiss et al., 1997). High dietary vitamin E increased concentrations of α-tocopherol in blood neutrophils at parturition. The high vitamin E treatment was 1,000 IU/day of vitamin E during the first 46 days of the dry period, 4,000 IU/day during the last 14 days of the dry period, and 2,000 IU/day during lactation.

The percentage of quarters with new infections at calving was not different (32.0%) between cows receiving treatments that contained low and intermediate concentrations of vitamin E but was reduced (11.8%) in cows receiving the high vitamin E treatment. Clinical mastitis affected 25.0, 16.7, and 2.6% of quarters during the first 7 days of lactation for cows receiving the low, intermediate, and high vitamin E treatments, respectively. Cows with plasma concentrations of α-tocopherol less than 3.0 µg/ml at calving were 9.4 times more likely to have clinical mastitis during the first 7 days of lactation than were cows with concentrations greater than 3.0 µg/ml (Weiss et al., 1997).

Many attempts have been made to control lipid oxidation in meats through the use of antioxidants. One such approach is through dietary supplementation of vitamin E, which functions as a lipid-soluble antioxidant in cell membranes (Linder, 1985), thus protecting phospholipids and even cholesterol against oxidation. Increased dietary levels of vitamin E result in higher tissue α-tocopherol concentrations and greater stability of these tissues toward lipid oxidation and thus, for example, increased shelf-life of pork (Soler-Velásquez et al., 1998; Corino et al., 1999; Lauridsen et al., 1999). Buckley and Connolly (1980) reduced the rate of rancidity development in frozen pork by including vitamin E in the feed (80 mg per day per animal) for 7 days before slaughter of the pigs. Likewise, meat from turkeys raised on vitamin E-supplemented diets was more resistant to rancidity development than meat from birds receiving control diets (Uebersax et al., 1978; Bartov et al., 1983).

Dramatic effects of vitamin E supplementation (500 IU per head daily) to finishing steers on the stability of beef color have been observed (Faustman et al., 1989a). Loin steaks of control steers discolored 2 to 3 days sooner than those of steers supplemented with vitamin E. Supplemental dietary vitamin E extended the color shelf-life of loin steaks from 3.7 to 6.3 days. This was most likely due to the increased α-tocopherol content of the loin tissue of the supplemented animals, which was approximately fourfold greater than that of the controls (Faustman et al., 1989a). Color is an extremely critical component of fresh red meat appearance and greatly influences the customer's perception of meat quality. Steaks from cattle supplemented with vitamin E were preferred over those from controls by 91% of Japanese survey participants (N = 10,941), and 58% of all participants identified muscle color as the most important factor in selecting beef products (Sanders et al., 1997).

In a subsequent report, Faustman et al. (1989b) observed that vitamin E stabilized the pigments and lipids of meat from the supplemented steers. Perhaps the vitamin E-supplemented steers were able to incorporate a greater amount of vitamin E into cellular membranes, where it can perform its antioxidant function. The effects of vitamin E as an in vivo lipid stabilizer and its effect on flavor and storage properties of various meats have been reviewed. Supplementing cattle with vitamin E resulted in steaks that exhibited superior lean color, less surface discoloration, more desirable overall appearance, and less lipid oxidation during retail display than control steaks (Sanders et al., 1997). Vitamin E also plays a role in controlling the color of veal calf meat. Combined feeding of monosodium phosphate and 100 IU of vitamin E per calf daily produced a light-colored veal without making calves anemic (Agboola et al., 1990).

Feeding supplemental vitamin E at levels of 1,000 to 2,000 mg of naturally occurring mixed tocopherols per cow per day increased the vitamin E content of milk and its stability against oxidized flavor (Krukovsky and Loosli, 1952; Neilsen et al., 1953). The vitamin E content of milk from cows fed stored feeds was lower than that of milk from cows on pasture, and their milk was more susceptible to development of oxidized flavor (Krukovsky et al., 1950).

Feeding supplemental vitamin E as dl-α-tocopheryl acetate, providing an equivalent of 500 mg of dl-α-tocopherol per cow per day, increased the vitamin E content and oxidative stability of milk (Dunkley et al., 1967). Nicholson et al. (1991) suggested that adequate Se improves the transfer of dietary tocopherol to milk.

The need for supplementation of vitamin E is dependent on the requirement of individual species, conditions of production, and available vitamin E in food or feed sources (see Natural Sources). The primary factors that influence the need for supplementation include (1) vitamin E- and/or Se-deficient concentrates and roughages; (2) excessively dry ranges or pastures for grazing livestock; (3) confinement feeding where vitamin E-rich forages are not included, or only forages of poor quality are provided; (4) diets that contain predominantly non–α-tocopherols and thereby are less biologically active; (5) diets that include ingredients that increase vitamin E requirements (e.g., unsaturated fats, waters high in nitrates); (6) harvesting, drying, or storage conditions of feeds that result in destruction of vitamin E and/or Se (see Natural Sources); (7) accelerated rates of gain, production, and feed efficiency that increase metabolic demands for vitamin E; and (8) intensified production that also indirectly increases vitamin E needs of animals by elevating stress, which often increases susceptibility to various diseases (McDowell and Williams, 1991; McDowell, 1992). After stress, livestock may have reductions in α-tocopherol concentrations in certain tissues. Supplemental vitamin E may be required after stress to restore α-tocopherol in tissues (Nockels et al., 1996). Based on health data, Weiss (1998) suggested the vitamin E requirement should be increased at least 500% and perhaps as much as 700% above NRC recommendations for dry cows and lactating cows.

Vitamin E-Se deficiencies are found in specific world regions and are characterized by low concentrations of feedstuffs. Regions that rely on concentrate importation from these areas deficient in vitamin E and/or Se (e.g., midwestern United States) likewise must provide these nutrients to livestock. Adverse conditions, such as poor weather (drought and early frost), molds, and insect infestation, will reduce the vitamin E value of feedstuffs. The vitamin E activity in blighted corn was 59% lower than that in sound corn, and the vitamin E activity in lightweight corn averaged 21% below that in sound corn (Hoffmann-LaRoche, 1994). Feed spoilage will also promote vitamin E-Se deficiencies; therefore, to prevent loss of vitamin E in diets, the producer should use fresh feed at all times because the vitamin is rapidly destroyed under hot, humid conditions. Also, the producer should use an antioxidant in the diet to prevent the destruction of the vitamin E (as well as other vitamins, e.g., vitamin A). Losses during storage increase as the duration and temperature of storage increase. Rate of oxidation of natural tocopherols is increased in diets containing increased levels of copper, iron, zinc, or manganese (Dove and Ewan, 1991).

In pet foods, the most important feed ingredient that will dictate the need for vitamin E supplementation is fat source and the stability of the fat source. Large amounts of PUFA can quickly precipitate vitamin E deficiency. Fats from oilseeds are normally not highly detrimental because the oils, in addition to containing high amounts of predominantly linoleic acid (18:2), likewise are sources of vitamin E. Fish oils, however, contain little vitamin E and are highly destructive to vitamin E stores and greatly increase the requirements of the vitamin. This can be a problem for cats, since their diets can be very high in fish and fish oils. The long-chain, highly unsaturated fatty acids in fish oil can quickly deplete the cat's body stores of vitamin E. A diet that contains high levels of fish oil may cause a threefold to fourfold increase in a cat's daily requirement for vitamin E. Pets should never be fed rancid fats as they will quickly bring about destruction of fat-soluble vitamins.

The ability of vitamin E to affect growth, health, and reproduction of animals is documented. A vitamin E supplementation program utilizing both parenteral and oral administration is often suggested, particularly when fresh green pasture is lacking. Mahan (1991) assessed the influence of low supplemental vitamin E (< 16 IU/kg) to sows and offspring in three parities. Smaller litter size, sow agalactia, and pig mortality during the first week after birth resulted from inadequate supplemental vitamin E to breeding sows.

Exercise has an influence on vitamin E requirements and needed supplementation (Davies et al., 1982; Valberg et al., 1993). Dietary levels of vitamin E greater than the 80 IU/kg dry matter, and potentially approaching 300 IU/kg dry matter, are required to maintain blood and muscle vitamin E concentrations in horses undergoing exercise conditioning. The level of vitamin E recommended by the NRC for working horses, 80 IU/kg dry matter, will not maintain serum vitamin E levels.

In humans, vitamin E supplements may protect overworked muscles during exercise. In a pair of studies, sedentary men took either a placebo or 530 mg of vitamin E every day for 7 weeks. They then performed a vigorous 45-minute workout on the treadmill. After the workout, blood samples from the men who took vitamin E contained smaller amounts of chemicals that promote inflammation. That effect, the researchers speculated, should limit both soreness and injury after strenuous exercise (Consumer Report on Health, 1993).

Good experimental evidence indicates a need for supplemental vitamin E in the diets of pregnant and lactating women, newborn infants (particularly premature infants), and older persons suffering from circulatory disturbances and intermittent claudication. Chronic diarrhea is also associated with reduced absorption of vitamin E (Liuzzi et al., 1998). Higher levels may be indicated for persons exposed to oxygen and environmental pollutants, such as ozone, nitrites, and heavy metals. Feeding LBW infants entails problems somewhat different from those of normal-weight infants. Because of their reduced absorption of fat, utilization of α-tocopherol is impaired; thus special effort is required to ensure adequate intake. The American Academy of Pediatrics

Committee on Nutrition (1977) recommended that formulas for these infants should provide 5 IU of water-soluble α-tocopherol daily.

There are human health benefits of consumption of higher levels of vitamin E (Vitamin E Research and Information Service, 1993; McDowell et al., 1996). Typical human vitamin E supplementation levels are 200 to 800 IU daily. The antioxidant nutrients, vitamin E, vitamin C, and β-carotene, have become the focus for their protective role in disease prevention, particularly cardiovascular disease (atherosclerosis) and cancer. Vitamin E also has a beneficial effect in preventing eye disorders, skin diseases, ulcers, and intermittent claudication (inadequate blood flow). Vitamin E may reduce atherosclerosis by preventing low-density lipoproteins from oxidizing and causing arterial injury.

Antioxidants influence the virulence of virus infections. In a healthy state, a virus would be benign or less virulent. Vitamin E deficiency may allow viruses to cause disease and may have important implications for enterovirus-induced inflammatory heart disease in adult human populations (Beck et al., 1994).

TOXICITY

Compared with vitamin A and vitamin D, both acute and chronic studies with animals have shown that vitamin E is relatively nontoxic but not entirely devoid of undesirable effects. Hypervitaminosis E studies in rats, chicks, and humans indicate maximum tolerable levels in the range of 1,000 to 2,000 IU/kg of diet (NRC, 1987).

Massive doses of vitamin E (5,000 mg of dl-α-tocopherol per kilogram of diet) caused reduced packed-cell volumes in trout (NRC, 1993). Administration of vitamin E to vitamin K-deficient rats, dogs, chicks, and humans exacerbated the coagulation defect associated with vitamin K deficiency (Corrigan, 1982). In chickens, the effects of vitamin E toxicity are depressed growth rate, reduced hematocrit, reticulocytosis, increased prothrombin time (corrected by injecting vitamin K), and reduced calcium and phosphorus in dry, fat-free bone ash (NRC, 1987).

In humans, isolated and inconsistent reports have appeared on the adverse effects from high intakes of dl-α-tocopheryl acetate, but most adults appear to tolerate these doses. Negative effects in human subjects consuming up to 1,000 IU of vitamin E per day included headache, fatigue, nausea, muscular weakness, and double vision. Large doses of α-tocopherol in anemic children suppress normal hematological response to parenteral iron administration (RDA, 1989).

216

■ REFERENCES

Adams, C.R. (1973). Effect of Processing on the Nutritional Value of Feeds, p. 142. National Adacemy of Sciences, Washington D.C.

Adamstone, F.B., Krider, J.L., and James, M.F. (1949). *Ann. N.Y. Acad. Sci. 52,* 260.

Agboola, H.A., Cahill, V.R., Conrad, H.R., Ockerman, H.W., Parker, C.F., Parrett, N.A., and Long, A.R. (1990). *J. Anim. Sci. 68,* 117.

American Academy of Pediatrics, Committee on Nutrition (1977). *Pediatrics 60,* 19.

Anderson, H.D., Elvehjem, C.A., and Gonce Jr., J.E. (1939). *Proc. Soc. Exp. Biol. Med. 42,* 750.

Anderson, H.D., Elvehjem, C.A., and Gonce Jr., J.E. (1940). *J. Nutr. 20,* 433.

Anderson, P.H., Berrett, S., and Patterson, D.S. (1976). *Vet. Rec. 99,* 316.

Andrews, E.D., Hartley, W.J., and Grunt, A.B. (1968). *N.Z. Vet. J. 16,* 3.

Baalsrud, K.J., and Overnes, G. (1986). *Eq. Vet. J. 18,* 472.

Badwey, J.A., and Karnovsky, M.L. (1980). *Ann. Rev. Biochem. 49,* 695.

Barton, C.R., and Allen, W.M. (1973). *Vet. Rec. 92,* 288.

Bartov, I., Basker, D., and Angel, S. (1983). *Poult. Sci. 62,* 1224.

Bauernfeind, J.C. (1969). *World Rev. Anim. Prod. 5,* 20.

Bauernfeind, J.C. (1980). *In* Vitamin E: A Comprehensive Treatise, p. 99 (L.J. Machlin, Ed.). Marcel Dekker, New York.

Beck, M.A. (1997). *J. Nutr. 127,* 966S.

Beck, M.A., Kolbeck, P.C., Kohr, L.H., Shi, Q., Morris, V.C., and Levander, O.A. (1994). *J. Nutr. 124,* 345.

Bell, J.G., Cowey, C.B., Adron, J.W., and Shanks, A.M. (1985). *Br. J. Nutr. 53,* 149.

Bendich, A. (1987). *In* Proc. Roche Technical Symposium: The Role of Vitamins on Animal Performance and Immune Response. RCD 7442. Hoffmann-La Roche Inc., Nutley, New Jersey.

Bendich, A., Gabriel, E., and Machlin, L.J. (1986). *J. Nutr. 116,* 675.

Bieri, J.G., and Prival, E.L. (1965). *Proc. Soc. Exp. Med. 120,* 554.

Blaxter, K.L. (1962). *Proc. Nutr. Soc. 21,* 211.

Bostedt, H. (1980). *Collegium Vet. 61,* 45.

Bragdon, J.H., and Levine, D.H. (1949). *Am. J. Pathol. 25,* 265.

Brownlee, N.R., Huttner, J.J., and Panganamala, R.V. (1977). *J. Lipid Res. 18,* 635.

Buckley, D.J., and Connolly, J.F. (1980). *J. Food Protect. 43,* 265.

Burkholder, W.J., and Swecker, W.S. (1990). *Semin. Vet. Med. Surg. (Small Anim.) 5*(3), 154.

Cavalier, S.J., and Gambetti, P. (1981). *Neurology 31,* 714.

Charmley, E. Hidiroglou, N., Ochoa, L., McDowell, L.R., and Hidiroglou, M. (1992). *J. Dairy Sci. 75,* 804.

Chavance, M., Herbeth, B., Fournier, C., Janot, C., and Vernhes, G. (1989). *Eur. J. Clin. Nutr. 43,* 827.

Chew, B.P. (1995). *J. Nutr. 125,* 1804S.

Chow, C.K. (1979). *Am. J. CLin. Nutr. 32,* 1066.

Chung, Y.K., and Mahan, D.C. (1995). *Korean J. Anim. Sci. 37,* 616.

Cipriano, J.E., Morrill, J.L., and Anderson, N.V. (1982). *J. Dairy Sci. 65,* 2357.

Codner, E.C., and Thatcher, C.D. (1993). *Compend. Cont. Educ. Small Anim. 15,* 411.

Coelho, M.B. (1991). Vitamin Stability in Premixes and Feeds: A practical approach, p. 56. BASF Technical Symposium, Bloomington, Minnesota.

Cohen, H., and Lapointe, M.R. (1980). *J. Assoc. Off. Anal. Chem. 63,* 1254.

Combs Jr., G.F., and Combs, S.B. (1986). The Role of Selenium. Academic Press, Inc., New York.

Consumer Report on Health. (1993). 5(4), 33.

Cordy, D.R. (1954). *Cornell Vet. 44,* 310.

Corino, C., Oriani, G., Pantaleo, L., Pastorelli, G., and Salvatori, G. (1999). *J. Anim. Sci. 71,* 1755.

Corrigan, J. (1982). *Ann. N.Y. Acad.Sci. 393,* 361.

Cort, W.M., Vincente, T.S., and Waysek, E.H. (1983). *J. Agric. Food Chem. 31,* 1330.

Creech, B.G., Feldman, G.L., Ferguson, I.M., Reid, R.L., and Couch, J.R. (1957). *J. Nutr. 62,* 83.

Davies, J.A., Quintanilha, A.T., Brooks, G.A., and Packer, L. (1982). *Biochem. Biophys. Res. Comm. 107,* 1198.

Dewes, H.F. (1981). *N.Z. Vet. J. 29,* 83.

Dierenfeld, E.S. (1989). *J. Zoo. Wildl. Med. 20,* 3.

Dierenfeld, E.S. (1994). *J. Nutr. 124,* 2579S.

Dierenfeld, E.S., and Dolensek, E.P. (1988). *Zoo Biol. 7,* 165.

Dierenfeld, E.S., and Traber, M.G. (1992). *In* Vitamin E in Health and Disease (L. Packer and J. Fuchs, eds.), p. 345. Marcel Dekker, New York.

Dill, S.G., and Rebhun, W.C. (1985). *Compend. Cont. Educ. Pract. Vet. 7,* S627.

Dove, C.R., and Ewan, R.C. (1990). *J. Anim. Sci. 68,* 2407.

Dove, C.R., and Ewan, R.C. (1991). *J. Anim. Sci. 69,* 1994.

Drouchner, W. (1976). *Ubers Terernahrung 4,* 93.

Dunkley, W.L., Ronning, M., Franke, A.A., and Robb, J. (1967). *J. Dairy Sci. 50,* 492.

Elvehjem, C.A., Gonce Jr., J.E., and Newell, G.W. (1944). *J. Pediatr. 24,* 436.

Erskine, R.J., Eberhart, R.J., Grasso, P.J., and Scholz, R.W. (1989). *Proc. Am. Assoc. Bovine Pract.* p. 119, Calgary, Alberta, Canada.

Evans, H.M. (1925). *Proc. Natl. Acad. Sci. U.S.A. 11,* 373.

Faustman, C., Cassens, R.G., Schaefer, D.M., Buege, D.R., and Scheller, K.K. (1989a). *J. Food Sci. 54(2),* 485.

Faustman, C., Cassens, R.G., Schaefer, D.M., Buege, D.R., Williams, S.N., and Scheller, K.K. (1989b). *J. Food Sci. 54(4),* 838.

Finch, J.M., and Turner, R.J. (1989). *Vet. Immunol. Immunopathol. 23,* 245.

Franklin, S.T., Sorenson, C.E., and Hammell, D.C. (1998). *J. Dairy Sci. 81,* 2623.

Friedrichsen, J.V., Arascott, G.H. and Willis, D.L. (1980). *Nutr. Rep. Int. 22,* 41.

Fritsche, K.L., and McGuire, S.O. (1996). *J. Nutr. Biochem. 7,* 623.

Gallo-Torres, H.E. (1980). *In* Vitamin E. A Comprehensive Treatise (L.S. Machlin, ed.), p. 193. Marcel Dekker, New York.

Gardner, H.W. (1989). *Free Radic. Biol. Med. 7,* 65.

Gatlin, D.M. III, Poe, W.E., and Wilson, R.P. (1986). *J. Nutr. 116*, 1061.

Gershoff, S.N., and Norkin, S.A. (1962). *J. Nutr. 77*, 303.

Gill, D.R., Smith, R.A., Hicks, R.B., and Ball, R.L. (1986). *Ok. Agra. Exp. Sta. Res. Rep. MP 118*, 240.

Gitter, M., and Bradley, R. (1978). *Vet. Rec. 103*, 24.

Glienke, L.R., and Ewan, R.C. (1974). *J. Anim. Sci. 39*, 975(Abstr).

Golub, M.S., and Gershwin, M.E. (1985). *In* Animal Stress (G.P. Moberg, ed.) *Am. J. Physiol. Soc.* Bethesda, Maryland.

Gullickson, T.W., Palmer, L.S., Boyd, W.L., Nelson, J.W., Olson, F.C., Calverley, C.E., and Boyer, P.D. (1949). *J. Dairy Sci. 32*, 495.

Guss, S.B. (1977). Management and Diseases of Dairy Goats, Dairy Goat Journal Publ. Corp., Scottsdale, Arizona.

Hadden, J.W. (1987). *Ann. N.Y. Acad. Sci. 496*, 39.

Haeger, K. (1974). *J. Clin. Nutr. 27*, 1179.

Hardy, B., and Frape, D.L. (1983). Micronutrients and Reproduction, No. 1895. Hoffmann-La Roche, Basel.

Hargis, A.M., Haupt, K.H., and Prieur, D.J. (1985). *Compend. Contin. Educ. Pract. Vet. 7*(4), 306.

Harris, P.L., and Embree, N.D. (1963). *Am. J. CLin. Nutr. 13*, 385.

Harrison, J.H., Hancock, D.D., and Conrad, H.R. (1984). *J. Dairy Sci. 67*, 123.

Hartley, W.J., and Grant, A.B. (1961). *Fed. Proc. Fed. Am. Soc. Exp. Biol. 20*, 679.

Harvey, J.D., and Bieber-Wlaschny, M. (1988). *Feedstuffs 60*(12), 15.

Hayes, K.C., and Rousseau, J.E. (1970). *Lab. Anim. Care 20*, 48.

Hayes, K.C., Nielsen, S.W., and Rousseau Jr., J.E. (1969). *J. Nutr. 99*, 196.

Heinzerling, P.H., Rollin, C.F., Nockels, C., Quarles, L., and Tengerdy, R.P. (1974). *Proc. Exp. Biol. Med. 146*, 279.

Helgebostad, A., and Ender, F. (1973). *Acta Agric. Scand. Suppl. 19*, 79.

Herdt, T.H., and Stowe, H.D. (1991). *Vet. Clin. North Am. Food Anim. Pract. 7*, 391.

Hidiroglou, M. (1989). *J. Dairy Sci. 72*, 1067.

Hidiroglou, M., and Charmley, E. (1991). *Am. J. Vet. Res. 52*, 640.

Hidiroglou, M., and Singh, K. (1991). *J. Dairy Sci. 74*, 2718.

Hidiroglou, M., Hoffman, I., and Jenkins, K.J. (1969). *Can. J. Physiol. Pharmacol. 47*, 953.

Hidiroglou, M., McAllister, A.J., and Williams, C.J. (1987). *J. Dairy Sci. 70*, 1281.

Hidiroglou, N, and McDowell, L. (1987). *Int. J. Vitam. Res. 57*, 261.

Hidiroglou, N., Laflamme, L.F., and McDowell, L.R. (1988a). *J. Anim. Sci. 66*, 3227.

Hidiroglou, N., McDowell, L.R., and Pastrana, R. (1988b). *Int. J. Vitam. Nutr. Res. 58*, 189.

Hidiroglou, N., McDowell, L.R., and Balbuena, O. (1989). *J. Dairy Sci. 72*, 1793.

Hidiroglou, N., Butler, G., and McDowell, L.R. (1990). *J. Anim. Sci. 68*, 782.

Hidiroglou, N., McDowell, L.R., Papas, A.M., Antapli, M., and Wilkinson, N.S. (1992a). *J. Anim. Sci. 70*, 2556.

Hidiroglou, N., Cave, N., Atwal, A.S., Farnsworth, E.R., and McDowell, L.R.

(1992b). *Ann. Rech. Vet. 23*, 337.

Hidiroglou, N., McDowell, L.R., Batra, T.R., and Papas, A.M. (1994). *Reprod. Nutr. Dev. 34*, 133.

Hill, G.M., Link, J.E., Meyer, L., and Fritsche, K.L. (1999). *J. Anim. Sci. 77*, 1762.

Hintz, H.F. (1996). *In* Vitamin E in Animal Nutrition and Management, (M.B. Coelho, ed.), 2nd Ed., p. 449, BASP Corporation, Mount Olive, New Jersey.

Hoekstra, W.G. (1975). *Fed. Proc. 34*, 2083.

Hoffmann-La Roche. (1972). Vitamin E, No. 1206. F. Hoffmann-La Roche & Co. Ltd., Basel, Switzerland.

Hoffmann-La Roche. (1991). Vitamin E for Ruminants. RCD 8361/191. Hoffmann-La Roche Inc., Nutley, New Jersey.

Hoffmann-La Roche. (1994). Vitamin Nutrition for Ruminants. RCD 87751/894. Hoffmann-La Roche Inc., Nutley, New Jersey.

Hove, E.L., Fry, G.S., and Schwarz, K. (1958). *Proc. Soc. Exp. Biol. Med. 98*, 27.

Hutchinson, L.J., Scholz, W., and Drake, T.R. (1982). *J. Am. Vet. Med. Assoc. 181*, 581.

Jacob, R.A. (1995). *Nutr. Res. 15*, 755.

Jager, F.C. (1977). *Nutr. Metabol. 14*, 210.

Jensen, L.S. (1968). *Proc. Soc. Exp. Biol. Med. 128*, 970.

Jensen, L.S., and McGinnis, J. (1957). *Poult. Sci. 36*, 212.

Jensen, S.K., Engberg, R.M., and Hedemann, M.S. (1999). *J. Nutr. 129*, 1355.

Jialal, I., and Grundy, S.M. (1993). *Circulation 88*, 2780.

King, R.L., Burrows, F.A., Hemken, R.W., and Bashore, D.L. (1967). *J. Dairy Sci. 50*, 943.

Kozicki, L., Silva, R.G., and Barnabe, R.C. (1981). *Vet. Med. 28*, 538.

Krukovsky, V.N., and Loosli, J.K. (1952). *J. Dairy Sci. 35*, 834.

Krukovsky, V.N., Whiting, F., and Loosli, J.K. (1950). *J. Dairy Sci. 33*, 791.

Langseth, L. (1995a). *Antiox. Vitam. Newsl. 11*, 1.

Langseth, L. (1995b). *Antiox. Vitam. Newsl. 12*, 1.

Langweiler, M., Sheffy, B.E., and Schultz, R.D. (1983). *Am. J. Vet. Res. 44*, 5.

Lauridsen, C., Nielsen, J.H., Henckel, P., and Sørensen, M.T. (1999). *J. Anim. Sci. 77*, 105.

Lee, R.W., Stuart, R.L., Perryman, K.R., and Ridenour, K.W. (1985). *J. Anim. Sci. 61*(Suppl. 1), 425.

Linder, M.C. (1985). *In* Nutritional Biochemistry and Metabolism (M.C. Linder, ed.). Elsevier Sci. Publ. Co., New York.

Liu, J.F., and Huang, C.J. (1995). *J. Nutr. 125*, 3071.

Liu, J.F., and Huang, C.J. (1996). *J. Nutr. 126*, 2227.

Liu, S.K., Dolensek, E.P., Adams, C.R. and Tappe, J.P. (1983). *J. Am. Vet. Med. Assoc. 183*, 1266.

Liu, S.K., Dolensek, E.P. and Tappe, J.P. (1985). *Heart Vessels 1*(Suppl.), 282.

Liuzzi, J.P., Cioccia, A.M., and Hevia, P. (1998). *J. Nutr. 128*, 2467.

Lopez-Bote, C.J., Rey, A.I., Sanz, M., Gray, J.I., and Buckley, D.J. (1997). *J. Nutr. 127*, 1176.

Machlin, L.J. (1991). *In* Handbook of Vitamins (L.J. Machlin, ed.), p. 99.

Marcel Dekker, Inc., New York.

Mahan, D.C. (1991). *J. Anim. Sci. 69*, 2904.

Mahan, D.C., and Vallet, J.L. (1997). *J. Anim. Sci. 75*, 2731.

Marin-Guzman, J., Mahan, D.C., Chung, Y.K., Pate, J.L., and Pope, W.F. (1997). *J. Anim. Sci. 75*, 2994.

Marin-Guzman, J., Mahan, D.C., Jones, L.S., and Pate, J.L. (1989). *Ohio Swine Res. Ind. Rep.* The Ohio State Univ., Anim. Sci. Dept. Series 89-1, p. 20.

Mason, R.M., Ostrum, P., and McDowell, L.R. (1985). *Florida Cattlemen, March*, 1993.

Maynard, L.A., Loosli, J.K., Hintz, H.F., and Warner, R.G. (1979). *In* Animal Nutrition, 7th Ed., p. 283. McGraw-Hill, New York.

McCay, P.B., Gibson, D.D., and Hornbrook, K.R. (1981). *Fed. Proc. 40*, 199.

McDowell, L.R. (1985). *In* Nutrition of Grazing Ruminants in Warm Climates (L.R. McDowell, ed.), p. 339. Academic Press, Orlando, Florida.

McDowell, L.R. (1992) Minerals in Animals and Human Nutrition. Academic Press, San Diego, California.

McDowell, L.R. (1997). Minerals for Grazing Ruminants in Tropical Regions, 3rd Ed. University of Florida, Gainesville.

McDowell, L.R., and Williams, S.N. (1991). *In* 2nd Annual Florida Ruminant Nutrition Symposium, p. 46. Gainesville, Florida.

McDowell, L.R., Froseth, J.H., Piper, R.C., Dyer, I.A., and Kroening, G.H. (1977). *J. Anim. Sci. 45*, 1326.

McDowell, L.R., Williams, S.N., Hidiroglou, N., Njeru, C.A., Hill, G.M., Ochoa, L., and Wilkinson, N.S. (1996). *Anim. Feed Sci. Tech. 60*, 273.

McGuire, S.O., Alexander D.W., and Fritsche, K.L. (1997). *J. Nutr. 127*, 1388.

McIntosh, G.H., Lawson, C.A., Bulman, F.H., and McMurchie, E.J. (1985). *Proc. Nutr. Soc. Australia 10*, 207.

McMurray, C.H., and Blanchflower, W.J. (1979). *J. Chromatogr. 178*, 525.

McMurray, C.H., and Rice, D.A. (1984). Vitamin E and Selenium Deficiency Diseases, No. 1953. Hoffmann-La Roche, Basel.

McMurray, C.H., Rice, D.A., and Blanchflower, W.J. (1980). *Proc. Nutr. Soc. 39*, 65(Abstr).

Meydani, S.N. (1995). *Nutr. Rev. 53*, 552.

Michel, R.L., Whitehair, C.K., and Keahey, K.K. (1969). *J. Am. Vet. Med. Assoc. 155*, 50.

Miller, W.H. Jr. (1989). *Vet. Clin. North Am. Small Anim. Pract. 19*(3), 497.

Moore, R.M., and Kohn, C.W. (1991). *Compend. Cont. Educ. Pract. Vet. 13*, 476.

Moore, T., Sharman, I.M., and Ward, R.J. (1957). *J. Sci. Food Agric. 8*, 97.

Morrow, J.L., McGlone, J.J., Tribble, L.F., and Stansbury, W.F. (1987). *Anim. Sci. Res. Rpt. Texas Tech.*, p. 14, Lubbock, Texas.

Morand-Fehr, P. (1981). *In* Goat Production, p. 193 (G. Gall, Ed.). Academic Press, New York.

Muller G.H., Kirk, R.W., and Scott, D.W. (1989). *In* Small Animal Dermatology, 4th Ed., p. 658. W.B. Saunders Co., Philadelphia.

Munson, T.O., Holzworth, J., Small, E., Witzel, S., Jones, T.C., and Luginbuhl, H. (1958). *J. Am. Vet. Med. Assoc. 133*, 563.

Muth, O.H. (1955). *J. Am. Vet. Med. Assoc. 126*, 355.

Neilsen, J., Fisher, A.N., and Pedersen, A.H. (1953). *J. Dairy Res. 20,* 333.

Nicholson, J.W., St. Laurent, A.M., McQueen, R.E., and Charmley, E. (1991). *Can. J. Anim. Sci. 71,* 143.

Njeru, C.A., McDowell, L.R., Wilkinson, N.S., Linda, S.B., Williams, S.N., and Lentz, E.L. (1992). *J. Anim. Sci. 70,* 2562.

Njeru, C.A., McDowell, L.R., Wilkinson, N.S., Linda, S.B., and Williams, S.N. (1994a). *J. Anim. Sci. 72,* 1636.

Njeru, C.A., McDowell, L.R., Wilkinson, N.S., Linda, S.B., Rojas, L.X., and Williams, S.N. (1994b). *J. Anim. Sci. 72,* 739.

Noble, R.E., Moore, J.H., and Harfoot, C.G. (1974). *Br. J. Nutr. 31,* 99.

Nockels, C.F. (1990). *In* Proc. National Feed Ingredients Association Nutrition Institute: Developments in Vitamin Nutrition and Health Applications, Kansas City, Missouri. National Feed Ingredients Association (NFIA), Des Moines, Iowa.

Nockels, C.F. (1991). Vitamin E requirement of beef cattle: Influencing factors. BASF Technical Symposium, p. 40. Bloomington, Minnesota.

Nockels, C.F., Odde, K.G., and Craig, A.M. (1996). *J. Anim. Sci. 74,* 672.

NRC. Nutrient Requirements of Domestic Animals. National Academy of Sciences-National Research Council, Washington, D.C.

(1977). Nutrient Requirements of Rabbits, 2nd Ed.

(1978). Nutrient Requirements of Nonhuman Primates.

(1982a). Nutrient Requirements of Mink and Foxes.

(1985a). Nutrient Requirements of Dogs, 2nd Ed.

(1985b). Nutrient Requirements of Sheep, 5th Ed.

(1986). Nutrient Requirements of Cats, 3rd Ed.

(1989a). Nutrient Requirements of Dairy Cattle, 6th Ed.

(1989b). Nutrient Requirements of Horses, 5th Ed.

(1993). Nutrient Requirements of Fish.

(1994). Nutrient Requirements of Poultry, 9th Ed.

(1995). Nutrient Requirements of Laboratory Animals, 4th Ed.

(1996). Nutrient Requirements of Beef Cattle, 7th Ed.

(1998). Nutrient Requirements of Swine, 10th Ed.

NRC. (1987). Vitamin Tolerance of Animals. National Academy of Sciences-National Research Council, Washington, D.C.

Obel, A.L. (1953). *Acta Pathol. Microbiol. Scand. Suppl. 94,* 5.

Ochoa, L., McDowell, L.R., Williams, S.N., Wilkinson, N., Boucher, J., and Lentz, E.L. (1992). *J. Anim. Sci. 70,* 2568.

Orstadius, K., Nordstrom, G., and Lannek, N. (1963). *Cornell Vet. 53,* 60.

Oski, F.A., and Barness, L.A. (1967). *J. Pediatr. 70,* 211.

Padh, H. (1991). *Nutr. Rev. 49,* 65.

Panganamala, R.V., and Cornwell, D.C. (1982). *Ann. N.Y. Acad. Sci. 393,* 376.

Pappenheimer, A.M. (1942). *Am. J. Pathol. 18,* 169.

Pappenheimer, A.M., and Goettsch,M. (1931). *J. Exp. Med. 53,* 11.

Pappu, A.S., Fatterpacker, P., and Sreenivasan, A. (1978). *Biochem. J. 172,* 115.

Peplowski, M.A., Mahan, D.C., Murray, F.A., Moxon, A.L., Cantor, A.H., and Ekstrom, K.E. (1981). *J. Anim. Sci. 51,* 344.

Piper, R.C., Froseth, J.A., McDowell, L.R., Kroening, G.H., and Dyer, I.A. (1975). *Am. J. Vet. Res. 36,* 273.

Poston, H.A., G.F. Combs Jr., and Leibovitz, L. (1976). *J. Nutr. 106*, 892.

Pruiett, S.P., Morrill, J.L., Blecha, F., Reddy, P.G., Higgins, J., and Anderson, N.V. (1989). *J. Anim. Sci. 67*(Suppl 1), 243.

Putnam, M.E. (1984). *Pig Vet. Soc. Proc. 9*, 178.

Putnam, M.E. (1986). *Mod. Vet. Pract. 67*, 121.

Rajaraman, V., Nonneche, B.J., Franklin, S.T., Hammell, D.C., and Horst, R.L. (1998). *J. Dairy Sci. 81*, 3278.

RDA. (1989). Recommended Dietary Allowances, 9th Ed., National Academy of Sciences-National Research Council, Washington, D.C.

Reddy, P.G., Morrill, J.J., and Frey, R.A. (1987a). *J. Dairy Sci. 70*, 123.

Reddy, P.G., Morrill, J.L., Minocha, H.C., and Stevenson, J.S. (1987b). *J. Dairy Sci. 70*, 993.

Reffett, J.K, Spears, J.W., and Brown, Jr., T.T. (1988). *J. Anim. Sci. 66*, 1520.

Rice, D.A., Blanchflower, W.J., and McMurray, C.H. (1981). *Vet. Rec. 109*, 161.

Riedel-Caspari, G., Schmidt, F.W., Gunther, K.D., and Wagner, K. (1986). *J. Vet. Med. 33*, 650.

Riis, R.C., Sheffy, B.E., and Loew, E. (1981). *Am. J. Vet. Res. 42*, 74.

Ringer, D.H., and Abrams, G.D. (1970). *J. Am. Vet. Med. Assoc. 157*, 1228.

Roquet, J., Nockels, C.F., and Papas, A.M. (1992). *J. Anim. Sci. 70*, 2542.

Rumsey, T.S. (1975). *Feedstuffs 47*, 30.

Sanders, S.K., Morgan, J.B., Wulf, D.M., Tatum, J.D., Williams, S.N., and Smith, G.C. (1997). *J. Anim. Sci. 75*, 2634.

Sarter, M., and Van Der Linde, A. (1987). *Neurobiol. Aging 8*, 297.

Scott, D.S., and Sheffy, B.E. (1987). *Companion Anim. Pract. 1*(4), 42.

Scott, D.W., and Walton, D.K. (1985). *J. Am. Anim. Hosp. Assoc. 21*, 345.

Scott, D.W., Walton, D.K., Manning, T.O., Smith, C.A., and Lewis, R.M. (1983). *J. Am. Anim. Hosp. Assoc. 19*, 481.

Scott, M.L. (1980). *Fed. Proc. Fed. Am. Soc. Exp. Biol. 39*, 2736.

Scott, M.L., Nesheim, M.C., and Young, R.J. (1982). Nutrition of the Chicken, p. 119. Scott, Ithaca, New York.

Sergeev, I.N., Aarkhapchev, Y.P., and Spirichev, V.B. (1990). *Biokhimiya-Engl. Tr. 55*, 1483.

Sheffy, B.E. (1979). *Compend. Cont. Ed. 1*, 759.

Sheffy, B.E., and Schultz, R.D. (1979). *Cornell Vet. 68*, 48.

Sheffy, B.E., and Williams, A.J. (1981). Animal Nutrition Events, p. 1. 1781 Hoffmann-La Roche, Basel, Switzerland.

Shimotori, N., Emerson, G.A., and Evans, H.M. (1940). *J. Nutr. 19*, 547.

Sitrin, M.D., Liberman, F., Jensen, W.E., Noronha, A., Milburn, C., and Addington, W. (1987). *Ann. Intern. Med. 107*, 51.

Smith, K., Hogan, J.S., and Weiss, W.P. (1997). *J. Anim. Sci. 75*, 1659.

Smith, K.L., and Conrad, H.R. (1987). Proc. Roche Technical Symposium. The Role of Vitamins on Animals Performance and Immune Response, p. 47. Daytona Beach, Florida.

Smith, K.L., Harrison, J.H., Hancock, D.D., Todhunter, D.A., and Conrad, H.R. (1984). *J. Dairy Sci. 67*, 1293.

Smith, P.J., Tappel, A.L., and Chow, C.K. (1974). *Nature (London) 247*, 392.

Smith, S.E. (1970). *In* Duke's Physiology of Domestic Animals, (M.J. Swenson, ed.), 8th Ed., p. 634. Cornell Univ. Press Ithaca, New York.

Sokol, R.J. (1989). *Free Radic. Biol. Med. 6*, 189.

Soler-Velásquez, M.P., Brendemuhl, J.H., McDowell, L.R., Sheppard, K.A., Johnson, D.D., and Williams, S.N. (1998). *J. Anim. Sci. 76*, 110.

Stephan, Z.F., and Hayes, K.C. (1978). *Fed. Proc. 73*, 706(Abstr).

Stephens, L.C., McChesney, A.E., and Nockels, C.F. (1979). *Br. Vet. J. 135*, 291.

Stuart, R.L. (1987). Proc. The Role of Vitamins on Animal Performance and Immune Response, p. 67. Hoffmann-La Roche, Nutley, New Jersey.

Sure, B. (1924). *J. Biol. Chem. 58*, 693.

Tanaka, K., Hashimoto, T., Tokumaru, S., Iguchi, H., and Kojo, S. (1997). *J. Nutr. 127*, 2060

Taylor, S.I., Lambden, M.P., and Tappel, A.L. (1976). *Lipids 11*, 530.

Tengerdy, R.P. (1980). *In* Vitamin E: A Comprehensive Treatise (L.J. Machlin, ed.). Marcel Dekker, New York.

Tengerdy, R.P. (1989). *Ann. N.Y. Acad. Sci. 570*, 335.

Thompson, J.N., and Scott, M.L. (1969). *J. Nutr. 97*, 335.

Tiege, J., Saxegaard, F., and Froslie, A. (1978). *Acta Vet. Scand. 19*, 133.

Tollersrud, S. (1973). *Acta Agric. Scand. Suppl. 19*, 124.

Tollerz, G., and Lannek, N. (1964). *Nature (London), 201*, 846.

Trapp, A.L., Keahey, K.K., Whitenack, D.L., and Whitehair, C.K. (1970). *J. Am. Vet. Med. Assoc. 157*, 289.

Turley, C.P., and Brewster, M.A. (1993). *J. Nutr. 123*, 1305.

Turner, R.J., and Finch, J.M. (1990). *J. Comparative Pathol. 102*, 16.

Uebersax, M.A., Uebersax, M.L., and Dawson, L.E. (1978). *Poult. Sci. 57*, 937.

Ullrey, D.E. (1969). Michigan State University Bulletin AH-SW-695, p. 16.

Ullrey, D.E. (1981). *J. Anim. Sci. 53*, 1039.

Ullrey, D.E. (1982). *Proc. Distill. Feed Conf. Distill. Feed Res. Counc. Cincinnati 37*, 81.

Ullrey, D.E., Miller, E.R., Ellis, D.J., Orr, D.E., Hitchcock, J.P., Keahey, K.K., and Trapp, A.L. (1971). *Mich. State Univ. Agr. Exp. Sta. Rep. Swine Res. 148*, 48.

Underwood, E.J. (1981). The Mineral Nutrition of Livestock. Commonwealth Agricultural Bureaux, London.

Valberg, S., Jonsson, L., Lindholm, A., and Holgrem. N. (1993). *Equine Vet. 25.* 11.

Van Kruiningen, J.J. (1967). *Gastroenterology 53*, 114.

Van Saun, R.J., Herdt, T.H., and Stowe, H.D. (1989). *J. Nutr. 119*, 1156.

Van Vleet, J.F. (1975). *J. Am. Vet. Med. Assoc. 166*, 769.

Van Vleet, J.F., Crawley, R.R., and Amstutz, H.E. (1977). *J. Am. Vet. Med. Assoc. 171*, 443.

Van Vleet, J.F., Runnels, L.J., Cook Jr., J.R., and Scheidt, A.B. (1987). *Am. J. Vet. Res. 48*, 1520.

Velásquez-Pereira, J., Risco, C.A., Chenoweth, P.J., McDowell, L.R., Prichard, D., Martin, F.G., Wilkinson, N.S., Williams, S.N., and Staples, C.R. (1998). *J. Anim. Sci. 76*, 2894.

Velásquez-Pereira, J., Risco, C.A., McDowell, L.R., Staples, C.R., Prichard, D., Chenoweth, P.J., Martin, F.G., Williams, S.N., Rojas, L.X., Calhoun, M.C., and Wilkinson, N.S. (1999). *J. Dairy Sci. 82*, 1240.

Vitamin E Research and Information Service. (1993). An Overview of Vitamin

E Efficacy in Humans. VERIS, LaGrange, Illinois, 24 pp.

Walter, W.D., and Jensen, L.S. (1963). *J. Nutr. 80*, 327.

Weiss, W.P. (1998). *J. Dairy Sci.* 81, 2493.

Weiss, W.P., Hogan, J.S., Smith, K.L., and Hoblet, K.H. (1990). *J. Dairy Sci. 73*, 381.

Weiss, W.P., Hogan, J.S., Todhunter, D.A., and Smith, K.L. (1997). *J. Dairy Sci. 80*, 1728.

Whanger, P.D. (1981). *In* Selenium in Biology and Medicine, (J.E. Spallholz, J.L. Martin, and H.E. Ganther, eds.), p. 230. AVI, Westport, Connecticut.

Whitehair, C.K., Vale, O.E., Loudenslager, M., and Miller, E.R. (1983). *Mich. State Univ. Agr. Exp. Sta. Res. Swine Rep. 456*, 9.

Worden, A.N. (1958). *Vet Rec. 70*, 189.

Wretlind, B.K., Orstadius, K., and Lindberg, P. (1959). *Zentralbl. Vet. Med. 6*, 963.

Williamson, H., Stowe, H.D., Bull, R.W., and Miller, E.R. (1993). *J. Anim. Sci. 71*, 2464.

Young, L.G., Lun, A., Pos, J., Forshaw, R.P., and Edmeades, D.E. (1975). *J. Anim. Sci. 40*, 495.

Young, L.G., Miller, R.B., Edmeades, D.M., Lun, A., Smith, G.C., and King, G.J. (1978). *J. Anim. Sci. 47*, 639.

VITAMIN K

INTRODUCTION

Vitamin K was the last fat-soluble vitamin to be discovered. For many years after its discovery, vitamin K appeared to be limited in its function to only the normal blood-clotting mechanism. However, vitamin K-dependent proteins have been identified that suggest roles for the vitamin in addition to that of blood coagulation. Because of the blood-clotting function, vitamin K was previously referred to as the "coagulation vitamin," "antihemorrhagic vitamin," and "prothrombin factor."

Vitamin K is indispensable for maintaining the function of the blood coagulation system in humans and all investigated animals. Even though vitamin K is synthesized by intestinal microorganisms, deficiency signs have been observed under field conditions. Poultry, and to a lesser degree pigs, are susceptible to vitamin K deficiency. In ruminants a deficiency can be caused by ingestion of spoiled sweet clover hay, which is a natural source of dicumarol (a vitamin K antagonist). In human nutrition, vitamin K is most required in infants because of insufficient intestinal synthesis and in adults in whom fat absorption is impaired.

HISTORY

This history of vitamin K discovery has been reviewed (McCollum, 1957; Almquist, 1975; Olson and Suttie, 1978; Loosli, 1991; Suttie, 1991). Hemorrhagic signs and symptoms frequently had been seen in infants, in patients with obstructive jaundice, in experimental animals maintained on purified diets, and in cattle eating moldy sweet clover hay. The presence of a dietary antihemorrhagic factor was first suspected in 1929, when Henrik Dam of Denmark fed chickens a purified low-fat diet in an attempt to determine whether they were able to synthesize cholesterol. He noted that chickens became anemic and developed subcutaneous and intermuscular hemorrhages and that blood taken from these animals clotted slowly. Hemorrhagic signs were reported by other workers using ether-extracted fish meal for chicks (McFarlane et al., 1931). Since the condition was prevented by unextracted fish meal, the curative factor was fat soluble. When the ether extracts were added back to the feed, the animals returned to normal. However, studies in a number of laboratories soon demonstrated that this disease could not be cured by administration of any of the known fat-soluble vitamins (A, D, and E) or other known physiologically active lipids.

Dam continued to study the distribution and lipid solubility of the active component in vegetable and animal sources, and in 1935 he proposed that the antihemorrhagic vitamin of the chick was a new fat-soluble vitamin that he called vitamin K, from the Danish word for coagulation (*koagulation*). At the same time, Almquist and Stokstad (1935) of California, described their success in curing the hemorrhagic disease with ether extracts of alfalfa and clearly pointed out that microbial action in fish meal and bran preparations could lead to development of antihemorrhagic activity. Of historical note, it is interesting that research journals of Almquist and Stokstad actually discovered what were later referred to as vitamins K_1 and K_2 in 1928. The paper reporting their results was delayed by university administrators, and when it was finally submitted to the journal *Science,* it was rejected. About that time, Dam's research was published. When Dam (with Doisey) later received the Nobel prize for the discovery of vitamin K, he had reportedly expected Almquist to share the prize. Doisey also contributed to the knowledge of the role of vitamin K in blood clotting (Loosli, 1991). Dam et al. (1936) demonstrated that prothrombin activity decreased in vitamin K-deficient chicks. At about the same time, the hemorrhagic condition resulting from obstructive jaundice (deficiency of bile) was shown to be due to poor absorption of vitamin K, and bleeding episodes were attributed to lack of plasma prothrombin (Suttie, 1991). This hemorrhagic condition was originally thought to be due solely to a lowered concentration of plasma prothrombin (factor II), but during the 1950s it was shown that the synthesis of three other clotting factors—VII, IX, and X—were also depressed in the deficient state.

A number of groups were involved in attempts to isolate and characterize this new vitamin, and Dam's collaboration with Karrer, of the University of Zurich, resulted in isolation of the vitamin from alfalfa as a yellow oil (Suttie, 1991). Research proceeded to show that a large number of chemical compounds possess some degree of vitamin K activity. The main source present in plants was referred to as K_1, and the form synthesized by microflora as K_2. The simplest source of vitamin K_3 is menadione, produced by laboratory synthesis. Vitamin K_1 was synthesized by three laboratories in 1939, while the structure of K_2 was elucidated in 1940 but was not synthesized until 1958 by Isler and coworkers in Switzerland.

It was only in 1974 that the metabolic role of vitamin K was elucidated, when γ-carboxyglutamate was found to be present in the vitamin K-dependent proteins but absent from the abnormal precursors that circulate in deficiency (Nelsestuen et al., 1974; Stenflo, 1974). In more recent years, four additional vitamin K-dependent proteins have been identified in plasma (C, S, Z, and M) and a major protein of the bone matrix (osteocalcin).

CHEMICAL STRUCTURE, PROPERTIES, AND ANTAGONISTS

The general term vitamin K is now used to describe not a single chemical entity but a group of quinone compounds that have characteristic antihemorrhagic effects. Vitamin K is a generic term for a homologous group of fat-soluble vitamins consisting of a 2-methyl-1,4-naphthoquinone, with the various isomers differing in the nature and length of the side chain (Fig. 5.1). When synthesized in the laboratory, it yields a mixture of cis- and trans-isomers; the cis-form has little, if any, vitamin K activity. Vitamin K extracted from plant material was named phylloquinone or vitamin K_1. Phylloquinone has a phytyl side chain composed of four isoprene units, the first of which contains a double bond.

Vitamin K-active compounds from material that had undergone bacterial fermentation were named menaquinones or vitamin K_2. The simplest form of vitamin K is the synthetic menadione (K_3), which is composed of the active nucleus (2-methyl-1,4 naphthoquinone) and has no side chain. The menaquinone family of K_2 homologs is a large series of vitamins containing unsaturated side chains that differ in number of isoprene units. Numerous natural analogs have been isolated, almost all of which are variations of the side chain at position 3. Some of these chains are quite long, with as many as 65 carbon atoms in some bacterial vitamin K forms, but none is specifically required for activity. Menaquinone-4 is synthesized in liver from ingested menadione or changed to a biologically active menaquinone by intestinal microorganisms.

229

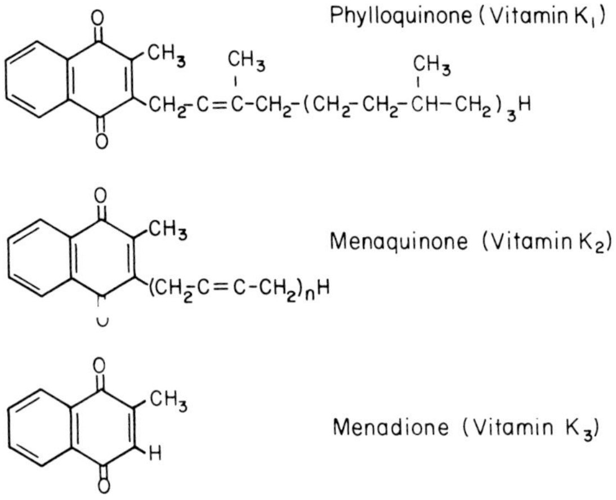

Phylloquinone (Vitamin K₁)

Menaquinone (Vitamin K₂)

Menadione (Vitamin K₃)

Fig. 5.1 Chemical structures of the vitamin K compounds.

Vitamin K is a golden yellow viscous oil. Natural sources of vitamin K are fat soluble, stable to heat, and labile to oxidation, alkali, strong acids, light, and irradiation. Vitamin K_1 is slowly degraded by atmospheric oxygen but fairly rapidly destroyed by light. In contrast to natural sources of vitamin K, some of the synthetic products, such as salts of menadione, are water soluble.

A number of vitamin K antagonists exist that increase the need for this vitamin. Vitamin K deficiency is brought about by ingestion of dicumarol (Fig. 5.2), an antagonist of vitamin K, or by feeding sulfonamides (in monogastric species) at levels sufficient to inhibit intestinal synthesis of vitamin K. Mycotoxins, toxic substances produced by molds, are also antagonists causing vitamin K deficiency. A hemorrhagic disease of cattle that was traced to consumption of moldy sweet clover hay was described in the 1920s. The destructive agent was found to be dicumarol, a substance produced from natural coumarins. Dicumarols are produced by molds, particularly those that attack sweet clover, thus giving rise to the term sweet clover disease (see Deficiency). During the process of spoiling, harmless natural coumarins in sweet clover are converted to dicumarol (bis-hydroxycoumarin), and when toxic hay or silage is consumed by animals, hypoprothrombinemia results, presumably because dicumarol combines with the proenzyme to prevent formation of the active enzyme required for the synthesis of prothrombin. It probably also interferes with synthesis of factor VII and other coagulation factors.

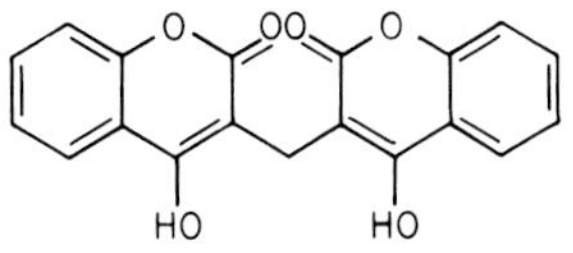

Dicumarol

3,3'-methyl-bis-(4-hydroxycoumarin)

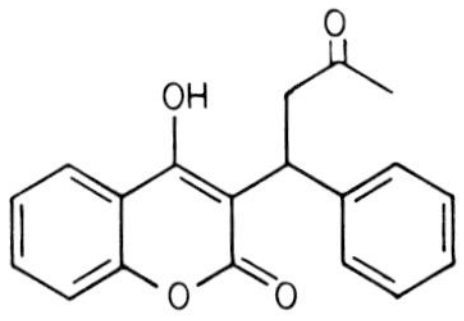

Warfarin

3-(α-acetonylbenzyl)-4-hydroxycoumarin

Fig. 5.2 Antagonists of vitamin K include coumarin derivatives.

Dicumarol serves as an anticoagulant in medicine to slow blood co-agulation in people with cardiovascular disease to avoid intravascular blood clots, just as vitamin K under other conditions increases coagula-tion time. Thus additional vitamin K will overcome this action by dicumarol. Goplen and Bell (1967) showed that in cattle, vitamin K_1 is much more potent than vitamin K_3 as an antidote to dicumarol. The most successful dicumarol for long-term lowering of the vitamin K-de-pendent clotting factors is warfarin (Fig. 5.2), which is widely used as a rodenticide. Concern has been expressed because of the identification of anticoagulant-resistant rat populations. Spread of this resistance led to synthesis of new and more effective coumarin derivatives (Hadler and Shadbolt, 1975; Suttie, 1991).

Because of the use of dicumarol derivatives as clinical anticoagu-lants, investigation of the mechanism of action of dicumarol has been of interest to vitamin K researchers (Suttie, 1991). Investigations have cen-tered on interconversion of vitamin K and its 2,3-epoxide as the site of coumarin action. One hypothesis is that metabolic effects of these com-pounds are the consequence of their inhibition of the microsomal epox-ide reductase (Bell, 1978). The epoxide apparently acts as a competitive inhibitor of vitamin K at its site of action, and a coumarin such as war-farin is an inhibitor of vitamin K action only to the extent that it in-creases the cellular ratio of oxide to the vitamin.

ANALYTICAL PROCEDURES

Vitamin K can be analyzed by a variety of color reactions or by di-rect spectroscopy. The chemical reactivity is a function of the naphtho-quinone nucleus, and other quinones also react with many of the available colorimetric assays. For spectroscopy to be successful, a significant amount of separation is often required to eliminate interfering substances present in crude extracts.

Improved procedures for vitamin K analyses have used high-pressure liquid chromatography (HPLC) as an analytical tool to investigate the vitamin as well as the interconversion of vitamin K to its 2,3-epoxide. The HPLC method is highly suitable for vitamin K analysis because of its high sensitivity, specificity, and accuracy (Manz and Maurer, 1982; Shino, 1988). In addition to feeds, phylloquinone concentrations in blood, milk, and selected tissues are now more commonplace.

The classic biological assay for the amount of vitamin K in an unknown source is a determination of the whole-blood clotting time of chicks. This assay measures prothrombin time since prothrombin is the most limiting vitamin K-dependent blood-clotting factor in chicks receiving vitamin K-deficient diets. Young chicks are raised on a vitamin K-deficient diet until their whole-blood clotting time is increased to four to seven times normal. The usual one-stage method for measuring prothrombin time consists of adding excess thromboplastin (obtained from chick brain or another source) and calcium to the blood and then measuring the time for the blood to clot. The response of chicks receiving a standard vitamin K preparation is compared to the prothrombin time obtained when a supplement containing an unknown quantity of vitamin K is added to the vitamin K-deficient basal diet (Scott et al., 1982; Weiser and Tagwerker, 1982).

METABOLISM

Absorption and Transfer

Like all fat-soluble vitamins, vitamin K is absorbed in association with dietary fats and requires the presence of bile salts and pancreatic juice for adequate uptake from the alimentary canal. Absorption of vitamin K depends on its incorporation into mixed micelles, and optimal formation of these micellar structures requires the presence of both bile and pancreatic juice. Thus, any malfunction of the fat-absorption mechanism, for example, biliary obstruction, will reduce availability of vitamin K. Unlike phylloquinone and the menaquinones, menadione bisulfites and phosphates are relatively water soluble and therefore are absorbed satisfactorily from low-fat diets. Male animals are more susceptible to dietary vitamin K deprivation than females, apparently as a result of stimulation of phylloquinone absorption by estrogens. The administration of estrogens increases absorption in both male and female animals (Jolly et al., 1977). The lymphatic system is the major route of transport of absorbed phylloquinone from the intestine in mammals but by portal circulation in birds, fishes, and reptiles. Shearer et al. (1970) demonstrated the association of phylloquinone with serum lipoproteins, but little is known of the existence of specific carrier proteins. The absorption of various forms of vitamin K has been studied and found to differ significantly. Ingested phylloquinone is absorbed by an energy-dependent process from the proximal portion of the small intestine (Hollander, 1973). In contrast to the active transport of phylloquinone, menaquinone is absorbed from the small intestine by a passive non–carrier-mediated process. Menadione can be absorbed from both the small intestine and the colon by a passive process and can be alkylated to a biologically active form (Hollander and Truscott, 1974).

Efficiency of vitamin K absorption has been measured at 10 to 70%, depending on the form in which the vitamin is administered. Some reports have indicated that menadione is completely absorbed, but phylloquinone only at a rate of 50%. Rats were found to excrete about 60% of ingested phylloquinone in the feces within 24 hours of ingestion but only 11% of ingested menadione (Griminger and Donis, 1960; Griminger, 1984a). However, 38% of ingested menadione but only a small amount of phylloquinone were excreted via the kidneys in the same period. The conclusion was that although menadione is well absorbed, it is poorly retained, while just the opposite is true for phylloquinone. Poor retention of menadione can be explained by the need to add, in the liver, a difarnesyl chain and thus transform it into menaquinone (vitamin K_2) with a 20-carbon chain (MK-4). Apparently there are quantitative limitations in this biosynthetic step. The menadione not converted is rapidly detoxified and excreted. The turnover of liver phylloquinone was found to be 2 to 4 times more rapid than menaquinone initially, but no difference was found between the sources at 48 hours (Will and Suttie, 1992). However, phylloquinone was much more effective than menaquinone in maintaining normal vitamin K status in rats at low dietary concentrations (0.2 μmol/kg diet), whereas at high dietary concentrations (5.6 μmol/kg diet) they were equally effective.

Konishi et al. (1973) administered radioactive menadione, phylloquinone, or menaquinone-4, to rats and found that radioactive menadione was spread over the whole body much faster than the other two compounds, but the amount retained in the tissues was low. Martius and Alvino (1964) utilized radioactive menadione to establish that it could

233

be converted to a more lipophilic compound that, on the basis of their limited characterization, appeared to be menaquinone-4. Therefore, they concluded that the vitamin K form of animal tissues was menaquinone-4. They found that when either a menaquinone or a phylloquinone was given to animals, the side chain was removed, probably by the microorganisms in the gut.

On the contrary, Griminger and Brubacher (1966) showed that a major portion of the phylloquinone they fed to chicks was absorbed and deposited in the liver intact, and that as such it had as good biological activity upon prothrombin synthesis as the menaquinone-4, which they found in the chick's liver following feeding of menadione. Therefore, menaquinone-4 is most likely produced only if menadione is fed, or if the intestinal microorganisms degrade the dietary K_1 or K_2 to menadione. The formation of menaquinone-4 is not obligatory for metabolic activity, since phylloquinone is equally active in bringing about synthesis of the K-dependent blood-clotting proteins (Scott et al., 1982).

Newborn infants have low vitamin K body stores, indicating poor placental transfer. Correlation of vitamin K between mothers and babies have suggested that the vitamin passes the placenta only in small quantities (Suzuki et al., 1989). The vitamin is frequently not detectable in the cord blood from mothers with normal plasma levels, and sometimes, levels from neonates are only half those of their mothers.

Storage and Excretion

About half of the total body pool of vitamin K is in the liver. A number of studies have shown that phylloquinone and menaquinones are specifically concentrated and retained in the liver. Menaquinone concentrations exceed those of phylloquinone in organs other than liver (Thijssen et al., 1996). Menadione is found to be widely distributed in all tissues and very rapidly excreted. Although phylloquinone is rapidly concentrated in liver, it does not have a long retention time (17 hours half-life) in this organ (Thierry et al., 1970; Shearer et al., 1996). Therefore, the inability to rapidly develop vitamin K deficiency in most species results from the difficulty in preventing absorption of the vitamin from the diet or from intestinal synthesis rather than from a significant storage of the vitamin.

Some breakdown products of vitamin K are excreted in the urine. One of the principal excretory products is a chain-shortened and oxidized derivative of vitamin K, which forms a γ-lactone and is probably excreted as a glucuronide. Vitamin K oxide has also been identified as a metabolite of vitamin K in rats (Matschiner et al., 1970). The principal metabolites of menadione are the sulfate and glucuronide of dihydrom-enadione (Losito et al., 1967). Some vitamin K is re-excreted into the intestine with bile, part of which is excreted in the feces. In humans, 20% of injected phylloquinone was excreted in the urine, and 40 to 50% was excreted in the feces via the bile (Shearer and Barkhan, 1973).

FUNCTIONS

Coagulation time of blood is the major function ascribed to vitamin K. Four vitamin K-dependent proteins involved in blood coagulation were discovered early in the investigations of the vitamin as a result of hemorrhagic disease caused by deficiency. The vitamin is required for the synthesis of the active form of prothrombin (factor II) and other plasma clotting factors (VII, IX, and X). These four blood-clotting proteins are synthesized in the liver in inactive precursor forms (zymogens) and then converted to biologically active proteins by the action of vitamin K (Suttie and Jackson, 1977). In deficiency, administration of vitamin K brings about a prompt response and return toward normal of depressed coagulation factors in 4 to 5 hours. In the absence of the liver, this response does not occur.

The blood-clotting mechanism can apparently be stimulated by either an intrinsic system, in which all the factors are in the plasma, or an extrinsic system. In the extrinsic system of coagulation, injury to the skin or other tissue frees tissue thromboplastin that, in the presence of various factors and calcium, changes prothrombin in the blood to thrombin. The enzyme thrombin facilitates the conversion of the soluble fibrinogen into an insoluble fibrin clot (Fig. 5.3). Fibrin polymerizes into strands and enmeshes the formed elements of the blood, especially the red blood cells, to form the blood clot (Griminger, 1984a). The final active component in both the intrinsic and extrinsic systems appears to activate the Stuart-Prower factor, which in turn leads to activation of prothrombin. The principal steps involved in blood clotting are presented in Fig. 5.3, illustrating the need for vitamin K at four different sites in these reactions.

It is recognized that vitamin K-deficient animals synthesize vitamin K-dependent proteins but in an inactive form, and vitamin K is needed to convert these inactive protein precursors to biologically active proteins (Suttie, 1980). Investigations related to vitamin K mechanisms revealed that prothrombin contained 10 residues of a previously unrecognized amino acid, γ-carboxyglutamic acid (Gla). Likewise, the Gla residues were found in the three other vitamin K-dependent proteins.

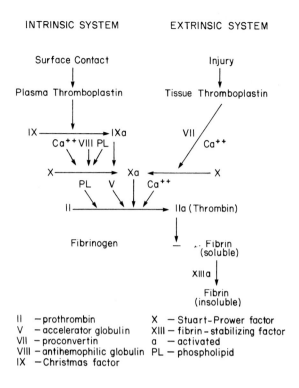

INTRINSIC SYSTEM   EXTRINSIC SYSTEM

Surface Contact   Injury

Plasma Thromboplastin   Tissue Thromboplastin

II — prothrombin   X — Stuart-Prower factor
V — accelerator globulin   XIII — fibrin-stabilizing factor
VII — proconvertin   a — activated
VIII — antihemophilic globulin PL — phospholipid
IX — Christmas factor

Fig. 5.3 Scheme involving blood clotting. The vitamin K-dependent factors (synthesis of each is inhibited by dicumarol) include factor IX, Christmas factor; factor X, Stuart-Prower factor; factor VII, proconvertin; and factor II, prothrombin.

The amino-terminal regions of these proteins are homologous, and the Gla residues are in essentially the same position in all of these clotting factors (Suttie and Olson, 1990).

The metabolic function of vitamin K is as the coenzyme in the carboxylation of protein-incorporated glutamate residues to yield γ-carboxyglutamate (Fig. 5.4), thus converting inactive precursor proteins to biological activity. Carboxylation allows prothrombin and the other procoagulant proteins to participate in a specific protein-calcium-phospholipid interaction that is necessary for their biological role (Suttie and Jackson, 1977). To participate in this reaction, vitamin K is converted to hydroquinone and is then reconstituted to the quinone form via vitamin K-epoxide.

Liver microsomes contain enzymes that oxidize the vitamin to its

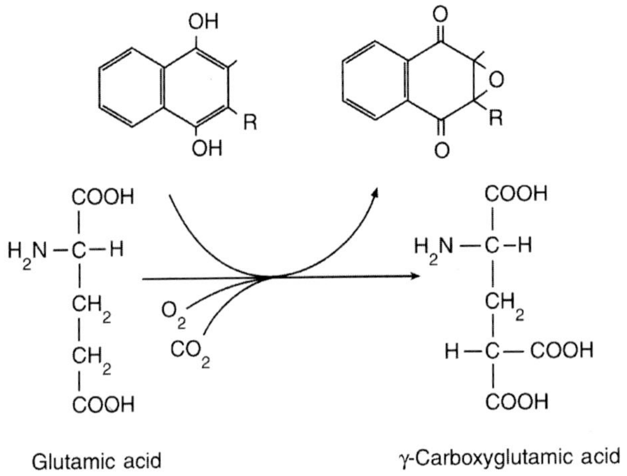

Fig. 5.4 The vitamin K-dependent carboxylation reaction. The enzyme carboxylates specific glutamic acid residues of a limited number of proteins to γ-carboxyglutamic acid residues.

2,3-epoxide and reduce the epoxide back to the reduced vitamin. The carboxylase activity and epoxidase activity appear to share a common oxygenated intermediate, and available data suggest that this may be a hydroperoxide of the vitamin. Evidence indicates that the role of vitamin K is to labilize the γ-hydrogen of the substrate for CO_2 attack rather than to activate or transfer the CO_2 (Suttie, 1980). Warfarin and other anticoagulants of the coumarin type interfere with 2,3-epoxide reductase and therefore with the reconstitution of the active form of vitamin K (see Chemical Structure, Properties, and Antagonists).

Four other vitamin K-dependent proteins have been identified in plasma (C, S, Z, and M). Proteins C and S play an anticoagulant rather than a procoagulant role in normal hemostasis (Suttie, 1990; Combs, 1992). Protein C inhibits coagulation, and stimulated by protein S, it promotes fibrinolysis. Also, a protein C-S complex can partially hydrolyze the activated factors V and VIII and thus inactivate them. Individuals with inherited deficiency of factor C are at high risk for thromboses. Protein S also has the potential to be involved in the regulation of bone turnover (Binkley and Suttie, 1995). Functions for proteins M and Z are unknown.

Continuing research has revealed that vitamin K-dependent reactions are present in most tissues and not just blood, and that a reasonably large number of proteins are subjected to this posttranslational car-

237

boxylation of specific glutamate residues to γ-carboxyglutamate residues (Vermeer, 1986; Ferland, 1998). Gla-containing proteins have been purified from kidney, liver mitochondria, spermatozoa, urine, chick chorioallantoic membrane, and snake venoms. Atherocalcin is a vitamin K-dependent protein in atherosclerotic tissue. A vitamin K-dependent carboxylase system has been identified in skin, which may be related to calcium metabolism in skin (de Boer-van den Berg et al., 1986). Two of the best characterized vitamin K-dependent proteins not involved in hemostasis are osteocalcin or bone Gla protein (BGP) and matrix Gla protein, which were initially discovered in bone. Osteocalcin is a protein containing three Gla residues that give the protein its mineral-binding properties. Osteocalcin appears in embryonic chick bone and rat bone matrix at the beginning of mineralization of the bone (Gallop et al., 1980). It accounts for 15 to 20% of the non-collagen protein in the bone of most vertebrates and is one of the most abundant proteins in the body. Osteocalcin is produced by osteoblasts, with synthesis controlled by 1,25-dihydroxy vitamin D. Matrix Gla protein-deficient mice have abnormal calcification leading to osteopenia, fractures, and premature death due to arterial calcification (Booth and Mayer, 1997).

As is true for other non-blood vitamin K-dependent proteins, the physiological role of osteocalcin remains largely unknown (Price, 1993). However, reduced osteocalcin content of cortical bone (Vanderschueren et al., 1990) and alteration of osteocalcin distribution within osteons (Ingram et al., 1994) are associated with aging. It remains unknown whether any of these findings are related to the age-related increased risk of fracture. Osteocalcin may play a role in the control of bone remodeling because it has been reported to be a chemoattractant for monocytes, the precursors of osteoclasts (Mundy and Poser, 1983). Serum osteocalcin has been shown to be a good predictor of bone turnover in pigs (Carter et al., 1996). This suggests a possible role for osteocalcin in bone resorption (Binkley and Suttie, 1995).

Several reports have indicated that warfarin treatment alters the functional properties of bone particles prepared from rats. However, vitamin K-deficient chick embryos were able to mobilize sufficient quantities of calcium for normal skeletal development, although they exhibited severe reduction in blood clotting and bone osteocalcin concentration (Lavelle et al., 1994).

Observations that vitamin K could be involved in the pathogenesis of bone mineral loss have been summarized (Binkley and Suttie, 1995): (1) low blood vitamin K in patients with bone fractures; (2) concentration of circulating under-γ-carboxylated osteocalcin associated with age, low bone-mineral density, and risk for hip fracture; (3) anticoagulant therapy associated with decreased bone density; and (4) vitamin K supplementation, which decreases bone loss and calcium excretion.

Vitamin K has been suggested as a protective factor against gastric mucosal lesions, but the mechanism of protection is unclear (Yonaga, 1990). The protective effect of vitamin K against the development of taurocholate-induced gastric lesions in mice increased with the dosage of the vitamin, but the vitamin's protective effect varied according to the differences in its chemical structure. Phylloquinone was the most effective, followed by menaquinone and then menadione.

Vitamin A activity has been related to the vitamin K-dependent protein matrix Gla protein. The consistent induction of matrix Gla protein in rat cultured cells and in animals administered retinoic acid suggest that this vitamin K-dependent protein may mediate some of the known actions of retinoic acid in differentiation and development (Cancela et al., 1993).

In animals, discoveries of active proteins that depend on vitamin K for their synthesis are becoming common. Discovery of a vitamin K-dependent protein in skeletal tissue suggested that distribution of γ-carboxyglutamic acid was much more widespread than was once realized. A number of pathological states result in an ectopic calcification of various tissues. Residues of Gla have been found in these lesions as well as in calcium-containing kidney stones. Microsomes from kidney cortex possess a vitamin K-dependent carboxylase activity. Proteins containing Gla residues all interact with Ca^{2+} or other divalent cations, but their physiological roles are not well understood. Although much is unknown concerning vitamin K function apart from blood coagulation, it is apparent that a reasonably large number of proteins may be involved.

REQUIREMENTS

Vitamin K requirement of mammals is met by a combination of dietary intake and microbial biosynthesis in the gut, which may involve intestinal microorganisms (such as *Escherichia coli*) as well as ruminal microbes. Ruminal microorganisms in particular synthesize large amounts of vitamin K, explaining why ruminants do not appear to need a dietary source of the vitamin. Animals that practice coprophagy, such as the rabbit, can utilize much of the vitamin K that is eliminated in the feces. In rats, most menaquinone absorbed results from fecal ingestion rather than dietary sources, or from direct synthesis and absorption from the intestine (Kindberg et al., 1987). Animal feces contain substantial amounts of the vitamin even when none is present in feed. Despite the intestinal synthesis, animals can be rendered deficient when fed vitamin K-free diets, and coprophagy is prevented if animals are maintained germ-free, or if a vitamin K antagonist is given. Difficulties in demonstrating dietary requirement in many species include the varying degrees to which they utilize vitamin K synthesized by intestinal bacteria and the degree to which different species practice coprophagy. Contrary to most animals, poultry have a limited ability for intestinal synthesis, so adequate dietary supplies are of greater importance (see Deficiency).

Chicks were also found to contain less hepatic vitamin K epoxide reductase (Will et al., 1992). Activity of this enzyme in chicks was about 10% of that in rats fed the same diets; the inability of chicks to effectively recycle the epoxide of vitamin K (phylloquinone 2,3 epoxide) seems to be the major factor in its high requirement for the vitamin.

Rats caged on litter obtain vitamin K, as well as B vitamins, by eating feces. Thus the practice was established of keeping experimental animals on wire screens to prevent this complication in vitamin feeding experiments. This practice was assumed to be successful until Barnes and coworkers (1957) showed, using a new technique, that rats may eat 50 to 65% of their feces even when maintained on wire screens. In a later experiment, in which rats were prevented by this new technique from eating feces, vitamin K deficiency developed uniformly with a vitamin K-free diet.

Because of microbial synthesis, a precise expression of vitamin K requirements is not feasible. However, attempts to determine the contribution of microbial synthesis have been made. In conventional rats, the vitamin requirement is 0.05 to 0.10 ppm, whereas in germ-free rats, the requirement is more than doubled, to about 0.25 ppm (Suttie and Olson, 1990). In humans, vitamin K homologs stored in liver indicate that about 40 to 50% of the daily requirement is derived from diet (mostly vitamin K_1), and the remainder from microbiological synthesis.

Estimated vitamin K requirements for various animals and humans are presented in Table 5.1. The daily requirement for most species ranges from 2 to 200 μg of vitamin K per kilogram of body weight. This requirement can be altered by age, sex, strain, anti-vitamin K factors, disease conditions, and any condition influencing lipid absorption or altering intestinal flora (see Deficiency and Supplementation sections). Rapid rate of feed passage (e.g., diarrhea) through the digestive tract may also influence vitamin K synthesis in animals. It is well known that antibiotic intake will reduce synthesis of intestinal vitamin K. In mice, a direct effect of antibiotic on vitamin K requirements has been shown.

■ Table 5.1 Vitamin K Requirements for Various Animals and Humans

Animal	Purpose or Class	Requirement[a]	Reference
Beef cattle	Adult	Microbial synthesis	NRC (1996)
Dairy cattle	Adult	Microbial synthesis	NRC (1989a)
Chicken	Leghorn, 0–18 weeks	0.5 mg/kg	NRC (1994)
	Laying (100-g intake)	0.5 mg/kg	NRC (1994)
	Broilers	0.5 mg/kg	NRC (1994)
Duck	All classes	4.0 mg/kg	NRC (1994)
Turkey	0–4 weeks	1.75 mg/kg	NRC (1994)
	8–12 weeks	1.0 mg/kg	NRC (1994)
	Breeding	1.0 mg/kg	NRC (1994)
Sheep	Adult	Microbial synthesis	NRC (1985b)
Swine	All classes	0.5 mg/kg	NRC (1998)
Horse	Adult	Microbial synthesis	NRC (1989b)
Goat	Adult	Microbial synthesis	NRC (1981)
Rabbit	Adult	2 mg/kg	NRC (1977)
Cat	Adult	0.1 mg/kg	NRC (1986)
Dog	Growing	1 mg/kg	NRC (1985a)
Fish	Lake trout	0.5–1 mg/kg	NRC (1993)
Rat	All classes	1.0 mg/kg	NRC (1995)
Guinea pig	Growing	5 mg/kg	NRC (1995)
Human	Infants	5–10 µg/day	RDA (1989)
	Children	15–30 µg/day	RDA (1989)
	Adults	45–80 µg/day	RDA (1989)

[a]Expressed as per unit of animal feed on either as-fed (approximately 90% dry matter) or dry basis (see Appendix, Tables A1a,b). Human data are expressed as µg/day.

Even in the absence of intestinal flora, administration of an antibiotic exacerbated vitamin K deficiency (Shirakawa et al., 1990).

Excess of vitamin A and calcium have been shown to influence vitamin K requirements. Rats fed excess retinol had two to three times the carboxylase activity of endogenous prothrombin precursors, which is an indicator of vitamin K deficiency (Lee and Morre, 1992). Hall et al. (1991) reported a hemorrhagic condition in pigs fed 2.7% dietary calcium. The condition was cured with vitamin K supplementation and was not produced in treatment with less dietary calcium.

The adult human requirement for vitamin K is extremely low, and there seems little possibility of a simple dietary deficiency developing in the absence of complicating factors (Suttie, 1991). In humans, since placenta transfer of vitamin K is poor, intestinal flora are insufficiently developed during the first days after birth to provide the vitamin and, because of the low vitamin K content of the mother's milk (e.g., 1 to 2 µg/L), prothrombin level is very low in the newborn. Breast-fed infants may ingest only 1 µg/day, which is only 20% of the requirement. Recommended daily requirements for adults range from 45 to 80 µg

(RDA, 1989). Depletion studies that included a clotting assay, under-carboxylated prothrombin, and a decrease in urinary γ-carboxyglutamic acid suggest vitamin K requirements for humans of about 1 μg/kg body weight daily (Suttie et al., 1988).

NATURAL SOURCES

There are two major natural sources of vitamin K: phylloquinones (vitamin K_1) in plant sources and menaquinones (vitamin K_2) produced by bacterial flora in animals. Vitamin K concentrations of various foods and feedstuffs are presented in Table 5.2. Green leaves are the richest natural source of vitamin K_1. Light is important for its formation, and parts of plants that do not normally form chlorophyll contain little vitamin K. However, natural loss of chlorophyll, as in the fall yellowing of leaves, does not bring about a corresponding change in vitamin K. In most green leafy vegetables, phylloquinone increased during plant maturation, and cabbage was found to contain three to six times more of the vitamin in the outer than the inner leaves (Ferland and Sadowski, 1992b).

Vitamin K is present in fresh, dark green vegetables and in an extract of pine needles. Cauliflower, broccoli, spinach, lettuce, and brussels

■ Table 5.2   Vitamin K Concentration of Various Foods and Feedstuffs (as-fed basis)

Food or Feedstuff	Vitamin K Level (ppm)
Alfalfa hay, sun cured	19.4
Alfalfa meal, dehydrated (20% protein)	14.2
Barley, grain	0.2
Cabbage (green)	4.0
Carrots	0.1
Corn, grain	0.2
Eggs	0.2
Fish meal, herring (mechanically extracted)	2.2
Liver (cattle)	1–2
Liver (swine)	4–8
Meat (lean)	1–2
Peas	0.1–0.3
Potatoes	0.8
Sorghum, grain	0.2
Soybean, protein concentrate (70.0% protein)	0.0
Spinach	6.0
Tomatoes	4.0

Sources: From NRC (1982b) and Marks (1975).

sprouts are excellent sources. Edible oils are good sources of vitamin K_1, and human requirements of the vitamin are met when soybean or rapeseed oil exceed 15% of the caloric content (Ferland and Sadowski, 1992a).

Most feeds containing very high levels of vitamin K are not usually fed to domestic animals, with the exception of alfalfa leaf meal, which is sometimes included in small amounts in the diets of poultry and other animals. Cereals and oil cakes contain only small amounts of vitamin K, while liver and fish meal are good animal sources of the vitamin. All feeds or foods of animal origin, including fish meal and fish liver oils, are much higher in vitamin K after they have undergone extensive bacterial putrefaction. Milk from cattle has been reported to be 10 times as rich as that of the human, and vitamin K content of cow's milk is known to vary significantly with the month of sampling. Both human colostrum (3.4 µg/L) and later produced milk (2.9 µg/L) were insufficient to meet infant requirements (Canfield et al., 1991). The effect of food processing and cooking on vitamin K content has not been carefully considered; however, limited data suggest that food vitamin K is relatively stable, with the greatest loss resulting from oxidation. Irradiation of beef has resulted in destruction of the vitamin. Ferland and Sadowski (1992a) reported that vitamin K_1 content of edible vegetable oils was stable to processing, decreased slightly with heat, and was rapidly destroyed by both daylight and fluorescent light. Amber glass containers protected the oils from the destructive effects of light.

The menaquinones (vitamin K_2) are produced by the bacterial flora in animals and are especially important in providing the vitamin K requirements of humans and most other mammals. However, the chick does not receive sufficient vitamin K from intestinal microbial synthesis (Scott et al., 1982). Type of diet, independent of vitamin K concentration, will influence total menaquinone synthesis. Rats fed a diet based on boiled white rice had less menaquinone production and more severe vitamin K deficiency than animals consuming diets based on autoclaved black-eye beans (Mathers et al., 1990).

Vitamin K production in the rumen of ruminants and subsequent passage along the small intestine, a region of active absorption, make such synthesized vitamin K highly available to the host. In nonruminants, the site of synthesis is in the lower gut, an area of poor absorption; thus availability to the host is limited unless the animal practices coprophagy, in which case the synthesized vitamin K is highly available.

DEFICIENCY

The major clinical sign of vitamin K deficiency in all species is impairment of blood coagulation. Clinical signs include low prothrombin levels, increased clotting time, and hemorrhaging. In its most severe form, vitamin K deficiency will cause subcutaneous and internal hemorrhages, which can be fatal. Deficiency can result from insufficient vitamin K in the diet, lack of microbial synthesis within the gut, inadequate intestinal absorption, or inability of the liver to use the available vitamin K.

Effects of Deficiency

Ruminants

Intestinal microorganisms provide vitamin K to preruminant animals. Nestor and Conrad (1990) studied vitamin K in preruminant veal calves and concluded that intestinal microorganisms synthesized sufficient menaquinone-4 to meet needs of the vitamin prior to rumen development.

Microorganisms in the rumen synthesize large amounts of vitamin K, and a deficiency is seen only in the presence of a metabolic antagonist, such as dicumarol from moldy sweet clover. Dicumarol is a fungus metabolite produced from substrates in sweet clover hay. The coumarin derivatives are not active in the fresh plant because they are bound to glycosides, but are active when sweet clover is improperly cured (Vermeer, 1984). This condition, referred to as sweet clover poisoning or hemorrhagic sweet clover disease, has been responsible for a large number of animal losses. Ruminants may die from hemorrhage following a minor injury, or even from apparently spontaneous bleeding. Dicumarol passes through the placenta in pregnant animals, and newborn animals may become affected immediately after birth.

All clinical signs of dicumarol poisoning relate to the hemorrhages caused by failure of blood coagulation. The first appearance of clinical disease after consumption of spoiled sweet clover varies greatly and depends to a large extent on dicumarol content of the particular sweet clover fed and animal age. If dietary dicumarol is low or variable, animals may consume it for months before signs of disease appear. In an experiment with calves, dicumarol poisoning was produced by feeding naturally spoiled, sweet clover hay that contained a minimum of 90 mg dicumarol per kilogram of hay (Alstad et al., 1985). The minimum time required to develop clinical signs of vitamin K deficiency in these calves was 3 weeks. In veterinary practice, another common cause of induced vitamin K deficiency is the accidental poisoning of animals with warfarin (a synthetic coumarin used as a rodent poison). Initial clinical signs may be stiffness and lameness from bleeding into muscles and articulations. Hematomas, epistaxis (nose bleed), or gastrointestinal bleeding may be observed. Death may occur suddenly, with little preliminary evidence of disease, and is caused by spontaneous massive hemorrhage or bleeding after injury, surgery, or parturition. DeHoogh (1989) reported that two possible early embryonic deaths occurred and one cow aborted from sweet clover poisoning.

Measurement of clotting time or prothrombin is considered a fairly good measure of vitamin K deficiency. In experimentally induced dicumarol poisoning (hemorrhagic sweet clover disease), Alstad et al. (1985) reported that normal prothrombin time is equal to or less than 20 seconds. Deficiency of vitamin K was characterized by prothrombin times longer than 40 to 60 seconds; with severe deficiency, prothrombin time can be as long as 5 to 6 minutes.

Swine

Schendel and Johnson (1962) were able to produce a vitamin K deficiency in baby pigs by using a sulfa drug and an antibiotic and by carefully minimizing coprophagy by cleaning the feces from wire bottom cases where the pigs were housed. Likewise, hemorrhagic disease occurred in piglets weaned at 5 to 6 weeks of age within 2 weeks after transfer onto flat decks (Hoppe, 1987). This vitamin K-responsive outbreak had occurred because (1) the diet was virtually free of vitamin K, (2) sulfonamide, a known vitamin K-antagonist, was included in the diet, and (3) flat deck-housing was used, which precludes intake of microbial vitamin K from feces or litter.

Hall et al. (1991) accidentally produced vitamin K deficiency characterized by increased blood clotting times and high death losses when feeding excess calcium (2.7%) without supplemental vitamin K. Either supplemental vitamin K or reduced dietary Ca prevented the disease condition.

Clinical and subclinical signs of vitamin K deficiency include increased prothrombin and blood-clotting time, internal hemorrhage, and anemia due to blood loss (Cunha 1977; Newsholme et al., 1985). Newborn pigs may be pale with loss of blood from the umbilical cord. Until recently, vitamin K deficiency under natural conditions was not expected, as it was thought that pigs synthesized most if not all of the vitamin that was required. However, in the late 1960s and early 1970s,

245

there were prevalent reports of a bleeding disease of young pigs on commercial diets that was successfully treated with vitamin K supplementation. Observations from Australia and New Zealand were of hemorrhaging in the navel of newborn pigs (Cunha, 1977).

A number of field trials in the United States have reported a hemorrhagic syndrome in growing pigs. In one study, hemorrhagic syndrome occurred 9 days after pigs were fed a standard diet, while those receiving either 2.5% dehydrated alfalfa meal or supplemental vitamin K remained in good health (Fritschen et al., 1970). Gross visible signs for hemorrhagic syndrome were large subcutaneous hemorrhages, blood in urine, and abnormal breathing. (Note: Field observation may not be the same as experiments.) Additional clinical signs from field observation are that some pigs will develop enlarged blood-filled joints and become lame, whereas others may have swelling along the body wall that are filled with unclotted blood. Hematomas (or blood swellings) in the ears also occur (Cunha, 1977). Hemorrhagic conditions in the growing pig have in some cases been associated with ingestion of molds, such as aspergillus or moldy materials, and have usually responded to vitamin K therapy.

Exactly why vitamin K supplementation is needed is not definitely known. Cunha (1977) and Scott et al. (1982) have summarized likely reasons for vitamin K deficiency under field conditions:

1. As confinement feeding has increased, less pasture and alfalfa, both of which are good sources of vitamin K, are used for production of higher energy and more efficient diets. Likewise, there has been a trend toward the use of solvent-extracted soybean meal and other oil seed meals, and higher-quality (less putrefied) fish meals, which are lower in vitamin K than the original expeller meals and somewhat putrid fish meals.

2. Hemorrhaging gastric ulcers, which occur frequently, may increase vitamin K needs.

3. Mycotoxins produced by certain molds may be present in the feed.

4. Antimetabolite (antivitamin K) may be in the feed and thus increase vitamin K needs.

5. Use of slatted floors lessens the opportunity for coprophagy since feces are an excellent source of vitamin K.

6. Use of sulfa drugs, antibiotics, and other medications may reduce intestinal synthesis of the vitamin.

7. Breed or strains of pigs may require more vitamin K. Increased litter size and rate of gain may also increase the need for vitamin K.

Poultry

Vitamin K deficiency causes a reduction in the prothrombin content of the blood and, in the chick, may reduce the quantity in the plasma to less than 2% of normal. Since the prothrombin content of the blood of normal, newly hatched chicks is only about 40% that of adult birds, very young chicks are readily affected by a deficiency of vitamin K. A carry-over from the parent hen to the chick has been demonstrated (Almquist, 1971). Therefore, breeder hen diets should be supplemented with vitamin K to ensure good chick health. To this point, laying hens fed a diet deficient in vitamin K produce eggs low in the vitamin, and when the eggs are incubated, the chicks produced have low reserves and prolonged blood-clotting time. Adverse effects on blood clotting are not apparent until after hatching, when hemorrhaging and mortality occur if trauma occurs. As a consequence, the chicks may bleed to death from an injury as slight as that caused by debeaking or wing banding (Fig. 5.5).

In very young chicks deficient in vitamin K, blood coagulation time begins to increase after 5 to 10 days of age, with clinical signs occurring most frequently in chicks 2 to 3 weeks after they begin consuming a vi-

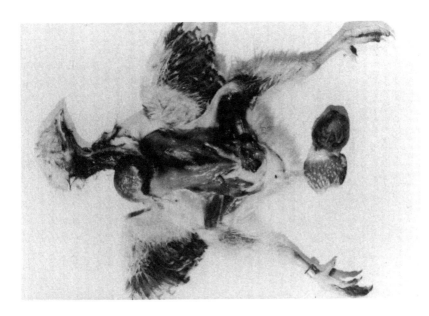

Fig. 5.5 Generalized hemorrhage due to severe vitamin K deficiency in a young chick. (Courtesy of M.S. Scott, Cornell University.)

tamin K-deficient diet. Hemorrhages often occur in any part of the body, either spontaneously or as the result of an injury or bruise. Postmortem examination usually reveals accumulations of blood in various parts of the body; sometimes there are petechial hemorrhages in the liver, and almost invariably there is erosion of the gizzard lining.

Even though inadequate dietary vitamin K alters bone osteocalcin, signs associated with the skeletal system are not as apparent as blood-clotting problems. One study found that although blood clotting was impaired and there was a reduction in bone γ-carboxyglutamic acid concentration, vitamin K deficiency did not functionally impair skeletal metabolism of laying hens and their progeny (Lavelle et al., 1994).

Borderline deficiencies of vitamin K often cause small hemorrhagic blemishes on the breast, legs, and wings; in the abdominal cavity and on the surface of the intestine (Fig. 5.6). Chicks show anemia that may be due in part to loss of blood, but also to the development of hypoplastic bone marrow. Even borderline deficiency of vitamin K is of economic importance in broiler production because the hemorrhagic areas that occur in the legs or throughout the body may result in a high percentage of condemnations during inspection at the processing plant (Scott et al., 1982). A condition manifested by numerous small hemorrhages scattered throughout all tissues has been reported frequently in the commercial broiler industry (Almquist, 1978).

A number of considerations influence the likelihood of vitamin K deficiency in poultry, including dietary sources of the vitamin, level of the vitamin in the maternal diet, intestinal synthesis, coprophagy, presence of sulfa drugs and other nonnutrients in the diet, and disease conditions. Chicks with coccidiosis, a disease that causes severe damage along the intestinal tract, may bleed excessively or fatally. When sulfaquinoxaline or certain other drugs are present in the feed or drinking water, or when coccidiosis is being treated, up to 10 times as much supplementary vitamin K is needed as when these drugs are absent (Scott et al., 1982). Antimicrobial agents suppress intestinal bacteria that synthesize vitamin K, and in their presence, the bird may be entirely dependent on dietary vitamin K (NRC, 1994). Arsanilic acid increases the need for dietary vitamin K in both breeder and chick diets.

In poultry, little intestinal synthesis occurs because of the short digestive tract. The young chicken's large intestine or colon, a major area of bacterial activity, comprises less than 6% of the total length of the intestinal tract, while the figure for the adult of the same species is 7% (Griminger, 1984b). In other domestic animals, the relative length varies from 13% for the dog to 28% for the rabbit. Also, poultry cannot uti-

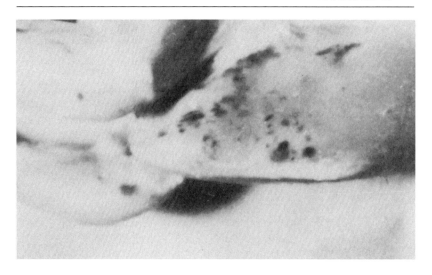

Fig. 5.6 Hemorrhagic blemishes in the muscle of a chicken fed a diet deficient in vitamin K. (Courtesy of M.L. Scott, Cornell University.)

lize the vitamin K synthesized by intestinal flora because the synthesis is taking place too close to the distal end of the intestinal tract to permit significant absorption.

Rapid rate of food passage through the digestive tract may also influence vitamin K synthesis in poultry. First defecation in pigs, for a specific portion of diet, may occur about 15 hours after feeding, but most of a given meal will be retained in the tract appreciably longer. A comparable period for chickens would be approximately 3 hours (Griminger 1984b).

Horses

There are no conclusive reports in the literature relating to vitamin K deficiency in the equine species (NRC, 1989b). Clinical responses of some "bleeders" to vitamin K therapy suggest that some horses may require additional supplies of vitamin K (Wakeman et al., 1975). However, it is generally assumed that phylloquinone in pasture or in good-quality hay and that synthesized by microorganisms of the cecum and colon are in sufficient quantities to meet requirements.

Other Animal Species

As a result of adequate dietary supplies and intestinal synthesis, vitamin K deficiency has not been reported in the guinea pig, and the mink has been little studied. Other species, including trout and channel catfish, have been reported to have limited response to supplemental vitamin K, with requirements determined only for trout (NRC, 1993) and juvenile marine shrimp (Shiau and Liu, 1994).

DOGS AND CATS

Vitamin K deficiency signs are only occasionally described for dogs; however, accidental intake of dicumarol types of rat poison, such as warfarin and diphenadione (vitamin K antagonist), will result in a hemorrhagic condition in dogs (Kerr, 1986; Mount and Kass, 1989). Clinical signs in dogs include paleness and evidence of slow but persistent bleeding from a number of sites, including gums, bowel, and several injection punctures (Kerr, 1986). Vitamin K deficiency has been demonstrated in adult dogs following diversion of bile from the intestine by means of a cholecystonephrostomy (NRC, 1985a). Vitamin K absorption from both diet and intestinal bacterial synthesis was apparently reduced. Some reports indicate that newborn pups suspected of vitamin K deficiency occasionally respond to vitamin K therapy. Vitamin K deficiency is rare in cats. However, vitamin K antagonism attributable to ingestion of rodenticides containing warfarin or related compounds is a cause of hemorrhaging in cats. Clinical signs of vitamin K deficiency could include hematomas in the elbows; hemorrhage in the conjunctiva; and extensive hemorrhage in and around the stifle joint, with necropsy revealing extensive hemorrhage in the bladder, sublumbar area, pelvic canal, and perineum (Maddison et al., 1990).

FISH

Information on intestinal vitamin K-synthesizing microflora in fish is lacking. However, cultured sardines fed a menadione-supplemented feed were rich in menaquinone-4, which indicates that menadione was converted to menaquinone-4 in the body. Vitamin K deficiency results in anemia and prolonged coagulation time in fish. Hemorrhages in channel catfish fed a vitamin K-deficient diet have been reported, while other studies of this species have found no benefit with supplemental dietary vitamin K (NRC, 1993). For trout, no growth or survival data for vitamin K deficiency have been reported. However, dietary sulfaguanidine, as well as cold water temperatures, have caused prolonged blood coagulation times. In shrimp, weight gain and feed efficiency were significantly higher in those fed menadione-supplemented diets than in controls.

FOXES

On farms where silver and blue foxes were born with subcutaneous hemorrhages, enrichment of diets of pregnant females with vitamin K was beneficial (NRC, 1982a).

LABORATORY ANIMALS

Vitamin K deficiency (manifested as prolonged blood-clotting time and hemorrhage) deveoped within 2 to 3 weeks in rats fed low dietary quantities of the vitamin; the process was accelerated by feeding sulfonamides or preventing coprophagy (NRC, 1995). Rats given a low-fiber diet based on boiled white rice developed signs of severe vitamin K deficiency within 23 days (Mathers et al., 1990). In mice, supplemental vitamin K corrected vaginal hemorrhages and fetal resorptions caused by feeding a vitamin K antagonist. Hypoprothrombinemia can be produced in adult male hamsters either by feeding a vitamin K-deficient diet or by treatment with vitamin K antagonists. Guinea pigs did not develop hemorrhages or abnormal clotting times when fed a purified diet without vitamin K (NRC, 1995). Deficiency was not in evidence due to the active intestinal flora and coprophagic habits.

NONHUMAN PRIMATES

An increase in prothrombin time of rhesus monkeys was demonstrated when vitamin K-deficient diets (soy protein based) were fed (Hill et al., 1964). Evidently, the vitamin K requirement is small (NRC, 1978), but vitamin K deficiency bleeding disorders are a particular risk for monkeys whose intestinal tracts do not harbor bacteria that can synthesize vitamin K (newborn animals and those receiving long-term, broad-spectrum antibiotic therapy).

RABBITS

When a vitamin K-deficient diet was fed to pregnant rabbits, the result was placental hemorrhage and abortion of young (NRC, 1977).

Humans

Primary vitamin K deficiency is uncommon in healthy adult humans because of the widespread distribution of vitamin K in plant and animal tissues and the microbial flora of the normal gut, which synthesize the menaquinones in amounts that may supply the bulk of the vitamin K requirement. Cases of acquired vitamin K deficiency do, however, occur in the adult population and, although relatively rare, they present a significant problem for some individuals. Hazell and Baloch (1970) observed that a relatively high percentage of older hospitalized adults have hypoprothrombinemia that responds to orally administered vitamin K.

Deficiency of vitamin K may result from inadequate intake, absorption, or utilization, or as a result of drugs that interfere with its activity. Deficiency can occur rapidly in patients with poor food intake who are on antibiotics, particularly in the postoperative period (Pineo et al., 1973).

The most common condition known to result in vitamin K deficiency occurs in patients who have a low dietary intake of vitamin K and are taking antibiotics. Patients with restricted food intake or who are on total parenteral nutrition and are taking antibiotics should be closely observed for vitamin K deficiency.

Vitamin K as a fat-soluble vitamin requires the presence of bile salts for its absorption in the upper small intestine; thus deficiency can be caused by biliary obstruction. In sprue, idiopathic steatorrhea, ulcerative colitis, and other conditions in which fats are not effectively absorbed, bleeding due to deficiency of vitamin K may occur. Severe bleeding during or, more frequently, a day or two after an operation for the relief of jaundice due to obstruction of the common bile duct was once a complication much feared by surgeons. Today it is recognized that this danger can be circumvented by giving vitamin K by injection prior to the operation.

Hemorrhagic disease of the human newborn can result from dietary lack of vitamin K. The condition can affect infants as old as 3 to 4 months. It is more common among breast-fed infants than those fed formulated diets. The disease involves intracranial hemorrhage and has high rates of associated death and central nervous system damage. Tulchinsky et al. (1993) reviewed hemorrhagic disease of the newborn in New York State and found that in 65% of 34 deaths, vitamin K had not been administered or was given only after onset of hemorrhage. As a result of this review, prophylactic vitamin K was made a mandatory newborn care procedure in the State Public Health Code.

Newborn infants represent a special case of vitamin K nutrition because (1) the placenta is a relatively poor organ for maternal-fetal transmission of lipids, and (2) the newborn baby has a sterile intestinal tract and, furthermore, is apt to be fed foods relatively free from bacterial contamination. Breast milk and clean cow's milk are very poor sources of the vitamin. Historically, it was once a mystery why cleanliness at times led to hemorrhage due to an apparent vitamin K deficiency in infants receiving breast milk. Hemorrhages did not occur in children who received milk under less sanitary conditions because many bacteria are capable of producing vitamin K. There is an increasing incidence of hemorrhagic disease in newborns due to maternal drug ingestion and rising popularity of breast-feeding.

Infants in the first week of life have less prothrombin in their blood than normal adults and have a prolonged prothrombin time. In normal infants, plasma prothrombin concentration and that of other vitamin K-dependent factors may decrease to levels as low as 30% of adult levels in the second and third days of life. Then, as food is taken and the gastrointestinal tract is colonized, these levels gradually climb to normal adult values over a period of weeks (Anonymous, 1985). Mild vitamin K deficiency is seen in all newborn infants and is particularly severe in premature infants. It is due to inadequate liver synthesis and is aggravated by decreased dietary intake and inadequate production by intestinal bacterial flora. The tendency to correlate the general low levels of prothrombin seen in all infants, and particularly in premature or low-birth-weight infants, with an insufficient hepatic level of vitamin K is only partially correct as part of the prothrombin deficiency is due to an inability of the immature liver to synthesize sufficient clotting factors (Suzuki, 1979).

Breast-fed infants are at higher risk of hemorrhage than are formula-fed babies because human milk contains only 1 to 2 μg of vitamin K per liter, whereas cow's milk contains 5 to 17 μg/L (Haroon et al., 1982). Furthermore, breast milk is sterile and delays (through the flora it encourages) colonization of the gut with vitamin K-synthesizing bacteria.

Assessment of Status

Measurement of blood-clotting time has been used to evaluate the body status of vitamin K (see Analytical Procedures), and although blood-clotting time is a fairly good measure of vitamin K deficiency, a more accurate measure is obtained by determining the prothrombin time. Prothrombin time is indicative of efficiency of conversion of prothrombin to thrombin and fibrinogen to fibrin. Prothrombin time in severely deficient chicks, for example, may be extended from normal, 17 to 20 seconds, to 5 to 6 minutes or longer.

Prolongation of the prothrombin time in the absence of liver disease indicates vitamin K deficiency, with further clarification by specific vitamin K-dependent factor assays or by the rapid response to administration of vitamin K. There are a number of one- and two-stage modified assays for prothrombin determination. Also, snake venom preparations (e.g., *Oxyuranus echis*) have been used to develop one-stage clotting assays for prothrombin (Carlisle et al., 1975).

Inadequate vitamin K results in lowered plasma concentrations of the vitamin K-dependent clotting factors—prothrombin (factor II), factor VII, factor IX, and factor X. Measurement of the plasma concentration of one of the vitamin K-dependent clotting factors is a good way to assess vitamin K status.

Recent advances in methodology have made it possible to routinely measure circulating phylloquinone as a method of evaluating vitamin K status. Levels below 0.5 ng/ml have been associated with impaired clotting functions. Assessing adequacy by using the rather insensitive prothrombin time required a large decrease in vitamin K activity in order to conclude that an apparent deficiency existed.

The ability to immunochemically detect circulating γ-carboxyglutamic acid residues is a basis for evaluating vitamin K status (Suttie, 1991). Restricted vitamin K for humans results in a functional clotting assay that detects undercarboxylated prothrombin in plasma and a decrease in urinary γ-carboxyglutamic acid (Suttie et al., 1988). Urinary excretion of γ-carboxyglutamate reflects functional vitamin K status, since γ-carboxyglutamate released by catabolism of proteins is neither reutilized nor metabolized. An increase in the extent of γ-carboxylation of the vitamin K-dependent bone protein (osteocalcin) by administering vitamin K to subjects with no other signs of vitamin K deficiency suggests that this might be one of the more sensitive criteria for determining vitamin K status (Bach, 1994; Binkley and Suttie, 1995). More sensitive methods than blood coagulation provide an opportunity to monitor much milder forms of vitamin K deficiency.

SUPPLEMENTATION

As long as natural dietary vitamin K sources (e.g., green leafy plants) are sufficiently high and/or bacterial synthesis in the intestinal tract remains functional, supplemental dietary vitamin K is not necessary. However, high sources of vitamin K, such as green leafy plants, are not usually fed to nongrazing domestic animals. An exception is alfalfa meal, which is sometimes included in small amounts in chicken and other animal feed. Therefore, a source of vitamin K needs to be added to the diets of animals that are not getting fresh greens, or their dried equivalent, and are not synthesizing sufficient amounts of this vitamin in their gastrointestinal tract.

Scott et al. (1982) reported that natural ingredients used in poultry

254

diets a few years earlier had probably contained sufficient vitamin K, while their current diets did not. The common feedstuffs used in past years, such as high levels of alfalfa meal, high-fat soybean and other oilseed meals, and putrefied fish meals, supplied ample vitamin K. Trends toward (1) reducing levels of alfalfa for production of higher-energy, higher-efficiency diets; (2) solvent extraction of soybean meals and other oilseed meals; (3) improved processing of fish meals, resulting in lower menaquinone levels because of less putrefaction; and (4) use of vitamin K-inhibiting drugs in feed and drinking water have had a combined effect that necessitates supplementation of most poultry feeds. Inadequate vitamin K under practical circumstances for poultry is most likely to occur during the starting period, and supplementation of the feed at this time is advantageous. Dietary changes affecting poultry vitamin K needs are similar for swine in confinement (see Deficiency); however, it is generally accepted that swine better utilize vitamin K from microbial synthesis.

Vitamin K antagonists will increase the vitamin K needs of livestock. In adjusting dietary vitamin K fortification levels, an appropriate margin of safety is needed to prevent deficiency and low optimum performance in livestock. Vitamin K antagonists include the following:

1. Use of certain antibiotics and sulfa drugs. Sulfonamides and broad-spectrum antibiotic drugs can virtually sterilize the lumen of the intestine. Nelson and Norris (1961) showed that the inclusion of 0.1% sulfaquinoxaline increased the chick's need for supplemental vitamin K by four to seven times. By altering the ruminal and/or intestinal microflora, an excellent source of vitamin K is lost.

2. Ingestion of an antimetabolite. Sweet clover contains high levels of dicumarol, which can decrease prothrombin levels. Although known to be potentially toxic, sweet clover hay is still fed to animals in certain parts of the world (e.g., the Northern Plains states of the U.S.). Under these conditions, vitamin K supplementation would be warranted, as it would when animals accidentally consume a dicumarol-based rat poison (e.g., warfarin). Warfarin, a synthetic antimetabolite, is a highly effective rat poison. Rats ingest large amounts of this extremely palatable antimetabolite and eventually die from internal hemorrhaging. Marks (1975) observed that the most common cause of vitamin K deficiency in veterinary practice is the accidental poisoning of domestic animals with warfarin. Aflatoxin (a mycotoxin) is a toxic substance produced by molds. Vitamin K supplements may be helpful in correcting the deficiency associated with aflatoxicosis.

The level of supplemental vitamin K should be adequate to meet the requirements under the wide variety of stress conditions encountered in practical poultry and swine production. Squibb (1964) obtained increased prothrombin times, indicating a higher vitamin K requirement in chicks during the early stages of Newcastle disease. Studies have shown an interrelationship between the severity of coccidiosis and vitamin K requirement and indicated that as much as 8 mg of vitamin K per kilogram of diet was needed at times for maximum growth and feed efficiency (Scott et al., 1982). Field reports with swine have indicated that hemorrhaging in stressed animals occurs at birth in the navel and following castration. Various reports have indicated that levels of 2 to as high as 16 g of vitamin K per ton of feed were needed because the lower levels were not effective under certain farm conditions (Cunha, 1977). Scott et al. (1982) concluded that coccidiosis possibly produces a triple stress on the vitamin K requirement by (1) reducing feed intake and thereby the supply of vitamin K, (2) injuring the intestinal tract and reducing absorption of the vitamin, and (3) treatment with sulfaquinoxaline or other coccidiostats that cause an increased requirement for vitamin K.

In vitamin K-deficient calves, normal prothrombin time was achieved within 6 to 8 days after intramuscular injection with phylloquinone at 0.22 to 1.1 mg/kg body weight. Vitamin K_1 dosages of 1.1, 2.2, and 3.3. mg/kg administered intramuscularly were effective in lowering prothrombin times to approximately normal values within 24 hours (Alstad et al., 1985). For confirmed cases of vitamin K deficiency, vitamin K_1 was shown to be much more potent than vitamin K_3 in cattle (Alstad et al., 1985).

Vitamin K_1 is not available to the feed industry because it is too expensive for this purpose; instead, water-soluble menadione (vitamin K_3) salts are used to provide vitamin K activity in feeds. Because of instability, menadione is not used in feed as the pure vitamin, but is formulated as an additional product with sodium bisulfite and its derivatives. Water-soluble derivatives of menadione, including menadione sodium bisulfite (MSB), menadione sodium bisulfite complex (MSBC), and menadione dimethyl-pyrimidinol bisulfite (MPB), are the principal forms of vitamin K included in commercial diets. The greatest menadione activity is in MSB (50%), followed by MPB (45.4%), and MSBC (33%) (Schneider and Hoppe, 1986). Sometimes MSB is coated with gelatin to increase stability, resulting in 25% menadione activity.

Stability of the naturally occurring sources of vitamin K is poor. However, stability of the water-soluble menadione salts is excellent in multivitamin premixes unless trace minerals are present (Frye, 1978).

Basic pH conditions also accelerate the destruction of menadione salts; thus soluble or slightly soluble basic mineral substances should not be included in multivitamin premixes containing menadione. Coelho (1991) concluded that vitamin K in the form of MSB or MSBC is very sensitive to moisture and trace minerals, sensitive to light and gastric pH, and moderately sensitive to reduction and acid pH. Choline chloride is particularly destructive to vitamin K, with an average monthly loss of 34 to 38% for MSBC and MPB when stored in a vitamin premix with choline (Coelho, 1991). Less water-soluble forms or coated K_3 forms exhibit superior stability compared to uncoated MSB. At higher temperatures, uncoated MSB preparations lost about 60% activity (Gropp and Mehringer, 1990). Heat, moisture, and trace minerals increase the rate of destruction of menadione salts in both pressure-pelleted and extruded feeds (Hoffmann-La Roche, 1981). For these reasons, greater quantities of vitamin K_3 are recommended in premixes that contain large quantities of choline chloride and certain trace elements, and especially when plain MSB is used or premixes are exported or stored for an extended period (Schneider and Hoppe, 1986).

Clinical use of vitamin K in human nutrition is largely limited to two forms: a water-soluble form of menadione (menadiol sodium diphosphate) and the more expensive phylloquinone. Some danger of hyperbilirubinemia has been associated with menadione usage (Suttie, 1991), whereas vitamin K in the form of phylloquinone is biologically more available. Griminger and Brubacher (1966) found four times as much vitamin K in eggs of hens fed phylloquinone as in eggs of hens fed an equivalent level of menadione.

Vitamin K supplementation has been found to have a definite value in human therapy (1) as a preoperative and postoperative measure to prevent risk of bleeding; (2) when absorption is impaired, as in obstructive jaundice, because bile is necessary for the absorption of vitamin K; and (3) in newborns with hemorrhagic disease. Surgical patients should be given supplemental vitamin K for loss of blood from operations, therapy with antibiotics, and fasting procedures. Phylloquinone is rapidly depleted by fasting; it may be difficult to prevent vitamin K deficiency by dietary phylloquinone alone during long-term fasting after surgery. In one study, plasma phylloquinone decreased rapidly from 1.16 to 0.36 nmol/L in 11 patients during postoperative fasting (Usui et al., 1990).

Low-dose maternal vitamin K_1 supplementation does not sufficiently increase vitamin K in breast milk (Greer et al., 1991; Pietschnig et al., 1993). Recommendations from various locations suggest oral supplementation of infants at birth with 1 mg (Birkbeck, 1988; Cornelissen et al., 1993; Groot and De-Groot, 1993). In babies at risk, intramuscular injection of 500 µg at birth, followed by 25 µg by mouth daily for 3 weeks, is recommended (Birkbeck, 1988). In a study involving 100 infants, the authors concluded that vitamin K is equally effective whether administered orally or intramuscularly (Malik et al., 1992). Intracranial hemorrhage due to vitamin K deficiency in breast-fed infants is dramatically decreased with vitamin K supplementation in newborns. Nevertheless, breast-fed infants with cholestasis or fat malabsorption remain at high risk of vitamin K deficiency and hemorrhage (Bancroft and Cohen, 1993).

TOXICITY

Toxic effects of the vitamin K family are manifested mainly as hematological and circulatory disorders. Not only is species variation encountered, but profound differences are observed in the ability of the various vitamin K compounds to evoke a toxic response (Barash, 1978). The natural forms of vitamin K, phylloquinone and menaquinone, are nontoxic at very high dosage levels. The synthetic menadione compounds, however, have shown toxic effects when given to humans, rabbits, dogs, and mice in excessive amounts. The toxic dietary level of menadione is at least 1,000 times the dietary requirement (NRC, 1987). Menadione compounds can be safely used at low levels to prevent the development of deficiency but should not be used as a pharmacological treatment for a hemorrhagic condition.

The parenteral LD_{50} of menadione or its derivatives is a few hundred milligrams per kilogram of body weight in some species. Dosages of 2 to 8 mg/kg body weight were reported to be lethal in horses (Rebhun et al., 1984), resulting in renal colic, hematuria, azotemia, and electrolyte abnormalities consistent with acute renal failure. At necropsy, lesions of renal tubular nephrosis were found. Also, 200 mg of menadione sodium bisulfite administered to horses intravenously resulted in depression, stiffness, colic, laminitis, and renal fibrosis and failure (Maxie et al., 1992).

In animal studies, oral ingestion of large amounts of vitamin K_1 (25 g/kg body weight) produced no fatalities, whereas menadione had an LD_{50} (in mice) equal to 500 mg/kg of diet (Molitor and Robinson, 1940). Anemia, hemoglobinuria, urobilinuria, and urobilinoguria were observed with oral doses of 25 to 50 mg/kg. These doses are approximately 125 times the recommended clinical dose (0.05 mg/kg) for humans. The anemia seen following excessive vitamin K_3 administration appears to be reversible following withdrawal (Richards and Shapiro, 1945).

Full-term infants appear to have a greater tolerance to vitamin K than premature infants. It is concluded that all vitamin K analogs are safe when administered in the proper dosage; however, the formulation with the greatest margin of safety is vitamin K_1.

■ REFERENCES

Almquist, H.J. (1971). *In* The Vitamins, (W.H. Sebrell Jr., and R.S. Harris, eds.),Vol. 3, 2nd Ed., p. 418. Academic Press, New York.
Almquist, H.J. (1975). *Am. J. Clin. Nutr. 28,* 656.
Almquist, H.J. (1978). *In* Handbook Series in Nutrition and Foods, Section E: Nutritional Disorders (M. Rechcigl Jr., ed.), Vol. 2, p. 195. CRC Press, Boca Raton, Florida.
Almquist, H.J., and Stokstad, L.R. (1935). *Nature (London) 136,* 31.
Alstad, A.D., Casper, H.H., and Johnson, L.J. (1985). *J. Am. Vet. Med. Assoc. 187,* 729.
Anonymous. (1985) *Nutr. Rev. 43,* 303.
Bach, A.V. (1994). Sensitivity of Various Indicies of Human Vitamin K Deficiency, M.S. Thesis, University of Wisconsin, Madison.
Bancroft, J., and Cohen, M.B. (1993). *J. Pediatr. 16,* 78.
Barash, P.G. (1978). *In* Handbook Series in Nutrition and Foods, Section E: Nutritional Disorders (M. Rechcigl Jr., ed.), Vol. 1, p. 97. CRC Press, Boca Raton, Florida.
Barnes, R.H., Fiala, G., McGehee, B., and Brown, A. (1957). *J. Nutr. 63,* 489.
Bell, R.G. (1978). *Fed. Proc. Fed. Am. Soc. Exp. Biol. 37,* 2599.
Binkley, N.C., and Suttie, J.W. (1995). *J. Nutr. 125,* 1812.
Birkbeck, J.A. (1988). *New Zealand Med. J., 101,* 421.
Booth, S.L., and Mayer, J. (1997). *Nutr. Rev. 55,* 282.
Cancela, M.L., Williamson, M.K., and Price, P.A. (1993). *Nutr. Res. 13,* 87.
Canfield, L.M., Hopkinson, J.M., Lima, A.F., Silva, B., and Garza, C. (1991). *Am. J. Clin. Nutr. 3,* 730.
Carlisle, T.L., Shah, D.V., Schlegel, R., and Suttie, J.W. (1975). *Proc. Soc. Exp. Biol. Med. 148,* 140.
Carter, S.D., Cromwell, G.L., Combs, T.R., Colombo, G., and Fanti, P. (1996). *J. Anim. Sci. 74,* 2719.
Coelho, M.B. (1991). Vitamin stability in premixes and feeds: A practical approach. BASF Technical Symposium, Bloomington, Minnesota.
Combs Jr., G.F. (1992). The Vitamins. Academic Press, San Diego, California.
Cornelissen, E., Kollee, L., Abreu, R., Motohara, K., Monnens, L., and De-Abreu, R. (1993). *Acta Paediatr. 82,* 656.
Cunha, T.J. (1977). Swine Feeding and Nutrition. Academic Press, Inc., New York.
Dam, H., Schonheyder, F., and Tage-Hansen, E. (1936). *Biochem. J. 30,* 1075.
De Boer-van den Berg, M.A.G., Verstijnen, C.P.H.J., and Vermeer, C. (1986). *J.*

Invest. Dermatol. 87, 377.

DeHoogh, W. (1989). *Bovine Pract. 24,* 173.

Ferland, G. (1998). *Nutr. Rev. 56,* 223.

Ferland, G., and Sadowski, J.A. (1992a). *J. Agric. Food Chem. 40,* 1869.

Ferland, G., and Sadowski, J.A. (1992b). *J. Agric. Food Chem. 40,* 1874.

Fritschen, R.D., Peo Jr., E.R., Lucas, L.E., and Grace, O.D. (1970). *J. Anim. Sci. 31,* 199(Abstr.).

Frye, T.M. (1978). *Proc. Roche Vitam. Nutr. Update Meet., Arkansas Nutr. Conf., Little Rock,* p. 54. Hoffmann-La Roche, Nutley, New Jersey.

Gallop, P.M., Lian, J.B., and Hauschka, P.V. (1980). *N. Engl. J. Med. 302,* 1460.

Goplen, B.P., and Bell, J.M. (1967). *Can. J. Anim. Sci. 47,* 91.

Greer, F.R., Marshall, S., Cherry, J., and Suttie, J.W. (1991). *Pediatrics 88,* 751.

Griminger, P. (1984a). *Feedstuffs,* 56(38), 26.

Griminger, P. (1984b). *Feedstuffs,* 56(39), 24.

Griminger, P., and Brubacher, G. (1966). *Poult. Sci. 45,* 512.

Griminger, P., and Donis, O. (1960). *J. Nutr. 70,* 361.

Groot, C.J., and De-Groot, C.J. (1993). *Voeding 54,* 10.

Gropp, J., and Mehringer, W. (1990). *Zeitschrift-fur Ernahrungswissenschaft 29,* 219.

Hadler, M.R., and Shadbolt, R.S. (1975). *Nature (London) 253,* 275.

Hall, D.D., Cromwell, G.L., and Stahly, T.S. (1991). *J. Anim. Sci. 69,* 646.

Haroon, Y., Shearer, M.J., Rahim, S., Gunn, W.G., McEnery, G., and Barkhan, P. (1982). *J. Nutr. 112,* 1105.

Hazell, K., and Baloch, K.H. (1970) *Gerontol. Clin. 12,* 10.

Hill, R.B., Schendel, H.E., Rama Rao, P.B., and Johnson, B.C. (1964). *J. Nutr. 84,* 259.

Hoffmann-La Roche. (1981). Rationale for Roche Recommended Vitamin Fortification—Dogs and Cats. RCD 5963/1280. Hoffmann-La Roche, Inc., Nutley, New Jersey.

Hollander, D. (1973). *Am. J. Physiol. 225,* 360.

Hollander, D., and Truscott, T.C. (1974). *J. Lab. Clin. Med. 83,* 648.

Hoppe, P.P. (1987). *Praktische Tierarzt 68,* 32.

Ingram, R.T., Park, Y.K., Clarke, B.L., and Fitzpatrick, L.A. (1994). *J. Clin. Invest. 93,* 989.

Jolly, D.W., Craig, C., and Nelson, T.E. (1977). *Am. J. Physiol. 232,* H12.

Kerr, M.C. (1986). *Vet. Rec. 119*(17), 435.

Kindberg, C., Suttie, J.W., Uchida, K., Hirauchi, K., and Nakao, H. (1987). *J. Nutr. 117,* 1032.

Konishi, T., Baba, S., and Sone, H. (1973). *Chem. Pharm. Bull. 21,* 220.

Lavelle, P.A., Lloyd, A.P., Gay, C.V., and Leach Jr., R.M. (1994). *J. Nutr. 124,* 371.

Lee, L., and Morre, D.M. (1992). *Korean J. Nutr. 25,* 492.

Loosli, J.K. (1991). *In* Handbook of Animal Science (P.A. Putnam, ed.), Academic Press, San Diego, California.

Losito, R., Owen, C.A., and Flock, E.V. (1967). *Biochemistry 6,* 62.

Maddison, J.E., Watson, A.D.J., Eade, I.G., and Exner, T. (1990). *J. Am. Vet. Med. Assoc. 197,* 1495.

Malik, S., Udani, R.H., Bichile, S.K., Agrawal, R.M., Bahrainwala, A.T., and

Tilaye, S. (1992). *Indian Pediatr. 29*, 857.

Manz, U., and Maurer, R. (1982). *Int. J. Vitam. Nutr. 52*, 248.

Marks, J. (1975). A Guide to the Vitamins. Their Role in Health and Disease, p. 73. Medical and Technical Publ., Lancaster, England.

Martius, C., and Alvino, C. (1964). *Biochem Z. 340*, 316.

Matschiner, J.T., Bell, R.G., Amelotti, J.M., and Knauer, T.E. (1970). *Biochim. Biophys. Acta 201*, 309.

Mathers, J.C., Fernandez, F., Hill, M.J., McCarthy, P.T., Shearer, M.J., and Oxley, A. (1990). *Br. J. Nutr. 63*, 639.

Maxie, G., Van Dreumel, T., McMaster, D., and Baird, J. (1992). *Can. Vet. J. 33*, 756.

McCollum, E.V. (1957). *In* A History of Nutrition, The Riverside Press, Cambridge, Massachusetts.

McFarlane, W.D., Graham, W.R., and Richardson, F. (1931). *Biochem. J. 25*, 358.

Molitor, H., and Robinson, H. (1940). *Proc. Soc. Exp. Biol. Med. 43*, 125.

Mount, M.E., and Kass, P.H. (1989). *Am. J. Vet. Res. 59*, 1704.

Mundy, G.R., and Poser, J.W. (1983). *Calcif. Tissue Int. 35*, 164.

Nelsestuen, G.L., Zytkovicz, T.H., and Howard, J.B. (1974). *J. Biol. Chem. 249*, 6347.

Nelson, T.S., and Norris, L.C. (1961). *J. Nutr. 73*, 135.

Nestor Jr., K.E., and Conrad, H.R. (1990). *J. Dairy Sci. 73*, 3291.

Newsholme, S.J., Cullen, J.S.C., Nel, P.W., and Reyers, F. (1985). *J. S. Afr. Vet. Assoc. 56*, 101.

NRC. Nutrient Requirements of Domestic Animals. National Academy of Sciences-National Research Council, Washington, D.C.
(1977). Nutrient Requirements of Rabbits, 2nd Ed.
(1978). Nutrient Requirements of Nonhuman Primates.
(1981). Nutrient Requirements of Goats.
(1982a). Nutrient Requirements of Mink and Foxes.
(1985a). Nutrient Requirements of Dogs, 2nd Ed.
(1985b). Nutrient Requirements of Sheep, 5th Ed.
(1986). Nutrient Requirements of Cats, 3rd Ed.
(1989a). Nutrient Requirements of Dairy Cattle, 6th Ed.
(1989b). Nutrient Requirements of Horses, 5th Ed.
(1993). Nutrient Requirements of Fish.
(1994). Nutrient Requirements of Poultry, 9th Ed.
(1995). Nutrient Requirements of Laboratory Animals, 4th Ed.
(1996). Nutrient Requirements of Beef Cattle, 7th Ed.
(1998). Nutrient Requirements of Swine, 10th Ed.

NRC. (1982b). United States-Canadian Tables of Feed Composition, 3rd Ed. National Academy of Sciences-National Research Council, Washington, D.C.

NRC. (1987). Vitamin Tolerance of Animals. National Academy of Sciences-National Research Council, Washington, D.C.

Olson, R.E., and Suttie, J.W. (1978). *Vitam. Horm. 35*, 59.

Pietschnig, B., Haschle, F., Vanura, H., Shearer, M., Veitl, V., Kellner, S., and Schuster, E. (1993). *Eur. J. Clin. Nutr. 47*, 209.

Pineo, G.F., Gallus, A.S., and Hirsh, J. (1973). *J. Can. Med. Assoc. 109,* 880.

Price, P.A. (1993). *J. Clin. Invest. 91,* 1268.

RDA. (1989). Recommended Dietary Allowances, 10th Ed. National Academy of Sciences-National Research Council, Washington, D.C.

Rebhun, W.C., Tennant, B.C., Dill, S.G., and King, J.M. (1984). *J. Am. Vet. Med. Assoc. 184,* 1237.

Richards, R.K., and Shapiro, S. (1945). *J. Pharmacol. Exp.Ther. 84,* 93.

Schendel, H.E., and Johnson, B.C. (1962). *J. Nutr. 76,* 124.

Schneider, J., and Hoppe, P.P. (1986). Bioavailability of Nutrients in Feed Ingredients, p. 1. National Feed Ingredients Association (NFIA), Des Moines, Iowa.

Scott, M.L., Nesheim, M.C., and Young, R.J. (1982). Nutrition of the Chicken, p. 119. Scott, Ithaca, New York.

Shearer, M.J., and Barkhan, P. (1973). *Biochim. Biophys. Acta 297,* 300.

Shearer, M.J., Barkhan, P., and Webster, G.R. (1970). *Br. J. Haematol. 18,* 297.

Shearer, M.J., Bach, A., and Kohlmeier, M. (1996). *J. Nutr. 126,* 1181S.

Shiau, S., and Liu, J. (1994). *J. Nutr. 124,* 277.

Shino, M. (1988). *Analyst, 113,* 393.

Shirakawa, H., Komai, M., and Kimura, S. (1990). *Inter. J. Vit. Nutr. Res. 60,* 245.

Squibb, R.L. (1964). *Poult. Sci. 43,* 1443.

Stenflo, J., Fernlund, P., Egan, W., and Roepstorff, P. (1974). *Proc. Natl. Acad. Sci. 71,* 2730.

Suttie, J.W. (1980). *Fed. Proc. Fed. Am. Soc. Exp. Biol. 39,* 2730.

Suttie, J.W. (1990). *Clin. Cardiol. 13,* 16.

Suttie, J.W. (1991). *In* Handbook of Vitamins, 2nd Ed. (L.J. Machlin, ed.), p. 145. Marcel Dekker, New York.

Suttie, J.W., and Jackson, C.M. (1977). *Physiol. Rev. 57,* 1.

Suttie, J.W., and Olson, R.E. (1990). *In* Nutrition Reviews. Present Knowledge in Nutrition (R.E. Olson, ed.), p. 122. Nutrition Foundation, Washington, D.C.

Suttie, J.W., Mummah-Schendel, L.L., Shah, D.V., Lyle, B.J., and Greger, J.L. (1988). *Am. J. Clin. Nutr. 47,* 475.

Suzuki, S. (1979). *J. Perinat. Med. 7,* 229.

Suzuki, S., Maki, M., Shirakawa, K., and Terao, T. (1989). *J. Perinat. Med. 17,* 305.

Thierry, M.J., Hermodson, M.A., and Suttie, J.W. (1970). *Am. J. Physiol. 219,* 854.

Thijssen, H.H.W., Drittij-Reijnders, M.J., and Fischer, M.A. (1996). *J. Nutr. 126,* 543.

Tulchinsky, T.J., Patton, M.M., Randolph, L.A., Meyer, M.R., and Linden, J.V. (1993). *Am. J. Publ. Health 83,* 1166.

Usui, Y., Tanimura, H., Nishimura,N., Kobayashi, N., Okanoue, T., and Ozawa, K. (1990). *Am. J. Clin. Nutr. 51,* 846.

Vanderschueren, D., Gevers, G., Raymaekers, G., Devos, P., and Dequeker, J. (1990). *Calcif. Tissue Int. 46,* 179.

Vermeer, C. (1984). *Mol. Cell. Biochem. 61,* 17.

Vermeer, C. (1986). *Haemostasis 16,* 239.

Wakeman, D.L., Ott, E.A., Crawford, B.H., and Cunha, T.J. (1975). Horse Production in Florida, p. 75. Bull.No. 188, Florida Dept. of Agricultural and Consumer Services, Gainesville, Florida.

Weiser, H., and Tagwerker, F. (1982). Optimization of the Vitamin K Bioassay of Vitamin K Forms for Feed Supplementation, No. 1794. Hoffmann-La Roche, Basel, Switzerland.

Will, B.H., and Suttie, J.W. (1992). *J. Nutr. 122,* 953.

Will, B.H., Usui, Y., and Suttie, J.W. (1992). *J. Nutr. 122,* 2354.

Yonaga, T. (1990). *Nutr. Res. 10,* 761.

THIAMIN

INTRODUCTION

Thiamin (also called thiamine, aneurin[e], and vitamin B_1) was the first vitamin to be discovered. Under most circumstances, there is little chance of thiamin deficiency for monogastric animals, including humans, when diets contain ample quantities of whole cereal grains or starchy roots. However, many thiamin antagonists in the food supply, and sensitivity of the vitamin to processing (e.g., heat), can lead to deficiency. Thiamin deficiency in humans has been a problem mostly in Asian countries, where highly milled (polished) rice is consumed, thus eliminating the thiamin-rich bran fraction of the grain. For years, it was accepted that ruminants did not require vitamin B supplementation because of adequate rumen microflora synthesis. Intensification of ruminant feeding, involving high-concentrate diets, and management systems with increased levels of production have resulted in nervous disorders that are responsive to thiamin supplementation.

HISTORY

Thiamin is considered to be the oldest vitamin, and the disease beriberi probably is the earliest documented deficiency disorder. Beriberi was prevalent in many world regions (particularly Asia) where diets were based on highly milled or polished rice. The early history of thiamin has been reviewed (Jansen, 1956; Williams, 1961; Sebrell and Harris, 1973; Loosli, 1991). Beriberi was recognized in China as early as 2697 B.C. Beriberi occurred sporadically until the middle of the nineteenth century, but after about 1870, with the introduction of the steam-powered rice mills, the incidence of the disease rose steeply, chiefly in prisons and barracks. In prisons in Java, a sentence of longer than 3 months was equivalent to capital punishment, because after that time nearly all prisoners developed beriberi and died. Beriberi was prevalent in armies and navies, particularly during times of war. In 1895, 26% of the entire Japanese army of 17,500 had beriberi. Infantile beriberi was the leading cause of death in some countries, with infants comprising 70 to 80% of all deaths from beriberi in the Philippines from 1912 to 1930.

No cure was found for beriberi until K. Takaki studied sailors in the Japanese Navy in the early 1880s, when the incidence of beriberi was 32%. By replacing some of the polished rice with other foods, Takaki was able to dramatically reduce the incidence of beriberi. He incorrectly thought that added dietary protein was responsible for preventing beriberi.

In the 1890s Eijkman, a Dutch investigator, produced paralysis in chickens fed boiled polished rice. He called the condition polyneuritis and observed that clinical signs were similar to beriberi symptoms in humans. In the course of experiments, Eijkman noticed by chance that both polyneuritis and beriberi could be both prevented and cured if rice bran was consumed with the polished rice. He mistakenly believed that the polished-rice diet produced a toxin that was counteracted by feeding rice polishings. The conclusion that beriberi was caused by a vitally important food constituent was formulated in 1901 by Grijns, who was Eijkman's successor.

Ten years later (1911), Funk, of the Lister Institute in London, obtained a potent anti-beriberi substance from rice bran (thiamin) that had the character of an amine. Thus the term vitamin(e), for vital amine, was coined. However, it was later found that many vitamins are not amines.

Around the same time (1910), Captain Edward B. Vedder, who was in the U.S. Army in Manila in the Philippines, became convinced that beriberi, which was very prevalent, was indeed caused by a nutritional deficiency; he began in earnest to pursue the isolation of the active factor. In 1912 Vedder and Chamberlain presented a paper on preventing and treating beriberi with rice polishings. This practice saved many from death due to infantile beriberi and was influential in establishing the deficiency theory for beriberi.

In 1860-61 the Burk and Wills expedition crossed the Australian continent from south to north. These explorers were the first Europeans to make this trip, but both died on the return trip as they consumed the Nardoo fern, which contained a high level of thiaminase activity (Earl and McCleary, 1994). In 1926 two Dutch chemists, Jansen and Donath, successors to Eijkman and Grijns in the Indonesian laboratory, succeeded in crystallizing thiamin in pure form. In 1936 Williams and colleagues, after many years of work, determined the chemical structure of thiamin and were able to synthesize the vitamin. Earlier in his career Williams had worked closely with Vedder in the Philippines toward the control of beriberi through better nutrition.

CHEMICAL STRUCTURE, PROPERTIES, AND ANTAGONISTS

Thiamin consists of a molecule of pyrimidine and a molecule of thiazole linked by a methylene bridge (Fig. 6.1); it contains both nitrogen and sulfur atoms. Thiamin is isolated in pure form as the white thiamin hydrochloride. The vitamin has a characteristic sulfurous odor and slightly bitter taste. Thiamin is very soluble in water, sparingly so in alcohol, and insoluble in fat solvents. It is very sensitive to alkali, in which the thiazole ring opens at room temperature when pH is above 7. In a dry state, thiamin is stable at 100°C for several hours, but moisture greatly accelerates destruction, and thus, it is much less stable to heat in fresh than in dry foods. Under ordinary conditions, thiamin hydrochloride is more hygroscopic (takes up moisture) than the mononitrate form. However, both products should be kept in sealed containers. Autoclaving destroys thiamin, an observation that played an important role in the discovery that what was originally considered to be a single vitamin was actually a member of the vitamin B complex (Maynard et al., 1979).

Substances with an anti-thiamin activity are fairly common in nature and include structurally similar antagonists as well as structure-altering antagonists and thiamin-degrading enzymes (thiaminases). The synthetic compounds pyrithiamine, oxythiamine, and amprolium (coccidiostat) are structurally similar antagonists, and their mode of action is competitive inhibition with biologically inactive compounds, thus interfering with thiamin at different points in metabolism. Synthetic thiamin antagonists are often used in studies of the pharmacodynamics of thiamin (Barclay and Gibson, 1982). Pyrithiamine blocks chiefly the esterification of thiamin with phosphoric acid, resulting in inhibition of the thiamin coenzyme cocarboxylase. Oxythiamin likewise displaces cocarboxylase from important metabolic reactions. Amprolium inhibits the absorption of thiamin from the intestine and blocks the phosphorylation of the vitamin.

Heat-stable thiamin antagonists occur in a number of plants (e.g., ferns and tea); these include polyphenols (e.g., caffeic acid and tannic acid), which oxidize the thiazole ring to yield the nonabsorbable thiamin

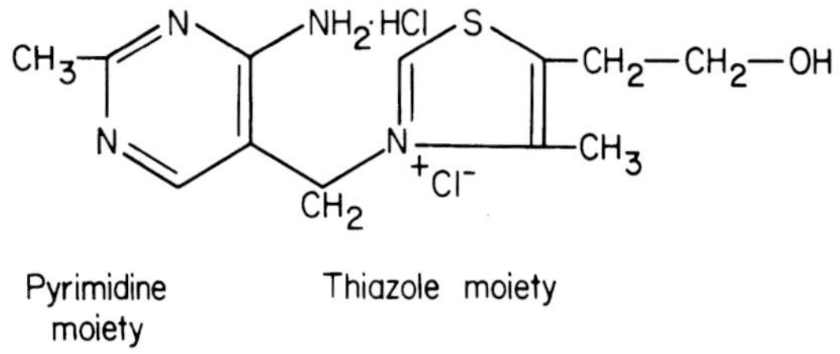

Pyrimidine
moiety

Thiazole moiety

Fig. 6.1 Structure of thiamin hydrochloride.

disulfide. Tall fescue (*Festuca arundinacea* Schreb.) toxicosis resembles diseases caused by enhanced rumen thiaminase activity (Lauriault et al., 1990). Thiamin supplementation has been found to reduce tall fescue (endophyte-infected) toxicosis (Lauriault et al., 1990; Dougherty et al., 1991).

Sulfur has been shown to be antagonistic to thiamin enzymes. The sulfite ion has been shown to cleave thiamin from enzymes at the methylene bridge between the pyrimidine and thiazole rings and analytically will mimic thiaminase. Sulfate increases thiamin-destroying activity in the rumen contents, and the destructive mechanism involves thermolabile factor(s); however, the ruminal synthesis of thiamin is not affected by sulfate (Olkowski et al., 1993).

Thiaminase activity destroys thiamin activity by altering the structure of the vitamin. The disease Chastek paralysis in foxes and other carnivores fed certain types of raw fish results from a thiaminase that splits the thiamin molecule into two components, thus inactivating it. Two types of thiaminase enzymes have been described (Brent and Bartley, 1984). Thiaminase II simply cleaves the vitamin at the methylene bridge between the thiazole and pyrimidine rings. Thiaminase I substitutes a nitrogen-containing ring for the thiazole ring. This leads to less thiamin, but it also gives rise to thiamin analogs composed of the pyrimidine ring of the original thiamin, and another ring from the "co-substrate." This created thiamin analog inhibits one or more thiamin-requiring reactions necessary for energy metabolism in the central nervous system (CNS) (Frye et al., 1991).

Since thiaminase is heat labile, the problem can be avoided in fish, for example, by cooking the fish at 83°C for at least 5 minutes. Many kinds of fish contain thiaminase, and thiamin deficiency has been reported in penguins, seals, and dolphins fed primarily fish diets in zoos (Maynard et al., 1979). Thiaminase is found mainly in herrings, sprats, stints, and various carp species—a total of some 50 species, most of which live in fresh water. Wild aquatic animals apparently do not develop thiamin deficiency even though they eat a diet primarily of fish, because fish must undergo some putrefaction to release the enzyme (Evans, 1975). In vitro and in vivo experiments have shown that 1 kg of fish can destroy up to 25 mg of thiamin. This degradation takes place within the first 30 minutes after ingestion, while still in the stomach. Certain microorganisms (bacteria and molds) also have been shown to produce thiaminases. A disease in horses known as bracken fern poisoning results from antagonism to thiamin.

ANALYTICAL PROCEDURES

Thiamin activity can be analyzed by biological, microbiological, and chemical methods. Biological methods are based on curative ability for polyneuritis in pigeons; bradycardia in rats; or growth in chicks, pigeons, and rats. Microbiological tests are fairly rapid, inexpensive, and very sensitive, but some organisms lack specificity for thiamin compared to the pyrimidine and thiazole moieties or the enzyme form of the vitamin. Chemical analytical analysis for thiamin is conducted by oxidative condensation of thiamin to thiochrome, which shows a characteristic blue fluorescence in ultraviolet light. The fluorometric thiochrome method is the procedure most widely used to estimate thiamin in foodstuffs and feeds. A promising method using high-performance liquid chromatography (HPLC) for routine determination of thiamin in foods has been developed (Ollilainen et al., 1993).

METABOLISM

Digestion, Absorption, and Transport

Thiamin is readily digested and released from natural sources. A precondition for normal absorption of thiamin is sufficient production of stomach hydrochloric acid. Phosphoric acid esters of thiamin are split in the intestine. Free thiamin is soluble in water and easily absorbed. Absorption occurs in the small intestine, particularly in the jejunum. In most species, absorption is negligible in the distal portion of the small intestine, and in the stomach and large intestines. Thus, thiamin synthesized by gut microflora in the cecum or large intestine is largely unavailable to the animal except by coprophagy. The horse, however, can absorb thiamin from the cecum. Ruminants can also absorb free thiamin from the rumen, but the rumen wall is not permeable for bound thiamin or for thiamin contained in rumen microorganisms.

The mechanism of thiamin absorption is not yet fully understood, but apparently both active transport and simple (passive) diffusion are involved (S'Klan and Trostler, 1977; Gubler, 1991). At low concentrations there is an active sodium-dependent transport against the electrochemical potential, whereas at high concentrations it diffuses passively through the intestinal wall. Absorption from the rumen is also believed to be an active mechanism.

Absorbed thiamin is transported via the portal vein to the liver with a carrier plasma protein, thiamin-binding protein (Rose, 1990). This binding protein is hormonally regulated (e.g., corticosteroid hormones) and is associated with thiamin transport into and out of the cell. In blood, 90% of total thiamin is in the cellular fraction (predominantly erythrocytes), while the plasma contains largely free unesterified thiamin. Thiamin is efficiently transferred to the fetus. In human placentas thiamin concentration was found to be 4.5 mmol/L in maternal plasma versus 45.9 mmol/L in venous cord plasma, indicating a massive retention by the fetus (Zempleni et al., 1992).

Phosphorylation

Thiamin phosphorylation can take place in most tissues, but does so particularly in the liver. Four-fifths of thiamin in animals is phosphorylated in liver under the action of adenosine triphosphate (ATP) to form the metabolically active enzyme form thiamin pyrophosphate (TPP; or thiamin diphosphate or cocarboxylase). Of total body thiamin, about 80% is TPP, about 10% is thiamin triphosphate (TTP), and the remainder is thiamin monophosphate (TMP) and free thiamin. Extracellular fluids, including serum, milk, and cerebrospinal fluid, contain only free (unesterified) thiamin and TMP, suggesting that these forms cross cell membranes while TPP and TTP cannot.

Storage and Excretion

In animal tissues, thiamin occurs mostly as phosphate esters. Although thiamin is readily absorbed and transported to cells throughout the body, it is not stored to any great extent. Thiamin content in individual organs varies considerably, with the vitamin preferentially retained in organs with high metabolic activity. During deficiency, thiamin is retained in greatest quantities in important organs such as the heart, brain, liver, and kidneys. The principal storage organs are the liver and kidney; however, approximately one-half of total thiamin is present in muscle (Tanphaichair, 1976). Thiamin is one of the most poorly stored vitamins. Mammals can exhaust their body stores within 1 to 2 weeks (Ensminger et al., 1983). Since thiamin is not stored in large amounts, it is relatively easy to develop severe deficiency in a short time, even in adult animals.

Thiamin intakes in excess of current needs are rapidly excreted. This means that the body needs a regular supply and that unneeded intakes are wasted. The pig is somewhat of an exception, however—for some unknown reason its tissues contain several times as much thiamin as other species studied. Thus it has a store that can meet body needs on a thiamin-deficient diet for as long as 2 months (Heinemann et al., 1946).

Absorbed thiamin is excreted in both urine and feces, with small quantities excreted in sweat. Urinary thiamin is mainly free thiamin and TMP. However, when subjects consume low-thiamin diets, the main urinary excretion is pyrimidine and thiazole, and further degradation of these substances has been identified (Brown, 1990). Fecal thiamin may originate from feed, synthesis by microorganisms, or endogenous synthesis (e.g., via bile or excretion through the mucosa of the large intestine). When thiamin is administered in large doses, urinary excretion first increases, then reaches a saturation level, and with additional thiamin the fecal concentration increases considerably (Bräunlich and Zintzen, 1976).

FUNCTIONS

Decarboxylation of α-Keto Acids and Transketolase Reactions

Thiamin in all cells functions principally as the coenzyme cocarboxylase or TPP. Thiamin monophosphate is completely inactive, and any coenzyme activity previously attributed to the triphosphate undoubtedly results from partial conversion to diphosphate by hydrolysis of the terminal phosphate ester bond by thiamin triphosphatase (Gubler, 1991).

The citric acid cycle (Krebs cycle or tricarboxylic acid cycle) is responsible for production of energy in the body. In this cycle, breakdown products of carbohydrates, fats, and proteins are brought together for further breakdown and for synthesis. The vitamins riboflavin, niacin, and pantothenic acid, as well as thiamin, play roles in the cycle. Thiamin is the coenzyme for all enzymatic decarboxylations of α-keto acids. Thus it functions in the oxidative decarboxylation of pyruvate to acetate,

271

which in turn is combined with coenzyme A for entrance into the tricarboxylic cycle.

In mammals, thiamin is essential in two oxidative decarboxylation reactions in the citric acid cycle that take place in cell mitochondria and one reaction in the cytoplasm (Fig. 6.2). These are essential reactions for utilization of carbohydrates to provide energy. Decarboxylation in the citric acid cycle removes carbon dioxide, and the substrate is converted into the compound having the next lower number of carbon atoms. In the mitochondria, reactions pyruvate dehydrogenase forms acetyl CoA from pyruvate and α-ketoglutarate dehydrogenase to convert α-ketoglutarate to succinyl CoA as follows:

$$\text{Pyruvate} \rightarrow \text{acetyl-CoA} + CO_2 \qquad (1)$$

$$\alpha\text{-Ketoglutaric acid} \rightarrow \text{succinyl-CoA} + CO_2 \quad (2)$$

It has been shown that decarboxylation of the three branched-chain α-ketoacids derived from the deamination of leucine, isoleucine, and valine are also oxidatively decarboxylated by a multienzyme complex analogous to those for pyruvic and α-ketoglutaric acids, but more specific for these branched-chain α-ketoacids (Gubler, 1991).

TPP is a coenzyme in the transketolase reaction that is part of the direction oxidative pathway (pentose phosphate cycle) of glucose metabolism that occurs not in mitochondria but in the cell cytoplasm in liver, brain, adrenal cortex, and kidney, but not skeletal muscle. Transketolase catalyzes transfer of C_2 fragments; hence with ribulose 5-phosphate as donor and ribose 5-phosphate as acceptor, sedoheptulose 7-phosphate and triose phosphate are formed. This is the only mechanism known for synthesis of ribose, which is needed for nucleotide formation of RNA and DNA synthesis and results in formation of nicotinamide adenine dinucleotide phosphate (NADP), which is essential for reducing intermediates from carbohydrate metabolism to form fatty acids. It can also supply intermediate sugars for glycolysis.

Other Functions

Thiamin has a vital role in nerve function, although the mechanism of action is unclear. It has been postulated that thiamin, probably as TPP, plays an essential role in nerve transmission, apart from its enzymatic role in the Krebs cycle and the pentose pathway. When nerves are stimulated, the levels of TPP and TTP decrease, and TMP and free thiamin are released into the surrounding medium. This is believed to in-

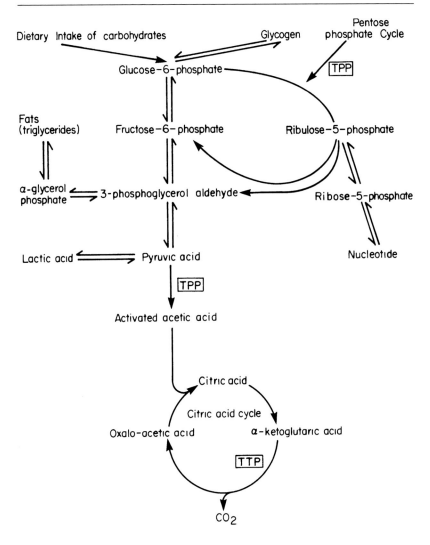

Fig. 6.2 Thiamin as thiamin pyrophosphate (TPP) in the metabolism of carbohydrates. (Modified from Bräunlich and Zintzen, 1976.)

volve sodium and potassium transport at the membrane (Barchi, 1976). Fatty acids and cholesterol are the major constituents of cell membranes, and effects on their synthesis would affect membrane integrity and function. Thiamin deficiency in cultured glial cells impairs their ability to synthesize fatty acids and cholesterol. The defect is related to reduced formation of key lipogenic enzymes. These changes could be the basis of degenerative changes seen in glial cells in early thiamin deficiency.

Stimulation of nerves by either electrical or chemical means has been found to result in the release of thiamin (as free thiamin and the monophosphate ester) that is associated with the dephosphorylation of its higher phosphate esters (Combs, 1992). The antagonist pyrithiamine can displace thiamin from nervous tissue and change the electrical activity of the tissue. Possible mechanisms of action of thiamin in nervous tissue include the following (Muralt, 1962; Cooper et al., 1963): (1) Thiamin is involved in the synthesis of acetylcholine, which transmits neural impulses; (2) thiamin participates in the passive transport of sodium of excitable membranes, which is important for the transmission of impulses at the membrane of ganglionic cells; and (3) the reduction in the activity of transketolase in the pentose phosphate pathway that follows thiamin deficiency reduces the synthesis of fatty acids and the metabolism of energy in the nervous system.

Thiamin has been shown to have a role in insulin biosynthesis. Isolated pancreatic islets from thiamin-deficient rats secreted less insulin than those from controls (Rathanaswami and Sundaresan, 1991). In thiamin-deficient rats the total pancreatic protein content was not altered when compared with control rats, whereas the pancreatic insulin content was decreased.

REQUIREMENTS

Many factors influence requirements for thiamin (Sebrell and Harris, 1973). Thiamin requirements in some species are difficult to establish because of vitamin synthesis by microflora in ruminants and most likely for all species in the lower intestine. More important than dietary effects on synthesis is the general conclusion that most of the synthesis apparently occurs too far down the intestinal tract for absorption. Intestinal synthesis, therefore, would be of greatest benefit to animals that practice coprophagy. However, in horses, there is considerable synthesis of thiamin in the digestive tract, with an estimated 25% of the free thiamin in the cecum absorbed (Linerode, 1966). In humans and most livestock species other than ruminants and horses, it is doubtful whether the amount of thiamin produced by intestinal synthesis and absorbed is large enough to make a significant contribution to body needs.

In ruminants, total feed thiamin and that available from ruminal synthesis have to be considered together, and the total need is yet to be defined. Animals with functional rumens are generally considered to

274

have no dietary thiamin requirements because of microbial synthesis. However, thiamin deficiency can be produced in lambs, calves, and other young ruminants that do not have a functional rumen. Thiamin deficiency can be produced as late as the sixth week of life, the preruminant period. Mixed rations consisting of milk, sources of high energy, and hay stimulate growth of the villi in the rumen, but milk alone retards development of the rumen mucosa and thus thiamin synthesis. Self-synthesis of thiamin becomes significant in calves only from the sixth week of life on, and this synthesis is still relatively weak at weaning after 5 months (Zintzen, 1974).

The self-synthesis of thiamin is subject to dietary composition in the rumen; synthesis is significantly enhanced by carbohydrates such as molasses, which are easily soluble, and by supplies of nitrogen, such as urea. When monogastric animals receive only marginal amounts of thiamin, they will develop deficiency signs earlier if their feed is also low in protein (Abe, 1969). In chickens, the amount of intestinal synthesis would depend on carbohydrate type present in the diet, synthesis being favored by cooked (dextrinized) starches versus glucose or sucrose (Scott et al., 1982). Some microorganisms in the rumen or intestine are detrimental to thiamin in that they may consume thiamin or produce thiaminases, thus making the ingested thiamin unavailable to the animal. Concentration of thiamin in the gastrointestinal tract (especially in the rumen) is more uniform than it is in the feed. The self-synthesis of thiamin is therefore high when the vitamin level in feed is low, and less when feed is rich in thiamin. Therefore, there must be some regulating mechanism that governs the concentrations of the vitamin in the rumen and maintains this within certain limits (Zintzen, 1974).

Diet composition can dramatically influence thiamin requirements. Inadequate dietary protein in the diets of lactating cows may decrease thiamin synthesis in the rumen and the amount of thiamin entering the duodenum (Breves et al., 1984). Since thiamin is specifically involved in carbohydrate metabolism (see Functions), level of dietary carbohydrate relative to other energy-supplying components influences thiamin requirement. The need for thiamin increases as consumption of carbohydrates increases. When thiamin is deficient, body reserves become depleted more rapidly when animals are being maintained on feed rich in carbohydrates than when they are receiving a diet rich in fat and protein. The "thiamin-sparing" effect of fats and protein has long been known. The survival time of thiamin-deficient pigs was increased by increasing fat levels to 28% of the diet (Ellis and Madsen, 1944). This indicated that the requirement for thiamin was decreased as the dietary energy from carbohydrate was replaced with higher levels of fat. If the chief source of energy for muscular work is carbohydrate, then thiamin requirements will increase. If fat or other noncarbohydrate materials serve as the energy source, the work will have less impact on the thiamin requirement. Thiamin status is influenced by folacin; rats deficient in folacin had decreased absorption of low doses of thiamin (NRC, 1995).

Thiamin requirements are obviously higher if feeds contain raw materials (e.g., fish) or additives with anti-thiamin action (see Chemical Structure, Properties, and Antagonists). Spoiled and moldy feeds may contain such antagonists or thiaminases. Chicks kept on feed infected with *Fusarium moniliforme* developed polyneuritis that could be cured with thiamin injections (Fritz et al., 1973). High dietary intakes of sulfur (Gooneratne et al., 1989) as well as substances in tall fescue (*Festuca arundinacea* Schreb.) (Edwin et al., 1968; Lauriault et al., 1990) were antagonistic to thiamin, resulting in higher requirements.

Disease conditions also result in increased thiamin requirements. When dietary thiamin is marginal, typical signs of thiamin deficiency are more likely to develop in infected animals than in normal animals. Endoparasites such as strongylids and coccidia compete with the host for thiamin contained in food. It has been shown experimentally that infection with these coccidia results in considerable reduction in thiamin blood levels. Thiamin levels were directly correlated to infection severity (McManus and Judith, 1972). Likewise, conditions such as diarrhea and malabsorption increased the requirement.

Size, genetic factors, and metabolic status affect thiamin requirements. Thiamin requirement is proportional to size. Conditions that increase the metabolic rate (e.g., rapid growth, fever, hyperthyroidism, pregnancy, and lactation) increase thiamin requirements. Light poultry breeds (Leghorn) seem to have higher thiamin requirements than heavy breeds (Thornton and Schutze, 1960), and leghorn hens deposit more thiamin in eggs than do heavy hens. Need for thiamin increases during gestation, during lactation, and in hyperthyroidism; during lactation, the rat needs five times the normal level. As an animal ages, its need for thiamin increases because efficiency of vitamin utilization likely diminishes.

Table 6.1 summarizes thiamin requirements for various livestock species and humans; a more complete listing is given in the appendix (Table A1). The recommended dietary allowance of 0.5 mg/100 kcal for thiamin is nearly four times the amount at which signs of deficiency were observed in humans and is well within the range observed to be consistent with good health (RDA, 1989). A minimum intake of 1 mg/day is recommended for individuals consuming 2,000 kcal/day. On a calorie basis, infant requirements are similar to those of adults.

In humans, additional factors that influence thiamin requirements include alcohol and drug consumption, smoking, and inborn errors of metabolism. Alcoholism results in less dietary thiamin intake as well as decreased absorption and utilization of the vitamin (Leevy, 1982). Drugs that cause nausea and lack of appetite, induce diuresis, or increase intestinal motility will reduce the availability of thiamin (Gubler, 1991). Strauss and Scheer (1939) reported a marked reduction in thiamin excretion in heavy smokers. Patients with thiamin-responsive inborn errors of metabolism respond to pharmacological doses of thiamin (Scriver, 1973).

■ Table 6.1　Thiamin Requirements for Various Animals and Humans

Animal	Purpose or Class	Requirement[a]	Reference
Beef cattle	Adult	Microbial synthesis	NRC (1996)
Dairy cattle	Calf	6.5 ppm milk replacer	NRC (1989a)
	Adult	Microbial synthesis	NRC (1989a)
Chicken	Leghorn, 0–12 weeks	1.0 mg/kg	NRC (1994)
	Leghorn, 12–18 weeks	0.8 mg/kg	NRC (1994)
	Laying (100-g intake)	0.7 mg/kg	NRC (1994)
	Broilers, 0–8 weeks	1.8 mg/kg	NRC (1994)
Japanese quail	All classes	2.0 mg/kg	NRC (1994)
Turkey	All classes	2.0 mg/kg	NRC (1994)
Sheep	Adult	Microbial synthesis	NRC (1985b)
Swine	Growing-finishing, 3–5 kg	1.5 mg/kg	NRC (1998)
	Growing-finishing, 5–120 kg	1.0 mg/kg	NRC (1998)
	Adult	1.0 mg/kg	NRC (1998)
Horse	Growing, maintenance, pregnant, and lactation	3.0 mg/kg	NRC (1989b)
	Working	5.0 mg/kg	NRC (1989b)
Goat	Adult	Microbial synthesis	NRC (1981)
Mink	Growing	1.2 mg/kg	NRC (1982a)
Fox	Growing	2.0 mg/kg	NRC (1982a)
Cat	Adult	5.0 mg/kg	NRC (1986)
Dog	Growing	0.75 mg/kg	NRC (1985a)
Fish	Catfish	1.0 mg/kg	NRC (1993)
	Pacific salmon	10–15 mg/kg	NRC (1993)
	Rainbow trout	1–10 mg/kg	NRC (1993)
Rat	All classes	4.0 mg/kg	NRC (1995)
Mouse	All classes	5.0 mg/kg	NRC (1995)
Human	Infants	0.3–0.4 mg/day	RDA (1989)
	Children	0.7–1.0 mg/day	RDA (1989)
	Adults	1.1–1.6 mg/day	RDA (1989)

[a]Expressed as per unit of animal feed on either as-fed (approximately 90% dry matter) or dry basis (see Appendix, Tables A1a,b). Human data are expressed as mg/day.

NATURAL SOURCES

In plant products, most thiamin occurs as free thiamin, while in animal products, phosphorylated forms (mostly TPP) predominate. Cereal grains and their by-products, soybean meal, and peanut meal are relatively rich sources of thiamin. Most foods are relatively low in thiamin. It is essentially absent in oils and fats and some highly refined foods, such as sugars, and the content in green vegetables, fruits, and sea foods is relatively low. Lean pork, liver, kidney, and egg yolk are animal products rich in thiamin. The content in lean pork can be doubled by increasing the thiamin intake of the pig (Heinemann et al., 1946). Thiamin content of typical feedstuffs is shown in Table 6.2.

Brewer's yeast is the richest known natural source of thiamin. Since the vitamin is present primarily in the germ and seed coats, by-products containing the latter are richer than the whole kernel, while highly milled flour is very deficient. Whole rice may contain 5 ppm of thiamin, with much lower and higher concentrations for polished rice (0.3 ppm) and rice bran (23 ppm), respectively (Marks, 1975). Wheat germ ranks next to yeast in thiamin concentration. The level of thiamin in grain rises as the level of protein rises; it depends on species, strain, and use of nitrogenous fertilizers (Aitken and Hankin, 1970; Zintzen, 1974). The content in hays decreases as plants mature and is lower in cured than in fresh products. Thiamin concentration is correlated with leafiness and greenness as well as protein content. In general, good-quality hay is a substantial source, and in a dry climate there is practically no loss in storage. Reddy and Pushpamma (1986) studied the effects of 1 year's storage and insect infestation on thiamin content of feeds. Thiamin losses were high in different varieties of sorghum and pigeonpea (40 to 70%) and lower in rice and chickpea (10 to 40%), with insect infestation causing further loss.

The presence of molds in feeds can result in substantial nutrient loss, including thiamin (Cook, 1990). The content of thiamin was reduced from 43 to 50% for two cultivars of wheat infested with *Aspergillus flavus* compared to the uncontaminated sound wheat (Kao and Robinson, 1973). Moldy feed analyses showed thiamin content of less than 0.1 mg/kg, whereas the same feed not contaminated with *Fusarium moniliforme* had a thiamin content of 5.33 mg/kg. The antagonistic factor could be destroyed by treatment with steam (Fritz et al., 1973).

Thiamin is susceptible to destruction by several factors involved with handling and processing of foods. Milk is not a rich source of thiamin,

■ Table 6.2   Thiamin Content in Foods and Feedstuffs

Energy-Protein Feed Sources (Plant)	mg/kg	Protein Sources (Animal)	mg/kg
Alfalfa meal	3.9	Blood meal, dried	0.2
Barley grain, dried	5.7	Chicken	0.4
Beans	6.0	Eggs, whole	3.4
Brewer's grains, dried	0.8	Fish meal, with solubles	2.0
Brewer's yeast, dried	95.2	Liver and glandular meal	2.6
Coconut meal, dried	0.8	Meat and bone meal	0.1
Corn (maize), yellow grain	3.5	Milk, cow's	0.4
Corn (maize), germ meal	10.9	Skim milk, dried	3.5
Corn (maize), dried gluten meal	2.1		
Cottonseed meal, solvent extracted	6.4		
Distiller's dried solubles	6.8		
Linseed meal, expeller extracted	5.1		
Millet, dried	4.5		
Oat grain	5.2		
Peanut meal	12.0		
Peas, dried	9.0		
Potatoes, sweet	0.9		
Potatoes, white	1.0		
Rice, bran	23.0		
Rice, grain	5.0		
Rice, polished	0.3		
Rye, dried	4.4		
Sesame meal	10.0		
Sorghum grain	3.9		
Sugarbeet pulp, dried	0.4		
Sugarcane molasses	1.2		
Wheat bran	8.0		
Wheat grain	5.5		
Wheat standard middlings, dried	12.0		
Whey, dried	8.0		

Sources: Modified from Bräunlich and Zintzen (1976), Marks (1975), and Scott et al. (1982).

with processing resulting in the following losses: pasteurization, 9 to 20%; sterilization, 30 to 50%; spray-drying, 10%; roller-drying, 15%; and condensing (canning), 40% (Gubler, 1991). Since thiamin is water soluble as well as unstable to heat, large losses in certain cooking operations result (McDowell, 1985). There was up to 40% loss after 8 months' storage of frozen meat. Roasting beef and pork and boiling vegetables resulted in 40 to 50% loss. Cooking with microwave leads to much smaller losses. In conventionally roasted pork and chicken, 48 to 96% of thiamin was retained, whereas microwave-treated samples showed retention as high as 88 to 96% (Uherová et al., 1993). Parboiled rice was found to contain more thiamin than regular rice at both the same levels of milling, because parboiling paddy rice results in inward diffusion of water-soluble vitamins to the endosperm (Grewal and Sangha, 1990).

DEFICIENCY

The classic diseases, beriberi in humans and polyneuritis in birds, represent a late stage of thiamin deficiency resulting from peripheral neuritis, perhaps caused by accumulation of intermediates of carbohydrate metabolism. Comparing signs of thiamin deficiency in various species, one sees that disorders affecting the CNS are the same in all species. This is explained by the fact that in all animals, the brain covers its energy requirement chiefly by the degradation of glucose and is therefore dependent on biochemical reactions in which thiamin plays a key role.

In addition to neurological disorders, the other main group of disorders involves cardiovascular damage. Clinical signs associated with heart function are slowing of heartbeat (bradycardia), enlargement of the heart, and edema. Less specific clinical signs include gastrointestinal problems, muscle weakness, easy fatigue, hyperirritability, and lack of appetite (anorexia). Of all nutrients, thiamin deficiency has the most marked effect on appetite. Animals consuming a low-thiamin diet soon show severe anorexia, lose all interest in food, and will not resume eating unless given thiamin. If the deficiency is severe, thiamin must be force-fed or injected to induce animals to resume eating. Table 6.3 lists clinical signs (and symptoms) associated with thiamin deficiency in various species. Animals developing thiamin deficiency most readily are chickens and pigeons; pigs, rats, mice, and rabbits are less readily depleted, probably because of endogenous thiamin production.

Effects of Deficiency

Ruminants

Young animals that do not have a fully developed rumen can be thiamin deficient, as shown in experiments with calves and lambs (McDonald, 1982). Clinical signs include apparent weakness that is usually first exhibited by poor leg coordination, especially of the forelimbs, and by inability to rise and stand. The head is frequently retracted (Fig. 6.3) along the shoulder, and the heart may develop arrhythmia. Specific signs are usually accompanied by anorexia and severe diarrhea, followed by dehydration and death (NRC, 1996). Signs in the calves can be either acute or chronic. In one study, acutely affected calves were anorectic, had severe diarrhea, and died within 24 hours. These signs appeared after 2 to 4 weeks on a low-thiamin diet (Johnson et al., 1948).

■ Table 6.3 Clinical Signs Associated with Thiamin Deficiency in Various Species

	General Signs	Cardiovascular Signs	Nervous Disorders	Other Signs
Human	Loss of appetite, tiredness/apathy, lack of concentration, irritable, anxiety states, depression	ECG changes, falling blood pressure, arrhythmia edema, hypotension, tachycardia	Muscular weakness, calf cramps, weakened reflexes, loss of feeling, neuritic symptoms, coma	Dyspnea
Hen	Loss of appetite, loss of weight, weakness	Bradycardia (from 300 down to 90–100/min), cyanosis, edema	Opisthotonos, leg weakness, muscular weakness, extension spasms, apathy, paresis	Sudden death, gonad damage, gut atony, diarrhea, hypothermia
Pigeon	Loss of weight	Heart failure, tachycardia	Leg weakness, opisthotonos, ataxia, paresis	Crop voiding (vomiting)
Mouse	Loss of appetite, loss of weight, weakness	Pathological changes in the myocardium	Hyperexcitability, ataxia, circumduction, hemorrhages in the mesencephalon, opisthotonos	Pathological changes in liver, testicles, skeletal muscle, diarrhea, hypothermia
Rat	Loss of appetite, disturbances of growth, general weakness	Bradycardia (from 500 down to 250–300/min), slackened pulse and reduced respiratory rate	Ataxia and cramps, paralysis circumduction, nodding of the head	Diarrhea, skin atony, hypothermia
Rabbit	—	—	Paralysis, cramps, opisthotonos	Coma
Cat	Loss of appetite, loss of weight	Myocardial damage	Ataxia, ventral flexion of the head	
Dog	Loss of appetite, loss of weight, weakness	Slow pulse	Paresis, cramps, opisthotonos	Gastrointestinal disorders, vomiting, hypothermia

■ Table 6.3 Continued

General Signs	Cardiovascular Signs	Nervous Disorders	Other Signs
Fox			
Loss of appetite, loss of weight	Pathological changes in the heart	Polyneuritis, ataxia, irritability, cramps, spastic paresis, paralysis	Groaning, pathological changes in the liver
Mink			
Loss of appetite, loss of weight	—	Polyneuritis, ataxia, cramps, convulsions, spastic paresis, paralysis, opisthotonos	Diarrhea, poor quality of pelt
Pig			
Loss of appetite, loss of weight, weakness, premature births, high mortality among the young	Slow pulse, cyanosis, heart failure, tachycardia, dilatation of the heart, edema, hemorrhages in the gastrointestinal wall and myocardium	—	Vomiting, dyspnea, diarrhea, skin atony, hypothermia, sudden death
Young Ruminant			
Loss of appetite, loss of weight, weakness	Cardiac arrhythmia, tachycardia	Hyperesthesia, polyneuritis, ataxia, convulsions, cramps, opisthotonos, spastic paresis, paralysis	Diarrhea, dyspnea, lachrymation, gnashing of the teeth, sometimes disorders of vision
Horse			
Loss of appetite, loss of weight, lusterless coat	Heart failure, tachycardia	Nervousness, ataxia, apathy, muscle tremors, cramps, coma	Diarrhea, constipation, dyspnea

Source: Modified from Bräunlich and Zintzen (1976).

282

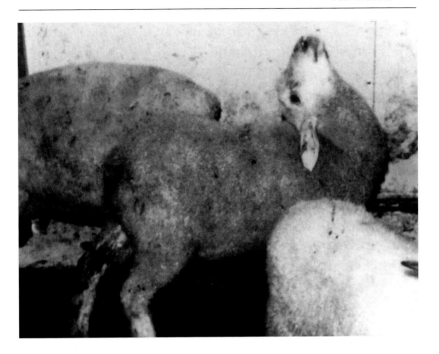

Fig. 6.3 Sheep with thiamin deficiency. Characteristics of the condition are
head bent backward (opisthotonos), cramp-like muscle contractions, disturbance of balance, and aggressiveness. (Courtesy of Michel Hidiroglou, Animal
Research Center, Ottawa, Ontario, Canada.)

Because of extensive ruminal thiamin synthesis, the general conclusion is that ruminants possessing a normally functioning rumen have no
dietary thiamin requirement. Despite the fact that rumen microbes synthesize thiamin, and feeds—particularly whole grains—contain thiamin,
deficiencies do develop in ruminants. In a number of world areas, a thiamin-responsive disease known as polioencephalomalacia (PEM) occurs
sporadically in cattle, sheep, and goats. Other names for PEM in different regions include cerebrocortical necrosis, cerebral necrosis, and forage poisoning.

The term PEM refers to a laminar softening or degeneration of brain
gray matter (Brent and Bartley, 1984). However, it is commonly used to
describe the CNS condition in ruminants. The condition affects mainly
calves and young cattle between 4 months and 2 years old, and lambs,
young sheep, and goats between 2 and 7 months old. The incidence of
PEM is reported to be between 1 and 20%, and mortality may reach
100%. Clinical signs in mild cases include dullness, blindness, muscle

tremors (especially of the head), and opisthotonos. The condition is characterized by circling, head pressing, and convulsions, and in severe cases, the animal collapses within 12 to 72 hours after onset of the disease (Fig. 6.4). Because of the circling, the condition is sometimes called "circling disease." The ears drop, and in the final stages, the limbs and head are extended. General twitching of the musculature of the ears and eyelids, waving of the head and neck, and grinding of the teeth with groaning sometimes occur. Without treatment, death usually comes within a few days. The main lesions in these animals are necrotic areas in both cerebral hemispheres.

PEM may run a short, acute course or may occur in a milder form and run a more protracted course. The condition, particularly in its mild form, probably is often not diagnosed and may occur more frequently than is recognized. Clinical signs of CNS disorders associated with PEM are more readily recognized than nonspecific signs such as scouring, reduced growth, and anorexia. However, these signs are exhibited at later stages of thiamin deficiency (Rammell and Hill, 1986). Thornber et al. (1979) reported that animals on thiamin-deficient diets may not show clinical signs of a CNS disorder for 3 to 5 weeks or longer, although depressed blood thiamin levels and other clinical signs may be observed. Without treatment, mortality is about 50% of animals with the mild form and possibly up to 100% in animals with acute PEM. The incidence and death rates are higher in young animals from 2 to 5 months of age than for animals older than 1 year.

High-sulfur diets are associated with thiamin deficiency and PEM (Gould, 1998). Gould et al. (1991) reported that steers with the highest rumen fluid sulfide concentrations coincided with the onset of clinical signs of PEM. Several cases of PEM occurred when gypsum had been used as a feed intake limiter. It would appear that the sulfate ion of gypsum, during its conversion to sulfide, must pass through sulfite, which may destroy thiamin. The sulfite ion apparently will cleave thiamin at the methylene bridge, mimicking thiaminase. In lambs, PEM was induced by administration of a sulfide solution; neurological clinical signs included stupor, visual impairment, and seizures (McAllister et al., 1992).

Feedlot cattle that received 0.72% sulfate had 50% less gains than controls, and 3 of 20 head developed PEM (Sadler et al., 1983). Supplementation of sheep fed diets high in sulfur (0.63%) had clinical signs of PEM, which were prevented with supplemental thiamin (243 ppm) (Olkowski et al., 1992). However, thiamin did not totally prevent development of microscopic brain lesions, which are characteristic of

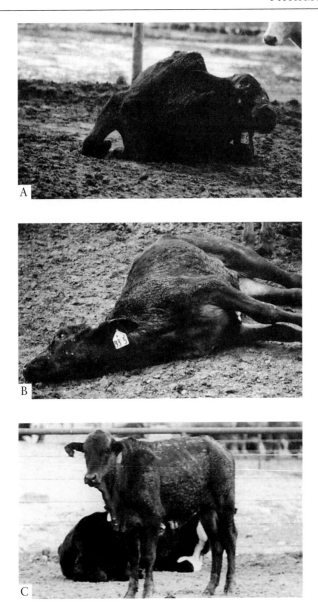

Fig. 6.4 (A and B). An animal with polioencephalomalacia, a disease of thiamin deficiency. Feedlot cattle suffering from this condition show dullness and sometimes blindness, with a series of nervous disorders such as circling, head pressing, and convulsions. Six to eight hours after thiamin injection, the same animal was able to stand (C). With continued thiamin treatment, in 3 to 5 days, the animal returned to almost normal, with slight brain damage. (Courtesy of B. Bock, University of Florida.)

PEM. In sheep, high sulfur intake was shown to have a detrimental effect on in vitro polymorphonuclear leukocyte function. This can mean that ruminants in areas where large quantities of sulfur are taken in with water and feed have compromised immune function due to lower copper and thiamin status and hence are at risk of increased susceptibility to infections (Olkowski et al., 1990). Field studies (Olkowski et al., 1991) found an inverse correlation between water sulfate content and blood thiamin in beef cattle. Cattle receiving water with less than 200 ppm of sulfate had higher blood thiamin than cattle receiving water with over 1,000 ppm of sulfate. Feedlot nutritionists have reported cases of PEM when high percentages of wet-milled corn by-products were fed. Sulfuric acid is used to steep corn in the wet-milling process; much of the sulfur then remains with the by-product.

Livestock grazing endophyte-infected (*Acremonium coenophiatum*) tall fescue develop tall fescue toxicosis. Clinical signs of fescue toxicity include reduced feed intake and growth, elevated body temperature, and ergot-like clinical signs with necrosis in the extremities. Smith et al. (1986) grazed cattle from April to September on high-endophyte fescue. The cattle exhibited typical signs of summer fescue toxicosis (reduced performance, elevated body temperature, and rough hair coat) compared to cattle grazing endophyte-free fescue. Following grazing, the cattle were fed corn:corn silage diets with and without supplemental thiamin. Dietary supplementation with 0.5 g of thiamin during the feedlot phase improved the daily weight gain by 0.19 kg/day.

Tall fescue toxicosis resembles conditions caused by enhanced rumen thiaminase activity (e.g., PEM) that may be treated with thiamin (Edwin et al., 1968; Lauriault et al., 1990). Responses to supplemental thiamin were found to be greater when cattle grazing endophyte-infected tall fescue were exposed to heat stress (Lauriault et al., 1990). Results suggest that oral thiamin supplementation may alleviate tall fescue toxicosis of beef cattle during warm weather. A contrary earlier report (Fontenot et al., 1988) found that feeding thiamin to cattle grazing moderately endophyte-infected fescue had no beneficial effect.

Zintzen (1974) concluded that PEM can be definitely established if the following four situations exist:

1. Case history: Animals have been maintained on high-energy feeds rich in carbohydrates, and other animals on the same farm have, from time to time, died after exhibiting CNS disorders.

2. Biochemical evidence: Blood pyruvate has steeply increased, and the activity of erythrocyte-transketolase has been reduced.

3. Diagnosis and therapy: Animals thought to have PEM react promptly to treatment with thiamin provided they are treated in the early stages of the disease.

4. Pathological changes: Necropsy shows typical pathological anatomical changes (bilateral cortical necrosis) in the brain.

Seasonal trends have been associated with PEM, which may be due to increased metabolic demands of gestation, lactation, and growth. Additionally, feeding high-concentrate diets may induce PEM. In goats in Bikaner, India, PEM was prevalent throughout the year, with the highest incidence in late winter (Lonkar et al., 1993). It was suggested that scarcity of grazing may have led the animals to consume plants containing substances with thiaminase activity.

Polioencephalomalacia generally occurs in feedlot cattle, frequently about 3 weeks after a ration change. Research suggests that PEM is associated with lactic acid acidosis, with both conditions related to adaptation to grain diets. Oltjen et al. (1962) reported that thiamin in the rumen is decreased by a reduction in rumen pH; a low ruminant pH is characteristic of cattle fed high-concentrate diets. Although little information is available on the direct addition of thiamin to finishing cattle diets, Brethour (1972) reported that in two trials, a combination of thiamin and sodium carbonate supplement increased feed intake by 5% and daily gain by 8%. In a third trial, thiamin administered alone gave an intermediate response to calves immediately after weaning.

PEM has caused significant economic losses in tropical countries, not only in feedlots where high-grain diets are provided, but also where high levels of molasses are fed. When molasses is provided (ad libitum) together with rations containing little crude fiber, a disease referred to as "molasses toxicity" or "molasses drunkenness" occurs. Clinical signs of this condition closely resemble PEM, and studies completed in Cuba have suggested that thiamin treatment, together with additional roughage, may be an effective cure (Losada et al., 1971).

A number of experiments have shown that PEM is caused by naturally occurring thiamin antagonists, in connection with reduced thiamin synthesis or destruction of the vitamin (see Chemical Structure, Properties, and Antagonists). Several researchers have reported that most field cases of PEM result from progressive thiamin deficiency, likely a result of gut and ruminal bacterial thiaminases (Frye et al., 1991). Clinical reports of PEM have shown that under high-concentrate feeding systems of beef cattle and lambs, thiaminase may become active in the rumen and cause thiamin deficiency in animals with functional rumens (Edwin

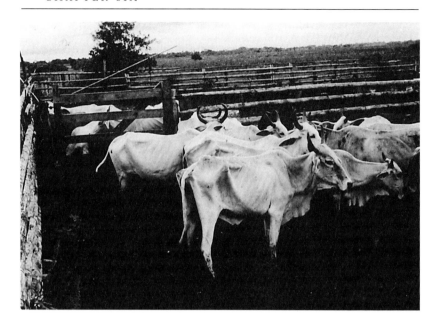

Fig. 6.5 A wasting disease (*secadera*) of cattle in the llanos of Colombia. The disease is characterized by emaciation in spite of the availability of good-quality forage. *Secadera* has been reported as thiamin deficiency because it has been alleviated with thiamin injections. However, the condition has also been controlled with a highly fortified complete mineral supplement. (L.R. McDowell, University of Florida.)

and Lewis, 1971). These thiaminases may be produced by microorganisms (bacteria and fungi) in contaminated feeds (Davies et al., 1968). Thiaminase I has been shown to increase in the feces when dairy cows were switched from a low- to high-concentrate diet (Soita and Brent, 1993). Amprolium's mode of action as a coccidiostat is apparently through inhibition of thiamin phosphorylation. Loew and Dunlop (1972) found that high levels of amprolium (considerably above the levels needed to prevent coccidiosis) could produce the physical signs and the histological lesions of PEM.

Both *Clostridium sporogenes* and *Bacillus thiaminolyticus* have been isolated from the rumen of PEM cases. Both organisms produce thiaminase type I. Thiaminases are found in certain plant species and are produced by microorganisms believed to be responsible for PEM. This has been a special problem in Australia, where PEM occurs under pasture conditions, apparently being derived from some of the fern species.

From Colombia, Mullenax (1983) reported a wasting disease

known as *secadera* (drying up) as thiamin deficiency because the condition had been alleviated within thiamin injections. Mullenax suggested that a fungus associated with native forages contains a thiaminase. On the contrary, Miles and McDowell (1983) reported that the wasting disease *secadera* (Fig. 6.5) can be successfully controlled with a highly fortified complete mineral supplement. It is possible that supplementation of this wasting disease is controlled by either thiamin or minerals through different mechanisms (McDowell, 1985).

Swine

Thiamin deficiency in swine reveals itself particularly in decreased appetite and body weight, vomiting, slow pulse, subnormal body temperature, nervous signs, postmortem heart changes, and sudden death because of heart failure. Animals consuming a low-thiamin diet soon show severe anorexia, lose all interest in food, and will not resume eating unless given thiamin. If the deficiency is severe, thiamin must be force-fed or injected to induce animals to resume eating. Heinemann et al. (1946) reported that pigs can utilize stored thiamin over a long period, as 56 days were required for the pigs in the study to lose their appetites after being placed on a thiamin-deficient diet. In another study, death occurred 74 days after pigs were placed on a thiamin-free but otherwise adequate diet (Loew, 1978). For young pigs, severe thiamin deficiency resulted in death at the age of 3 to 4 weeks.

First signs of thiamin deficiency in pigs are reduced feed consumption and vomiting, with a sharp reduction in weight gains (Miller et al., 1955). Functional and structural cardiac changes are the main findings in experimentally deficient swine; in contrast to clinical reports, nervous system lesions were not detected. Electrocardiographically demonstrable changes in heart tissue were seen in enlarged hearts obtained from pigs on thiamin-deficient diets (Fig. 6.6). Microscopically, it is possible to recognize inflammations and necrotic changes in the myocardial fibers.

Thiamin-deficient animals have elevated plasma pyruvate concentrations (Miller et al., 1955), since with deficiency of the vitamin there is an accumulation of intermediates of carbohydrate metabolism. The red blood cell enzyme transketolase is lowered in thiamin-deficient pigs, with this enzyme used as an indicator of thiamin status (see Deficiency, Assessment of Status).

Poultry

Poultry are more susceptible to neuromuscular effects of thiamin deficiency than most mammals. In chickens and turkeys, there is loss of

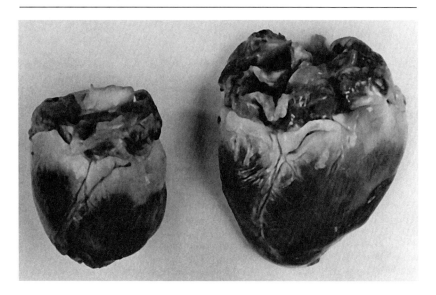

Fig. 6.6 Enlarged heart on right is due to thiamin deficiency. Heart on left is from a similar pig fed the same diet plus thiamin. (Courtesy of T.J. Cunha and Washington State University.)

appetite, emaciation, impairment of digestion, general weakness, opisthotonos or stargazing, and frequent convulsions, with polyneuritis as a late or terminal extreme clinical sign. Deficient birds can rapidly detect and discriminate against feeds that do not provide the vitamin (Hughes and Wood-Gush, 1971) and are high in carbohydrate content (Thornton and Shutze, 1960).

Early signs of thiamin deficiency are lethargy and head tremors. Chicks fed very low thiamin (0.4 ppm) survived for only 7 to 10 days, apparently only a few days after the supply of thiamin in the yolk sac was exhausted (Gries and Scott, 1972). Some chicks developed nervous disorders, apathy, and tremor as early as the third or fourth day of life. These signs increased in severity up to ataxia, inability to stand, and high-grade opisthotonos or twisting of the neck. Severity of the spasms increased when the chicks were frightened. Chicks that showed these high-grade nervous disorders died within a few hours. Cardiac abnormalities have also been reported in acutely thiamin-deficient chicks (Sturkie et al., 1954). Paralysis of the crop, manifested as delayed emptying, accompanied the general neuropathy of experimental thiamin deficiency in chicks (Naidoo, 1956). Deficiency in pigeons resulted in crop voiding (vomiting).

In mature chickens, polyneuritis is observed approximately 3 weeks after they are fed a thiamin-deficient diet (Scott et al., 1982). As the deficiency progresses, paralysis of the muscles occurs, beginning with the flexors of the toes and progressing upward, affecting the extensor muscles of the legs, wings, and neck. The chicken sits on its flexed legs and draws back the head in a stargazing (opisthotonos) position (Fig. 6.7). Retraction of the head is due to paralysis of the anterior neck muscles. At this stage, the chicken soon loses the ability to stand or sit upright and falls to the floor, where it may lie with the head still retracted.

Acutely deficient pigeons developed vomiting, emaciation, leg weakness, and opisthotonos, the last of which appeared between 7 and 12 days after beginning the thiamin-free diet (Swank, 1940). Chronic deficiency due to a diet partially inadequate in thiamin resulted in leg weakness but no opisthotonos. Evidence of cardiac failure was also noted. The lesions produced in thiamin-deficient pigeons were reported to be identical to those found in Wernicke's encephalopathy (polioencephalitis) in humans (Lofland et al., 1963). Mycotoxinin-duced polyneuritis in pheasants was eliminated within hours after intraperitoneal injection of thiamin (Cook, 1990). In thiamin-deficient

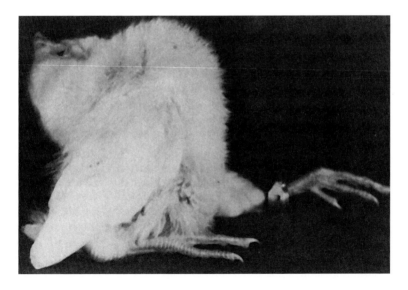

Fig. 6.7 Polyneuritis in a thiamin-deficient chick. Muscle paralysis causes extended legs and retraction of the head. (Courtesy of M.L. Scott, Cornell University.)

turkeys, onset of anorexia was rapid, and by the fourth day, deficient birds had significantly lower feed consumption (Remus and Firman, 1990).

In chickens with thiamin deficiency, body temperature drops to as low as 36°C, and respiratory rate progressively decreases (Scott et al., 1982). There is adrenal gland hypertrophy that apparently results in tissue edema, particularly in the skin. Atrophy of genital organs also occurs in chickens affected with chronic thiamin deficiency, being more pronounced in the testes than in the ovaries. The heart shows a slight degree of atrophy.

The hen transfers thiamin to the egg in proportion to dietary content (Polin et al., 1963). Inadequate thiamin to the breeder flock will result in high mortality of embryos prior to hatching and of chicks that hatch with polyneuritis (Polin et al., 1962; Charles et al., 1972).

Horses

Under normal circumstances the natural diet plus synthesis by microorganisms in the gut probably meet the thiamin needs of horses (NRC, 1989b). Thiamin synthesis in the intestinal tract of horses was inferred by Carroll et al. (1949), who found the following concentrations of thiamin (mg/kg dry matter) in the diet and intestinal contents: diet, 1.1; duodenum, 0.5; ileum, 2.2; cecum, 7.1; anterior large colon, 17.8; and anterior small colon, 7.8. Linerode (1966) estimated that 25% of the free thiamin in the cecum is absorbed by the horse. However, absorption of microbially synthesized thiamin in the intestine may not meet total needs.

Horses fed experimental diets low in thiamin exhibited anorexia, loss of weight, incoordination (especially in the hind legs), lower blood thiamin, elevated blood pyruvic acid, and dilated and hypertrophied heart (Carroll et al., 1949). Incoordination and other nervous signs were alleviated by feeding thiamin, indicating that this species requires a dietary source of this vitamin. A lack of thiamin causes reproductive failure in both sexes.

Because of generally adequate thiamin dietary supplies and intestinal synthesis, deficiency results under practical conditions only when thiaminase-containing plants are provided (see Chemical Structure, Properties, and Antagonists). Ingestion of sufficient quantities of the thiaminase-containing bracken fern *Pteridium aquilinum* was shown to readily cause thiamin deficiency in horses (Kingsbury, 1964). The signs in affected horses included weight loss, incoordination, lethargy, cardiac irregularities, muscular twitching and tremors, and prostration; death usually followed convulsions. Anorexia was not apparent until other signs became severe. Treatment with thiamin was successful if given before terminal stages. The horsetail (*Equisetum arvense*) and star thistle (*Centaurea solstitialis*) may act in the same way as bracken fern.

Diniz et al. (1984) observed incoordination, staggering, and muscular tremors in 27 mules 2 months after introduction to bracken-infested pasture. Eight died, and the rest recovered after removal from the pasture and injection with 100 mg of thiamin. Generalized congestion, pulmonary edema, and serosal and mucosal hemorrhages were noted at necropsy.

Other Animal Species

DOGS AND CATS

The main clinical signs for thiamin deficiency in dogs and cats are anorexia and nervousness, leading to spasms and finally to death (NRC, 1985a; Davidson, 1992). Thiamin deficiency in cats and dogs has been associated with feeding meat preserved with sulfur dioxide (Studdert and Labuc, 1991).

Of all the domestic animals, the cat is most often reported to be clinically thiamin deficient. This might well be expected as domesticated cats often consume fish, and thiaminase may be present in many cat foods (NRC, 1986). However, these are usually heat-treated, which would be expected to inactivate thiaminase. Most cases have been the result of feeding cats diets that contained a large proportion of raw fish (Hoffmann-La Roche, 2000). Experimental studies with cats have produced signs of thiamin deficiency within 23 to 40 days of consuming diets composed solely of raw carp or raw salt-water herring (Smith and Proutt, 1944). Subcutaneous administration of thiamin to affected cats resulted in recovery in all cases.

In thiamin-deficient cats, anorexia and sometimes vomiting occur within 2 weeks of ingestion of a thiamin-deficient diet, followed by the sudden development of neurological disorders including abnormal posture, ataxia, and seizures, culminating in progressive weakness and death. Affected cats often show ventroflexion of the head when suspended by the rear legs, or somersaulting when the cat leaps (Hoffmann-La Roche, 1998). Affected kittens also have dilated pupils. Postural abnormalities likely develop and may include a spastic gait, curling up when lifted, or a head tilt. Seizures or abnormal behavior, dilated pupils, stupor, or opisthotonos (spasms causing head and heels to bend backward) may also be observed (Shell, 1995).

Depending on the severity of the case, deficiency signs in cats can be alleviated by administration of thiamin; however, hemorrhages that occur in the periventricular gray matter of the brain because of thiamin deficiency can permanently affect the animal. Cats that recovered from experimentally induced thiamin deficiency were found to have significantly greater difficulty learning or remembering maze tasks (Ralston Purina, 1987).

Thiamin deficiency in dogs results from animals consuming diets in which marginal thiamin concentrations were destroyed in food processing, or thiaminases were sufficiently high in the diet. A group of sled dogs fed a diet of frozen, uncooked carp developed clinical signs of thiamin deficiency after 6 months. The addition of oatmeal, a dry dog food, and 100 mg of thiamin daily to the affected dogs resulted in complete recovery within 2 months (Houston and Hulland, 1988).

Pathological changes in dogs due to thiamin deficiency predominately involve the nervous system and heart. The pattern of pathological changes depends on the period of induction; acute deficiency tends to involve the brain and produce severe neurological signs, whereas chronic deficiency produces pathological changes in the heart and peripheral nerves. Dogs sometimes show cardiac hypertrophy (enlargement), with slowing of the heart rate and signs of congestive heart failure, including labored breathing and edema.

FISH

Thiamin deficiency signs in fish are similar to those observed in mammals and birds. The principal signs are anorexia, arrest of growth, and neurological disturbances. Fish swim restlessly, twist around with spasmodic jerks of the body, and often collide with the walls of the tank (Bräunlich and Zintzen, 1976). The slightest disturbances trigger fright reactions that may result in sudden death. The surface of the body and the fins are discolored and the liver is pale. Neurological disorders such as hyperirritability due to thiamin deficiency have been reported in salmonids, channel catfish, Japanese eel, and Japanese parrot fish (NRC, 1993).

Chinook salmon reared on a thiamin-inadequate diet exhibited poor appetite, muscle atrophy, instability, and loss of equilibrium, followed by convulsions and death. Freshwater eels developed deficiency after consuming thiaminase-containing clams (Hashimoto et al., 1970). The main cause of thiamin deficiency in commercial fish production is dietary provision of raw fish.

FOXES AND MINK

Thiamin deficiency is also a problem in pelt animal farming and is manifested as Chastek paralysis. The disease occurs in mink and foxes and is induced by feeding these animals certain types of raw fish (see Chemical Structure, Properties, and Antagonists). Clinical signs of thiamin deficiency in mink are reported as anorexia, weight loss, and emaciation, followed later by nervous disorders such as involuntary movements, unsteady gait, muscular spasms, and attacks of cramp or general paralysis. When affected animals are touched, they exhibit extension spasms in the hind limbs. The terminal phase is characterized by opisthotonos and unconsciousness, and animals die in a characteristic contorted position. Histological examination shows brain hemorrhages and lesions of the neural pathways (Bräunlich and Zintzen, 1976). In foxes, clinical signs include anorexia and abnormal gait, followed by severe ataxia, inability to stand, hyperesthesia, constant moaning, and convulsions (Long and Shaw, 1943).

LABORATORY ANIMALS

Thiamin deficiency can be induced readily in rats and produces abnormalities of the central and peripheral nervous system and the heart and results in poor reproductive performance (NRC, 1995). Anorexia and weight loss are prominent. Deficient rats have ataxia, impaired "righting" reflex, and drowsiness, which were reversed by injection of thiamin hydrochloride. Chronic thiamin deprivation leads to selective neuropathological damage in the brain.

Mice deficient in thiamin had violent convulsions—especially when held a few seconds by the tail—cartwheel or circular movements, brain hemorrhages, decreased food intake, poor growth, early mortality, silver-streaked muscle lesions, and testicular degeneration (NRC, 1995). Exposure of thiamin-deficient mice to ethanol resulted in brain damage that was more severe than either treatment alone (Phillips, 1987).

Reduced food intake and weight losses, followed by CNS disorders, occurred in young, thiamin-deficient guinea pigs. An unsteady gait appeared, with some retraction of the head as the condition progressed. Death was reported within 4 weeks (Reid and Bieri, 1967; NRC, 1995). In hamsters, low thiamin intake was associated with chronically deficient animals with depressed growth and more rapid induction of tumors after applications of a chemical carcinogen (Salley et al., 1962).

NONHUMAN PRIMATES

The reported clinical signs of thiamin deficiency in rhesus monkeys include weight loss, apathy, weakness, loss of reflexes, paralysis, incoordination, convulsions, prostration, heart failure, and death (Blank et al., 1975; NRC, 1978). Focal necrosis of myocardial fibers is a relatively constant finding and has been associated with abnormalities in the electrocardiogram (Rinehart and Greenberg, 1949).

RABBITS

Rabbits fed a thiamin-free diet, along with a thiamin antagonist (neopyrithiamin), developed ataxia, flaccid paralysis, convulsions, and coma, followed by death (Reid et al., 1963; NRC, 1977). The rabbit differed from nearly all other species in not developing anorexia. Apparently, intestinal synthesis and coprophagy prevented the usual signs from developing.

CROCODILES

Suspected thiamin deficiency was reported in farmed saltwater crocodiles (*Crocodylus porosus*) in northern Australia (Jubb, 1992). Disease conditions were noted in 4 of 11 clutches of crocodile hatchlings. Sudden loss of righting reflex was the outstanding feature of the disease. Affected hatchlings would be found floating or lying on their sides or backs, listless, with jaws open and unable to right themselves (Fig. 6.8).

Humans

Classic beriberi has been known since the earliest recorded times in the Far East, where it is endemic because of prevalent consumption of polished rice. Beriberi was the primary health problem in Indonesia, Malaysia, Japan, and the Philippines as recently as the 1940s. In 1947 the Philippine mortality rate from beriberi was 132 per 100,000 population—second only to tuberculosis. Through rice enrichment with thiamin, this rate was reduced to 14 per 100,000 by 1960.

In beriberi, both cardiac and nervous functions are usually disturbed. The disease occurs in a wet form, characterized by edema (Fig. 6.9) and cardiovascular symptoms, and a dry form, characterized by peripheral neuritis, paralysis, and muscular atrophy. However, the forms merge, making it hard to differentiate the two. The chronic form may last for years; cardiac symptoms may appear suddenly (shoshin beriberi) and result in death within a short time. It is generally believed that the more serious the nervous lesions, the greater the muscular pain and

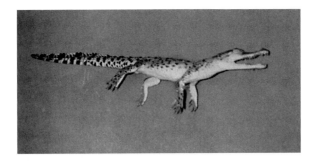

Fig. 6.8 A 2-month-old saltwater crocodile hatchling with suspected thiamin deficiency, floating on its side in shallow water. The listless appearance and open jaws are also characteristic of the disease. (Courtesy of T.F. Jubb, Department of Western Australia, Kununurra.)

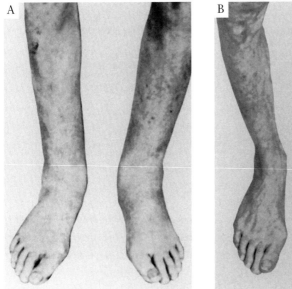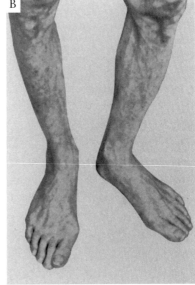

Fig. 6.9 Thiamin deficiency in a man. (A) Swelling of the legs, with pitting in ankle region, marks beginning of so-called wet beriberi. (B) The same patient 4 days after a single intravenous injection of 50 mg of thiamin. During this period, the patient's excretion of fluid exceeded intake by 10.5 lb. His general nutritional state improved as a result of increased appetite. (Courtesy of Alan T. Forrester, *Vitamin Manual*, The Upjohn Company, Kalamazoo, Michigan.)

weakness and the less likely the development of acute beriberi. The heart is saved from extreme insufficiency by forcing the patient into complete rest at an early stage in the attack.

General symptoms of beriberi include anorexia, heart enlargement, tachycardia (versus bradycardia in animals), lassitude and muscle weakness, paresthesia, loss of knee and ankle reflex with subsequent foot and wrist drop, ataxia due to muscle weakness, and dyspnea on exertion (Tang et al., 1989; Gubler, 1991). The "squat test" illustrates the neurological damage, as beriberi patients are unable to rise from a squatting position.

The signs and symptoms vary depending on age, individual, diet, duration and severity of the deficiency, and abruptness of onset. Peripheral neuropathy (dry beriberi) is a symmetrical impairment, with loss of sensory, motor, and reflex function affecting the distal segments of limbs more severely than the proximal ones, and with less cardiac involvement. Disturbances of the higher nervous centers, nystagmus, and ophthalmoplegia are frequent. In advanced stages, patients exhibit general muscular atrophy, ataxia, mental confusion, and defective short-term memory.

The sequence of symptoms is variable, but beriberi often begins with numbness in feet, heaviness of legs, prickly sensations, and itching. Muscles become tender, and squeezing the calf of the leg causes pain. Cardiac symptoms develop at some stage and are characterized by palpitation, epigastric pain, coldness of extremities, and enlargement of the heart. Later symptoms and clinical signs include edema of ankles, puffiness of face, digestive disturbances, anorexia, nausea, and vomiting.

Infantile beriberi, common in the Orient, is an acute form of the disease. It is probably an important cause of the high infant mortality in Southeast Asia. Nursing mothers, who provide milk deficient in thiamin, may or may not show mild signs of deficiency. The condition usually occurs in the first few months of life and begins with anorexia, regurgitation, abdominal distention, and colicky pain. Oliguria is followed by edema, and there is dyspnea, with a peculiar cry or grunt thought to be caused by edema of the vocal cords. Later, cardiovascular signs and congestive failure increase and nervous signs appear, with muscular twitching, coma, and death. Cardiac failure is often the cause of death. Each phase may last only a few hours, and the whole course of the condition only a day or two.

Beriberi has been largely eliminated in most countries where fortification of rice is practiced, but is still prevalent in those countries where unfortified polished rice is widely used. More recent incidences of beriberi or low thiamin status have been reported in Gambia (Tang et al., 1989), Indonesia (Djoenaidi et al., 1992), Lithuania (Piktelite et al., 1992), Poland (Pardo et al., 1991), and Turkey (Wetherilt et al., 1992). In countries where large amounts of fish are eaten raw, human thiamin deficiency may occur. Elsewhere, poverty, alcoholism, food faddism, or poorly prepared food may result in inadequate thiamin ingestion. A variety of malabsorptive disorders can jeopardize nutritional status with respect to thiamin. Severe polyneuropathy developed in one patient after jejunoileal bypass surgery (Glad et al., 1978), and thiamin blood status was found more depleted in patients with Crohn's disease (Kuroki et al., 1993).

Studies have suggested that some degree of thiamin deficiency is widespread in the elderly (Marks, 1975). This may result mostly from generally poor appetite and eating habits or low income. However, it has been demonstrated that old rats require more thiamin per gram of food eaten than young rats, and transport of thiamin across the intestine is significantly lower in older than younger rats (Gubler, 1991).

Blass and Gibson (1978) have reported decreased levels of pyruvate dehydrogenase activity in the brain of patients with Alzheimer's disease. Tucker et al. (1990) found a decrement in alpha-wave activity in the electroencephalographic indices of older persons with low thiamin status, suggesting subtle neuropsychological impairment with mild thiamin deficiency.

The most frequently encountered type of thiamin deficiency in developed countries is associated with alcoholism (Wernicke's syndrome), resulting from inadequate intake of thiamin. Thiamin deficiency in chronic alcoholism has a triple origin: (1) inadequate intake resulting from appetite loss, or decreased intake of a balanced diet for economic and/or other reasons; (2) decreased absorption; and (3) decreased utilization. The signs of this syndrome range from mild confusion to coma and include ophthalmoplegia, cerebellar ataxia, psychosis, confabulation and severely impaired retentive memory, and cognitive function. Blass and Gibson (1977) showed that at least some patients with Wernicke's syndrome have a genetically determined abnormal transketolase that, in effect, requires a higher concentration of the coenzyme to saturate the apoenzyme.

Some Japanese studies (Zintzen, 1974) have indicated that the structure-altering antagonists of thiamin (see Chemical Structure, Properties, and Antagonists) produced by bacteria and fungi are main causes of beriberi, since they are involved in up to 70% of all cases. Bacillary and clostridial species that produce these antagonists have been isolated from intestinal flora of Japanese people tested. They may be consumed with contaminated food, such as moldy rice.

Assessment of Status

In thiamin deficiency determination, there is no question about the specificity of such signs as polyneuritis and Chastek paralysis, but these are terminal stages. The problem of identifying the early stages by any specific sign is an unsolved one for thiamin and for several other of the B vitamins. When thiamin deficiency is acute, the specific effects of the deficiency cannot be distinguished from some unspecific effects, such as those of anorexia (Zintzen, 1974). In humans, thiamin deficiency can be tentatively diagnosed on a clinical basis, particularly with careful inquiry into the patient's dietary habits or other conditions that might predispose to deficiency, and confirmed by positive results of thiamin supplementation.

Some specific criteria that are suitable for the assessment of the thiamin status include (1) concentration of thiamin in blood and urine, (2) levels of products of intermediate metabolism that are dependent on the enzyme function of thiamin, and (3) activities of enzymes in which thiamin is a coenzyme.

Thiamin concentrations are decreased in blood and urine when this vitamin is deficient. Clinical signs of deficiency were noted when less than 7% of a 1-mg dose of thiamin was excreted in the urine in a dose-retention test (Horwitt et al., 1948). Urinary excretion of thiamin reflects thiamin saturation or depletion because the vitamin is excreted promptly when ingested in excess of needs. Both blood levels and urinary excretion of thiamin are only a reflection of the immediately preceding intake and other factors and may not be a reliable index of tissue stores, distribution, or biochemical functioning and hence are of limited value for interpretation of actual thiamin status.

Thiamin is needed for pyruvate metabolism, and with deficiency, abnormally high concentrations of pyruvic and lactic acids in the blood indicate thiamin inadequacy. For a calf on a deficient diet, urinary excretion of thiamin drops to very low levels in 20 to 25 days, and increased pyruvate excretion follows. Blood pyruvate and lactate levels increase suddenly to 400 and 500% of normal as the deficiency develops (NRC, 1989a). However, the measurements of these levels often cannot be used to detect mild thiamin deficiency. Also these tests are not entirely specific, because toxicity by minerals such as arsenic and antimony will also inhibit the utilization of pyruvate. Increased pyruvate can also result from a number of pathological conditions, such as those arising from increased adrenal gland activity. Acute polyneuritis has been shown to develop before rise of blood pyruvate in pigeons.

So far, the best criterion for determining thiamin status is activity of enzymes that depend on the vitamin as a coenzyme. These enzymes include pyruvate decarboxylase, α-ketoglutarate decarboxylase, and transketolase. Transketolase activity measurement is the most convenient, feasible, specific, and sensitive of tests for thiamin deficiency. Blood (particularly the red cell) transketolase activity is a reliable index of the availability of coenzyme TPP, and thus correlated well with the degree of deficiency in both animals and humans (Brin, 1962; Takeuchi et al., 1990; Lonkar et al., 1993; Rains et al., 1997). Transketolase is an excellent indicator in that it is useful in detecting marginal thiamin deficiency.

Diagnosis of thiamin deficiency in ruminants initially depended upon recognition of the clinical signs in live animals, followed by confirmatory brain histopathology or clinical response to thiamin administration (Rammell and Hill, 1986). Moreover, sick animals react so promptly to treatment with thiamin (sometimes within hours) that early treatment with thiamin is even used for confirming the diagnosis of PEM. The best transketolase assay for assessing thiamin deficiency is based on the so-called TPP effect, which is the percent of increase in transketolase activity following addition of excess TPP to the sample. Values of 120 to 250% have been reported for animals diagnosed with PEM (Edwin et al., 1979). It has been suggested that fecal thiaminase I is an indicator of thiaminase presence in the digestive tract, and high levels of this fecal enzyme may be correlated to PEM (Soita and Brent, 1993).

SUPPLEMENTATION

Thiamin is found in most feedstuffs, but in widely differing concentrations. Good thiamin sources are cereals, milling by-products, oil extraction residues, and yeast (see Natural Sources). The thiamin content of most common feeds should be three to four times greater than the required amounts for most species (Brent, 1985). For swine and poultry consuming typical diets (e.g., corn-soybean meal), thiamin is one of the vitamins least likely to be deficient. Likewise, under normal feeding and management conditions, and in the absence of antimetabolites, thiamin deficiency should theoretically not occur in either young or adult ruminants.

Drying and processing can lower the concentrations of available thi-

301

amin in feedstuffs because thiamin is heat labile. For example, it was reported that use of high-moisture barley treated with sulfur dioxide resulted in destruction of 61% of dietary thiamin (Gibson et al., 1987). Treatment of feed ingredients with sulfur dioxide inactivates thiamin. This process was used to produce deficient diets in early studies to determine the pig's thiamin requirement (NRC, 1998).

Utilization of available thiamin in feedstuffs may be limited and may be impaired by thiamin antagonists and processing methods (e.g., heat); therefore, it is common practice to add supplemental thiamin to poultry and pig feeds principally as low-cost insurance. Thiamin supplementation should normally be considered not for grazing ruminants but rather for animals that might develop PEM as a result of consuming high-concentrate diets. Grazing ruminants would not normally receive supplemental thiamin unless evidence is provided that consumed pastures contain antagonists. An example would be thiamin incorporated into diets for livestock grazing potentially toxic tall fescue pastures during midsummer when toxicosis is likely to be severe. Thiamin may be supplied to cattle at the daily rate of 1 g per head (Lauriault et al., 1990). Johnson and Krautmann (1989) reported that 500 mg of thiamin per head per day, for the first 30 days that cattle are in the feed yard, reduced the effects of thermal stress.

Subclinical deficiencies of thiamin can result in reduced synthesis of other B-vitamins since some rumen bacteria require thiamin to grow. Mathison (1986) reported one feedlot trial in which a significant response to supplemental thiamin was observed. In this trial, transketolase was numerically reduced in the controls. Thiamin did not increase gain in two subsequent trials, although there appeared to be a reduction in bloat in one trial. A concurrent field survey, conducted in Alberta, Canada, showed that 2.7% of 645 cattle sampled had marginal levels of TPP. In acute PEM, 1 g/day of injected thiamin is indicated until the animals are eating, then 500 mg/day can be supplemented in the diet for 7 to 14 days (Mathison, 1986). A level of 4 to 6 mg/kg diet in high-grain diets was suggested to help prevent subclinical deficiency.

Thiamin supplementation should be greatly modified if diets contain anti-thiamin substances, such as thiaminases from fish or moldy feeds. As an example, in free-range farming, pigs may occasionally suffer from bracken poisoning, as the roots contain anti-thiamin substances. The animals can be saved by timely thiamin injections.

For mink, the thiamin requirement is estimated to be 1.2 mg/kg dry feed. In Scandinavia, however, due to the risk of destruction of thiamin when mink are fed on fish, much higher dosages (up to 6 mg/kg) are rec-

ommended (Bräunlich and Zintzen, 1976). Other fish eaters, for example, seals, may also develop thiamin deficiency (Geraci, 1974). It has
been calculated and confirmed by determinations of blood transketolase
activity that a seal weighing 80 kg and consuming 4 to 6 kg of fish per
day has a daily thiamin requirement of 100 to 150 mg.

Intentionally added nonnutrient substances to diets are sometimes
of concern, such as the coccidiostat amprolium, a thiamin antimetabolite. A mild thiamin deficiency from amprolium added to a standard
commercial hen feed caused a reduction in the feed intake and egg-lay-
ing performance and an increase in the mortality of embryos and chicks.
These phenomena could be prevented or effectively counteracted by
high thiamin doses in the feed. At recommended levels, amprolium apparently does not interfere with the thiamin metabolism of the chicken
(Scott et al., 1982). Sometimes other thiamin antagonists, such as the
free bisulfite present in certain menadione sulfite forms or other forms
of sulfur, are added to the feed.

Animals with clinical signs of thiamin deficiency and/or other indicators of thiamin insufficiency (e.g., transketolase activity) should be
given thiamin at therapeutic doses. Since thiamin deficiency causes
anorexia, injection of the vitamin is preferred to oral doses when deficiency is severe. In calves weighing less than 50 kg, clinical signs were
prevented with 0.65 mg of thiamin-HCl per kilogram of liquid diet fed
at 10% of live weight (65 mg/kg live weight) (Johnson et al., 1948). Animals with PEM need to be rapidly provided with supplemental thiamin.
Levels of thiamin to be administered intravenously or intramuscularly
for 3 days have been recommended for lambs and calves (100 to 400
mg/day) and for sheep and cattle (500 to 2,000 mg/day) (Zintzen, 1974).

For general maintenance following the treatment of mild cases (or
as a prophylactic measure when a herd is at risk), 5 to 10 mg of thiamin
should be added to 1 kg of dry feed. Feeds should be enriched with thiamin in a concentration such that each animal will receive 100 to 500
mg daily. Likewise, roughage should be added to the daily ration at a
level of 1.5 kg/100 kg body weight. For therapeutic purposes, 6.6 to 11
mg/kg body weight repeated every 6 hours for 24 hours has been suggested for goats (Smith, 1979).

The administration of thiamin to animals with PEM generally produces rapid results, sometimes in a matter of hours. When recognition
of the disease has been delayed and irreversible necroses have already
developed in the brain, treatment with the vitamin may be useless. The
prospects of achieving satisfactory treatment of animals incapable of
standing are very limited. Although treatment improves the condition of

such animals, relapses and permanent damage are probable due to irreversible changes in the CNS. Without doubt, PEM is the most important disease arising from thiamin deficiency in ruminants. It is also noteworthy that thiamin can be used effectively as a support in the treatment of the two metabolic disorders of rumen—acidosis and ketosis. Even though treatment with thiamin can be therapeutically successful, it does not follow that deficiency of thiamin contributes to the etiology of these two diseases (Zintzen, 1974).

In horses, parenterally administered thiamin in high doses (1,000 mg intramuscularly) has a marked sedative effect that is particularly noticeable in nervous and excited horses (Bräunlich and Zintzen, 1976). Intramuscular or intravenous injections of 1,000 to 2,000 mg of thiamin also have a digitalis-like effect on the heart. Thiamin is also used in doses of 200 to 300 mg for the alleviation of muscle cramps (myoglobinuria, melanuric colic, spastic constipation).

Effects of thiamin supplements on exercising horses were explored by Topliff et al. (1981), who proposed that 4 mg of thiamin per kilogram of air-dry diet may not be sufficient. It may be prudent to ensure that the diets of performance horses contain 5 mg of thiamin per kilogram of diet dry matter (NRC, 1989b).

Thiamin sources available for addition to feed are the hydrochloride and mononitrate forms. Because of its lower solubility in water, the mononitrate form is preferred for addition to premixes; it has somewhat better stability characteristics in dry products than the hydrochloride (Bauernfeind, 1969).

Stability of thiamin in feed premixes can be a problem. More than 50% of the thiamin was destroyed in premixes after 1 month at room temperature (Verbeeck, 1975). When thiamin was observed in premixes without minerals, no losses were encountered when kept at room temperature for 6 months. After 6 months only 27% of the activity of thiamin hydrochloride remained in a vitamin premix that also contained choline and trace minerals (Coelho, 1991).

For humans in developed countries, a number of foods have been fortified with thiamin (e.g., bread enrichment) for many years. Rice enrichment in the Far Eastern countries has dramatically reduced incidence of beriberi. It has even been suggested that addition of thiamin to alcoholic beverages might help prevent the serious effects of thiamin deficiency in heavy consumers as well as in alcoholics. However, Crane and Price (1983) conclude that the addition of thiamin to beer in the form of alkyl disulfides is not a practical or effective method of enrichment and offers no special advantage. In world regions where beriberi is still endemic, a good case could be made for routine administration of thiamin to all patients in whom heart failure is present without clear evidence of the cause (Djoenaidi et al., 1992).

TOXICITY

Thiamin in large amounts is not toxic, and usually the same is true of parenteral doses. Excess thiamin is easily cleared by the kidneys. Dietary intakes of thiamin up to 1,000 times the requirement are apparently safe for most animal species (NRC, 1987). Intolerance to thiamin is relatively rare in humans; daily oral doses of 500 mg have been administered for as long as a month with no ill effects. However, there were several reports of toxic reactions following repeated parenteral injections of large doses. These were anaphylactic reactions resulting from sensitization to the vitamin. Parenteral doses of thiamin at 100 times the recommended intake produced headache, convulsions, weakness, paralysis, cardiac arrhythmia, and allergic reactions (Combs, 1992).

Lethal doses with intravenous injection were 125, 250, 300, and 350 mg/kg body weight for mice, rats, rabbits, and dogs, respectively (Gubler, 1991). Vasodilation, fall in blood pressure, bradycardia, respiratory arrhythmia, and depression resulted when animals were given thiamin in large doses intravenously.

■ REFERENCES

Abe, T. (1969). *J. Vitaminol. 15,* 339.

Aitken, F. C., and Hankin, R. G. (1970). Vitamins in Feeds for Livestock, Commonwealth Bureau of Animal Nutrition, Techn. Comm. No. 25, Central Press, Aberdeen.

Barchi, R. L. (1976). Thiamine (C. J. Gubler, M. Fujiwara, and P. M. Dreyfus, eds.) p. 282. John Wiley and Sons, New York.

Barclay, L. L., and Gibson, G. E. (1982). *J. Nutr. 112,* 1899.

Bauernfeind, J. C. (1969). *World Rev. Anim. Prod. 5*(21), 20.

Blank, N. K., Vick, N. A., and Schulman, S. (1975). *Acta Neuropathol. 31,* 137.

Blass, J. P., and Gibson, G. E. (1977). *N. Engl. J. Med. 297,* 1367.

Blass, J. P., and Gibson, G. E. (1978). Advances in Neurology, Vol. 21. R. A. P. Kark, R. N. Rosenberg, and L. J. Schut (Eds.). Raven Press, p. 181-198, New York.

Bräunlich, K., and Zintzen, H. (1976). Vitamin B_1 No. 1593. Hoffmann-La Roche, Basel, Switzerland.

Brent, B. E. (1985). *Feed Management 36*(12), 8.

Brent, B. E., and Bartley, E. E. (1984). *J. Anim. Sci. 59,* 813.

Brethour, J. R. (1972). *J. Anim. Sci. 35,* 260(Abstr.).

Breves, G., Brandt, M., Hoeller, H., and Rohr, K. (1984). *J. Agr. Sci. Camb. 96*, 587.

Brin, M. (1962). *Ann. N.Y. Acad. Sci. 98*, 528.

Brown, M. L. (1990). *In* Present Knowledge in Nutrition (M. L. Brown, ed.), 6th Ed., p. 142. International Life Sci. Inst., Washington, D.C.

Carroll, F. D., Gross, H., and Howell, C. E. (1949). *J. Anim. Sci. 8*, 290.

Charles, O. W., Roland, D. A., and Edwards Jr., H. M. (1972). *Poult. Sci. 51*, 419.

Coelho, M. B. (1991). Vitamin stability in premixes and feeds: A practical approach, p. 56. BASF Technical Symposium, Bloomington, Minnesota.

Combs Jr., G. F. (1992). The Vitamins. Academic Press, San Diego, California.

Cook, M. E. (1990). *In* Proc. 1990 Natl. Feed Ingred. Assoc. Nutr. Inst. Development in Vitamin Nutrition and Health Applications, Kansas City, Missouri. National Feed Ingredients Association (NFIA), Des Moines, Iowa.

Cooper, J. R., Roth, R. H., and Kini, M. M. (1963). *Nature (London) 199*, 609.

Crane, S., and Price, J. (1983). *J. Nutr. Sci. Vitaminol. 29*, 381.

Davidson, M. G. (1992). *Vet. Rec. 130(5)*, 94.

Davies, E. T., Pill, A. H., and Austwick, P. K. A. (1968). *Vet. Rec. 83*, 681.

Diniz, J. M. F., Bashe, J. R., and deCamargo, N. J. (1984). *Arquivo Brasileiro de Med. Vet. Zootech. 36*, 512.

Djoenaidi, W., Notermans, S. L. H., and Dunda, G. (1992). *Eur. J. Clin. Nutr. 46*, 227.

Dougherty, L. T., Lauriault, L. M., Bradley, N. W., Gay, N., and Cornelius, P. L. (1991). *J. Anim. Sci. 69*, 1008.

Earl, J.W., and McCleary, B.V. (1994). *Nature 368*, 683.

Edwin, E. E., and Lewis, G. (1971). *J. Dairy Res. 38*, 79.

Edwin, E. E., Lewis, G., and Allcroft, R. (1968). *Vet. Rec. 83*, 176.

Edwin, E. E., Markson, L. M., and Shreeve, J. (1979). *Vet. Rec. 104*, 4.

Ellis, N. R., and Madsen, L. L. (1944). *J. Nutr. 27*, 253.

Ensminger, A. H., Ensminger, M. E., Konlande, J. E., and Robson, J. R. K. (1983). *In* Foods and Nutrition Encyclopedia, Vol. I, A-H, p. 1,208. Pegus Press, California.

Evans, W. C. (1975). *Vit. Horm. 33*, 467.

Fontenot, J. P., Allen, V. G., and Brock, A. (1988). Grazing low and high endophyte infected fescue by cattle and effects of thiamin supplementation. Anim.-Sci. Research Rep., Virginia Agricultural Experiment Station No. 8:108, Blacksburg, Virginia.

Fritz, J. C., Mislivec, P. B., Pla, G. W., Harrison, B. N., Weeks, C. E., and Dantzman, J. G. (1973). *Poult. Sci. 52*, 1523.

Frye, T. M., Williams, S. N., and Graham, W. (1991). *Vet. Clin. North Am. Food Anim. Pract. 7*, 217.

Geraci, J. R. (1974). *J. Am. Vet. Med. Assoc. 165*, 801.

Gibson, D. M., Kennelly, J. J., and Aherne, F. X. (1987). *Can. J. Anim. Sci. 67*, 841.

Glad, B. W., Hodges, R. E., and Michas, C. A. (1978). *Am. J. Med. 65*, 69.

Gooneratne, S. R., Olkowski, A. A., and Christensen, D. A. (1989). *Can. J. Vet. Res. 53*, 462.

Gould, D.H. (1998). *J. Anim. Sci. 76*, 309

Gould, D. H., McAllister, M. M., Savage, J. C., and Hamar, D. W. (1991). *Am. J. Vet. Res. 52,* 1164.

Grewal, P. K., and Sangha, J. K. (1990). *J. Sci. Food Agric. 52,* 387.

Gries, C. L., and Scott, M. L. (1972). *J. Nutr. 102,* 1269.

Gubler, C. J. (1991). *In* Handbook of Vitamins (L. J. Machlin, ed.), 2nd Ed., p. 233. Marcel Dekker, Inc., New York.

Hashimoto, Y., Arai, S., and Nose, T. (1970). *Bull. Jap. Soc. Sci. Fish 36,* 791.

Heinemann, W. W., Ensminger, M. E., Cunha, T. J., and McCulloch, E. C. (1946). *J. Nutr. 31,* 107.

Hoffmann-La Roche. (2000). Vitamins for Dogs and Cats, Nutley, New Jersey

Horwitt, M. K., Liebert, E., Kreisler, O., and Wittman, P. (1948). Investigations of Human Requirements for B-Complex Vitamins Bulletin No. 116. National Academy of Sciences, Washington, D.C.

Houston, D. M., and Hulland, T. J. (1988). *Can. Vet. J. 29,* 383.

Hughes, B. L., and Wood-Gush, D. G. M. (1971). *Physiol. Behav. 6,* 331.

Jansen, B. C. P. (1956). *Nutr. Abstr. Rev. 26,* 1.

Johnson, A. B., and Krautmann, B. A. (1989). *In* Proceedings of the 24th Pacific Northwest Animal Nutrition Conference, Boise, Idaho.

Johnson, B. C., Hamilton, T. S., Nevens, W. B., and Boley, L. E. (1948). *J. Nutr. 35,* 137.

Jubb, T. F. (1992). *Vet. Rec. 131,* 347.

Kao, C., and Robinson, R. J. (1973). *J. Food Sci. 37,* 261.

Kingsbury, J. M. (1964). Poisonous Plants of the United States and Canada. p. 105. Prentice-Hall, Englewood Cliffs, New Jersey.

Kuroki, F., Iida, M., Tominaga, M., Matsumoto, T., Hirakawa, K., Sugiyama, S., and Fujishima, M. (1993). *Di. Dis. Sci. 38,* 1614.

Lauriault, L. M., Dougherty, C. T., Bradley, N. W., and Cornelius, P. L. (1990). *J. Anim. Sci. 68,* 1245.

Leevy, C. M. (1982). *Ann. N.Y. Acad. Sci. 378,* 316.

Linerode, P. A. (1966). Studies on the Synthesis and Absorption of B Complex Vitamins in the Equine. Ph.D. Dissertation, Ohio State University, Wooster.

Loew, F. M. (1978). *In* Handbook Series in Nutrition and Food, Section E: Nutritional Disorders, (M. Rechcigl Jr., ed.) Vol. 2, p. 3. CRC Press, Boca Raton, Florida.

Loew, F. M., and Dunlop, R. H. (1972). *Am J. Vet. Res. 32,* 2195.

Lofland, H. B., Goodman, H. O., Clarkson, R. B., and Prichard, R. W. (1963). *J. Nutr. 79,* 188.

Long, J. B., and Shaw, J. N. (1943). *North Am. Vet. 24,* 234.

Lonkar, P. S., Sharma, S. N., Yadav, J. S., and Prasad, M. C. (1993). *Indian Vet. J. 70,* 873.

Loosli, J. K. (1991). *In* Handbook of Animal Science (P.A. Putnam, ed.), p. 25. Academic Press, San Diego, California.

Losada, H., Dixon, F., and Preston, T. R. (1971). *Rev. Cubana Cienc. Agric. 5,* 369.

Marks, J. (1975). A Guide to the Vitamins. Their Role in Health and Disease. Medical and Technical Publishing Co., Ltd., p. 73. Lancaster, England.

Mathison, G. W. (1986). *In* Proc., 21st Northwest Animal Nutrition Conference, p. 107. Vancouver, Canada.

Maynard, L. A., Loosli, J. K., Hintz, H. F., and Warner, R. G. (1979). Animal Nutrition. McGraw-Hill Book Co., New York.

McAllister, M. M., Gould, M. M., and Hamar, D. W. (1992). *J. Compar. Pathol.* *106,* 267.

McDonald, J. W. (1982). *Aust. Vet. J. 58,* 212.

McDowell, L. R. (1985). *In* Nutrition of Grazing Ruminants in Warm Climates (L. R. McDowell, ed.), p. 359. Academic Press, Orlando, Florida.

McManus, E. C., and Judith, F. R. (1972). *Poult. Sci. 51,* 1835.

Miles, W. H., and McDowell, L. R. (1983). *World Anim. Rev. 46,* 2.

Miller, E. R., Schmidt, D. A., Hoefer, J. A., and Luecke, R. W. (1955). *J. Nutr. 56,* 423.

Mullenax, C. (1983). *Carta Ganadera* 20(10), 7.

Muralt, A. (1962). *Ann. N.Y. Acad. Sci. 98,* 499.

Morris, H. P. (1947) *Vitam. Horm. 5,* 175.

Naidoo, D. (1956). *Acta Psychiatr. Neurol. Scand. 31,* 205.

NRC. Nutrient Requirements of Domestic Animals. National Academy of Sciences-National Research Council, Washington, D.C.

(1977). Nutrient Requirements of Rabbits, 2nd Ed.

(1978). Nutrient Requirements of Nonhuman Primates.

(1981). Nutrient Requirements of Goats.

(1982a). Nutrient Requirements of Mink and Foxes.

(1985a). Nutrient Requirements of Dogs, 2nd Ed.

(1985b). Nutrient Requirements of Sheep, 5th Ed.

(1986). Nutrient Requirements of Cats, 3rd Ed.

(1989a). Nutrient Requirements of Dairy Cattle, 6th Ed.

(1989b). Nutrient Requirements of Horses, 5th Ed.

(1993). Nutrient Requirements of Fish.

(1994). Nutrient Requirements of Poultry, 9th Ed.

(1995). Nutrient Requirements of Laboratory Animals, 4th Ed.

(1996). Nutrient Requirements of Beef Cattle, 7th Ed.

(1998). Nutrient Requirements of Swine, 10th Ed.

NRC. (1987). Vitamin Tolerance of Animals. National Academy of Sciences-National Research Council, Washington, D.C.

Olkowski, A. A., Gooneratne, S. R., and Christensen, D. A. (1990). *Res. Vet. Sci. 48,* 82.

Olkowski, A. A., Rousseaux, C. G., and Christensen, D. A. (1991). *Can. J. Anim. Sci. 71,* 825.

Olkowski, A. A., Gooneratne, S. R., Rousseaux, C. G., and Christensen, D. A. (1992). *Res. Vet. Sci. 52,* 78.

Olkowski, A. A., Laarvold, B., Patience, J. F., Francis, S. I., and Christensen, D. A. (1993). *Int. J. Vit. Nutr. Res. 63,* 38.

Ollilainen, V., Vahteristo, L., Uusi-Rauva, A., Varo, P., Koivistoinen, P., and Huttunen, J. (1993). *J. Food Compos. Anal. 6,* 152.

Oltjen, R. R., Sirny, R. J., and Tillman, A. D. (1962). *J. Nutr. 77,* 269.

Pardo, B., Sygnowska, E., Rywik, S., Kulesza, W., and Waskiewicz, A. (1991). Appetite, Academic Press, p. 1. London, England.

Phillips, S. C. (1987). *Acta Neuropathol. 73,* 171.

Piktelite, O. S., Aleinik, S. I., Yakushina, L. M., Blazheevich, N. V., Isaeva, V. A.,

Alekseeva, I. H., Glinka, E. Y., and Grishchenko, N. L. (1992). *Voprosy-Pitaniyay 4*, 32.

Polin, D., Wynosky, E. R., and Porter, C. C. (1962). *Proc. Soc. Exp. Biol. Med. 110*, 844.

Polin, D., Ott, W. H., Wynosky, E. R., and Porter, C. C. (1963). *Poult. Sci. 42*, 925.

Rains, T.M., Emmert, J.L., Baker, D.H., and Shay, N.F. (1997). *J. Nutr. 127*, 167.

Ralston Purina. (1987). Nutrition and Management of Dogs and Cats. Ralston Purina Co., St. Louis, Missouri.

Rammell, C. G., and Hill, J. H. (1986). *N Z Vet. J. 34*, 202.

Rathanaswami, P., and Sundaresan, R. (1991). *Biochem. Int. Marrickville 24*(6), 1057.

RDA. (1989). Recommended Dietary Allowances, 10th Ed., National Academy of Sciences-National Research Council, Washington, D.C.

Reddy, M. U., and Pushpamma, P. (1986). *Nutr. Rep. Int. 34*, 393.

Reid, J. M., Hove, E. L., Braucher, P. F., and Mickelsen, O. (1963). *J. Nutr. 80*, 381.

Reid, M. E., and Bieri, J. G. (1967). *Proc. Soc. Exp. Biol. Med. 126*, 11.

Remus, J. C., and Firman, J. D. (1990). *J. Nutr. Biochem. 1*, 636.

Rinehart, J. F., and Greenberg, L. D. (1949). *Arch. Pathol. 48*, 89.

Rose, R. (1990). *In* Proc. 1990 Natl. Feed Ingred. Assoc. Nutr. Inst. Developments in Vitamin Nutrition and Health Applications Kansas City, Missouri. National Feed Ingredients Association (NIFA), Des Moines, Iowa.

Sadler, W. C., Mahoney, J. H., Puch, H. C., Williams, D. L., and Hodge, D. E. (1983). *Anim. Sci. Abstr.* p. 467.

Salley, J. J., Eshleman, J. R., and Morgan, J. H. (1962). *J. Dent. Res. 41*, 1405.

Scott, N. L., Nesheim, M. C., and Young, R. J. (1982). Nutrition of the Chicken, p. 119. Scott, Ithaca, New York.

Scriver, C. R. (1973). *Metabolism, 22*, 1319.

Sebrell, W. H., and Harris, R. S. (1973). The Vitamins: Chemistry, Physiology, Pathology and Methods Vol. V., p. 98. Academic Press, New York.

Shell, L.G. (1995). *Feline Pract. 23*, 27.

S'Klan, D., and Trostler, N. (1977). *J. Nutr. 107*, 357.

Smith, D.C., and Proutt, L.M. (1944). *Proc. Soc. Exp. Biol. Med. 56*, 1.

Smith, M. C. (1979). *J. Am. Vet. Med. Assoc. 174*, 1328.

Smith, W. L., Gay, N., Boling, J. A., and Crowe, M. W. (1986). *J. Anim. Sci. 63*(Suppl. 1), 296.

Soita, H. W., and Brent, B. E. (1993). *J. Anim. Sci. 71*(Suppl. 1), 278.

Strauss, L. H., and Scheer, P. (1939). *Int. Z. Vitam. Forsch 9*, 39.

Studdert, V. P., and Labuc, R. H. (1991). *Aust. Vet. J. 68*, 54.

Sturkie, P. D., Singsen, E. P., Matterson, L. D., Kozeff, A., and Jungherr, E. L. (1954). *Am. J. Vet. Res. 15*, 457.

Swank, R. L. (1940). *J. Exp. Med. 71*, 683.

Takeuchi, T., Jung, E. H., Nishino, K., and Itokawa, Y. (1990). *Int. J. Vitam. Nutr. Res. 60*(2), 112.

Tang, C. M., Rolfe, M., Wells, J. C., and Cham, K. (1989). *Lancet 2*(8656), 206.

Tanphaichair, V. (1976). *In* Nutrition Reviews Present Knowledge in Nutrition

(D. M. Hegsted, C. O. Chichester, W. J. Darby, K. W. McNutt, R. M. Stalvey, and E. H. Stotz, eds.). The Nutrition Foundation Inc., New York.

Thornber, E. J., Dunlop, R. H., Gawthorne, J. M., and Huxtable, C. R. (1979). *Res. Vet. Sci. 26,* 378.

Thornton, P. A., and Schutze, J. E. (1960). *Poult. Sci. 39,* 192.

Topliff, D. R., Potter, G. D., Kreider, J. L., and Creagor, C. R. (1981). *In* Proc. 7th Eq. Nutr. Physiol. Soc. Symp., p. 167. Warrenton, Virginia.

Tucker, D. M., Penland, J. G., Sandstead, H. H., Milne, D. B., Heck, D. G., and Klevay, L. M. (1990). *J. Food Sci. 52,* 93.

Uherová, R., Hozová, B., and Smirnov, V. (1993). *Food Chem. 46,* 293.

Verbeeck, J. (1975). *Feedstuffs 47*(36), 4.

Wetherilt, H., Ackurt, F., Brubacher, G., Okan, B., Aktas, S., and Turdu, S. (1992). *Int. J. Vitam. Nutr. Res. 62,* 21.

Williams, R. R. (1961). Toward the Conquest of Beriberi. Harvard University Press, Cambridge, Massachusetts.

Zempleni, J., Link, G., and Kubler, W. (1992). *Int. J. Vitam. Nutr. Res. 62,* 165.

Zintzen, H. (1974). Vitamin B (Thiamine) in the Nutrition of the Ruminant, No. 1460. Hoffmann-La Roche, Basel, Switzerland.

RIBOFLAVIN

INTRODUCTION

After isolation of thiamin (vitamin B_1) as the "vitamin B" factor that prevented beriberi and polyneuritis, riboflavin (vitamin B_2) was the first growth factor to be characterized from the remaining B-complex vitamins. Riboflavin in the form of flavin mononucleotide (FMN) and flavin adenine dinucleotide (FAD) functions as a coenzyme in diverse enzymatic reactions. The vitamin is required in the metabolism of all plants and animals, and every plant and animal cell contains the vitamin.

Because of microbial ruminal synthesis, adult ruminants apparently do not require dietary riboflavin. Young ruminants, prior to development of the rumen, and other species require dietary sources of riboflavin because of their very limited synthesis by intestinal flora. Riboflavin is one of the vitamins most likely to be deficient in typical swine and poultry diets based on grains and plant protein supplements (e.g., soybean meal). Likewise, human diets low in animal protein products (especially milk and egg products) and leafy vegetables are likely to be deficient in riboflavin.

HISTORY

The historical aspects of riboflavin were reviewed by McCollum (1957), Wagner-Jauregg (1972), Sharman (1977), Scott et al. (1982), and Loosli (1991). In 1915, it was known that a water-soluble factor or factors promoted growth and prevented beriberi in rats. In 1920, it was found that heating feedstuffs (e.g., yeast) destroyed the beriberi preventive effect more readily than the growth-promoting effect. Therefore, it was determined that this water-soluble B vitamin contained two essen-

7

tial factors, one of which was more stable to heat than the other. The less stable factor was labeled vitamin F (B_1 or thiamin) and the heat-stable factor vitamin G (B_2 or riboflavin).

The biological importance of certain yellow pigments became apparent in 1932, when Warburg and Christain (Germany) isolated an oxidative enzyme ("old yellow enzyme") from yeast that was yellow with green fluorescence. They split it into a protein and a nonprotein (pigment) fraction. This was the first identification of a prosthetic or activating group of an enzyme. Thus, riboflavin was found in a coenzyme before it was discovered in free form. The yellow enzyme was found necessary for oxidation of glucose-6-phosphate.

In 1933, Kuhn (Germany) isolated a yellow pigment from egg white that showed green fluorescence and had oxidative properties. Kuhn suggested that this growth factor for rats be given the name *flavin*. Therefore, the terms *ovoflavin* from eggs, *lactoflavin* from milk, *hepatoflavin* from liver, and *uroflavin* from urine were used. Pure crystalline flavin compounds were found to contain ribose, and thus, the name riboflavin became popular.

In 1934–1935, riboflavin was synthesized by two groups—Kuhn's in Germany and Karrer's in Switzerland. At the same time, Györgi in Germany proved that the biological activity of the synthetic form was the same as that of the natural vitamin. The synthesis of FMN was accomplished in 1936 by Kuhn and Rudy. In 1938, Warburg discovered FAD as the coenzyme of D-amino acid oxidase. Other flavin-dependent enzymes were discovered thereafter at a rapid rate.

CHEMICAL STRUCTURE, PROPERTIES, AND ANTAGONISTS

Riboflavin consists of a dimethylisoalloxazine nucleus combined with the alcohol of ribose as a side chain. All flavins are isoalloxazines, which are 10-substituted derivatives of alloxazine, the parent tricyclic ring system, with nitrogens in positions 1, 3, 5, and 10. Riboflavin exists in three forms: as the free riboflavin and as the coenzyme derivatives FMN (also called riboflavin 5-phosphate) and FAD (Fig. 7.1). The coenzyme derivatives are synthesized sequentially from riboflavin. In the first step, catalyzed by flavokinase, riboflavin reacts with adenosine triphosphate (ATP) to form FMN; then FMN combines with a second molecule of ATP to form FAD in a reaction catalyzed by the enzyme FAD pyrophosphorylase.

Riboflavin is an odorless, bitter orange-yellow compound that melts

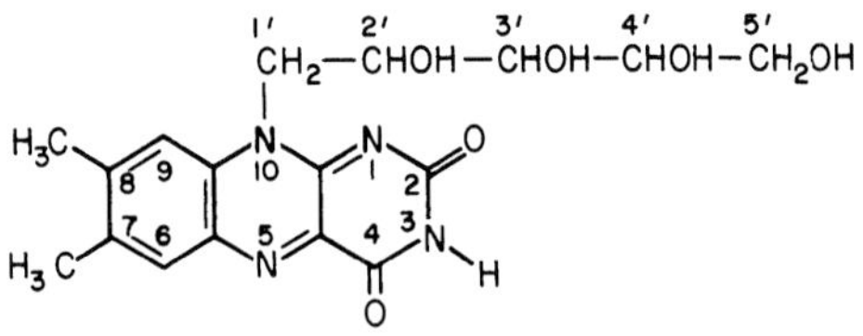

Riboflavin (7,8 dimethyl-10-(D,1'-ribityl)-isoalloxazine)

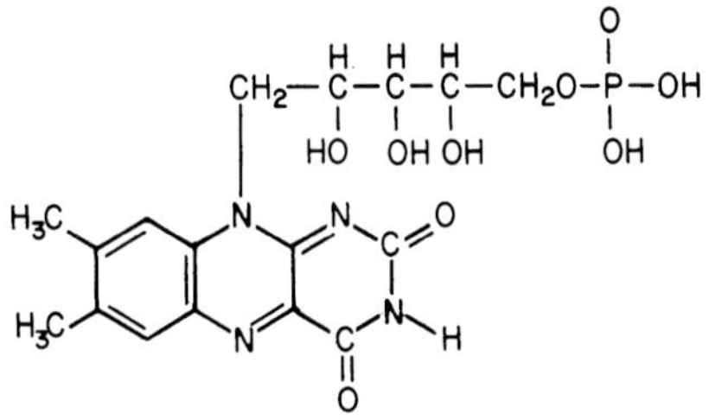

Flavin mononucleotide (FMN, riboflavin 5-phosphate)

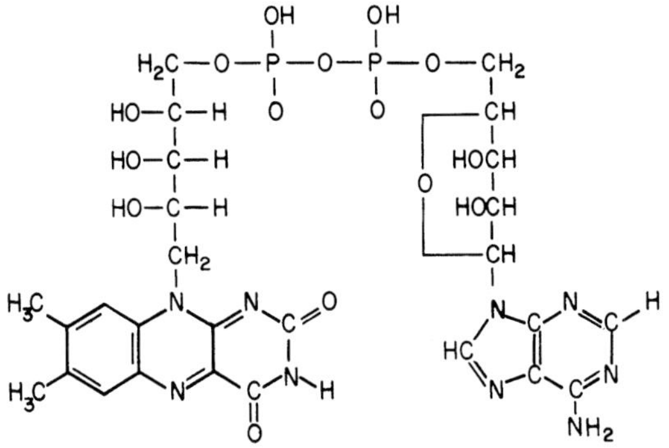

Flavin adenine dinucleotide (FAD)

Fig. 7.1 Structures of riboflavin, flavin mononucleotide (FMN), and flavin adenine dinucleotide (FAD).

at about 280°C. Its empirical formula is $C_{17}H_{20}N_4O_6$, with an elemental analysis of carbon 54.25%, hydrogen 5.36%, and nitrogen 14.89%. Riboflavin is only slightly soluble in water but readily soluble in dilute basic or strong acidic solutions. It is quite stable to heat in neutral and acid, but not alkaline solutions; very little is lost in cooking. Aqueous solutions are unstable to visible and ultraviolet light, and instability is increased by heat and alkalinity. When dry, it is not affected appreciably by light, but in solution, it is quickly destroyed.

Loss in milk during pasteurization and exposure to light is 10 to 20%. Much larger losses (50 to 70%) can occur if bottled milk is left standing in bright sunlight for more than 2 hours. Poultry mashes left exposed to direct sunlight for several days and frequently stirred are subject to some loss. In alkaline solution, light splits off ribityl residue, rapidly forming lumiflavin (7,8,10-trimethylisoalloxazine). In acid or neutral solution, light decomposition produces lumichrome (7,8-dimethylalloxazine).

Many flavins—which differ structurally and functionally from riboflavin, FMN, and FAD—have been discovered, with physiological roles often unknown. Antiriboflavin compounds may result from chemical changes in either the isoalloxazine nucleus or the ribityl side chain. A number of synthetic homologs of riboflavin exist. The antagonist D-galactoflavin, 7,8-dimethyl-10-(d-l′-dulcityl) isoalloxazine, has been used experimentally in animals and humans to hasten the development of riboflavin deficiency (Cooperman and Lopez, 1991). The phenothiazines (e.g., chlorpromazine, used in the treatment of schizophrenia) and the tricyclic antidepressant drugs (e.g., imipramine) are structural analogues of riboflavin and inhibit flavokinase. In experimental animals, administration of these drugs at doses equivalent to those used clinically results in increased urinary excretion of riboflavin, with reduced tissue concentrations of FMN and FAD, despite feeding diets providing more riboflavin than is needed to meet requirements (Pinto et al., 1981).

ANALYTICAL PROCEDURES

Analytical methods for riboflavin determination in feeds and biological tissues employ fluorometric or microbiological assays. The first assays measured the biological response in the rat and the chicken, but riboflavin can be assayed more readily by chemical or microbiological methods, so animal assays have given way to these. Growth and production of lactic acid by *Lactobacillus casei* are dependent on presence of riboflavin in the medium. Turbidity from the growth of the bacteria can be read in a colorimeter after 16 to 24 hours of incubation at 37°C.

Riboflavin rarely occurs free in nature, so natural products usually must be treated with acid or enzymes to liberate the riboflavin. If FMN or FAD are to be measured, special nonhydrolytic extraction procedures are required. Unique properties of riboflavin allowing for successful fluorometric analysis include the following (Scott et al., 1982): (1) Riboflavin gives off an intense greenish fluorescence, with intensity proportional to the concentration; (2) it is stable to heat and acid, allowing release from proteins; and (3) it is stable to oxidizing agents (e.g., potassium permanganate) needed to destroy other fluorescing materials. Because riboflavin is readily destroyed by blue or violet light, operations must be done in dim light or in amber or red glassware. Also, at a pH of greater than 7.0, dilute solutions may be destroyed by alkali even on clean glassware.

A high-performance liquid chromatographic (HPLC) methodology has been developed to determine riboflavin in plant (Fernando and Murphy, 1990) and animal (Li et al., 1993) sources that compares with fluorometric procedures. Using HPLC, it is possible to simultaneously determine the three principal forms of the vitamin, riboflavin, FMN, and FAD in foods (Russell and Vanderslice, 1991).

METABOLISM

Digestion, Absorption, and Transport

Riboflavin is found in feeds as FAD, FMN, and free riboflavin. Riboflavin covalently bound to protein is released by proteolysis digestion. Phosphorylated forms (FAD, FMN) of the riboflavin are hydrolyzed by phosphatases in the upper gastrointestinal tract to free the vitamin for absorption. For the rat, the ribityl side chain and the NH group at position 3 of the isoalloxazine moiety are essential for riboflavin binding to the small intestine brush border membrane (Casirola et al., 1994). Free riboflavin enters mucosal cells of the small intestine after apparently being absorbed in all parts of the small intestine. In a comparison between jejunal and ileal cells from guinea pigs, cells from both portions of the small intestine transported riboflavin almost equally (Hegazy and Schwenk, 1983). Cells from deficient animals have a greater maximal absorption uptake of riboflavin (Rose et al., 1986). At low concentrations, riboflavin absorption is an active Na^+-dependent carrier-mediated process (Hegazy and Schwenk, 1983). However, Said et al. (1993a,b) suggest that the carrier-mediated system in the rabbit is Na^+- and pH-independent in nature and transports the substrate rather by an electroneutral process. At high concentrations, riboflavin is absorbed by passive diffusion, proportional to concentration (Middleton, 1990). In mucosal cells, much of the riboflavin is phosphorylated to FMN by fla-

315

vokinase. Riboflavin enters the blood as both FMN and the free vitamin. In tissues, most of the FMN is then converted to the other coenzyme FAD by FAD-pyrophosphorylase.

Transport of flavin by blood plasma is known to involve both loose association with albumin and tight associations with some globulins (McCormick, 1990). A genetically controlled riboflavin-binding protein is present in serum and eggs. There is a hereditary recessive disorder in chickens—renal riboflavinuria—in which the riboflavin-binding protein is absent (White, 1996). Eggs become riboflavin deficient, and embryos generally do not survive beyond the fourteenth day of incubation (Clagett, 1971). Also, if riboflavin-binding protein is in excess, it can diminish riboflavin availability to the chicken embryo (Lee and White, 1996). Presumably, the lack of the specific vitamin transport protein prevents adequate transfer of dietary riboflavin to the developing fetus, and riboflavin losses occur via maternal urine.

In addition to poultry, specific binding proteins have been found in serum from pregnant cows and rats, human fetal blood, and uterine secretions in the pig. Riboflavin-carrier proteins were induced by estrogens and synthesized in liver (Durgakumari and Adiga, 1986). Rivlin (1984) suggested there may be physiological mechanisms in pregnancy that facilitate transfer of riboflavin from maternal stores to the fetus in a manner that is fundamentally similar to that in the laying hen. Riboflavin was efficiently transferred to the fetus. In human placenta, riboflavin concentration was 8.7 mmol/L in maternal plasma versus 40.6 mmol/L for venous cord plasma, indicating favorable retention by the fetus (Zempleni et al., 1992).

Much of the control of riboflavin utilization is at the level of flavocoenzyme formation. Hormonal control affects riboflavin metabolism, and specific binding proteins can be greatly increased by estrogen administration (Rivlin, 1984). Thyroid hormones enhance conversion of riboflavin into its coenzyme derivatives and hypothyroidism decreases it. The major site of thyroid hormone control appears to be flavokinase, and physiological doses of thyroxine increase hepatic activity of this enzyme (Rivlin, 1984). Adrenocorticotropic hormone and aldosterone both increase rate of formation of flavin coenzymes from riboflavin.

Tissue Distribution, Storage, and Excretion

Animals do not appear to have the ability to store appreciable amounts of riboflavin; the liver, kidney, and heart have the richest concentrations. Liver, the major site of storage, contains about one-third of the total body flavins. A significant amount of free riboflavin exists in retinal tissue, but its function is unclear. Free riboflavin constitutes less than 5% of the stored flavins, with 70 to 90% in the form of FAD. Intakes of riboflavin above current needs are rapidly excreted in urine, primarily as free riboflavin. The kidney excretes both riboflavin and FMN, the latter being dephosphorylated in the bladder. Minor quantities of absorbed riboflavin are excreted in feces, bile, and sweat.

FUNCTIONS

Riboflavin is required as part of many enzymes essential to utilization of carbohydrates, fat, and protein. More than 100 enzymes are known to bind FAD or FMN in animal and microbial systems. Riboflavin and related natural flavins participate in numerous and diverse reactions, perhaps more than for any other vitamin-coenzyme group. FMN and FAD, which contain riboflavin, function as prosthetic groups that combine with specific proteins to form active enzymes called flavoproteins. Most flavoproteins contain the FAD form, and a few contain FMN. Riboflavin in these coenzyme forms acts as an intermediary in the transfer of electrons in biological oxidation-reduction reactions. The enzymes that function aerobically are called oxidases, and those that function anaerobically are called dehydrogenases. The general function is in oxidation of substrate and generation of energy (ATP). By involvement in the hydrogen transport system, flavoproteins function by accepting and passing on hydrogen, undergoing alternate oxidation and reduction. Collectively, the flavoproteins show great versatility in accepting and transferring one or two electrons with a range of potentials. Many flavoproteins contain a metal (e.g., iron, molybdenum, copper, zinc), and the combination of flavin and metal ion is often involved in the adjustments of these enzymes in transfers between single- and double-electron donors. Xanthine oxidase contains the metals molybdenum and iron. It converts hypoxanthine to xanthine and the latter to uric acid. It also reacts with aldehydes to form acids, including the conversion of retinal (vitamin A aldehyde) to retinoic acid.

Flavoproteins may either accept H^+ directly from the substrate (the material being oxidized) or catalyze the oxidation of some other enzyme by accepting hydrogen from it, for example, from the niacin-containing coenzymes, nicotinamide adenine dinucleotide (NAD), and nicotinamide adenine dinucleotide phosphate (NADP). About 40 flavoprotein enzymes may be arbitrarily classified into three groups:

a. $NADH_2$ dehydrogenases—enzymes whose substrate is a reduced pyridine nucleotide, and the electron acceptor is a member of the cytochrome system or some other acceptor besides oxygen.

b. Oxidases (true)—enzymes that accept electrons from substrate and pass them directly to oxygen; they cannot reduce cytochromes. Oxygen is reduced to H_2O_2.

c. Dehydrogenases—enzymes that accept electrons directly from substrate and can pass them to one of the cytochromes.

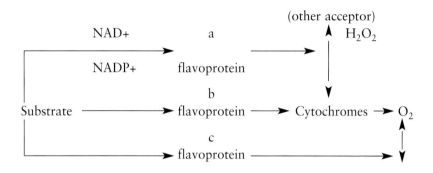

The main function of FMN and FAD is transferring hydrogen between the niacin-containing coenzymes, NAD and NADP, the iron porphyrin cytochromes, and directly from the substrate (Fig. 7.2). The sequence of electron acceptors in the early stages of the respiratory chain indicates that coenzyme Q (ubiquinone) acts between flavoprotein and cytochrome b. Thus these enzymes are a part of the chain that carries hydrogen from substrates (carbohydrates, amino acids, lipids, etc.) to molecular oxygen, forming water. These flavoprotein pathways are the most important means of electron transport for both mitochondria and microsomes (Scott et al., 1982).

Approximately 40 flavoprotein enzymes participate in electron transfer from metabolites and pyridine nucleotides to molecular oxygen and include the following:

1. Aerobic dehydrogenases (simple oxidases not containing metals)
    (a) D and L amino acid oxidases
    (b) Glycolic acid oxidase
    (c) Glucose oxidase
    (d) Warburg's old yellow enzyme
2. Oxidases (containing copper, iron, molybdenum, or zinc)
    (a) Cuproflavoprotein in butyryl-CoA-dehydrogenase

1) Succinate dehydrogenase (mitochondrial dehydrogenase)

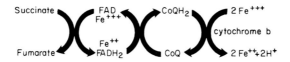

2) Lipoyl dehydrogenase (mitochondrial dehydrogenase)

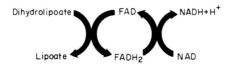

3) NADH dehydrogenase of mitochondria

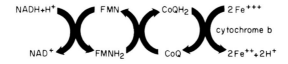

4) NADPH-cytochrome c reductase of microsomes

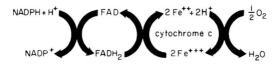

Fig. 7.2 Examples of hydrogen transfer involving flavoproteins. (Modified from Scott et al., 1982.)

    (b) Xanthine oxidase (flavoprotein containing iron and molybdenum)
    (c) Molybdoflavoprotein in aldehyde oxidase
    (d) DPNH-cytochrome reductase (iron-containing flavoprotein)
3. Anaerobic dehydrogenases
    (a) Lipoyl dehydrogenase
    (b) Acyl-CoA dehydrogenases and electron-transferring flavoprotein

319

(c) Succinic dehydrogenase-fumaric reductase
(d) Others
    Choline dehydrogenase
    α-Glycerophosphate dehydrogenase
    L-Galactone-γ-lactone dehydrogenase
    L-Lactate dehydrogenase
    D-Lactate cytochrome reductase
    Pyridine nucleotide-cytochrome *c* reductases

Riboflavin functions in flavoprotein-enzyme systems to help regulate cellular metabolism, and is also specifically involved in metabolism of carbohydrates. Riboflavin is also an essential factor in amino acid metabolism as part of amino acid oxidases. These oxidize α-amino acids to corresponding amino acids that decompose to give ammonia and α-keto acid. There are distinct enzymes oxidizing D-amino acids (prosthetic group FAD) and L-amino acids (prosthetic group FMN). An FAD-dependent hydroxylase is involved in the conversion of tryptophan to niacin.

Among the enzymes that require riboflavin is the FMN-dependent oxidase responsible for conversion of phosphorylated pyridoxine (vitamin B_6) to a functional coenzyme. In view of the widespread deficiency of riboflavin in Nigeria, and the involvement of riboflavin in vitamin B_6 metabolism, it is speculated that riboflavin status may account for the high occurrence of vitamin B_6 deficiency in young adults (Ajayi et al., 1989). Riboflavin deficiency also results in a decrease in the conversion of the vitamin B_6 coenzyme pyridoxal phosphate to the main vitamin B_6 urinary excretory product of 4-pyridoxic acid (Kodentsova et al., 1993).

Riboflavin deficiency had an effect on iron metabolism, with less iron absorbed and an increased rate of iron loss due to an accelerated rate of small intestinal epithelial turnover (Powers et al., 1991, 1993). In Gambian men, riboflavin deficiency reduced iron utilization with hemoglobin levels increased after riboflavin supplementation (Fairweather-Tait et al., 1992).

Riboflavin plays a role in fat metabolism (Cooperman and Lopez, 1991), and a FAD flavoprotein is an important link in fatty acid oxidation. This includes the acyl-coenzyme A dehydrogenases, which are necessary for the stepwise degradation of fatty acids. An FMN flavoprotein is required for synthesis of fatty acids from acetate. Thus, flavoproteins are necessary for both degradation and synthesis of fatty acids.

The fluidity of red blood cell membranes isolated from riboflavin-deficient rats was significantly lower than that of the controls. This decreased fluidity was accompanied by an increase in the activity of the membrane-bound enzyme acetylcholinesterase. This study demonstrated that a decrease in cells' ability to cope with peroxidative damage as a result of riboflavin deficiency may lead to changes in the fluidity and function of membranes (Levin et al., 1990). There was increased plasma lipid peroxidation in riboflavin-deficient, malaria-infected children (Das et al., 1990). It was proposed that riboflavin deficiency restricts regeneration of reduced glutathione, making the parasitized erythrocytes more vulnerable to destructive lipid peroxidation and increasing plasma lipid hydroperoxides. Elevated riboflavin levels were reported to provide protection against oxidative damage caused by oxidized forms of hemeproteins (Christensen, 1993).

Although riboflavin is present mostly as flavoprotein enzymes FAD and FMN, the retina contains free riboflavin in relatively large amounts. The function it fulfills there is still not clear. In avascular tissues such as the cornea, it is thought that oxidation takes place by means of a riboflavin-containing enzyme. In riboflavin deficiency, the body attempts oxygenation by vascularization (Marks, 1975).

REQUIREMENTS

Riboflavin requirements vary with heredity, growth, environment, age, activity, health, other dietary components, and synthesis by host. Riboflavin requirements for selected animals and humans are presented in Table 7.1. The majority of species have a requirement between 1 and 4 mg/kg of diet (dry basis). Where sufficient data are available, studies indicate that riboflavin requirements decline with animal maturity and increase for reproductive activity. Chicks receiving diets only partially deficient in riboflavin may recover spontaneously, indicating that requirement rapidly decreased with age (Scott et al., 1982). However, Deyhim et al. (1992) reported that 3.6 ppm dietary riboflavin for growing broilers was satisfactory through 4 weeks, but that benefits were obtained by exceeding the 3.6 ppm recommendation through 8 weeks. Several studies have indicated that the riboflavin requirement for prevention of leg paralysis is higher than that for growth (Ruiz and Harms, 1988).

Based upon sow farrowing performance and concentration of erythrocyte glutathione reductase (an indicator of riboflavin status) concentration, Frank et al. (1984) estimated the available riboflavin requirement for pregnancy to be about 6.5 mg daily. Using the same criteria, the suggested lactational requirement was about 16 mg daily (Frank et al., 1985,

■ Table 7.1 Riboflavin Requirements for Various Animals and Humans

Animal	Purpose or Class	Requirement[a]	Reference
Beef cattle	Adult	Microbial synthesis	NRC (1996)
Dairy cattle	Calf	6.5 ppm milk replacer	NRC (1989a)
	Adult	Microbial synthesis	NRC (1989a)
Goat	Adult	Microbial synthesis	NRC (1981)
Chicken	Leghorn, 0–6 weeks	3.6 mg/kg	NRC (1994)
	Leghorn, 6–18 weeks	1.8 mg/kg	NRC (1994)
	Laying (100-g intake)	2.5 mg/kg	NRC (1994)
	Broilers, 0–8 weeks	3.6 mg/kg	NRC (1994)
Duck (Pekin)	All classes	4.0 mg/kg	NRC (1994)
Japanese quail	All classes	4.0 mg/kg	NRC (1994)
Turkey	0–4 weeks	4.0 mg/kg	NRC (1994)
Sheep	Adult	Microbial synthesis	NRC (1985b)
Swine	Growing-finishing, 3–20 kg	3.0–4.0 mg/kg	NRC (1998)
	Growing-finishing, 20–120 kg	2.0–2.5 mg/kg	NRC (1998)
	Adult	3.75 mg/kg	NRC (1998)
Horse	All classes	2.0 mg/kg	NRC (1989b)
Mink	Growing	1.5 mg/kg	NRC (1982a)
Fox	Growing	1.25–4.0 mg/kg	NRC (1982a)
Cat	Growing	1.0 mg/kg	NRC (1986)
Dog	Growing	2–4 mg/kg	NRC (1985a)
Fish	Catfish	9.0 mg/kg	NRC (1993)
	Pacific salmon	7–25 mg/kg	NRC (1993)
	Rainbow trout	2.7–15 mg/kg	NRC (1993)
Rat	All classes	3.0 mg/kg	NRC (1995)
Mouse	All classes	7.0 mg/kg	NRC (1995)
Human	Infants	0.4–0.5 mg/day	RDA (1989)
	Children	0.8–1.2 mg/day	RDA (1989)
	Adults	1.3–1.8 mg/day	RDA (1989)

[a]Expressed as per unit of animal feed on either as-fed (approximately 90% dry matter) or dry basis (see Appendix, Tables A1a,b). Human data are expressed as mg/day.

1988). Massive riboflavin supplementation (10 to 160 mg/d) increased the percentage of sows farrowed but did not increase litter size (Pettigrew et al., 1996). Frank et al. (1988) suggested that first-litter gilts have a higher requirement for riboflavin than the second litter sow based on needs for both maternal growth and reproduction.

Increased dietary fat or protein increases requirements for riboflavin in rats and chickens. It was assumed that high urinary riboflavin excretion during periods of negative nitrogen balance for a number of species was a reflection of impaired riboflavin utilization or retention. However, Turkki and Holtzapple (1982) suggested, in studies with rats, that the effect of protein on riboflavin requirement is related to rate of growth and not to protein intake per se.

Microbial biosynthesis of riboflavin has been shown to occur in the gastrointestinal tract of a number of animal species and thus affects requirements. However, utilization of this endogenously synthesized riboflavin varies from species to species. Within a single species, utilization depends on diet composition and incidence of coprophagy. Carbohydrates such as starch, cellulose, or lactose are absorbed slowly and therefore exposed for a longer time to the intestinal bacteria, resulting in an increased riboflavin synthesis. Dextrose, fat, or protein as chief dietary constituents decrease intestinal production, thereby increasing dietary riboflavin requirements. Young rats fed a riboflavin-free, purified diet with sucrose as the only carbohydrate will cease to grow. However, when sucrose is replaced by starch, sorbitol, or lactose, growth is comparable to that of rats supplied with riboflavin (Haenel et al., 1959). For humans, diets with increased carbohydrates and decreased fat are suggested to reduce riboflavin requirements (Boisvert et al., 1993). Antibiotics, such as tetracycline, penicillin, and streptomycin, reduce the requirements of several animal species for riboflavin. They may stimulate microorganisms that synthesize riboflavin or inhibit microorganisms in the gut that compete for riboflavin.

Because of microbial ruminal synthesis of riboflavin, ruminants have no dietary requirements. Nevertheless, diet composition influences total microbial synthesis. Data of Miller et al. (1983a) also suggested a greater riboflavin ruminal synthesis with an increased proportion of dietary concentrates. Buziassy and Tribe (1960) measured increased synthesis of riboflavin with diets containing more protein. These authors also noted that ruminal synthesis was reduced with higher dietary intakes of the vitamin. Confirmation of net synthesis in the rumen is illustrated by McElroy and Goss (1940) in which the secretion of riboflavin in milk was equivalent to approximately 10 times the intake of the vitamin.

Temperature extremes apparently have an effect on riboflavin requirement. With pigs, riboflavin requirements were substantially higher at a low environmental temperature (Seymour et al., 1968). At environmental temperatures below 11°C, feed required per unit of gain increased, and rate of gain decreased with decreasing temperature. On the contrary, Onwudike and Adegbola (1984) reported riboflavin requirements to be higher for chickens in a tropical environment. A dietary level of 4.1 ppm riboflavin was adequate for egg laying with 5.7 ppm for hatchability, compared to 2.5 ppm for the NRC (1994) requirement. When requirement comparisons between animals residing at different environmental temperatures are calculated, total feed intakes must be considered.

Requirements of humans for riboflavin have been determined from experimental studies with adults and infants. Riboflavin allowance for human infants and adults ranges from 0.4 to 1.8 mg/day (RDA, 1989). Levels are to be increased by 0.3 mg during pregnancy, and by 0.5 mg during the first 6 months of lactation and possibly should be related to energy expenditure (Roe et al., 1982). A level of 0.5 mg per 1,000 kcal was estimated to be the minimum requirement for adults to maintain a normal urinary excretion. On a similar basis, the infant's minimum daily requirement was estimated as 0.6 mg per 1,000 kcal.

A number of factors influence riboflavin requirements including drugs (see Section III), disease, alcohol, heavy metals, and exercise (Cooperman and Lopez, 1991). Riboflavin absorption is decreased in hyperthyroidism and increased in hypothyroidism. There is an increased urinary excretion of riboflavin observed in diabetics (Cole et al., 1976). Riboflavin in blood is significantly decreased in patients with Crohn's disease (Kuroki et al., 1993). Alcohol may antagonize the utilization of FAD from foods (Combs, 1992). Divalent metals (e.g., copper, iron and zinc) form chelates with riboflavin and FMN, reducing absorption of the vitamin. Exercise has been shown to increase riboflavin requirements of both young and old individuals (Belko et al., 1985; Trebler-Winters et al., 1992).

NATURAL SOURCES

Riboflavin is synthesized by green plants, yeasts, fungi, and some bacteria. Rapidly growing, green, leafy vegetables and forages, particularly alfalfa, are a good source, with the vitamin richest in the leaves. Cereals and their by-products have a rather low content, in contrast to their supply of thiamin. Oil meals are fair sources. While grains and protein meals contain some riboflavin, they should not be relied on as the sole source of the vitamin. Riboflavin concentrates obtained from whey and distiller's solubles are important commercial sources, particularly for animal feeds. Although fruits and vegetables are moderately good sources of this vitamin, they are not consumed in sufficient quantities to meet daily requirements (Cooperman and Lopez, 1991). Riboflavin concentration in various foods and foodstuffs is shown in Table 7.2.

Riboflavin is more bioavailable from animal products than plant sources. Flavin complexes in plants are more stable to digestion and thus less digestible than animal sources (Combs, 1992). Singh and Deodhar (1992) concluded that milk factor(s) enhanced intestinal uptake of riboflavin in rat intestine. Bioavailability of riboflavin was less for chicks fed corn-soybean than purified amino acid diets; riboflavin bioavailabil-

■ Table 7.2   Riboflavin in Foods and Feedstuffs (ppm, dry basis)

Alfalfa hay, sun cured	13.4	Linseed meal, solvent extracted	3.2
Alfalfa leaves, sun cured	23.1	Liver, cattle	92.2
Barley, grain	1.8	Milk, skim, cattle	20.5
Bean, navy (seed)	2.0	Molasses, sugarcane	3.8
Blood meal	2.2	Oat, grain	1.7
Brewer's grains	1.6	Peanut meal, solvent extracted	9.8
Buttermilk (cattle)	33.1	Rice, bran	2.8
Chicken, broilers (whole)	15.6	Rice, grain	1.2
Citrus pulp	2.7	Rice, polished	0.6
Clover hay, ladino (sun cured)	17.2	Rye, grain	1.9
Copra meal (coconut)	3.7	Sorghum, grain	1.4
Corn, gluten meal	1.8	Soybean meal, solvent extracted	3.2
Corn, yellow grain	1.4	Soybean seed	3.1
Cottonseed meal,		Spleen, cattle	15.3
solvent extracted	5.3	Timothy hay, sun cured	10.1
Eggs	3.0	Wheat, bran	4.6
Fish meal, anchovy	8.2	Wheat, grain	1.6
Fish meal, menhaden	5.2	Yeast, brewer's	38.1
Fish, sardine	5.8	Yeast, torula	47.6

Source: NRC (1982b).

ity in the corn-soybean meal diet was 59.1% (Chung and Baker, 1990). Fermentation significantly increased the proportions of riboflavin present in the free form, resulting in a greater bioavailability of the vitamin in curd than in milk (Raghvendar et al., 1993).

For human diets, milk, eggs, liver, heart, kidney, and muscle meat are rich sources. Riboflavin content of milk, such as that of cows and goats, is many times higher than content in their feed because of rumen synthesis. Human milk contains about 0.5 mg riboflavin/L, while cow's milk is three times higher (e.g., 1.7 mg/L). For humans in the United States, it has been estimated that milk and milk products contribute almost one-half of dietary riboflavin in the diet, with meat, eggs, and legumes contributing about 25%. Fruits, vegetables, and cereal grains contribute about 10% each (Hunt, 1975).

Riboflavin is one of the more stable vitamins, but it can be easily destroyed by ultraviolet rays or sunlight. Appreciable amounts may be lost upon exposure to light; up to one-half the riboflavin content is lost in cooking eggs and pork chops in light and most of the vitamin in milk stored in clear glass or plastic bottles. However, processes like pasteurization, evaporation, and condensation have little effect on riboflavin content of milk. Sun-drying of fruits and vegetables is likely to lead to substantial losses of vitamin activity. The practice of adding sodium bicarbonate to make vegetables appear fresher accelerates the photodegradation of riboflavin (Rivlin, 1984). Riboflavin in meat is relatively stable during cooking, canning, and dehydration. There is no significant loss of riboflavin from microwave heating (Sigman-Grant et al., 1992). Milling of rice and wheat results in considerable loss of riboflavin, since most of the vitamin is in the germ and bran, which are removed during this process. About one-half the riboflavin content is lost when rice is milled, and whole wheat flour contains about two-thirds more riboflavin than white flour (Cooperman and Lopez, 1991). However, converted or parboiled rice, in which the whole brown rice is steamed, thereby driving the vitamins in the germ and aleurone layers into the endosperm prior to milling, retains more riboflavin than whole rice (Grewal and Sangha, 1990).

DEFICIENCY

Effects of Deficiency

Animals and humans are unable to synthesize riboflavin within tissues; therefore, requirements are met principally by dietary sources, with some intestinal microbial synthesis. Since riboflavin plays many essential roles in the release of food energy and the assimilation of nutrients, it is understandable why deficiency is reflected in a wide variety of signs that vary among species. However, it is not possible to relate signs to specific biochemical roles that have been established. A decreased growth rate and lowered feed efficiency are common signs in all species affected. Typical clinical signs often involve the eyes, the skin, and the nervous system. Riboflavin deficiency would not be expected in young nursing animals, as milk is a rich source of the vitamin.

Ruminants

Riboflavin is not required in the diet of adult ruminants because ruminal microorganisms synthesize this vitamin in adequate amounts. Apparently no response to supplemental riboflavin has been reported in animals with a functional rumen. Confirmation of net synthesis in the rumen can be obtained from work such as that of McElroy and Goss (1940), in which secretion of riboflavin in milk was shown to be equivalent to approximately 10 times dietary intake. Miller et al. (1983b) reported that cattle on a concentrate-silage diet synthesize approximately 38 mg of riboflavin in the rumen. A dairy cow producing 21 kg milk per day loses about 36 mg of riboflavin in milk alone, much more than the amount consumed in the diet. Beef cattle and other lactating ruminants that have a much lower loss of riboflavin due to lowered milk production are even less likely to be deficient in the vitamin. Impaired riboflavin synthesis or destruction was reported in sheep with ruminal acidosis, reflected by plasma riboflavin decreasing from 9.5 to 0.09 mg/ml (Basoglu et al., 1993).

Riboflavin deficiencies have been demonstrated in young ruminants whose rumen flora is not yet established. Failure to provide riboflavin results in redness of the buccal mucosa, lesions in the corners of the mouth, loss of hair, and excessive tear and saliva production (Radostits and Bell, 1970). Less specific signs are anorexia, diarrhea, and reduced growth.

Swine

Typical swine diets based largely on grains are often borderline to deficient in riboflavin. Signs of riboflavin deficiency in the young growing pig include anorexia, slow growth (Fig. 7.3), rough hair coat, dermatitis, alopecia, abnormal stiffness, unsteady gait, scours, ulcerative colitis, inflammation of anal mucosa, vomiting, cataracts, light sensitivity, and eye lens opacities (Cunha, 1977; NRC, 1998). Reduced feed intake was demonstrated in gilts given a lactation diet containing 1.3 mg/kg of riboflavin. These gilts consumed 30% less feed than gilts receiving 2.3 to 5.3 mg/kg of riboflavin (Frank et al., 1988). Typical clinical signs often involve the eye, the skin, and the nervous system. In severe riboflavin deficiency of pigs, researchers have observed increased blood neutrophil granulocytes, decreased immune response, discolored liver and kidney tissue, fatty liver, collapsed follicles, degenerating ova, and degenerating myelin of the sciatic and brachial nerves (NRC, 1998).

In riboflavin-deficient swine, reproduction is impaired (Fig. 7.4). Cunha (1977) summarized the clinical signs for gilts fed a riboflavin-deficient diet during reproduction and lactation as follows: (1) erratic or, at times, complete loss of appetite; (2) poor gains; (3) parturition 4 to 16 days premature; (4) one case of death of fetus in advanced stage with resorption in evidence; (5) all pigs either dead at birth or within 48 hours thereafter; (6) enlarged front legs in some pigs due to gelatinous edema in the connective tissue and generalized edema in many others; and (7) two hairless litters. The longer the period on riboflavin-deficient diets, the more severe the deficiency signs became. Christensen (1980) likewise reported resorption of fetuses and premature farrowing for riboflavin-deficient sows.

Riboflavin deficiency has led to anestrus (Esch et al., 1981). Deficiency of riboflavin in postpubertal gilts has led to a cessation of ovarian cyclicity without overt signs of deficiency. Gilts fed a riboflavin-de-

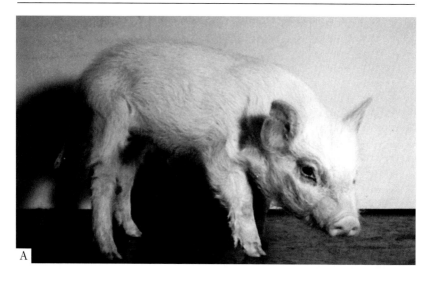

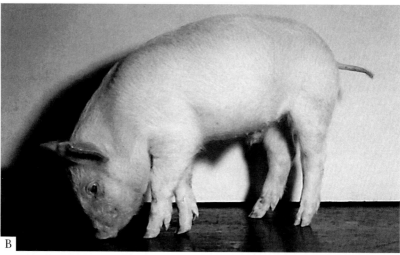

Fig. 7.3 (A) Riboflavin deficiency in a pig that received no dietary riboflavin. Note the rough hair coat, poor growth, and dermatitis. (B) Pig that received adequate riboflavin. (Courtesy of R.W. Luecke, Michigan Agricultural Experiment Station, East Lansing, Michigan, and *J. Nutr.* 52 [1954], 409.)

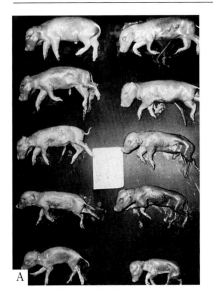
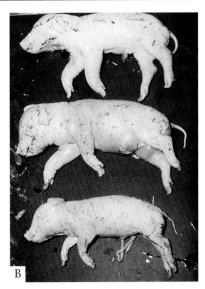
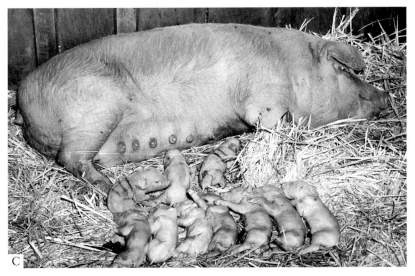

Fig. 7.4 Riboflavin deficiency. (A) All of the pigs in this litter were born dead; some were in the process of resorption. A few had edema and enlargement of front legs as a result of gelatinous edema. (B) Pigs from a litter in which gelatinous edema was more pronounced. (C) Seven of the ten pigs farrowed were born dead, and the other three were dead within 48 hours. The sow received a riboflavin-deficient diet for a shorter period than the sows farrowing the other two litters. (Courtesy of T.J. Cunha and Washington State University.)

ficient diet averaged progressively longer intervals between consecutive estrus periods until becoming anestrus 63 days after the beginning of the study. Riboflavin supplementation to gilts on a corn-soybean diet resulted in improved conception rate, embryonic survival, litter size, and live piglets at birth (Bazer and Zavy, 1988). Teratogenic effects in newborn pigs have been observed, including skeletal abnormalities, shortened bones, and fusions between ribs (Zintzen, 1975).

Poultry

Only a few of the feedstuffs fed to poultry contain enough riboflavin to meet the requirements of young growing poultry. The most critical requirements for riboflavin are those exhibited by the young chick and the breeder hen. The characteristic sign of riboflavin deficiency in the chick is "curled-toe" paralysis. However, it does not develop when there is absolute deficiency, or when the deficiency is very marked, because the chicks die before it appears. Chicks are first noted to be walking on their hocks with their toes curled inward. Deficient chicks do not move about except when forced to do so, and their toes are curled inward (Fig. 7.5) both when walking and when resting on their hocks (Scott et al., 1982). Legs become paralyzed, but the birds may otherwise appear normal.

Changes in the sciatic nerve produces curled-toe paralysis in growing chicks. There is a marked enlargement of sciatic and brachial nerve sheaths, with the sciatic nerve reaching a diameter four to six times normal size. Histological examinations of affected nerves showed definite degenerative changes in myelin sheaths which, when severe, may pinch the nerve, producing a permanent stimulus that causes curled-toe paralysis (Scott et al., 1982). Severe cases showed edema, nerve fiber separation, swelling in interstitial tissue, and leukocyte infiltration in the nerves. Ultrastructurally, the myelin sheaths of the affected nerves were twisted, separated, or fractured (Gao et al., 1993). When the curled-toe deformity is long standing, irreparable damage occurred in the sciatic nerve, and administration of riboflavin no longer cured the condition. Retarded growth, splay and hock-resting postures, and leg paralysis rather than curled-toe paralysis have been reported in some studies as the predominant signs of riboflavin deficiency in chicks (Ruiz and Harms, 1988; Chung and Baker, 1990).

Other signs of riboflavin deficiency are retardation of growth (Figs. 7.6 and 7.7), diarrhea after 8 to 10 days, and high mortality after about 3 weeks. When chicks are fed a diet deficient in riboflavin, their appetite is fairly good, but they grow very slowly and become weak and emaciated. There is no apparent impairment of feather growth; on the con-

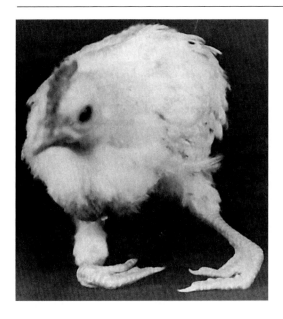

Fig. 7.5 Curled-toe paralysis in a riboflavin-deficient chick. (Courtesy of M.L. Scott, Cornell University.)

trary, main wing feathers often appear to be disproportionately long.

Signs of riboflavin deficiency in the poult and duckling differ from those in the chick. In the poult, dermatitis appears in about 8 days; the vent becomes encrusted, inflamed, and excoriated; growth is retarded or completely stopped by about the seventeenth day; and deaths begin to occur about the twenty-first day. In the duckling, clinical signs include diarrhea and cessation of growth.

In laying poultry, hatchability of incubated eggs is first reduced, and subsequently, egg production is decreased, roughly in proportion to degree of deficiency. Embryonic mortality typically has two peaks, and often a third peak. These are, respectively, on the fourth and twentieth days and on the fourteenth day of incubation. Embryos that fail to hatch from eggs of hens receiving low-riboflavin diets are dwarfed and exhibit pronounced micromelia; some embryos are edematous. The down fails to emerge properly, resulting in a typical abnormality termed "clubbed" down, which is most common in neck areas and around the vent. The nervous systems of these embryos show degenerative changes much like those described for riboflavin-deficient chicks. When dietary riboflavin provided to breeder hens was decreased from 9.7 to 1.7 mg/kg, embryo mortality increased to 83.3% and hatchability to 3.1%; decreasing riboflavin from 9.7 to 7.0, or 4.4 mg/kg had no effect on these variables (Flores-Garcia and Scholtyssek, 1992).

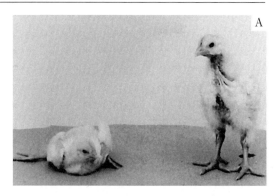

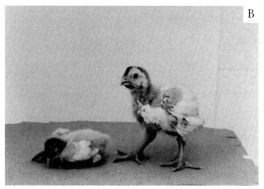

Fig. 7.6 Riboflavin deficiency in chicks. (A) The chick at left was fed a corn-soybean meal diet without supplemental riboflavin; it exhibited the predominant type of paralysis observed at the zero level of riboflavin supplementation. Both chicks are female. (B) Same as in (A), but the chicks are male. (Courtesy of N. Ruiz and R. Harms, University of Florida.)

Chicks fed a diet only marginally deficient in riboflavin often recover spontaneously. The condition is curable in the early stages, but in its acute stage, it is irreversible (NRC, 1994). There is increasing evidence that vigor and livability of the baby chick are directly tied to amount of riboflavin in the hen's diet (Anonymous, 1969).

Horses

It is generally felt that riboflavin synthesis in the cecum and colon provides some of the horse's requirement. When Carroll et al. (1949) fed a diet containing 0.4 mg of riboflavin per kilogram of dry matter, riboflavin concentrations (mg/kg of ingesta dry matter) in the various intestinal sections were as follows: duodenum, 3.8; ileum, 1.1; cecum, 7.0; anterior large colon, 9.2; and anterior small colon, 12.2. Horses fed low-riboflavin diets demonstrated anorexia, sporadic but severe weight loss, general weakness, and poor growth (Pearson et al., 1944).

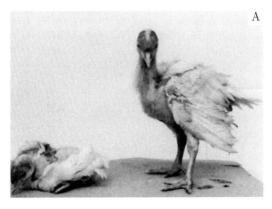

A

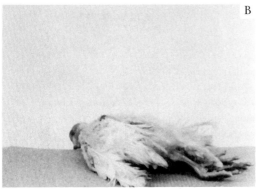

B

Fig. 7.7 Riboflavin deficiency in turkeys at 21 days of age. (A) The turkey at left was fed a corn-soybean basal diet without supplemental riboflavin. (B) Severe leg paralysis and poor feathering in a turkey poult fed the riboflavin-deficient diet. (Courtesy of N. Ruiz and R. Harms, University of Florida.)

Other Animal Species

DOGS AND CATS

Riboflavin-deficient dogs exhibit low growth rates, anemia, and corneal lesions (NRC, 1985a). The animals collapse, become comatose, and die. During the deficiency state, dermatitis develops on the chest, abdomen, inner thigh, axilla, and scrotum. In the final stages of the deficiency disease, muscular weakness develops and progresses within a few days to ataxia, followed by collapse, coma, and death (Hoffmann-La Roche, 2000).

Cats deficient in the vitamin develop cataracts, fatty livers, testicular hypoplasia, and alopecia with epidermal atrophy (NRC, 1986). Riboflavin deficiency manifests itself in cats after 4 to 8 weeks with anorexia, weight loss, and death. Anorexia resulting in weight loss and death is the principal deficiency sign in cats (Gershoff et al., 1959).

Chronic riboflavin deficiency in cats results in hair loss extending to the chest and feet, cataracts, and alopecia with epidermal atrophy.

FISH

Signs of riboflavin deficiency in fish are species specific (NRC, 1993). The only common signs are anorexia and poor growth. The first sign of riboflavin deficiency observed in salmonids (Halver, 1957; Steffens, 1970) appeared in the eyes and included photophobia, cataracts, corneal vascularization, and hemorrhages. Lack of coordinated swimming and dark skin color were also reported for riboflavin-deficient chinook salmon (Halver, 1957) and rainbow trout (Steffens, 1970). Additional signs of riboflavin deficiency in trout include slow growth, anorexia, inefficient conversion of feed, and opaque lens and cornea (NRC, 1993).

Channel catfish fed riboflavin-deficient diets developed deficiency signs including anorexia, poor growth, short-body dwarfism, and cataracts. Common carp exhibited nervousness, photophobia, and hemorrhages, with the initial deficiency signs of anorexia and nervousness. Signs of deficiency in Japanese eels were poor growth, anorexia, hemorrhage in fins and abdomen, photophobia, and lethargy (NRC, 1993).

FOXES AND MINK

Riboflavin deficiency in foxes results in decreased growth rate, signs of muscular weakness, chronic spasms, coma, opacity of the cornea, and decreased pigment production in the fur (Fig. 7.8). Foxes on a riboflavin-deficient diet show signs similar to those seen in riboflavin-deficient dogs. Mink on a riboflavin-deficient diet exhibit anorexia, weight loss, extreme weakness, and poor breeding results (NRC, 1982a).

LABORATORY ANIMALS

Classic signs of riboflavin deficiency in rats are dermatitis, alopecia, weakness, and decreased growth. Corneal vascularization and ulceration, cataract formation, anemia, myelin degeneration of sciatic nerves and spinal cord, fatty liver, congenital abnormalities, and metabolic abnormalities of hepatocytes may occur (Fig. 7.9) (NRC, 1995). Riboflavin deficiency in rats brings about an acceleration of the erythrocyte life cycle (Gaetani and D'Aquino, 1987). In mice, signs of riboflavin deficiency include poor performance, myelin degeneration in the spinal cord, corneal vacularization with ulceration, and lowered resistance to *Salmonella* infection (NRC, 1995). Riboflavin-deficient guinea pigs exhibit poor growth; rough hair coat; pale feet, nose, and ears; corneal vas-

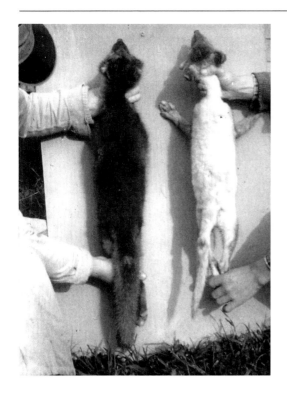

Fig. 7.8 Riboflavin defi-
ciency in foxes. After 7
weeks on a riboflavin-
deficient diet, the 12-
week-old blue fox at
right showed depigmen-
tation, shedding of fur,
and dermatitis. The lit-
termate at left was fed
a diet supplemented
with riboflavin. (Cour-
tesy of H. Rimeslatten,
Agriculture College of
Norway, Vollebekk.)

cularization; skin atrophy; myelin degeneration of the spinal cord; and
early death (NRC, 1995).

NONHUMAN PRIMATES

In the rhesus monkey, signs of riboflavin deficiency include "freckled"
dermatitis; incoordination; faulty grasping reflex; impaired vision; scanty
hair coat; and hypochromic, normocytic anemia. Deficiency in cebus
monkeys results in weight loss, dermatitis, alopecia, ataxia, and sudden
death, but no anemia (NRC, 1978). If not supplemented with riboflavin,
the monkeys may suddenly collapse and die. Deficiency in the baboon is
characterized by apathy, dermatitis, anemia, gingivitis, diarrhea, and adrenal cortical hemorrhage; skin lesions develop after 8 to 12 weeks.

RABBITS

Olcese et al. (1948) found that rabbits grew normally when fed pantothenic acid- and riboflavin-deficient diets; furthermore, these rabbits
excreted amounts of these vitamins greatly in excess of dietary intakes.

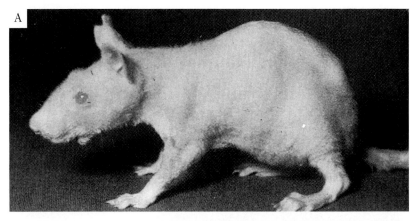

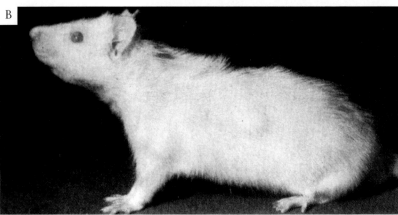

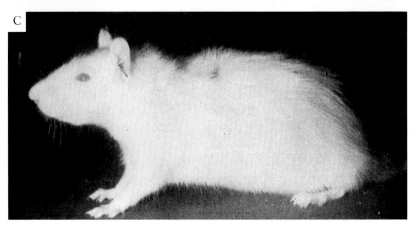

Fig. 7.9 Riboflavin deficiency in the rat, exhibited by (A) generalized dermatitis, growth failure, and marked keratitis of the cornea. (B) After 1 month of treatment with riboflavin, growth resumed, and ocular and skin lesions practically disappeared. (C) After 2 months of treatment, the rat showed no signs of deficiency. (Courtesy of Alan T. Forrester, *Scope Manual on Nutrition*, The Upjohn Company, Kalamazoo, Michigan.)

HUMANS

Riboflavin deficiency signs have been observed in humans consuming nutritionally poor diets and under experimental conditions. As in animals, riboflavin deficiency is believed to retard growth in humans, although no growth experiments have been undertaken. Clinically, riboflavin deficiency in humans is usually observed in conjunction with deficiencies of other B vitamins. The reason for the multiplicity of vitamin deficits is that dietary deficiencies tend to be multiple because the food sources are similar, and various metabolic functions involve a number of vitamin interrelationships.

Clinical features of riboflavin deficiency include seborrheic dermatitis around the nose and mouth; soreness and burning of the lips, mouth, and tongue; photophobia; burning and itching of the eyes; superficial vascularization of the cornea; cheilosis; angular stomatitis; glossitis; anemia; and neuropathy (Fig. 7.10) (Rivlin, 1984).

Clinical signs of glossitis begin with flattening, followed by disappearance of the tongue filiform papilla. The fungiform papillae become enlarged, the tongue color changes to a beefy red, the tongue is sore, and loss of taste sensation develops (Cooperman and Lopez, 1991). Dermatitis due to riboflavin deficiency begins most often in the nasolabial fold and is scaly and oily. Similar lesions may also appear around the eyes and on the ears. Dermatitis of the scrotum or vulva is frequently present (Marks, 1975). Corneal vascularization due to riboflavin deficiency always occurs in the entire circumference of the cornea and is nearly always bilateral. Corneal vascularization may be a result of the oxygen requirement of the corneal epithelium. Cells of the cornea have no hemoglobin supply but maintain integrity by intracellular oxidative processes that depend on riboflavin activity. Tears are a rich source of riboflavin. Foy and Mbaya (1977) stated that in vitamin A deficiency the tear ducts are blocked with keratin, and vascularization of the cornea follows from lack of tears. Thus, such patients should be given both vitamin A and riboflavin.

One of the first systemic experimental studies in humans resulted in cheilosis in 10 of 18 women consuming a low-riboflavin diet during a 94- to 130-day period (Sebrell and Butler, 1938). Cheilosis began with pallor of the lips in the angles of the mouth, followed by maceration. Within a few days, superficial transverse fissures appeared in the angles of the mouth.

In more recent studies, volunteers were fed a purified diet deficient only in riboflavin, along with the riboflavin antagonist galactoflavin

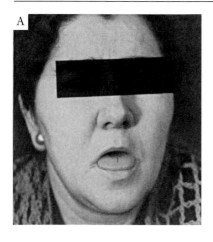
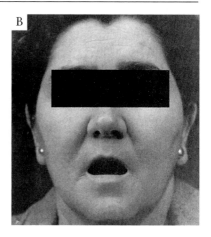

Fig. 7.10 (A) Riboflavin deficiency manifested as fissures at angle of mouth. (B) Complete eradication after treatment with riboflavin therapy. (Courtesy of Alan T. Forrester, *Scope Manual on Nutrition*, The Upjohn Company, Kalamazoo, Michigan.)

(Cooperman and Lopez, 1991). Additional clinical signs of riboflavin included anemia with reticulocytopenia after 3 to 9 weeks on the diet. This anemia was normocytic and normochromic and included leukopenia and thrombocytopenia, with morphological bone marrow changes. Peripheral neuropathy of the hands and feet occurred, characterized by hyperesthesia, coldness, and pain. There was also decreased perception to touch, pain, temperature, vibration, and position.

In developing countries, individuals consuming diets low in green leafy vegetables and animal products (e.g., especially milk products) are at high risk for riboflavin deficiency. Biochemical reflections of suboptimal intake and even minor signs of deficiency are common in many parts of the world. Reports from the 1980s include infants in New Guinea (Oppenheimer et al., 1983) and children and pregnant women in Gambia (Bates et al., 1983, 1984) and Nigeria (Ajayi, 1984, 1985). Incidences of riboflavin deficiency or low status in the 1990s were reported in Bangladesh (Hassan and Ahmad, 1992), China (Brun et al., 1990; Shaw, 1993), Egypt (Calloway et al., 1993), Lithuania (Piktelite et al., 1992), the Philippines (Kuizon et al., 1992), Thailand (Vudhivai et al., 1990), and Turkey (Wetherilt et al., 1992). In China (Brun et al., 1990), more than two-thirds of the population surveyed were in the medium- or high-risk category for riboflavin deficiency, while 89.9% of children surveyed in Turkey (Wetherilt et al., 1992) were at risk. Deficiency is encountered almost invariably in combination with deficits of other water-soluble vitamins. In fact, classic deficiency symptoms such as glossitis and dermatitis may have resulted from other complicating deficiencies (McCormick, 1990).

Widespread riboflavin deficiency may result in vitamin B_6 deficiencies. Severe riboflavin deficiency can affect the conversion of vitamin B_6 to its coenzyme (Anonymous, 1981b). The similar skin lesions seen in riboflavin and vitamin B_6 deficiencies reflect impaired maturation of collagen, which has been attributed to the need for pyridoxal 5′-phosphate (enzyme form of vitamin B_6), the formation of which from the 5′-phosphates of pyridoxine and pyridoxamine requires riboflavin operating as FMN with this oxidase (Prasad et al., 1983). Dual deficiencies of riboflavin and vitamin B_6 have been reported in Nigeria, Thailand, and Turkey; as an example, 89.9% of Turkish children were deficient in riboflavin and 83.4% deficient in vitamin B_6 (Wetherilt et al., 1992).

Overt clinical signs of riboflavin deficiency are rarely seen among inhabitants of developed countries. However, the so-called subclinical stage of the deficiency, characterized by a change in biochemical indices, is common. For Italy, Mobarhan et al. (1982) reported marginal deficiency in 18% of people over 65 years of age and 12% of children. The deficiency resulted in a shortened life span of erythrocytes. Riboflavin deficiency with biochemical changes, but not necessarily with clinical signs, was observed in women taking oral contraceptive agents, diabetics, children and adolescents from low socioeconomic backgrounds, children with chronic heart disease, and the aged (Cooperman and Lopez, 1991). In addition to major clinical signs of deficiency, retarded intellectual development has been observed in children, and even minor degrees of riboflavin deficiency in adults produced marked deterioration of personality (Sterner and Price, 1973).

Assessment of Status

Several methods have been used to assess nutritional status of riboflavin. These include clinical signs, blood and urine levels of the vitamin, and measurement of enzymatic coenzyme activity. The most certain way of identifying a riboflavin deficiency seems to be to cause a remission of the clinical signs in question by feeding riboflavin alone. Measuring riboflavin excretion in the urine is of some value, with the limitation that daily output of riboflavin is usually an estimate of dietary intake. Riboflavin red blood cell content appears to be a better measure on the basis of human studies. For the laying hen, riboflavin concentration in egg albumen is an excellent status indicator of the vitamin

(Squires and Naber, 1993). The estimated minimum critical egg albumen riboflavin concentrations needed to support maximum reproductive function are between 1.9 and 2.9 ppm.

The most rapid and dramatic biochemical method of determining riboflavin status is loss of erythrocyte glutathione reductase (EGR) activity, an FAD-containing enzyme. The ratio of EGR activity in erythrocytes with and without added FAD is considered the activity coefficient. Experimental studies—including those with livestock, laboratory animals, humans, and even fish—have shown that EGR activity is a very sensitive and specific indicator of riboflavin deficiency (Frank et al., 1988; Boisvert et al., 1993; Pettigrew et al., 1996).

SUPPLEMENTATION

Riboflavin is one of the vitamins most likely to be deficient for both nonruminant animals and humans. Before their rumens are developed, young ruminants (up to 2 months of age), if early weaned or dependent on milk replacer, have a dietary need for riboflavin. Cereal grains, though poor sources of riboflavin, are important for people in many developing countries where cereals constitute the major dietary component. Often, individuals in developing countries do not have the economic resources to consume the major dietary sources of riboflavin of meat, milk, and dairy products.

Supplementation and education programs for humans need to be implemented in developing countries to ensure adequate riboflavin intake. Growing children and pregnant-lactating mothers are groups at risk of deficiency. In India, children who received 5 mg of riboflavin daily for 1 year had elevated EGR levels, improved hand steadiness, and reduced incidence of glossitis (Prasad et al., 1990). Additional risk groups for whom supplemental riboflavin is required are people who exercise, alcoholics, diabetics, drug users, patients with chronic heart disease, patients on diuretics or undergoing hemodialysis, preterm infants, and people with other disease conditions (see Requirements).

Swine and poultry diets based on grains and plant protein sources are likewise often borderline deficient in riboflavin. Only a few feedstuffs fed to poultry and swine contain enough riboflavin to meet the requirements of growth and reproduction. The trend toward confinement feeding and use of less pasture and/or alfalfa in swine diets has increased need for riboflavin supplementation; both are excellent sources of the vitamin (Cunha, 1977).

Swine and poultry in confinement become more dependent on adequate vitamin (including riboflavin) and trace mineral supplementation, because least-cost feed formulation (e.g., using principally corn and soybean meal) limits the number of riboflavin-rich feed ingredients (milk fermentation and fish by-products and dehydrated alfalfa). The greater the variety of feed ingredients, the lower the chance of vitamin and trace element deficiencies for animals and humans alike.

Riboflavin is commercially available as a crystalline compound produced by chemical synthesis or fermentation. Most of the commercially available riboflavin is made by bacterial synthesis, a cheap and convenient way to produce crystalline riboflavin. It is available to the feed, food, and pharmaceutical industries as a high-potency U.S. Pharmacopeia (USP) or feed-grade powder, spray-dried powders, and dry dilutions. The water-soluble, riboflavin 5-phosphate salt is available for liquid oral and parenteral pharmaceuticals. High-potency USP or feed-grade powders are electrostatic, hygroscopic, and dusty; thus they do not flow freely, and they show poor distribution in feeds. In contrast, dilution of riboflavin as a spray-dried powder or dry dilution product, or including it in a premix, reduces its electrostacity and hygroscopicity for better flowability and distribution in feeds (Adams, 1978). Diluted riboflavin is added to feeds to increase its mixing properties.

Riboflavin is remarkably stable during heat processing (see Chemical Structure, Properties, and Antagonists; Natural Resources). However, considerable loss may occur if foods are exposed to light during cooking, and some losses occur in feed administered to animals out of doors. Only the portion of the feed exposed to light would be destroyed; therefore, this may be of little significance as only the top of concentrate mixtures in automatic feeders would be affected. In dry form, riboflavin is extremely resistant to oxidation even when heated in air for long periods. While it has been shown that field-cured alfalfa hay exposed to moisture can lose a significant amount of its riboflavin content in a relatively short time, under common circumstances riboflavin has good stability when added to mixed feeds (Anonymous, 1969).

Riboflavin is stable in multivitamin premixes (Frye, 1978). Up to 26% of riboflavin in pet food is lost during extrusion (Anonymous, 1981a). Storage losses of riboflavin in pelleted feeds are slight, but after pellets are in water for 20 minutes for fish feeding, about 40% of riboflavin may be lost (Goldblatt et al., 1979). One report demonstrated a 98% retention of riboflavin after 6 months in a vitamin premix; however, retention was only 59% when the premix contained choline and trace minerals (Coelho, 1991).

TOXICITY

A large body of evidence has accumulated indicating that treatment with riboflavin in excess of nutritional requirements has very little toxicity for experimental animals or for humans (Rivlin, 1978). Most data from rats suggest that dietary levels between 10 and 20 times the requirement (possibly 100 times) can be tolerated safely (NRC, 1987). When massive amounts of riboflavin are administered orally, only a small fraction of the dose is absorbed; the remainder is excreted in the feces. Toxicity is lacking probably because the transport system necessary for the absorption of riboflavin across the gastrointestinal mucosa becomes saturated, limiting riboflavin absorption (Christensen, 1973). Also, capacity of the tissues to store riboflavin and its coenzyme derivatives appears to be limited when excessive amounts are administered. No case of riboflavin toxicity in humans has been reported, and oral doses per kilogram of body weight of 340 mg for mice, 10 g for rats, and 2 g for dogs produced no toxic effects (Cooperman and Lopez, 1991).

Riboflavin is somewhat more toxic when administered parenterally. Only when doses of 600 mg/kg body weight were administered intraperitoneally to rats were ill effects evident (Unna and Greslin, 1942). Then anuria developed, and at autopsy, crystals were apparent in the collecting tubules and renal pelvis. Rainbow trout, like other animals, were insensitive to excess dietary riboflavin, as levels of 600 mg/kg of diet produced no undesirable effect on growth (Hughes, 1984).

■ REFERENCES

Adams, C. R. (1978). Proc. Roche Vitamin Nutrition Update Meeting, Arkansas Nutrition Conference p. 54. RCD 5483/1078. Hoffmann-La Roche, Nutley, New Jersey.
Ajayi, O. A. (1984). *Hum. Nutr. Clin. Nutr. 38,* 149.
Ajayi, O. A. (1985). *Hum. Nutr. Clin. Nutr. 39,* 383.
Ajayi, O. A., Maja, S. O., and Onabolu, Y. O. (1989). *Nutr. Res. 9,* 1339.
Anonymous (1969). Riboflavin No. 1170. Hoffmann-La Roche, Basel, Switzerland.
Anonymous (1981a). Rationale for Roche Recommended Vitamin Fortification RCD 5963/1280. Hoffmann-La Roche, Nutley, New Jersey.
Anonymous (1981b). *Nutr. Rev. 39,* 331.
Basoglu, A., Turgut, K., Eksen, M., Tras, B., Maden, M., Ok, M., Bas, A. L., and Kececi, T. (1993). *Vet. Fakultesi. Dergisi-Selcuk. Universitesi. 9,* 31.
Bates, C. J., Flewitt, A., Prentice, A. M., Lamb, W. H., and Whitehead, R. G.

(1983). *Hum. Nutr. Clin. Nutr. 37,* 427.

Bates, C. J., Prentice, A. M., and Watkinson, M. (1984). *Hum. Nutr. Clin. Nutr. 38,* 363.

Bazer, F. W., and Zavy, M. T. (1988). *J. Anim. Sci. 66*(Suppl. 1), 324(Abstr.).

Belko, A. Z., Meredith, M. P., and Kalkwarf, H. J. (1985). *Am. J. Clin. Nutr. 41,* 270.

Boisvert, W. A., Mendoza, I., Castaneda, C., Portocarrero, L. de, Solomons, N. W., Gershoff, S. N., and Russell, R. M. (1993) *J. Nutr. 123,* 915.

Brun, T. A., Chen, J., Campbell, T. C., Boreham, J., Feng, Z., Parpia, B., Shen, T. F., and Li, M. (1990). *Eur. J. Clin. Nutr. 44,* 195.

Buziassy, C., and Tribe, D. E. (1960). *Aust. J. Agric. Res. 11,* 989.

Calloway, D. H., Murphy, S. P., Beaton, G. H., and Lein, D. (1993). *Am. J. Clin. Nutr. 58,* 376.

Carroll, F. D., Goss, H., and Howell, C. E. (1949). *J. Anim. Sci. 8,* 290.

Casirola, D., Kasai, S., Gastaldi, G., Ferrari, G., and Matsui, K. (1994). *J. Nutr. Sci. Vitaminol. 40,* 289.

Christensen, H. N. (1993). *Nutr. Rev. 51,* 149.

Christensen, K. (1980). *Livestock Prod. Sci. 7,* 569.

Christensen, S. (1973). *Acta Pharmacol. Toxicol. 32,* 1.

Chung, T. K., and Baker, D. H. (1990). *Poult. Sci. 69,* 1357.

Clagett, C. O. (1971). *Fed. Proc. Am. Soc. Expt. Biol. 30,* 127.

Coelho, M. B. (1991). Vitamin Stability in Premixes and Feeds: A Practical Approach, p. 56. BASF Technical Symposium, Bloomington, Minnesota.

Cole, H. S., Lopez, R., and Cooperman, J. M. (1976). *Acta Diabet. Latina 13,* 25.

Combs Jr., G. F. (1992). The Vitamins. Academic Press, San Diego, California.

Cooperman, J. M., and Lopez, R. (1991). *In* Handbook of Vitamins (L.J. Machlin, ed.) 2nd Ed., p. 299. Marcel Dekker, Inc., New York.

Cunha, T. J. (1977). Swine Feeding and Nutrition. Academic Press, New York.

Das, B. S., Thurnham, D. I., Patnaik, J. K., Das, D. B., Satpathy, R., and Bose, T. K. (1990). *Am. J. Clin. Nutr. 51,* 859.

Deyhim, F., Belay, T., and Teeter, R. G. (1992). *Nutr. Res. 12,* 1123.

Durgakumari, B., and Adiga, P. R. (1986). *Mol. Cell. Endocrinol. 44,* 285.

Esch, M. W., Easter, R. A., and Bahr, J. M. (1981). *Biol. Reprod. 25,* 659.

Fairweather-Tait, S. J., Powers, H. J., Minski, M. J., Whitehead, J., and Downes, R. (1992). *Ann. Nutr. Metab. 36,* 34.

Fernando, S. M., and Murphy, P. A. (1990). *J. Agr. Food Chem. 38,* 163.

Flores-Garcia, W., and Scholtyssek, S. (1992). Proc. 19th World's Poultry Congress, Vol. 1, p. 622. Beekbergen, Netherlands.

Foy, H., and Mbaya, V. (1977). *Prog. Food Nutr. Sci. 2,* 357.

Frank, G. R., Bahr, J. M., and Easter, R. A. (1984). *J. Anim. Sci. 59,* 1567.

Frank, G. R., Bahr, J. M., and Easter, R. A. (1985). *J. Anim. Sci. 61*(Suppl. 1), 315.

Frank, G. R., Bahr, J. M., and Easter, R. A. (1988). *J. Anim. Sci. 66,* 47.

Frye, T. M. (1978). Proc. Roche Vitamin Nutrition Update Meeting, Arkansas Nutrition Conference, p. 70. RCD 5483/1078. Hoffmann-La Roche, Nutley, New Jersey.

Gaetani, S., and D'Aquino, M. (1987). *Nutr. Rept. Intern. 35,* 93.

Gao, Q. Y., Zhu, X. P., Cao, X. D., and Ma, X. X. (1993). *Acta Vet. Zootech. Sinica 24,* 469.

Gershoff, S.N., Andrus, S.B., and Hegsted, D.M. (1959). *J. Nutr. 68,* 75.

Goldblatt, M. J., Conklin, D. E., and Brown, W. D. (1979). *Proc. World Symp. Finfish Nutr. Fishfeed Technol. 2,* 117.

Grewal, P. K., and Sangha, J. K. (1990). *J. Sci. Food and Agr. 52,* 387.

Haenel, H., Ruttloff, H., and Ackermann, H. (1959). *Biochem. Ztschr. 331,* 209.

Halver, J. E. (1957). *J. Nutr. 62,* 225.

Hassan, N., and Ahmad, K. U. (1992). *Ecol. Food Nutr. 28,* 131.

Hegazy, E., and Schwenk, M. (1983). *J. Nutr. 113,* 1702.

Hoffmann-La Roche. (2000). *In* Vitamins for Dogs and Cats. Nutley, New Jersey.

Hughes, S. G. (1984). *J. Nutr. 114,* 1660.

Hunt, S. M. (1975). *In* Riboflavin (R.S. Rivlin, ed.), p. 199, Plenum Press, New York.

Kodentsova, V. M., Yakushina, L. M., Vrzhesinskaya, O. A., Beketova, N. A., and Spirichev, V. B. (1993). *Voprosy-Pitaniya 5,* 32.

Kuizon, M. D., Natera, M. G., Alberto, S. P., Perlas, L. A., Desnacide, J. A., Avena, E. M., Tajaon, R. T., and Macapinlac, M. P. (1992). *Eur. J. Clin. Nutr. 46,* 257.

Kuroki, F., Iida, M., Tominaga, M., Matsumoto, T., Hirakawa, K., Sugiyama, S., and Fujishima, M. (1993). *Di. Dis. Sci. 38,* 1614.

Lee, C.M., and White, H.B. (1996). *J. Nutr. 126,* 523.

Levin, G., Cogan, U., Levy, Y., and Mokady, S. (1990). *J. Nutr. 120,* 857.

Li, L. P., Chen, W. L., and Cui, J. T. (1993). *Chinese J. Chrom. 11,* 49.

Loosli, J. K. (1991). *In* Handbook of Animal Science, (P.A. Putnam, ed.), p. 25. Academic Press, San Diego, California.

Marks, J. (1975). A Guide to the Vitamins. Their Role in Health and Disease. Medical and Technical Publishing Co., Ltd., p. 73. Lancaster, England.

McCollum, E. V. (1957). *In* A History of Nutrition p. 291. The Riverside Press, Cambridge, Massachusetts.

McCormick, D. B. (1990). *In* Nutrition Reviews, Present Knowledge in Nutrition (M.L. Brown, ed.), 6th Ed., p. 146. International Life Sci. Inst., Washington, D.C.

McElroy, L. W., and Goss, H. (1940). *J. Nutr. 20,* 527.

Middleton, H. M. (1990). *J. Nutr. 120,* 588.

Miller, B. L., Goodrich, R. D., and Meiske, J. C. (1983a). *J. Anim. Sci. 57*(Suppl. 1), 454(Abstr.).

Miller, B. L., Plegge, S. D., Goodrich, R. D., and Meiske, J. C. (1983b). Minnesota Beef Report B-299, p. 1. University of Minnesota, St. Paul.

Mobarhan, S., Maiani, G., Zanacchi, E., Ferrini, A. M., Scaccini, C., Sette, S., and Ferro-Luzz, A. (1982). *Clin. Nutr. 360,* 71.

NRC. Nutrient Requirements of Domestic Animals. National Academy of Sciences-National Research Council, Washington, D.C.
 (1978). Nutrient Requirements of Nonhuman Primates.
 (1981). Nutrient Requirements of Goats.
 (1982a). Nutrient Requirements of Mink and Foxes.

344

(1985a). Nutrient Requirements of Dogs, 2nd Ed.
(1985b). Nutrient Requirements of Sheep, 5th Ed.
(1986). Nutrient Requirements of Cats, 3rd Ed.
(1989a). Nutrient Requirements of Dairy Cattle, 6th Ed.
(1989b). Nutrient Requirements of Horses, 5th Ed.
(1993). Nutrient Requirements of Fish.
(1994). Nutrient Requirements of Poultry, 9th Ed.
(1995). Nutrient Requirements of Laboratory Animals, 4th Ed.
(1996). Nutrient Requirements of Beef Cattle, 7th Ed.
(1998). Nutrient Requirements of Swine, 10th Ed.
NRC. (1982b). United States-Canadian Tables of Feed Composition, 3rd Ed. National Academy of Sciences-National Research Council, Washington, D.C.
NRC. (1987). Vitamin Tolerance of Animals. National Academy of Sciences-National Research Council, Washington, D.C.
Olcese, O., Pearson, P. B., and Schweigert, B. S. (1948). *J. Nutr. 35*, 577.
Onwudike, O. C., and Adegbola, A. A. (1984). *Trop. Agr. (Trinidad) 61*, 205.
Oppenheimer, S. J., Bull, R., and Thurnham, D. J. (1983). *P N G Med. J. 26*, 17.
Pearson, P. B., Sheybani, M. K., and Schmidt, H. (1944). *J. Anim. Sci. 3*, 166.
Pettigrew, J. E., El-Kandelgy, S. M., Johnston, L. J., and Shurson, G. C. (1996). *J. Anim. Sci. 74*, 2226.
Piktelite, O. S., Aleinik, S. I., Yakushina, L. M., and Blazheevich, N. V. (1992). *Voprosy-Pitaniya 4*, 32.
Pinto, J., Huang, Y. P., and Rivlin, R. S. (1981). *J. Clin. Invest. 67*, 1500.
Powers, H. J., Weaver, L. T., Austin, S., Wright, A. J. A., and Fairweather-Tait, S. J. (1991). *Br. J. Nutr. 65*, 487.
Powers, H. J., Weaver, L. T., Austin, S., and Beresford, J. K. (1993). *Br. J. Nutr. 69*, 553.
Prasad, P., Lakshmi, A. V., and Bamji, M. S. (1983). *Biochem. Med. 30*, 333.
Prasad, P., Bamji, M. S., Lakshmi, A. V., and Satyanarayana, K. (1990). *Nutr. Res. 10*, 275.
Radostits, O. M., and Bell, J. M. (1970). *Can. J. Anim. Sci. 50*, 405.
Raghvendar, S., Deodhar, A. D., and Singh, R. (1993). *Indian J. Dairy Sci. 46*, 525.
RDA. (1989). Recommended Dietary Allowances, 10th Ed., National Academy of Sciences-National Research Council, Washington, D.C.
Rivlin, R. S. (1978). *In* Handbook Series in Nutrition and Food, Section E: Nutritional Disorders (M. Rechcigl Jr., ed.), Vol. 1, p. 25. CRC Press, Boca Raton, Florida.
Rivlin, R. S. (1984). *In* Nutrition Reviews, Present Knowledge in Nutrition (R.E. Olson, ed.), p. 285. The Nutrition Foundation, Washington, D.C.
Roe, D. A., Bogusz, S., Sheu, J., and McCormick, D. B. (1982). *Am. J. Clin. Nutr. 35*, 495.
Rose, R. C., McCormick, D. B., Li, T. K., Lumeng, L., Haddad, J. G., and Spector, R. (1986). *Fed. Proc. Am. Soc. Expt. Biol. 45*, 30.
Ruiz, N., and Harms, R. H. (1988). *Poult. Sci. 67*, 794.
Russell, L. F., and Vanderslice, J. T. (1991). *Food Chem. 43(2)*, 151.
Said, H. M., Hollander, D., and Mohammadkhani, R. (1993a). *Biochim. Bio-*

phys. Acta 1148, 263.

Said, H. M., Mohammadkhani, R., and McCloud, E. (1993b). *Proc. Soc. Exp. Biol. Med. 202,* 428.

Scott, N. L., Nesheim, M. C., and Young, R. J. (1982). Nutrition of the Chicken. Scott, Ithaca, New York.

Sebrell, W. H., and Butler, R. E. (1938). *Public Health Rep. 53,* 2282.

Seymour, E. W., Speer, V. C., and Hays, V. W. (1968). *J. Anim. Sci. 27,* 389.

Sharman, I. (1977). *Endeavour 1,* 97.

Shaw, N. S. (1993). *Nutr. Res. 13,* 147.

Sigman-Grant, M., Bush, G., and Anantheswaran, R. (1992). *Pediatrics 90,* 412.

Singh, R., and Deodhar, A. D. (1992). *Ann. Nutr. Metab. 36,* 279.

Squires, M. W., and Naber, E. C. (1993). *Poult. Sci. 72,* 483.

Steffens, W. (1970). *Int. Rev. Ges. Hydrobiol. 59,* 255.

Sterner, R. T., and Price, W. R. (1973). *Am. J. Clin. Nutr. 26,* 150.

Trebler-Winters, L. R., Yoon, J. S., Kalkwarf, H. J., Davies, J. C., Berkowitz, M. G., Haas, J., and Roe, D. A. (1992). *Am. J. Clin. Nutr. 56,* 526.

Turkki, P. R., and Holtzapple, P. G. (1982). *J. Nutr. 112,* 1940.

Unna, K., and Greslin, J. G. (1942). *J. Pharmacol. Exp. Ther. 76,* 75.

Vudhivai, N., Pongpaew, P., Prayurahong, B., Kwanbunjan, K., Migasena, P., Chitwattanakorn, M., Hempfling, A., and Schelp, F. P. (1990). *Int. J. Vitam. Res. 60,* 75.

Wagner-Jauregg, T. (1972). *In* The Vitamins (W.H. Sebrell and R. S. Harris, eds.), p. 3. Academic Press, New York.

Wetherilt, H., Ackurt, F., Brubacher, G., Okan, B., Aktas, S., and Turdu, S. (1992). *Int. J. Vitam. Nutr. Res. 62,* 21.

White, H.B. (1996). *J. Nutr. 126,* 1303S.

Zempleni, J., Link, G., and Kubler, W. (1992). *Int. J. Vitam. Nutr. Res. 62,* 165.

Zintzen, H. (1975). A Guide to the Nutritional Management of Breeding Sows and Pigs. No. 1465. Hoffmann-La Roche, Basel, Switzerland.

NIACIN

INTRODUCTION

After isolation of thiamin and riboflavin from the vitamin B complex, niacin was the third B vitamin to be established and is sometimes referred to as vitamin B_3. Niacin exerts its major physiological effects through its role in the enzyme system for cell respiration. Niacin deficiency results in the disease pellagra in humans and blacktongue in dogs, and in 1937, scientists discovered that this vitamin would cure these conditions. Soon after, niacin was found to be a dietary essential for pigs, poultry, and other nonruminant animals.

Although the need for niacin for simple-stomached animals has been established, exact requirements are difficult to determine since the vitamin can be synthesized from the amino acid tryptophan. In many species, a single deficiency of only niacin does not exist; rather the deficiency condition is an inadequate intake of both niacin and tryptophan. The vitamin can also be considered a drug when administered at pharmacological levels.

HISTORY

Niacin has been known to organic chemists since 1867, long before its importance as an essential nutrient was recognized. The history of niacin and the significance of its deficiency have been reported (Harris, 1919; McCollum, 1957; Darby et al., 1975; Hankes, 1984; Anonymous, 1987; Loosli, 1991). As early as 1911 to 1913, Funk had isolated it from yeast and rice polishings in the course of an attempt to identify the water-soluble anti-beriberi vitamin. But interest in niacin was lost when it was found ineffective in curing pigeons of beriberi. Although Funk found that niacin did not cure beriberi, cures were more rapid when it was administered in conjunction with the concentrates containing the anti-beriberi vitamin (thiamin). Warburg and coworkers first demonstrated a biochemical function for nicotinic acid when they isolated it from an enzyme in 1935 and showed that it functioned as part of a hydrogen transport system.

Niacin deficiency in humans has been equated with pellagra, the disease considered a condition of the corn (maize)-eating population. Corn was brought to Spain by Columbus from America. Pellagra was not recognized until 1735 when Gaspar Casal, physician to Philip V of Spain, observed it in northern Spain. The local people had called it *mal de la rosa*, and Casal associated the disease with poverty and spoiled corn. The popularity of corn, and thus pellagra, spread eastward from Spain to southern France, Italy, Romania, Russia, and Egypt. Although the disease was first reported in Spain, most of the important early studies of the disease came from Italy. Pellagra was so prevalent in northern Italy that the first pellagra hospital was established at Legano in 1784.

Babcock, of Columbia, South Carolina, who established the identity of U.S. pellagra as the same disease in Italy, studied the case records of the South Carolina State Hospital and concluded that the disease occurred there as early as 1828. Most cases occurred in low-income groups, whose diet was limited to cheap foodstuffs. Diets characteristically associated with the disease were referred to as the three Ms—meal (corn), meat (back fat), and molasses—plus poverty.

In Spartanburg, South Carolina, a Public Health Service Hospital for the care and study of pellagra was in operation from 1917 to 1919. However, the hospital was closed in 1919 because there were no cases of pellagra, emphasizing the relationship between poverty and pellagra. Pellagra virtually disappeared from the southern United States as a result of the great increase in the price of cotton during and at the end of World War I. Prosperity made a wider choice of food available to all. Pellagra rapidly reappeared when the price of cotton fell and poverty again forced greater reliance on corn-based diets.

The word pellagra means rough skin, which would be dermatitis. Other descriptive names for the condition were *mal del sol* (illness of the sun) and "corn bread fever." After the turn of the century in the United States, particularly the South, it was common for 20,000 deaths to occur annually from pellagra. It was estimated that for every death due to pellagra, there were at least 35 cases of the disease. Even as late as 1941, which was 5 years after the cause of pellagra was known, 2,000 deaths due to the disease were reported. Clinical signs and mortality from pellagra could be referred to as the four Ds: dermatitis (of areas exposed to the sun), diarrhea, dementia (mental problems), and death. Several mental institutions in the United States, Europe, and Egypt were primarily devoted to care of pellagrins (Darby et al., 1975).

In 1914, Voegtlin reported the earliest study which proved that human pellagra is unquestionably caused by a dietary deficiency. He tested the effects on pellagrins receiving two contrasting diets; those receiving eggs, meat, and milk were cured, while those remaining on corn-based diets still had the disease. Also in 1914, Goldberger, a bacteriologist in the United States Public Health Service, was assigned the task of identifying the cause of pellagra. In his studies he observed that the disease was associated with poor diet and poverty and that well-fed persons did not contract the disease. In orphanages, prisons, and mental institutions in South Carolina, Georgia, and Mississippi the therapeutic value of good diets was demonstrated. Goldberger, his wife, and 14 volunteers constituted a "filth squad" who ingested and were injected with various biological materials and/or excreta from pellagrins, thus demonstrating the noninfectious nature of pellagra. At this time researchers and physicians did not want to believe that pellagra resulted from poor nutrition, but rather from an infection based on the popularity of the "germ theory" of disease. An important step toward the isolation of the preventive factor for pellagra was discovery of a suitable laboratory animal for testing its potency in various concentrated preparations. It was found that a pellagra-like disease (blacktongue) could be produced in dogs.

After it had been established that pellagra was a disease of nutritional deficiency, the next step was to discover the missing nutrient. Additional dietary protein was shown to be beneficial, so it was concluded that pellagra was due to protein deficiency. This view and, later, that it was more specifically due to a deficiency of the amino acid tryptophan, was held for some time. Following discovery that a crude extract of liver was effective in curing pellagra, and therefore was a source of the preventive factor, Elvehjem and colleagues (1937) isolated nicotinamide from liver as the factor that would cure blacktongue in dogs. Reports of the dramatic therapeutic effects of niacin in human pellagra quickly followed from several clinics.

In 1945, Krehl and coworkers found that tryptophan was as active as niacin in treatment of pellagra. Positive proof that tryptophan was converted to nicotinic acid was published by Heidelberger, who showed that the L-[^{14}C]tryptophan was converted to ^{14}C-labeled nicotinic acid in the rat. The conversion of tryptophan to niacin explained why foods rich in animal protein (e.g., milk) prevented and cured pellagra.

CHEMICAL STRUCTURE, PROPERTIES, AND ANTAGONISTS

Chemically, niacin ($C_6H_5O_2N$) is one of the simplest vitamins. The two forms of niacin—nicotinic acid and nicotinamide—correspond to 3-pyridine carboxylic acid and its amide, respectively (Fig. 8.1). The term niacin is used as a generic descriptor of pyridine 3-carboxylic acid and derivatives exhibiting the same qualitative biological activity of nicotinamide. There are antivitamins or antagonists for niacin. These compounds have the basic pyridine structure, with two of the important antagonists of nicotinic acid being 3-acetyl pyridine and pyridine sulfonic acid. Nicotinic acid and nicotinamide (niacinamide) possess the same vitamin activity; the free acid is converted to the amide in the body. Nicotinamide functions as a component of two coenzymes: nicotinamide adenine dinucleotide (NAD) and nicotinamide adenine dinucleotide phosphate (NADP) (Fig. 8.1).

Both nicotinic acid and nicotinamide are white, odorless, crystalline solids soluble in water and alcohol. They are very resistant to heat, air, light, and alkaline conditions and thus are stable in foods. Niacin is also stable in the presence of the usual oxidizing agents. However, it will undergo decarboxylation at a high temperature when in an alkaline medium. Nicotinic acid readily forms salts with metals such as aluminum, calcium, copper, and sodium. When in acid solution, niacin readily forms quaternary ammonium compounds, such as nicotinic acid hydrochloride, which is soluble in water. When in a basic solution, nicotinic acid readily forms carboxylic acid salts.

ANALYTICAL PROCEDURES

The most sensitive method for the determination of niacin and closely related compounds is microbiological. *Lactobacillus plantarum* responds to both forms of the vitamin, whereas *Leuconostoc mesenteroides* measures only nicotinic acid. Niacin must be freed from bound forms before assay. Since niacin is very stable to strong acids, it can be released by acid hydrolysis. Chemical methods of analysis are less sensitive than microbiological procedures and generally require more extensive extraction methods. The cyanogen bromide method of analysis is based on the reaction of pyridine derivatives with cyanogen bromide, forming a colored compound that can be used for quantitative measurement of the vitamin. The active coenzyme forms of niacin, the pyridine

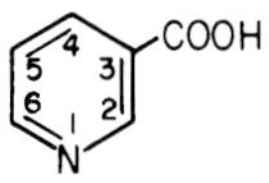

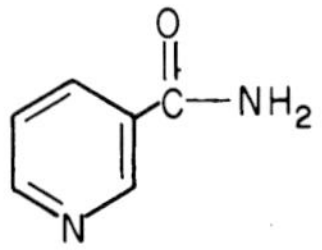

Nicotinic acid

(Pyridine-3 carboxylic acid)

Niacinamide

(3-pyridinecarboxylic acid amide)

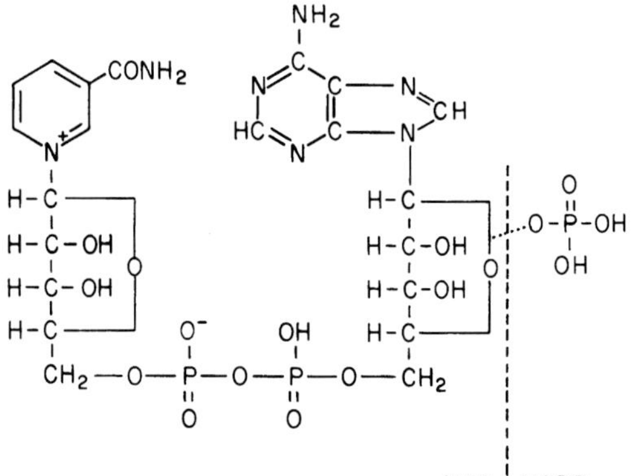

NAD ¦ NADP

Fig. 8.1 Chemical structures of nicotinic acid, nicotinamide, nicotinamide adenine dinucleotide (NAD), and nicotinamide adenine dinucleotide phosphate (NADP).

nucleotides NAD and NADP, can be determined by an enzyme-cycling colorimetric procedure (Nisselbaum and Green, 1969) or high-performance liquid chromatography (HPLC) (Stocchi et al., 1987). Bioassay procedures for niacin present two major difficulties in that (1) tryptophan in the diet is converted to niacin in the tissues, and (2) niacin is synthesized by intestinal bacteria to varying degrees. Chicks, puppies, and weanling rats have been used for biological niacin assay.

METABOLISM

Absorption, Transport, and Storage

Nicotinic acid and its amide are readily and very efficiently absorbed by diffusion at either physiological or pharmacological doses. At low concentrations absorption occurs as an Na$^+$-dependent facilitated diffusion, but at higher concentrations passive diffusion predominates. By employing the gastrointestinal tube technique, niacin was shown to be equally well absorbed from both the stomach and upper small intestine in humans (Bechgaard and Jespersen, 1977). In a steady-state situation, approximately 85% of a dose of 3 g of niacin per day was recovered from the urine of humans, and absorption was considered almost complete. In cattle studies, nicotinamide was more rapidly absorbed from the rumen than nicotinic acid (Erickson et al., 1991). This may have been due to differences in the dissociation constants of the compounds, with significance of ruminal fermentation and metabolism unknown.

Niacin in foods occurs mostly in its coenzyme forms, which are hydrolyzed during digestion, yielding nicotinamide, which seems to be absorbed without further hydrolysis in the gastrointestinal tract. The intestinal mucosa is rich in niacin conversion enzymes such as NAD glycohydrolase (Henderson and Gross, 1979). Nicotinamide is released from NAD in the liver and intestines by glycohydrolases for transport to tissues that synthesize NAD as needed. In the gut, mucosa nicotinic acid is converted to nicotinamide (Stein et al., 1994). Nicotinamide is the primary circulating form of the vitamin and is converted into its coenzyme forms in the tissues.

The tissue content of niacin and its analogs, NAD and NADP, is variable, dependent on the diet and a number of other factors, such as strain, sex, age, and treatment of animals (Hankes, 1984). Although niacin coenzymes are widely distributed in the body, no true storage occurs. Liver contains the greatest niacin concentration, but the amount stored is not great.

Excretion

Urine is the primary pathway of excretion of absorbed niacin and its metabolites. At high dosages, the half-life of both nicotinic acid and nicotinamide is determined mainly by rate of excretion of the unchanged compound in urine and not by metabolic change. When low dosages are used, both compounds are excreted principally as metabolites rather than as unchanged compounds.

The principal excretory product in humans, dogs, rats, and pigs is the methylated metabolite N'-methylnicotinamide or one of two oxidation products of this compound, 4-pyridone or 6-pyridone of N'-methylnicotinamide. On the other hand, in herbivores niacin does not seem to be metabolized by methylation, but large amounts are excreted unchanged. In the chicken, however, nicotinic acid is conjugated with or-nithine as either α- or δ-nicotinyl ornithine or dinicotinyl ornithine. The excretion of these metabolites is measured in studies of niacin require-ments and metabolism. Such studies are complicated by the fact that the kinds and relative amounts of these products vary with the species and level of niacin intake.

Tryptophan-Niacin Conversion

The amino acid tryptophan is a precursor for the synthesis of niacin in the body, and there is considerable evidence that synthesis can take place in the intestine. Investigations indicate that urinary excretion of the metabolite N'-methylnicotinamide is much larger when tryptophan is administered by stomach tube than when injected parenterally. There is also evidence that synthesis occurs in the developing chick embryo. The extent to which the metabolic requirement for niacin can be met from tryptophan will depend, first, on the amount of tryptophan in the diet and its bioavailability and, second, on the efficiency of the conver-sion of tryptophan to niacin. The pathway of tryptophan conversion to nicotinic acid mononucleotide in the body is shown in Fig. 8.2. Protein, energy, vitamin B_6, and riboflavin nutritional status and hormones affect one or more steps in the conversion sequence shown in Fig. 8.2, and hence can influence the yield of niacin from tryptophan. In addition, copper, iron, and magnesium all have roles in the transformation. Iron is required by two enzymes for the conversion of tryptophan to niacin with a deficiency reducing tryptophan utilization (Oduho et al., 1994). It is suggested that pellagra is not simply a disease of niacin deficiency, but more appropriately a disease of tryptophan metabolism (Anony-mous, 1987).

At low levels of tryptophan intake, the efficiency of conversion is high. It decreases when niacin and tryptophan levels in the diet are in-creased. When animals have received inadequate levels of tryptophan, increasing amounts of dietary tryptophan are used first to restore nitro-gen balance, next to restore blood pyridine nucleotides, and then to be excreted as niacin metabolites. Under starvation or energy restriction, efficiency of conversion increases, while pregnant women can convert tryptophan to niacin more efficiently than other adults (Narasinga Rao and Gopalan, 1984). A threefold increase in conversion efficiency was reported in pregnant women during the third trimester (Wertz et al., 1958). This increase presumably was due to the stimulation by estrogen of tryptophan oxygenase, a suggested rate-limiting enzyme in the path-

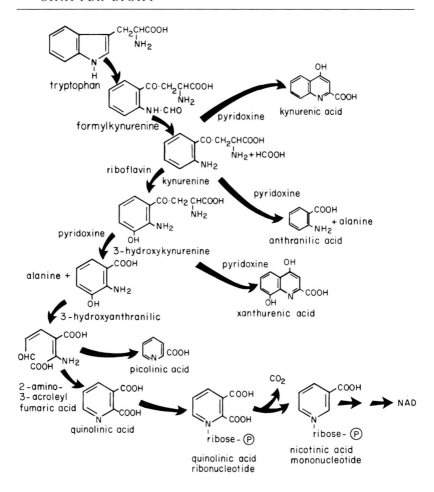

Fig. 8.2 Conversion of tryptophan to nicotinic acid mononucleotide plus some side reactions.

way (Rose and Braidman, 1971). Another factor that may affect this conversion ratio is amino acid imbalance due to excess leucine in the diet (see Deficiency, Humans).

Animal species differ widely in ability to synthesize niacin from tryptophan. According to a variety of experiments, approximately 60 mg of tryptophan is estimated to be equivalent to 1 mg of niacin in humans, while the rat is more efficient, with a conversion rate of 35 to 50 mg of tryptophan required. Conversion efficiency of tryptophan to niacin in the chick is estimated to be 45:1 (Baker et al., 1973; Chen and

Austic, 1989) and relatively efficient, while in the turkey it is inefficient, with conversions ranging from 103 to 119:1 (Ruiz and Harms, 1990c). Conversion efficiency is probably due to inherent differences in liver levels of picolinic acid carboxylase, the enzyme that diverts one of the intermediates (2-amino-3-acroleyl fumaric acid) toward the glutaryl-CoA pathway instead of allowing this compound to condense to quinolinic acid, the immediate precursor of nicotinic acid. Picolinic acid carboxylase in livers of various species (Table 8.1) has a very close inverse relationship to experimentally determined niacin requirements. The cat has been shown to have 30 to 50 times as much picolinic acid carboxylase activity as the rat. Thus, the cat has so much of this enzyme that it cannot convert any of its dietary tryptophan to niacin. The cat, therefore, has an absolute requirement for niacin itself. Conversely, the rat diverts very little of its dietary tryptophan to carbon dioxide and water and thus is very efficient in converting tryptophan to niacin. The duck has a very high niacin requirement (approximately two times that of chickens), with considerably higher levels of picolinic acid carboxylase activity (Scott et al., 1982).

FUNCTIONS

The major function of niacin is in the coenzyme forms of nicotinamide, NAD and NADP. Enzymes containing NAD and NADP are important links in a series of reactions associated with carbohydrate, protein, and lipid metabolism. They are especially important in the metabolic reactions that furnish energy to the animal. The coenzymes act as an intermediate in most of the H^+ transfers in metabolism, including more than 200 reactions in the metabolism of carbohydrates, fatty acids, and amino acids. These reactions are of paramount importance for normal tissue integrity, particularly of the skin, gastrointestinal tract, and nervous system.

The NAD- and NADP-containing enzymes play an important role in biological oxidation-reduction systems by virtue of their capacity to serve as hydrogen-transfer agents. Hydrogen is effectively transferred from the oxidizable substrate to oxygen through a series of graded enzymatic hydrogen transfers. Nicotinamide-containing enzyme systems constitute one such group of hydrogen-transfer agents. In electron transport, oxidation of reduced NAD or NADP is carried out by a second hydrogen-carrying system, the riboflavin coenzymes (see Chapter 7, Fig. 7.2). The nicotinamide moiety of the coenzyme operates in these

■ Table 8.1   Liver Picolinic Acid Carboxylase Activity Among Species

Species	Units/g liver (wet basis)
Cat	50,500
Lizard	29,640
Duck	17,330
Frog	13,720
Turkey	9,230
Cow	8,300
Pig	7,120
Pigeon	6,950
Chicken (high niacin-requiring strain)	5,380
Rabbit	4,270
Mouse	4,200
Guinea pig	3,940
Chicken (strain with low niacin requirement)	3,200
Human	3,180
Hamster	3,140
Toad	3,050
Rat	1,570

Sources: Modified from Ikeda et al. (1965), DiLorenzo (1972), and Scott et al. (1982).

systems by reversibly alternating between an oxidized quaternary pyridinium ion and a reduced tertiary amine. The transfer of hydrogen is reversible and stereospecific.

Some of these enzymes show a strict specificity for either NAD or NADP, while others utilize these coenzymes equally well. Important metabolic reactions catalyzed by NAD and NADP are summarized below:

1. Carbohydrate metabolism—(a) glycolysis (anaerobic oxidation of glucose) and (b) the Krebs cycle.
2. Lipid metabolism—(a) glycerol synthesis and breakdown, (b) fatty acid oxidation and synthesis, and (c) steroid synthesis.
3. Protein metabolism—(a) degradation and synthesis of amino acids and (b) oxidation of carbon chains via the Krebs cycle.
4. Photosynthesis.
5. Rhodopsin synthesis (see Chapter 2, Fig. 2.6).

NAD is specific for hydrogenases involved in passing electrons on to oxygen via the electron-transport system in the tricarboxylic acid cycle. Here NAD serves as the electron acceptor in three of the four dehydrogenation steps. As a hydrogen acceptor, NADH is formed which in turn functions as a hydrogen donor to the respiratory chain for ATP production; NAD as well participates as a codehydrogenase, with enzymes involved in the oxidation of fuel molecules such as glyceraldehyde 3-phosphate, lactate, alcohol, 3-hydroxybutyrate, pyruvate, and α-ketoglutarate dehydrogenases. NADP also participates in dehydrogenation reactions, particularly in the hexose monophosphate shunt of glucose metabolism. Reduced NADP has an important role in the synthesis of fats and steroids and is contained in the alcohol-dehydrogenase system, the lactic acid-dehydrogenase system, and other systems.

Both NAD and NADP are involved in degradation and synthesis of amino acids. NAD has a role, as the source of ADP-ribose for the ADP-ribosylation of proteins and poly(ADP-ribose). ADP-ribosyltransferases are enzymes of the cytosol, plasma membrane, and nuclear envelope, which catalyze the transfer of ADP-ribose onto arginine, lysine, or asparagine residues in acceptor proteins to form N-glycosides.

Niacin-dependent poly(ADP-ribose) is involved in the post-translational modification of nuclear proteins. The poly ADP-ribosylated proteins seem to function in DNA repair, DNA replication, and cell differentiation (Carson et al., 1987). In the event of DNA strand breaks, ADP-ribose subunits, cleaved from NAD^+, are covalently linked to amino acid residues, and the polymer is subsequently elongated and branched. Poly(ADP-ribose) is synthesized in response to DNA strand breaks. Rat data have shown that even mild niacin deficiency decreases liver poly(ADP-ribose) concentrations and that poly(ADP-ribose) levels are also altered by food restriction (Rawling et al., 1994). Zhang et al. (1993) suggested that severe niacin deficiency may increase the susceptibility of DNA to oxidative damage, likely due to lower availability of NAD. Turnover rates of protein in Japanese quail have been related to niacin deficiency, and a high turnover rate due to the deficiency was primarily attributed to enhanced degradation rate of proteins rather than enhanced synthesis rate of proteins (Park et al., 1991).

Niacin was found to be part of the glucose tolerance factor, an organochromium complex isolated from yeast that potentiates the insulin response (Mertz, 1975). The role of the niacin moiety in the glucose tolerance factor is unknown because free niacin has no similar effect.

REQUIREMENTS

Niacin requirements for various animals and humans are presented in Table 8.2. Niacin requirements vary widely, generally because (1) niacin is synthesized from tryptophan, and (2) much of dietary niacin is in a bound form unavailable to humans and animals.

■ Table 8.2 Niacin Requirements for Various Animals and Humans

Animal	Purpose or Class	Requirement[a]	Reference
Beef cattle	Adult	Microbial synthesis	NRC (1996)
Dairy cattle	Calf	2.6 ppm milk replacer	NRC (1989a)
	Adult	Microbial synthesis	NRC (1989a)
Chicken	Leghorn, 0–6 weeks	27.0 mg/kg	NRC (1994)
	Leghorn, 6–18 weeks	11.0 mg/kg	NRC (1994)
	Laying (100-g intake)	10.0 mg/kg	NRC (1994)
	Broilers, all classes	25–30 mg/kg	NRC (1994)
Duck (Pekin)	All classes	55 mg/kg	NRC (1994)
Japanese quail	All classes	20–40 mg/kg	NRC (1994)
Turkey	All classes	40–60 mg/kg	NRC (1994)
Sheep	Adult	Microbial synthesis	NRC (1985b)
Swine	Growing-finishing, 3–5 kg	20 mg/kg	NRC (1998)
	Growing-finishing, 5–120 kg	7–15 mg/kg	NRC (1998)
	Adult	10.0 mg/kg	NRC (1998)
Horse	Adult	Microbial synthesis	NRC (1989)
Goat	Adult	Microbial synthesis	NRC (1981b)
Fox	Growing	10 mg/kg	NRC (1982a)
Cat	Growing	40 mg/kg	NRC (1986)
Dog	Growing	450 μg/kg body wt.	NRC (1985a)
Fish	Catfish	14 mg/kg	NRC (1993)
	Pacific salmon	150–200 mg/kg	NRC (1993)
	Rainbow trout	1–10 mg/kg	NRC (1993)
Rat	All classes	15 mg/kg	NRC (1995)
Mouse	All classes	15 mg/kg	NRC (1995)
Human	Infants	5–6 mg/day	RDA (1989)
	Children	9–13 mg/day	RDA (1989)
	Adults	17–20 mg/day	RDA (1989)

[a]Expressed as per unit of animal feed on either as-fed (approximately 90% dry matter) or dry basis (see Appendix, Tables A1a,b). Human data are expressed as mg/day.

Some species, such as the cat, mink, and most fish, apparently lack the ability to convert tryptophan to niacin. For species that have the capacity to synthesize niacin from tryptophan, it is impossible to set the niacin requirement unless the tryptophan level is specified and it is known that the diet is adequate in vitamin B_6, since this vitamin is needed in synthesis of niacin from tryptophan. However, the vitamin B_6 level is adequate in most practical livestock diets. Riboflavin is required for synthesis of niacin from tryptophan as well as for conversion of vitamin B_6 to the functional coenzyme (pyrodoxal phosphate), which is needed for niacin synthesis (see Metabolism; Chapter 7, Functions). Likewise, many other nutrients and hormones affect conversion of niacin from tryptophan (see Metabolism).

Cunha (1982) listed a number of factors that influence niacin requirements for livestock, as follows:

1. Genetic differences, which can influence niacin needs, such as selection for meatier, faster-growing animals and increased production levels.

2. Ability to synthesize niacin from tryptophan (see Metabolism).

3. Increased stress and subclinical disease level on the farm because of closer and more frequent contact between animals in confinement.

4. Trend toward more intensified operations that may lessen opportunity for coprophagy and will reduce access to pasture.

5. Newer methods of handling and processing feeds that may affect niacin and tryptophan level and availability.

6. Various nutrient interrelationships, including amino acid imbalances.

7. Trend toward earlier weaning, which increases the need for higher vitamin levels in milk-substitute diets (prestarter and starter feeds).

8. Molds and antimetabolites in feeds that can increase certain nutrient needs.

The type of carbohydrate consumed may influence niacin requirements. For maximal growth, tilapia fingerlings required 26 ppm niacin when fed a glucose diet compared to 121 ppm for those fish fed a dextrin (from corn) diet (Shiau and Suen, 1992).

Niacin requirements of ruminants are unknown; the vitamin is normally synthesized in adequate quantities in the rumen. Niacin supplementation has been shown to be beneficial in beef cattle receiving high-concentrate diets and in high-producing dairy cows. In a review, Olentine (1984) summarized the factors affecting ruminant niacin requirements as follows:

1. Protein balance—excess of leucine, arginine, and glycine increases the requirement.

2. High tryptophan content of feeds—as tryptophan content increases, niacin requirements decrease.

3. Energy content—high-energy rations require more niacin per unit of feed.

4. Antibiotics—depending on the product, niacin requirements are increased.

5. Dietary rancidity—if fat is rancid, niacin requirements are increased.

6. Gastrointestinal synthesis—niacin is synthesized in the gastric and intestinal regions.

7. Availability of niacin and tryptophan in feedstuffs—cereal grains and other feedstuffs have varying degrees of niacin and tryptophan availability.

Human niacin requirements are based on niacin intake of pellagrins and on human depletion and repletion studies. Most food tables for humans list niacin as niacin equivalents (NEs), which represent the sum of milligrams of niacin (nicotinic acid plus nicotinamide) plus 1/60 mg of tryptophan (conversion rate of tryptophan to niacin). Niacin equivalents range from 13 to 19 mg for adults or 6.6 mg/1,000 kcal (RDA, 1989). This amount provides for differences in various diets consumed in terms of the bioavailability of niacin and the contribution of tryptophan. The Food and Agriculture Organization/World Health Organization Expert Group recommended an intake of 6.6 mg NE per 1,000 kcal for all age groups (Narasinga Rao and Gopalan, 1984). The RDA (1989) provided an increase of 2 and 5 mg NE for pregnancy and lactation, respectively.

Exercise (Haralambie, 1976), diabetes mellitus (Vague et al., 1987), and genetic disorders such as Hartnup's disease (Halvorsen and Halvorsen, 1963) can increase niacin requirements in humans. In Hartnup's disease there is impaired intestinal absorption of tryptophan (Halvorsen and Halvorsen, 1963), but in diabetes there are elevated concentrations of picolinic acid carboxylase, resulting in less efficient conversion of niacin from tryptophan (Ikeda et al., 1965).

NATURAL SOURCES

Niacin is widely distributed in foods of both plant and animal origin (Table 8.3). Large quantities of niacin are found in brewer's yeast and meats. Animal and fish by-products, distiller's grains and yeast, various distillation and fermentation solubles, and certain oil meals are good sources. Leafy materials, especially pasture grass, are fair sources. Milk, dairy products, fruits, and eggs are poor sources. Niacin is present in uncooked foods mainly as the pyridine nucleotides NAD and NADP, but some hydrolysis of these nucleotides to free forms may occur during food preparation.

Most species can use the essential amino acid tryptophan and synthesize niacin from it (see Metabolism and Requirements sections). Because tryptophan can give rise to body niacin, both niacin and tryptophan content should be considered in expressing niacin values of foods. However, since there is a preferential use of tryptophan for protein synthesis before any becomes available for conversion to niacin (Kodicek et al., 1974), it seems unlikely, given the low tryptophan content in many feedstuffs, that tryptophan conversion greatly contributes to the niacin supply.

Niacin is often present in feeds in a bound form that is not available.

■ Table 8.3   Niacin in Foods and Feedstuffs (mg/kg, dry basis)

Alfalfa hay, sun cured	42	Molasses, sugarcane	49
Alfalfa leaves, sun cured	53	Oat, grain	16
Barley, grain	94	Pea seeds	36
Bean, navy (seed)	28	Peanut meal, solvent extracted	188
Blood meal	34	Potato	37
Brewer's grains	47	Rice, bran	330
Buttermilk (cattle)	9	Rice, grain	39
Chicken, broilers (whole)	230	Rice, polished	17
Citrus pulp	23	Rye, grain	21
Clover hay, ladino (sun cured)	11	Sorghum, grain	43
Copra meal (coconut)	28	Soybean meal, solvent extracted	31
Corn, gluten meal	55	Soybean seed	24
Corn, yellow grain	28	Spleen, cattle	25
Cottonseed meal, solvent extracted	48	Timothy hay, sun cured	29
Fish meal, anchovy	89	Wheat, bran	268
Fish meal, menhaden	60	Wheat, grain	64
Fish, sardine	81	Whey	11
Linseed meal, solvent extracted	37	Yeast, brewer's	482
Liver, cattle	269	Yeast, torula	525
Milk, skim, cattle	12		

Source: NRC (1982b).

The niacin in cereal grains and their by-products is in a bound, complex form that is virtually unavailable, at least to simple-stomached animals (Luce et al., 1967). It seems that much of this niacin is also unavailable to rumen microorganisms. Any dietary niacin escaping degradation in the rumen will also likely be unavailable for absorption in the lower gut.

Initial evidence of bound forms of niacin stemmed from observed discrepancies between niacin values in cereals determined colorimetrically before and after hydrolysis with dilute NaOH. Microbiological assays similarly indicated that about 20% more niacin was obtained in dilute alkaline extracts of cereals than in aqueous or acid extracts.

Two types of bound niacin were initially described: (1) a peptide with molecular weight of 12,000 to 13,000, the so-called niacinogens, and (2) a carbohydrate complex with a molecular weight of approximately 2,370 (Darby et al., 1975). The name niacytin has been used to designate this latter material from wheat bran. A number of bound forms of niacin are apparently present in cereals. Ghosh et al. (1963), using a microbiological assay, reported that 85 to 90% of the total nicotinic acid in cereals is in a bound form. Mason et al. (1973) reported that bound niacin is linked to the macromolecules, of which about 60% were polysaccharides and 40% peptides or glycopeptides. Lack of niacin availability may be due to a blocking effect of these molecules, which prevent access of digestive enzymes to the niacin-macromolecule bond, and therefore free niacin would not be available for absorption.

About 40% of the total niacin in oilseeds is in bound form, while only a small proportion of the niacin in pulses, yeast, crustacea, fish, animal tissue, or milk is bound. Using a rat assay procedure, Carter and Carpenter (1982) showed that in eight samples of mature cooked cereals (corn, wheat, rice, and milo), only about 35% of the total niacin was available. In the calculation of the niacin content of formulated diets, probably all niacin from cereal grain sources should be ignored or at least given a value no greater than one-third of the total niacin.

Some bound forms of niacin are biologically available, but the niacin in corn is particularly unavailable and is implicated in the etiology of pellagra in societies that consume large quantities of the grain. Pellagra occurs in Mexico less frequently than one might expect; there the custom is to treat the maize with limewater before making tortillas, and in this way the nicotinic acid is liberated. Boiling releases niacin in sweet corn, a traditional way of treating corn used by the Hopi Indians (Kodicek et al., 1974). In immature seeds, niacin occurs as part of biologically available coenzymes necessary for seed metabolism. Binding of niacin to carbohydrate by ester linkages may cause it to be retained in the mature seed until it is utilized; the vitamin availability for man and animal is thus impaired (Wall and Carpenter, 1988). In rat growth assays for available niacin, corn harvested immaturely ("milk stage") gave values from 74 to 88 µg/g, whereas corn harvested at maturity gave assay values of 16 to 18 µg/g (Carpenter et al., 1988).

Beverages including tea and coffee also can contribute significantly to niacin intake. Roasted coffee contains more niacin than does raw coffee because the trigonelline present in raw coffee is converted to nicotinic acid when the coffee is roasted. In several Central and South American countries, absence of pellagra among those whose staple is maize is attributed to widespread consumption of coffee.

DEFICIENCY

Effects of Deficiency

Niacin deficiency is characterized by severe metabolic disorders in the skin and digestive organs. The first signs to appear are loss of appetite, retarded growth, weakness, digestive disorders, and diarrhea. The deficiency is found in both human and animal populations that are overly dependent on foods (particularly corn) low in available niacin and its precursor, tryptophan.

Ruminants

Young ruminants prior to the development of the rumen would be expected to suffer B-vitamin deficiencies, including niacin, when diets contain insufficient quantities of these vitamins. However, early studies with lambs and calves failed to produce deficiency when niacin-free diets were fed. Ability to produce niacin deficiency is dependent on use of a low-tryptophan milk diet. From these studies, it may be concluded that a dietary requirement of niacin for young ruminants does not exist as long as the level of tryptophan is maintained near 0.2% of the diet. In calves, a diet free of niacin and low in tryptophan produced deficiency signs of sudden anorexia, severe diarrhea, inability to stand, and dehydration, followed by sudden death. Supplementation with 2.6 mg of nicotinic acid per liter of milk offered ad libitum twice daily prevented the deficiency (Hopper and Johnson, 1955).

Synthesis of niacin in the rumen of cattle has been demonstrated and may be under metabolic control; that is, more niacin is synthesized when small amounts are provided in the diet and vice versa (Porter, 1961). Adult ruminants synthesize adequate niacin by microorganisms and/or conversion from tryptophan. However, the synthesizing ability appears to be low, since production responses from niacin supplementation can be demonstrated in both sheep and cattle. Niacin supplementation is especially beneficial to stressed animals, such as beef cattle being adapted to high-grain diets or lactating cows that have just calved.

BEEF CATTLE

The addition of niacin to beef cattle diets has been shown to significantly improve average daily gain and feed efficiency. Feeder calves responded positively in rate and efficiency of gain in the 29-day adaptation study by gaining an additional 8.3 kg with 70 ppm added niacin (Byers, 1979). Byers (1979, 1981) summarized 14 beef cattle studies demonstrating improved gains and feed efficiency by 9.7 and 10.9%, respectively. Growth from all trials was especially beneficial during the adaptation of cattle to feedlot diets (i.e., during the first 40 days).

Niacin appears to be effective in enhancing acclimation and adaptation to urea-supplemented diets. However, niacin stimulation of microbial protein production occurs regardless of dietary nitrogen source, but is greatest when natural protein rather than nonprotein nitrogen (urea) is fed (Brent and Bartley, 1984). This may be partly due to the synthesis of niacin from tryptophan. Minimal amounts of niacin supplied via microbial synthesis and diet become adequate in the later stages of the feedlot period, whereas earlier they are insufficient to meet demands. The large response exhibited during the feedlot adaptation phase indicates that supplemental niacin assists in overcoming shipping stress and allows for a more rapid adjustment to feedlot conditions and changing diets. Summaries of beef cattle studies over the total feeding period (73 to 176 days) indicate that 50 or 100 ppm of niacin is more effective than higher levels of 150, 250, or 500 ppm, with respect to gain.

DAIRY COWS

Niacin has been assumed to be synthesized in adequate amounts in the rumen to meet the needs of the dairy cow; however, evidence suggests that this may not be true for the high-producing dairy cow in early lactation. The effect of niacin on milk production and composition has been found to be variable, but it appears that niacin (5 to 6 g per cow per day) may have a beneficial effect on milk production early in the lactation period and when given to ketotic cows.

One report indicated that about 50% of dairy cows in high-production herds go through borderline ketosis during early lactation (Emery et al., 1964). The concentration of serum β-hydroxybutyrate was reduced from 1.24 to 0.74 mmol/L after 5 days, when 10 g of niacin was given to cows with ketosis (Flachowsky et al., 1988). Fronk and Schultz (1979) indicated that treating ketotic dairy cows with 12 g of nicotinic acid daily had a beneficial effect on the reversal of both subclinical and clinical ketosis. Other studies indicate that 6 g of niacin may be sufficient (Hoffmann-La Roche, 1994).

Other workers have reported that supplemental niacin increased microbial protein synthesis. Enhanced production of microbial protein might explain increased milk production, weight gain, and feed efficiency observed when urea-containing diets were supplemented with 250 to 500 mg/kg niacin (Cunha, 1982). Daily niacin supplementation of 3 to 6 g in early lactation dairy cows resulted in slight increases in milk production. In a study involving six dairy herds, Jaster et al. (1983) found that milk production of niacin-supplemented cows peaked earlier, and milk production of high-producing cows in first lactation was greater when they received supplemental niacin. In these herds there was only a slight increase in milk fat percentage. Klippel et al. (1993) reported that supplemental niacin decreased milk short- and medium-chain fatty acids and increased monounsaturated fatty acids.

In one study, increased dry matter intake of 0.8 kg per cow was reported with added niacin in diets based on soybean meal. An increase in 1 kg of dry matter can support 2.5 kg of higher milk yield or minimize weight loss, improving energy status (Hutjens, 1990). Part of this greater dry matter intake response could be related to less subclinical ketosis.

Horner et al. (1986) reported that feeding whole cottonseed and most other dietary fat sources to dairy cows resulted in a reduction of milk protein percentage and protein yield. Diets supplemented with 0.03% niacin (6 g niacin/20.45 kg dry matter) increased milk protein percentage compared to diets with 15% whole cottonseed. The authors concluded that milk protein depression with whole cottonseed was alleviated by niacin because of stimulation of mammary casein synthesis. Another study showed no beneficial effect of niacin on milk casein synthesis in cows fed whole cottonseed, which probably was due to their late stage of lactation (Lanham et al., 1992). Feeding cows niacin has been shown to correct fat-induced milk protein depression (Driver et al., 1990; Cervantes et al., 1996).

LAMBS

Mizwicki et al. (1975) observed that 500 ppm of supplemental niacin improved feed efficiency of lambs fed a high-concentrate diet containing urea. Supplementation studies (100 ppm niacin) with growing and finishing lambs revealed increased performance, with evidence that niacin stimulates rumen microbial protein synthesis (Shields and Perry, 1982). These studies indicated that supplemental niacin (1) increased nitrogen utilization, (2) improved the percentage of absorbed nitrogen retained, (3) reduced urinary nitrogen excretion, and (4) reduced the percentage of nitrogen found as urea nitrogen. All these positive changes point toward improved protein metabolism. Dittrich et al. (1993) indicated that supplemental niacin for lambs increased digestibility of crude fiber and improved wool production.

Swine

One would expect niacin to be deficient in typical swine diets, particularly when corn is fed, because corn is low in available niacin and tryptophan. Wide variation has been observed in the severity of clinical signs of niacin deficiency in pigs with similar breeding and environmental backgrounds. Occasionally, animals appear to thrive with no niacin, and other animals appear to vary in their requirement (Cunha, 1977). Young pigs require a dietary source of niacin when fed diets deficient in tryptophan (Luecke et al., 1948). However, niacin deficiency is less likely in pigs that weigh more than 27 kg (Luecke et al., 1948), and, more recently, Ivers and Veum (1993) found no benefit from niacin supplementation in 5-week-old pigs (7.5 kg) fed low-protein corn-soybean meal diets. During reproduction and lactation, it was not possible to produce niacin deficiency in sows fed a purified diet with either 18 or 26.1% casein (Ensminger et al., 1951). Ivers et al. (1993) reported no benefit from supplemental niacin in sow and litter performance when sows were fed corn-soybean meal-oat diets containing 12.8% crude protein. Evidently, the diets used in these studies contained enough tryptophan and/or synthesis of niacin by bacteria in the intestinal tract to supply niacin needs, or the experiment was not long enough for niacin deficiency to develop.

As mentioned earlier, niacin deficiency is characterized by severe metabolic disorders in the skin and digestive organs. Signs include poor appetite, decreased rate of gain (Fig. 8.3), stomatitis, normocytic anemia, and achlorhydria, followed by diarrhea, occasional vomiting, and

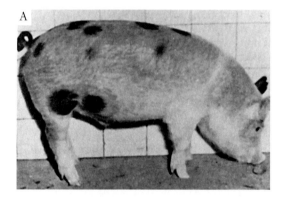

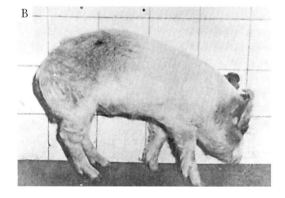

Fig. 8.3 Niacin deficiency. (A) Pig that has received adequate niacin; (B) pig that has not received adequate niacin. The difference in growth and condition is due to the addition of niacin in a diet containing 80% ground yellow corn. (Courtesy of D.E. Becker, Illinois Agriculture Experiment Station.)

an exfoliate type of dermatitis and hair loss (Cunha, 1977). Degenerative changes in the nervous system are reported to occur in the ganglion cells in the posterior root, with extensive chromatolysis in the dorsal root (Wintrobe et al., 1945).

Niacin-deficient pigs have inflammatory lesions of the gastrointestinal tract. Ulcerative necrotic lesions of the large intestine swarm with fusiform bacteria and spirochetes (Fig. 8.4). Diarrhea with foul-smelling feces particularly involves the large intestine, which thickens, is very red, and appears weak and "rotten." Enteric conditions may be due to niacin deficiency, bacterial infection, or both. Niacin-deficient pigs respond readily to niacin therapy, but there is no benefit for infectious enteritis. However, adequate dietary niacin probably allows the pig to maintain its resistance to bacterial invasion.

Poultry

There is good evidence that poultry—even chick and turkey embryos—are able to synthesize niacin, but that rate of synthesis may be too slow for optimal growth. Broilers from 3 to 7 weeks of age are reported not to require supplemental niacin while fed a corn-soybean meal diet, but the vitamin is required from 1 to 21 days of age (Ruiz and Harms, 1990a,b). It has been claimed that before a marked deficiency of niacin can occur in the chicken, there must first be a deficiency of tryptophan. Chicks at hatch have considerable tryptophan contained in the protein of the yolk; thus niacin deficiency will not readily occur unless the feed is low for both the amino acid and the vitamin (NRC, 1994).

Experiments using diets containing a limited amount of tryptophan have shown that the chick requires niacin and that deficiency causes enlargement of the tibiotarsal joint, bowing of the legs, poor feathering,

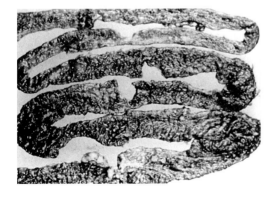

Fig. 8.4 Intestine from niacin-deficient pig shows thickened and hemorrhagic mucous membrane and denuded areas. (Courtesy of R.W. Luecke, Michigan State University.)

and dermatitis on the feet and head (Scott et al., 1982). The main clinical signs of niacin deficiency in young chicks is enlargement of the hock joint and bowing of the legs, similar to signs of perosis (Figs. 8.5 and 8.6). The main difference between this condition and the perosis of manganese or choline deficiency is that in niacin deficiency the Achilles tendon rarely slips from its condyles.

Niacin deficiency in the chick is characterized by appetite loss and growth failure. The deficiency results in blacktongue, a condition characterized by inflammation of the tongue and mouth cavity. Beginning at about 2 weeks of age, the entire mouth cavity, as well as the esophagus, becomes distinctly inflamed; growth is retarded, and feed consumption is reduced. Weight loss occurs, and both egg production and hatchability are reduced in niacin-deficient laying hens. Shell quality is improved with niacin supplementation (Leeson et al., 1991). Death loss can be affected. Jackson (1992) reported that 30 ppm of dietary niacin significantly decreased the mortality rate of layers compared to 10 ppm.

Turkey poults, pheasant chicks, ducklings, and goslings all expressed perosis as the primary niacin deficiency sign (NRC, 1994). Signs in turkeys and ducks, while similar to those of chickens, are much more severe. Compared to the chick, the turkey poult, duckling, pheasant chick, and gosling have higher requirements for niacin. This higher requirement is related to the less efficient conversion of tryptophan to niacin by these species (see Metabolism). Ducks receiving low-niacin diets show severely bowed legs and ultimately become too crippled and weak to walk. Niacin deficiency in the turkey is also characterized by severe bowing of the legs and enlargement of the hock joint. Goslings fed purified rations develop perosis and hock deformities that are preventable with administration of nicotinic acid (Briggs et al., 1953).

Horses

No requirements for niacin have been established for the horse, and deficiency has not been reported (NRC, 1989b). Synthesis of niacin by microflora in the lower digestive tract, as well as tissue synthesis from tryptophan, should likely preclude niacin deficiency. Microbial synthesis in the horse intestine was shown by Carroll et al. (1949), who fed a diet containing 3 mg of nicotinic acid per kilogram of dry matter and found the following nicotinic acid concentrations (ppm dry matter) in ingesta: duodenum, 55; ileum, 58; cecum, 121; anterior large colon, 96; and anterior small colon, 119.

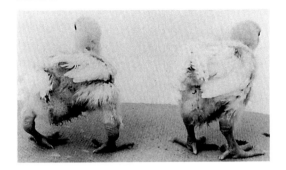

Fig. 8.5 Leg disorders in niacin-deficient broiler chicks. The bird on the left, with bowed legs, was fed a corn-soybean meal diet without supplemental niacin. (Courtesy of N. Ruiz and R. Harms, University of Florida.)

Other Animal Species

DOGS AND CATS

The similarity of niacin deficiency signs in dogs and humans is important because the dog became the laboratory animal used to identify the vitamin deficiency. Signs of deficiency in the dog are collectively known as blacktongue (canine pellagra). The condition occurs in dogs fed a diet primarily of flaked corn (maize) with little material of animal origin. Clinical signs include anorexia, apathy, retarded growth, weight loss, and drooling of thick ropy saliva (Fig. 8.7). There is severe cheilosis, glossitis, and gingivitis. Necrotic patches and ulcers may be seen on the oral mucosa, and there is a foul odor. The inflammatory changes may extend to the esophagus and eventually to the large intestine. There is bloody diarrhea, inflammation, and hemorrhagic necrosis of the duodenum and jejunum, with shortening and clubbing of villi and inflammation and degeneration of the mucosa of the large intestine. Uncorrected deficiencies lead to dehydration, emaciation, and death (NRC, 1985a). Because of burning or itching, animals scratch or bite at the skin, producing a traumatic dermatitis. Death generally occurs within 10 days of the onset of clinical signs.

Virtually no niacin is synthesized from tryptophan in the cat (see Metabolism). Niacin-deficient cats exhibit weight loss, anorexia, weakness, and apathy (NRC, 1986). There is drooling of thick saliva with a foul odor. The oral cavity is characterized by ulceration of the upper palate, and the tongue is fiery red, with ulceration and congestion along the anterior border. The fur may be unkempt, and diarrhea occurs. The deficiency can be associated with respiratory disease, which contributes to an early death.

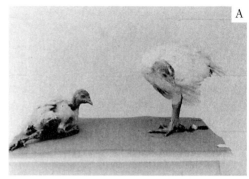

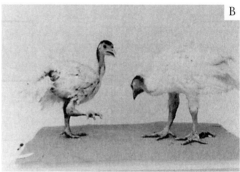

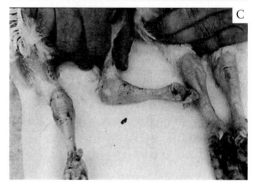

Fig. 8.6 Niacin deficiency in turkey poults. (A and B) The birds on the left side, which were fed a corn-soybean meal without supplemental niacin, showed perosis-like signs. (C) Comparison of the legs of the poults in B. (Courtesy of N. Ruiz and R. Harms, University of Florida.)

FISH

In fish species studied, tryptophan is not an adequate precursor to niacin, and the vitamin deficiency develops rapidly in many fish fed a niacin-deficient diet. Signs of niacin deficiency in trout and salmon include anorexia, reduced growth, poor feed conversion, photosensitivity or sunburn, intestinal lesions, muscular weakness and spasms, and increased mortality (NRC, 1993). Channel catfish and common carp deficient in niacin show skin and fin lesions, hemorrhages, deformed jaws,

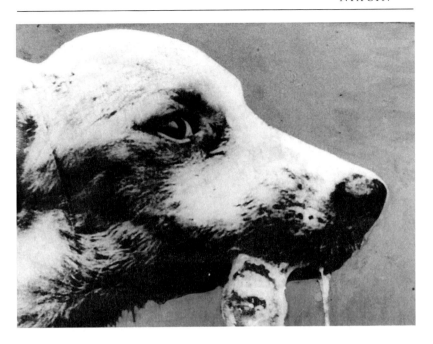

Fig. 8.7 Niacin-deficient dog with blacktongue exhibits drooling of thick, ropy saliva. (Courtesy of V. Ramadus Murthy, National Institute of Nutrition, Jamasi-Osmania, Hyderabad, India.)

anemia, exophthalmia, and high mortality rate (NRC, 1993). Niacin-deficient tilapia grew poorly, and skin, fin, and mouth lesions and hemorrhages developed; the snout was deformed and edema occurred (Shiau and Suen, 1992). Japanese eels exhibited reduced growth, ataxia, skin lesions, and dark coloration.

FOXES AND MINK

The mink is similar to the cat concerning niacin metabolism, with very inefficient conversion of tryptophan to niacin. Young mink fed a deficient diet displayed nonspecific signs, including weight loss, weak voice, general weakness, and bloody diarrhea (NRC, 1982a). Foxes fed a niacin-deficient diet exhibited anorexia, weight loss, and typical blacktongue, characterized by severe inflammation of the gums and fiery redness of the lips, tongue, and gums (NRC, 1982a).

LABORATORY ANIMALS

Laboratory rodents often do not show characteristic signs of niacin deficiency but exhibit nonspecific signs of appetite loss and growth re-

CHAPTER EIGHT

tardation (NRC, 1995). It is difficult to produce niacin deficiency in rats because compared to other species, rats are very efficient in converting tryptophan to niacin; 33 to 40 mg of tryptophan yield 1 mg of niacin. Rats fed niacin- and tryptophan-deficient diets develop behavioral changes, convulsions, diarrhea, rough hair coat, and alopecia. Niacin-deficient guinea pigs exhibit poor growth; reduced appetite; pale feet, nose, and ears; drooling, anemia, and a tendency toward diarrhea. Niacin deficiency has not been reported in the mouse, gerbil, hamster, or vole (NRC, 1995).

NONHUMAN PRIMATES

Niacin deficiency in the rhesus monkey is characterized by weight loss, apathy, anemia, skin pigmentation, and bloody diarrhea (NRC, 1978). Inefficient conversion of tryptophan to niacin has been suggested.

RABBITS

Substantial synthesis of niacin occurs in the intestinal tract of rabbits fed niacin-deficient diets. Niacin deficiency in rabbits has resulted in pronounced loss of appetite, followed by emaciation and diarrhea (NRC, 1977).

Humans

Traditionally, niacin deficiency in humans has been equated with pellagra. Symptoms of deficiency can be considered under three headings: (1) skin changes; (2) lesions of the mucous membranes of the mouth, tongue, stomach, and intestinal tract; and (3) changes of nervous origin.

The earliest symptom of pellagra is inflammation and soreness of the mouth, followed by bilateral symmetrical erythema on all parts of the body exposed to sunlight. Therefore, common sites are the extensor surfaces of the extremities, face, and neck (Fig. 8.8). The lesions are also found at sites of constant irritation, such as under the breast, scrotum, axilla, and perineum. A characteristic feature of these photosensitive lesions is their clear-cut demarcation from the adjoining, unaffected parts. The appearance of the dermatosis varies with the severity of the disease and from patient to patient.

Gastrointestinal symptoms often include glossitis and stomatitis, and the tongue has a characteristic swollen and beefy-red appearance. There is also anorexia, abdominal discomfort, and diarrhea. A burning

372

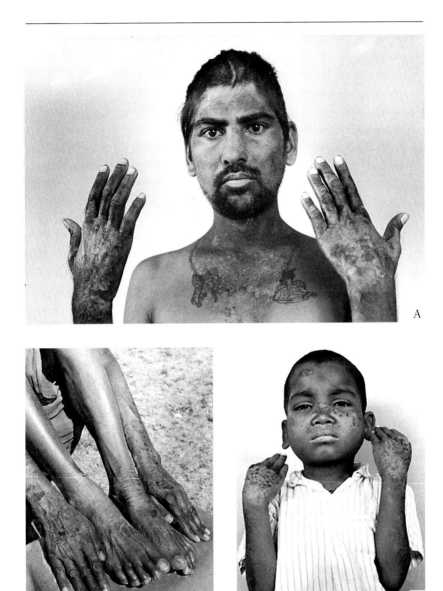

Fig. 8.8 Niacin deficiency: typical dermal lesions associated with pellagra. Dermatitis is severe when sunlight reacts with exposed skin. (A) Dermal lesions around neck have been referred to as Casal's necklace. (B) Affected hands and feet of a pellagrin. (C) Affected hands of a child. (Courtesy of V. Ramadus Murthy, National Institute of Nutrition, Jamasi-Osmania, Hyderabad, India.)

or raw sensation of the mouth, stomach, and rectum has been described. Angular stomatitis, cheilosis, atrophy of the lingual papillae, and glossitis are commonly seen. However, it is not known whether these are manifestations of niacin deficiency or are due to the associated deficiency of riboflavin and other members of the vitamin B-complex group.

Early mental symptoms include lassitude, lack of ambition, apprehension, depression, morbid fears, and memory loss, and these may be succeeded by disorientation, confusion, hysteria, and sometimes maniacal outbursts. More general symptoms, such as headache, irritability, inability to concentrate, and apathy, may also occur. Insomnia is a very common complaint. Various psychoses, such as manic-depressive syndromes, severe paranoia, and hallucinations, may necessitate confinement in a psychiatric institution. A considerable percentage of the patients in such institutions have been reported to be pellagrins, which bears testimony to the serious nature of the mental changes that occur (Gopalan and Rao, 1978).

As with deficiencies of the other B vitamins, pellagra often accompanies poverty, chronic alcoholism, dietary peculiarities, fever, hyperthyroidism, pregnancy, and the stress of injury or surgical procedures. Its incidence is much greater during the spring than any other season. In the advanced stages, pellagra can be diagnosed by the classic "three D's"— dermatitis, diarrhea, and dementia (death being the "fourth D"). Recognition of the disease in an early stage must depend on reliable medical and dietary history and thorough physical examination.

Pellagra has been endemic in certain areas of Italy, Spain, Romania, Egypt, and the southeastern United States. However, it has almost disappeared from industrialized countries except for its occurrence in some alcoholics. Hereditary disorders of schizophrenia and Hartnup disease involve impaired niacin function and are treated with high doses of the vitamin. Prolonged treatment with isoniazid also may lead to niacin deficiency by competition of the drug with pyridoxal phosphate, a coenzyme required in the tryptophan-to-niacin pathway. As mentioned earlier, pellagra has been considered a disease of the corn-eating population and has practically disappeared from all affluent societies. It is still encountered in parts of China, among the Bantus of South Africa, in the Middle East, in Yugoslavia, and in the corn-eating population of India (Gopalan and Rao, 1978).

Poverty and resulting diet selection can greatly influence incidence of pellagra. The social and economic upheaval of the U.S. Civil War (1860–1865) led to a corn-based diet for large sections of the population, and it was not until the United States entered World War II that increasing employment and a rise in the general standard of living solved the dietary problem. When cotton prices were high, more money was available to buy foods that prevent pellagra (e.g., animal products) versus subsisting on low-cost corn products. Pellagra was unknown in southern Africa until the outbreak of rinderpest in 1897, which led to widespread death of cattle and a major change in the dietary habits of the Bantu. From being a meat-eating and milk-drinking community they became, and have remained, largely maize eaters, and pellagra continues to be a major problem of public health nutrition in South Africa.

It had been accepted that the low tryptophan and unavailable niacin in corn was responsible for pellagra (see Natural Sources). However, identification of pellagra in populations subsisting on sorghum, a millet in which niacin is not so low or biologically unavailable, raised serious doubts regarding this concept (Gopalan, 1969). Pellagra is endemic among the poor communities of India where the millet *Sorghum vulgare* is the staple food. The effect of a high intake of leucine, and possibly an isoleucine-leucine imbalance, was suggested as causing pellagra in sorghum-eating as well as corn-eating populations (Gopalan, 1969). Later studies, however, showed conclusively that excess leucine does not cause pellagra, nor does it impact the metabolism of tryptophan to niacin (Manson and Carpenter, 1978; Lowry and Baker, 1989). One study indicated that concomitant vitamin B_6 deficiency, either primary or brought about by leucine toxicity, may also have an important role (Rao et al., 1975). Because iron is required by two enzymes in the tryptophan-to-niacin pathway, pellagra in populations having endemic anemia may be due not only to inadequate intake of bioavailable niacin but also to inadequate intakes of bioavailable iron (Oduho et al., 1994).

Assessment of Status

A functional biochemical test for assessing body reserves has had only limited success. Determination of blood serum levels of niacin or niacin-dependent enzymes has not proved to be a reliable or acceptable method for evaluating niacin status. However, although NAD in liver was not affected in niacin-deficient quail, the level of pectoral muscle NAD was markedly reduced (Park et al., 1991). In humans, erythrocyte NAD may serve as a sensitive indicator for the assessment of niacin status (Fu et al., 1989). Biochemical assessment of niacin nutritional status is usually based on measurement of urinary metabolites. Measurement of niacin metabolites would be dependent on species, as marked differences in type of metabolites exist among species (see Metabolism). In humans and most monogastric species, niacin is excreted largely as methylated products. Excreted niacin metabolites in a healthy, well-nourished adult human include 4 to 6 mg of N'-methylnicotinamide. One of the testing procedures widely used in human population surveys is the estimation of urinary excretion of N'-methylnicotinamide during a period of 4 to 5 hours after administering a test dose of 50 mg of niacinamide (Narasinga Rao and Gopalan, 1984).

SUPPLEMENTATION

Niacin supplementation must be considered as a possibility for all classes of livestock and in particular in swine and poultry diets. Much of the niacin in common feeds (plant sources) is in a bound form that is not available to animals (see Natural Sources). Although the bioavailability of niacin is suggested to be 100% in soybean meal, it is likely zero in wheat and sorghum and varies from 0 to 30% in corn. In formulating swine and poultry diets, therefore, niacin values for corn and other cereal grains and their by-product feeds should be almost disregarded. It is best to assume that these feeds provide no available niacin for the pig or chick (Cunha, 1982).

The pig and chick and most species can use the essential amino acid tryptophan to synthesize niacin, but they cannot convert niacin back to tryptophan. Therefore, if a diet contains enough niacin, the tryptophan is not depleted for niacin synthesis. Most monogastric diets do not contain large excesses of tryptophan, particularly diets based on corn. Tryptophan concentrations not only are low in corn, but are largely unavailable. Therefore, one should make sure that monogastric diets are adequate in niacin since it is very inexpensive, and it would be poor economics to satisfy niacin needs with the more expensive tryptophan (Cunha, 1982). Also, some species, such as the cat, mink, and fish, apparently lack the ability to convert tryptophan to niacin.

The most critical time for supplementation is during early growth, when requirements are the highest (Table 8.3). Evidence is lacking regarding the need to supplement practical diets of mature poultry (Scott et al., 1982) and swine (Ivers et al., 1993) with niacin. However, niacin requirements as recommended by the National Research Council for young swine and poultry may be insufficient. Cunha for swine and Scott for poultry have recommended higher niacin requirements as a reasonable safety factor (Cunha, 1982). Higher niacin levels are mainly recommended when subclinical disease level, stress, and higher production rates are encountered. For poultry, recommended levels are generally 12 to 25% higher than the NRC recommendations. Increased swine requirements are approximately double those of the NRC for growing swine under stressful conditions, with breeding animals needing a four-fold increase (Cunha, 1982). Producers must judge their own livestock operations in relation to stress conditions for animals and other factors that may require higher niacin supplementation levels.

Addition of niacin to a milk replacer is recommended at a level of 2.6 ppm because of lack of synthesis in the undeveloped rumen. Inclusion in diets of growing heifers cannot be justified by evidence (Schultz, 1983).

Supplementation of niacin for ruminants can be beneficial. If tryptophan is present in large amounts, the microorganisms can probably synthesize considerable niacin. However, in urea diets the microbes do not have enough tryptophan to draw upon and hence use exogenous sources of niacin. Supplementation appears to be of greatest benefit to stressed animals, such as beef cattle entering the feedlot, dairy cows immediately postpartum, and cows suffering from subclinical ketosis. Stressed sheep with ruminal acidosis had decreased plasma nicotinic acid from 7.01 to 0.42 µg/ml within 24 hours (Basoglu et al., 1993). Recommended supplemental niacin levels are estimated to be 50 to 100 ppm niacin for finishing beef cattle and 3 to 12 g daily for milking cows.

Niacin appears to be effective in enhancing acclimation and adaptation to urea-supplemented diets. Minimal amounts of niacin supplied via microbial synthesis and diet become adequate in the later stages of the feedlot period, whereas earlier they were insufficient to meet demands. The large response during the feedlot adaptation phase indicates that supplemental niacin assists in overcoming shipping stress and allows for a more rapid adjustment to feedlot conditions and changing diets. Summaries of beef cattle studies over the total feeding period (73 to 176 days) indicate that 50 to 100 ppm of niacin is more effective than higher levels of 150, 250, or 500 ppm with respect to gain.

Brent and Bartley (1984) found that a higher milk production response from niacin was greater for early postpartum cows than for those in midlactation. Niacin response in early postpartum cows might be partially explained via reduction in ketosis. Di Costanzo et al. (1997) reported that niacin did not significantly increase milk production but decreased skin temperatures during periods of mild or severe heat stress.

Although general results of field experiments on niacin supplementation for lactating cows are positive for both milk production and fat test, the somewhat erratic results and the occasional lack of statistical significance make it difficult to give an unqualified recommendation to include niacin in diets of all dairy cows in early lactation. However,

377

enough positive evidence is available to recommend it for herds with above-average incidence of ketosis and fat cow problems. For individual cows with positive tests indicating subclinical ketosis, a level of 12 g per day is recommended. When used as a general diet additive, a level of 6 g per day is suggested, starting 2 weeks before calving. This recommendation to start before calving is based on the evidence that it inhibits lipid mobilization and thus may prevent abnormal deposition of fat in the liver at calving time. Most evidence suggests that feeding be continued 8 to 12 weeks after calving (Schultz, 1983).

Niacin supplementation is important for human populations that depend primarily on corn and sorghum in their diets. Likewise, pellagra was found in war-torn nations of the Sahel and southeastern parts of Africa. Although the condition is largely eliminated in the more technologically advanced countries, it still is found as an undiagnosed complication of malnutrition in today's urban society (Bosco, 1980). Niacin deficiency is usually found in people with chronically bad dietary habits; people who consume low-calorie, low-protein, high-fat, and high-carbohydrate diets; alcoholics; and people with diseases that interfere with digestion and absorption. A large amount of wine (750 ml) markedly impairs liver protein metabolism, which is counteracted with supplemental nicotinamide (Volpi et al., 1997). Also, some individuals with metabolic defects (e.g., Hartnup disease, deviation of niacin-tryptophan metabolism) require supplemental niacin at levels higher than normally consumed in typical foods. Cases of pellagra were reported on isoniazid therapy, which responded to combined vitamin B_6 and niacin treatment (DiLorenzo, 1967).

Pharmacological effects from massive supplemental doses of niacin have been reported in humans. Large doses of nicotinic acid (but not the amide) produce vascular dilatation or "flushing," with accompanying sensation of burning of the face and hands. Large doses of nicotinic acid (3 g or more per day) administered orally result in a significant reduction of serum cholesterol and β-lipoprotein cholesterol (Narasinga Rao and Gopalan, 1984; Basu and Mann, 1997). The administration of nicotinic acid in the Coronary Drug Project was associated with a reduction in recurrent myocardial infarctions and in long-term total mortality (Canner et al., 1986). Nicotinic acid given as a drug in doses of 1.5 to 3 g/day decreased concentrations of total and low-density lipoprotein cholesterol and increased concentrations of high-density lipoprotein cholesterol. Niacin has also been used in treatment of schizophrenia. However, according to a review of all the relevant individual controlled studies, there is no evidence that nicotinic acid is an antipsychotic agent (Petrie and Ban, 1975). Nicotinamide has been shown to have a positive role in the reduction of insulin-dependent diabetes mellitus (Behme, 1995). Studies with rats revealed that pharmacological levels of niacin interfered with methionine metabolism, which was counteracted with simultaneous administration of niacin and vitamin B_6 (Basu and Mann, 1997). Beneficial effects of pharmacological doses of niacin must be weighed against the long-term effects of high doses, including laboratory evidence of diabetes, hepatic injury, and activation of peptic ulcer.

Niacin is supplied in two forms—niacinamide and nicotinic acid—both of which provide available niacin. In studies with chicks, relative to nicotinic acid used as a standard (100%), nicotinamide activity was 124%. Nicotinamide in NAD was utilized with an efficiency of 95% relative to nicotinamide per se (Oduho and Baker, 1993). Crystalline products are used in feeds and pharmaceuticals, and dry dilutions in feeds. An additional source of supplemental niacin is from the vitamin K supplement menadione nicotinamide bisulfite (MNB). Results with chicks suggest that MNB is fully effective as a source of vitamin K and niacin activity (Oduho et al., 1993).

Commercially produced niacin is quite stable compared to most other vitamins. Synthetic niacin and the amide were found to be stable in premixes with or without minerals for 3 months (Verbeeck, 1975). Gadient (1986) reported niacin to be insensitive to heat, oxygen, moisture, and light. The retention of niacin activity in pelleted feeds after 3 months at room temperature should be 95 to 100% as a general rule. One report demonstrated 98% retention of niacin after 6 months in a vitamin premix; however, retention was only 58% when the premix contained choline and trace minerals (Coelho, 1991).

TOXICITY

Harmful effects of niacin occur at levels far in excess of requirements. Nonruminant animals can tolerate oral exposures of at least 10 to 20 times their normal requirements. Limited research indicates that nicotinic acid and nicotinamide are toxic at dietary intakes greater than about 350 mg/kg of body weight per day (NRC, 1987). Short-term intravenous administration of niacin at a dose of 2.5 g/kg was needed before 50% of test mice died. Respective values for subcutaneous and oral routes of administration were 2.8 and 4.5 g/kg in mice. Nicotinamide is two to three times more toxic than the free acid (Waterman, 1978).

High levels of nicotinic acid, such as 3 g/day in humans, can cause vasodilation, itching, heat sensation, nausea, vomiting, headache, and occasional skin lesions. The substance can also cause more serious problems, including abnormally high blood sugar levels, elevated uric acid levels (which people with gout must avoid), peptic ulcers, and liver damage. Niacin therapy was discontinued in eight children because of flushing, abdominal pain, vomiting, headache, or elevated serum aminotransferase levels. It is suggested that although niacin treatment for children is efficacious, adverse effects are common (Colletti et al., 1993). In dogs, oral administration of 2 g of nicotinic acid per day (133 to 145 mg/kg of body weight) produced bloody feces in a few dogs, followed by convulsions and death (NRC, 1987).

■ REFERENCES

Anonymous (1987). *Nutr. Rev. 45*(5), 142.
Baker, D. H., Allen, N. K., and Kleiss, A. J. (1973). *J. Anim. Sci. 36,* 299.
Basoglu, A., Turgut, K., Eksen, M., Tras, B., Maden, M., Ok, M., Bas, A. L., and Kececi, T. (1993) *Vet. Fakultesi. Dergisi 2,* 31.
Basu, T. K., and Mann, S. (1997). *J. Nutr. 127,* 117.
Bechgaard, H., and Jespersen, S. (1977). *J. Pharm. Sci. 66,* 871.
Behme, M. T. (1995). *Nutr. Rev. 53,* 137.
Bosco, D. (1980). The People's Guide to Vitamins and Minerals from A to Zinc. Beaverbooks, Ltd., Ontario, Canada.
Brent, B. E., and Bartley, E. E. (1984). *J. Anim. Sci. 59,* 813.
Briggs, G. M., Hill, E. G., and Canfield, T. H. (1953). *Poult. Sci. 32,* 678.
Byers, F. M. (1979). *Anim. Nutr. Health, 35,* 20.
Byers, F. M. (1981). *Anim. Nutr. Health 36,* 36.
Canner, P. L., Berge, K. G., and Wenger, N. K. (1986). *J. Am. Cell. Cardiol. 8,* 1245.
Carpenter, K. J., Schelstraete, M., Vilicich, V. C., and Wall, J. S. (1988). *J. Nutr. 118,* 165.
Carroll, F. D., Gross, H., and Howell, C. E. (1949). *J. Anim. Sci. 8,* 290.
Carson, D. A., Seto, S., and Wasson, D. B. (1987). *J. Immunol. 138,* 1904.
Carter, E. G. A., and Carpenter, K. J. (1982). *J. Nutr. 112,* 2091.
Cervantes, A., Smith, T. R., and Young, J. W. (1996). *J. Dairy Sci. 79,* 105.
Chen, B. J., and Austic, R. E. (1989). *Poult. Sci. 68(Suppl. 1),* 27(Abstr.).
Coelho, M. B. (1991). Vitamin Stability in Premixes and Feeds: A Practical Approach, p. 56. BASF Technical Symposium, Bloomington, Minnesota.
Colletti, R. B., Neufeld, E. J., Roff, N. K., McAuliffe, T. L., Baker, A. L., and Newburger, J. W. (1993). *Pediatrics 92,* 78.
Cunha, T. J. (1977). Swine Feeding and Nutrition. Academic Press, Inc., New York.
Cunha, T. J. (1982). Niacin in Animal Feeding and Nutrition. National Feed Ingredients Association (NFIA), Fairlawn, New Jersey.
Darby, W. J., McNutt, K. W., and Todhunter, E. N. (1975). *Nutr. Rev. 33,* 289.
Di Costanzo, A., Spain, J. N., and Spiers, D. E. (1997). *J. Dairy Sci. 80,* 1200.

DiLorenzo, P. A. (1967). *Acta Dermatol. Venereol. 47*, 318.

DiLorenzo, R. N. (1972). Studies on the Genetic Variation in Tryptophan-Nicotinic Acid Conversion in Chicks. Ph.D. Dissertation, Cornell Univ., Ithaca, New York.

Dittrich, A., Suss, R., and Geissler, C. (1993). *In* Symposium, Vitamine und weitere Zusatzstoffe bei Mensch und Tier: 4, G. Flachowsky and R. Schubert (eds.), p. 176. Jena, Germany.

Driver, L. S., Grummer, R. R., and Schultz, L. H. (1990). *J. Dairy Sci. 73*, 463.

Emery, R. S., Burg, N., Braur, L. D., and Blank, G. N. (1964). *J. Dairy Sci. 47*, 1074.

Ensminger, M. E., Colby, R. W., and Cunha, T. J. (1951). Wash. Agric. Exp. Stn. Circ. 134, Pullman, Washington.

Erickson, P. S., Murphy, M. R., McSweeney, C. S., and Trusk, A. M. (1991). *J. Dairy Sci. 74*, 3492.

Flachowsky, G., Lober, U., Ast, H., Wolfram, D., and Matlhey, M. (1988). *Wiss. Z. Karl-Marx-Univ. Leipzig Math.-Naturwiss R. 37*, 55.

Fronk, T. J., and Schultz, L. H. (1979). *J. Dairy Sci. 62*, 1804.

Fu, C. S., Swendseid, M. E., Jacob, R. A., and McKee, R. W. (1989). *J. Nutr. 119*, 1949.

Gadient, M. (1986). *In* Proc. Maryland Nutrition Conference for Feed Manufacturers, p. 73. College Park, Maryland.

Ghosh, H. P., Sarkar, P. K., and Guha, B. C. (1963). *J. Nutr. 79*, 451.

Gopalan, C. (1969). *Lancet 1 (7587)*, 197.

Gopalan, C., and Rao, K. S. J. (1978). *In* Handbook Series in Nutrition and Food, Section E: Nutritional Disorders Volume 3 (M. Rechcigl Jr., ed.), p. 23. CRC Press, Inc.,West Palm Beach, Florida.

Halvorsen, K., and Halvorsen, S. (1963). *Pediatrics 31*, 29.

Hankes, L. V. (1984). *In* Handbook of Vitamins (L. J. Machlin, ed.), p. 329. Marcel Dekker, New York.

Haralambie, G. (1976). *Nutr. Metab. 20*, 1.

Harris, H. F. (1919). Pellagra. MacMillan, New York.

Henderson, L. M., and Gross, C. J. (1979). *J. Nutr. 109*, 654.

Hoffmann-La Roche (1994). Vitamin Nutrition for Ruminants, RCD 8361/191. Hoffmann-La Roche Inc., Nutley, New Jersey.

Hopper, J. H., and Johnson, B. C. (1955). *J. Nutr. 56*, 303.

Horner, J. L., Coppock, C. E., Schelling, G. T., Labore, J. M., and Nave, D. H. (1986). *J. Dairy Sci. 69*, 3087.

Hutjens, M. F. (1990). *In* Proc. 1990 Natl. Feed Ingred. Assoc. Nutr. Inst.: Developments in Vitamin Nutrition and Health Applications. National Feed Ingredients Association (NIFA), Des Moines, Iowa.

Ikeda, M., Tsuji, H., Nakamura, S., Ichiyama, A., Nishizuka, Y., and Hayaishi, O. (1965). *J. Biol. Chem. 240*, 1395.

Ivers, D. J., Rodhouse, S. L., Ellerseick, M. R., and Veum, T. L. (1993). *J. Anim. Sci. 71*, 651.

Ivers, D. J., and Veum, T. L. (1993). *J. Anim. Sci. 71*, 3383.

Jackson, M. (1992). Feeding Layers: Nutritional Considerations. Multi-State Poultry Meeting, Indianapolis, Indiana.

Jaster, E. H., Hartwell, G. F., and Hutjens, M. F. (1983). *J. Dairy Sci. 66*, 1046.

Klippel, M., Mockel, P., and Flachowsky, G. (1993). *In* Symposium Vitamine und weitere Zusatzstoffe bei Mensch und Tier: 4, G. Flachowsky and R. Schubert (eds.), p. 194. Jena, Germany.

Kodicek, E., Ashby, D. R., Muller, M., and Carpenter, K. J. (1974). *Proc. Nutr. Soc. 33*, 105A.

Lanham, J. K., Coppock, C. E., Brooks, K. N., Wilks, D. L., and Horner, J. L. (1992). *J. Dairy Sci. 75*, 184.

Leeson, S., Caston, L. J., and Summers, J. D. (1991). *Poult. Sci. 70*, 1231.

Loosli, J. K. (1991). *In* Handbook of Animal Science (P.A. Putnam, ed.), Academic Press, San Diego.

Lowry, K. R., and Baker, D. H. (1989). *FASEB J. 3*, A666(Abstr.).

Luce, W. G., Peo, E. R., and Hudman, D. B. (1967). *J. Anim. Sci. 26*, 76.

Luecke, R. W., McMillen, W. N., Thorp Jr., F., and Tull, C. (1948). *J. Nutr. 36*, 417.

Manson, J. A., and Carpenter, K. J. (1978). *J. Nutr. 108*, 1883.

Mason, J. B., Gibson, N., and Kodicek, E. (1973). *Br. J. Nutr. 30*, 297.

McCollum, E. V. (1957) *In* A History of Nutrition, p. 302. Riverside Press, Cambridge, Massachusetts.

Mertz, W. (1975). *Nutr. Rev. 33*, 129.

Mizwicki, K.L., Owens, F. N., Issacson, H. R., and Shockey, B. (1975). *J. Anim. Sci. 41*, 411(Abstr.).

Narasinga Rao, B. S., and Gopalan, C. (1984). *In* Nutrition Reviews, Present Knowledge in Nutrition (R. E. Olson, ed.), p. 318. The Nutrition Foundation, Inc., Washington, D.C.

Nisselbaum, J. S., and Green, S. (1969). *Anal. Biochem. 27*, 212.

NRC. Nutrient Requirements of Domestic Animals. National Academy of Sciences-National Research Council, Washington, D.C.
(1977). Nutrient Requirements of Rabbits, 2nd Ed.
(1978). Nutrient Requirements of Nonhuman Primates.
(1981). Nutrient Requirements of Goats.
(1982a). Nutrient Requirements of Mink and Foxes.
(1985a). Nutrient Requirements of Dogs, 2nd Ed.
(1985b). Nutrient Requirements of Sheep, 5th Ed.
(1986). Nutrient Requirements of Cats, 3rd Ed.
(1989a). Nutrient Requirements of Dairy Cattle, 6th Ed.
(1989b). Nutrient Requirements of Horses, 5th Ed.
(1993). Nutrient Requirements of Fish.
(1994). Nutrient Requirements of Poultry, 9th Ed.
(1995). Nutrient Requirements of Laboratory Animals.
(1996). Nutrient Requirements of Beef Cattle, 7th Ed.
(1998). Nutrient Requirements of Swine, 10th Ed.

NRC. (1982b). United States-Canadian Tables of Feed Composition, 3rd Ed. National Academy of Sciences-National Research Council, Washington, D.C.

NRC. (1987). Vitamin Tolerance of Animals. National Academy of Sciences-National Research Council, Washington, D.C.

Oduho, G. W., and Baker, D. H. (1993). *J. Nutr. 123*, 2201.

Oduho, G. W., Chung, T. K., and Baker, D. H. (1993). *J. Nutr. 123*, 737.

Oduho, G. W., Han, Y., and Baker, D. H. (1994). *J. Nutr. 124*, 444.

Olentine, C. (1984). *Feed Manage. 35*(4), 18.

Park, I. K., Shin, S., and Marquardt, R. R. (1991). *Int. J. Biochem. 23*(10), 1005.

Petrie, W. M., and Ban, T. A. (1975). *Drugs 30*, 58.

Porter, J. W. G. (1961). *In* Digestive Physiology and Nutrition of the Ruminant (D. Lewis, ed.), p. 226. Butterworth, London.

Rao, S. B., Raghuram, T. C., and Krishnaswamy, K. (1975). *Nutr. Metab. 18*, 318.

Rawling, J. M., Jackson, M., Driscoll, E. R., and Kirland, J. B. (1994). *J. Nutr. 124*, 1547.

RDA. (1989). Recommended Dietary Allowances, 10th Ed., National Academy of Sciences-National Research Council, Washington, D.C.

Rose, D. P., and Braidman, I. P. (1971). *Am. J. Clin. Nutr. 24*, 673.

Ruiz, N., and Harms, R. H. (1990a). *Poult. Sci. 69*, 433.

Ruiz, N., and Harms, R. H. (1990b). *Poult. Sci. 69*, 2231.

Ruiz, N., and Harms, R. H. (1990c). *Poult. Sci. 69*, 446.

Schultz, L. H. (1983). *In* Proceedings Eighteenth Annual Pacific Northwest Animal Nutrition Conference p. 69. Oregon State Univ., Corvallis, Oregon.

Scott, N. L., Nesheim, M. C., and Young, R. J. (1982). Nutrition of the Chicken, p. 119. Scott, Ithaca, New York.

Shiau, S. Y., and Suen, G. S. (1992). *J. Nutr. 122*, 2030.

Shields, D. R., and Perry, T. W. (1982). Effect of Supplemental Niacin on Protein Utilization by Lambs National Feed Ingredients Association (NFIA), Fairlawn, New Jersey.

Stein, J., Daniel, H., Whang, E., Wenzel, U., Han, A., and Rehner, G. (1994). *J. Nutr. 124*, 61.

Stocchi, V., Cucchiarini, L., Canestrari, F., Piacentini, M., and Fornaini, G. (1987). *Anal. Biochem. 167*, 181.

Vague, P., Vialettes, B., Lassman-Vague, V., and Vallo, J. (1987). *Lancet 1 (8533)*, 619.

Verbeeck, J. (1975). *Feedstuffs 47*(36), 4.

Volpi, E., Lucidi, P., Cruciani, G., Monarchia, F., Reboldi, G., Brunetti, P., Bolli, G.B., and De Feo, P. (1997). *J. Nutr. 127*, 2199.

Wall, J. S., and Carpenter, K. J. (1988). *Food Technol. 42*(10), 198.

Waterman, R. A. (1978). *In* Handbook Series in Nutrition and Food, Section E: Nutritional Disorders Volume 1, (M. Rechcigl Jr., ed.), p. 29, CRC Press, Inc., West Palm Beach, Florida.

Wertz, A. W., Lojkin, M. E., Bouchard, B. S., and Derby, M. B. (1958). *J. Nutr. 64*, 339.

Wintrobe, M. M., Stein, H. J., Follis, R. H., and Humphreys, S. (1945). *J. Nutr. 30*, 395.

Zhang, J. Z., Henning, S. M., and Swendseid, M. E. (1993). *J. Nutr. 123*, 1349.

VITAMIN B₆

INTRODUCTION

Vitamin B_6 refers to a group of three compounds: pyridoxol (pyridoxine), pyridoxal, and pyridoxamine. Their activities are equivalent in animals but not in various microorganisms. Vitamin B_6 acts as a component of many enzymes that are involved in the metabolism of proteins, fats, and carbohydrates. The vitamin is particularly involved in various aspects of protein metabolism.

Common feed ingredients for typical poultry and swine diets contain adequate amounts of vitamin B_6. Although such conditions are rare, vitamin B_6 can be deficient for poultry and swine in a few situations. Although animal diets are generally adequate in vitamin B_6, there is evidence of low vitamin B_6 status in the human population, especially in young and pregnant or lactating women. Vitamin B_6 deficiency in humans may be induced by long-term drug therapy, increased requirements resulting from malignancies, and numerous disease conditions.

HISTORY

The early history of vitamin B_6 has been summarized by McCollum (1957), Snell (1986), and Loosli (1991). Clinical signs of what was later to be known as vitamin B_6 deficiency were described in 1926 by Goldberger and Lillie in their attempts to produce pellagra in experimental animals. Rats developed a severe dermatitis called acrodynia (painful extremities). This dermatitis was also referred to as rat pellagra and was characterized by skin lesions, especially on the limbs and trunk, and by swelling of the paws and ears. These signs were easily distinguished from

385

those of riboflavin. In 1934 György first recognized vitamin B_6 as a distinct vitamin and showed that it prevented rat acrodynia and that the condition was not prevented by vitamin B_1 (thiamin), vitamin B_2 (riboflavin), or vitamin B_3 (niacin). Two years later Lepkowsky and associates showed the vitamin to be an essential nutrient for chickens.

Isolation of the vitamin in crystalline form was accomplished independently in five different laboratories in 1938. The vitamin was first isolated from rice bran and yeast. The structure of the vitamin was first explained by Kuhn and coworkers, who named it "adermin," because it was believed that skin dermatitis was the only clinical sign of the deficiency. The term was discarded when evidence accumulated for nondermal clinical signs for the vitamin deficiency. In view of the chemical structure of the compound (pyridine structure), György proposed pyridoxine as the vitamin name, and this proposal was widely adopted. However, by 1945 subsequent bacterial studies identified two additional compounds—pyridoxal and pyridoxamine. Thus, by official action of the Society of Biological Chemists and the American Institute of Nutrition, the original term B_6 became the approved name for this vitamin.

In 1939 chemical synthesis was accomplished by two independent laboratories. Therefore, only 5 years elapsed between the discovery of the vitamin and its chemical synthesis. The speed of isolation indicates the intense efforts expended in the mid-1930s to identify new vitamins. The principal coenzyme form of vitamin B_6 pyridoxal 5′phosphate (originally called codecarboxylase) was discovered in bacteria by Umbreit in 1944.

CHEMICAL STRUCTURE, PROPERTIES, AND ANTAGONISTS

Vitamin B_6 is a relatively simple compound with three substituted pyridine derivatives that differ only in functional group in the 4-position: alcohol (pyridoxine or pyridoxol), aldehyde pyridoxal, and amine pyridoxamine (Fig. 9.1). Pyridoxine is the predominant form in plants, whereas pyridoxal and pyridoxamine are the forms generally found in animal products. These three forms have equal activity when administered parenterally to animals but are not equivalent when administered to various microorganisms. Two additional vitamin B_6 forms found in foods are the coenzyme forms of pyridoxal phosphate (PLP) and pyridoxamine phosphate. Various forms of vitamin B_6 found in animal tissues are interconvertible, with vitamin B_6 metabolically active mainly as PLP and to a lesser degree as pyridoxamine phosphate.

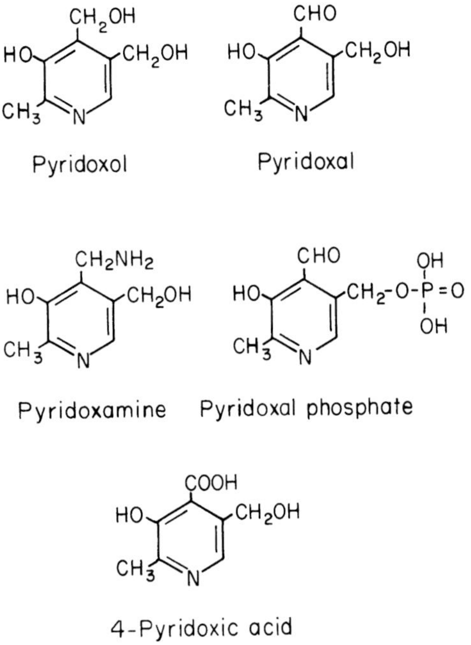

Pyridoxol

Pyridoxal

Pyridoxamine   Pyridoxal phosphate

4-Pyridoxic acid

Fig. 9.1 Structural formulas of pyridoxol, pyridoxal, pyridoxamine, pyridoxal phosphate, and 4-pyridoxic acid.

Various forms of vitamin B$_6$ can be destroyed by heat and alkali, and exposure to light, especially in neutral or alkaline media, is highly destructive. Forms of vitamin B$_6$ are colorless crystals soluble in water and alcohol as both free bases and commonly available hydrochlorides. Commercial preparation of vitamin B$_6$ is almost exclusively the hydrochloride salt of the alcohol form, pyridoxine hydrochloride.

Several vitamin B$_6$ antagonists exist that either compete for reactive sites of apoenzymes or react with PLP to form inactive compounds. The majority of natural antagonists are substituted hydrazines and hydroxylamines, that is, substances that form hydrozones or oximes with pyridoxal or PLP. Antagonists frequently react with pyridoxal kinase, thus preventing the phosphorylated form of the vitamin. Deoxypyridoxine is a powerful antagonist to vitamin B$_6$ and is commonly employed in experiments to accelerate the vitamin deficiency. Fortunately, this antivitamin does not occur in nature. A particularly important binding compound of vitamin B$_6$ is isonicotinic acid hydrazide (isoniazid), which is used in tuberculosis treatment. Isoniazid is a strong inhibitor of pyridoxal kinase and results in anemia in humans, probably by inhibiting the synthesis of δ-aminolevulinic acid and thus of heme. Isoniazid has been extensively used in experiments designed to clarify functions of various enzymes that are dependent on PLP (Price et al., 1957).

The antihypertensive drugs thiosemicarbizide and hydralazine have also been shown to interfere with vitamin B_6 usage. Penicillamine, which is used to remove body copper in copper poisoning and Wilson's disease, is also known to complex PLP. L-Dopa, an antiparkinsonism drug, has been shown to be a vitamin B_6 antagonist. Other drugs also form thiazalidine compounds or inhibit pyridoxine kinase, the enzyme that is needed in formation of PLP (Rothschild, 1982). Oral contraceptives (estrogen component) were shown to be antagonistic to vitamin B_6, resulting in deficiency of the vitamin (Salkeld et al., 1973). Presence of a vitamin B_6 antagonist in flax (linseed oil meal) is of particular interest to animal nutritionists. This substance was identified in 1967 as hydrazic acid and was found to have antibiotic properties (Parsons and Klostermann, 1967). Pesticides (e.g., carbaryl, propoxur, or thiram) can be antagonistic to vitamin B_6. Feeding a diet enriched with vitamin B_6 prevented disturbances in the active transport of methionine in rats intoxicated with pesticides (Witkowska et al., 1992). The response of sensitive persons to administration of large doses of monosodium glutamate ("Chinese restaurant syndrome") was eliminated by vitamin B_6 treatment (Folkers et al., 1981), indicating an antagonist to the vitamin. High doses (more than 2 g) of niacin have been used as lipid-lowering agents for humans. Niacin at these large dosages was found to interfere with vitamin B status (Basu and Mann, 1997).

ANALYTICAL PROCEDURES

Methods of analysis for vitamin B_6 must be capable of detecting all forms of the vitamin (Gregory, 1988). In biological systems the vitamin is usually bound to protein, and therefore extraction procedures are required. Bioassay using rat or chick growth has the advantage over microbiological procedures in that it measures all biologically active forms and does not require extraction of bound forms of the vitamin. However, rat and chick bioassay methods are expensive and time-consuming and have been largely replaced by other techniques.

The standard method for quantitation of vitamin B_6 in foods is microbiological assay. *Saccharomyces uvarum* (formerly *S. carlsbergensis*) is the organism commonly used in the microbiological method. This yeast organism, along with *Streptococcus faecalis* and *Lactobacillus casei,* makes it possible to differentiate between alcohol, amine, and aldehyde vitamin forms. Disadvantages in microbiological methods include the following: (1) The procedure is time consuming, (2) variability exists in growth response of various microorganisms to the vitamin, (3) microorganisms can mutate, (4) microbiologically unavailable complexes of the vitamin may be formed, and (5) microbial growth may be retarded by substances in the food extract.

Gas-liquid chromatography is used to analyze vitamin B$_6$, but mainly in pure standards. Combinations of chromatographic separation methods with fluorometric determinations may be used successfully for enriched foods and feeds. Vanderslice et al. (1980) developed a high-pressure liquid chromatography (HPLC) anion-exchange system that quantitatively separated phosphorylated and unphosphorylated forms of vitamin B$_6$ in pork, hamburger, carp, and nonfat dry milk. Methods using HPLC with fluorometric detection can serve as a simple and reliable method for the analysis of vitamin B$_6$ in foods and feeds (Van Schoonhoven et al., 1994).

METABOLISM

Digestion, Absorption, and Transport

Utilization of dietary vitamin B$_6$ by animals necessitates digestion and absorption of the five forms known to occur in foods: pyridoxine, pyridoxal, pyridoxamine, PLP, and pyridoxamine phosphate. Digestion would first involve splitting the vitamin, as it is bound to proteins of foods. Vitamin B$_6$ is absorbed mainly in the jejunum, but also in the ileum, by passive diffusion. Absorption from the colon is insignificant, even though colon microflora synthesize the vitamin. However, Durst et al. (1989) administered vitamin B$_6$ in the cecum to sows and concluded that the vitamin was absorbed at this location. Vitamin B$_6$ compounds are mainly absorbed from the diet in the dephosphorylated forms, but phosphorylated forms can be absorbed to a very limited extent (Mehansho et al., 1979). The small intestine is rich in alkaline phosphatases for the dephosphorylation reaction.

After absorption, B$_6$ compounds rapidly appear in liver, where they are mostly converted into PLP, considered to be the most active vitamin form in metabolism. Unlike PLP, pyridoxamine phosphate is involved only in several metabolic reactions. It is widely accepted that the synthesis of PLP and pyridoxamine phosphate from the three unphosphorylated forms is mediated by pyridoxal kinase and pyridoxamine phosphate (pyridoxine phosphate) oxidase. Pyridoxamine phosphate and PLP are also interconvertible through aminotransferases (formerly referred to as the transaminases). Sakurai et al. (1992) reported that a physiological dose of pyridoxamine was rapidly transformed to pyridoxal in the intestinal tissues and then released in the form of pyridoxal into the portal blood.

Both niacin (as the NADP-dependent enzyme) and riboflavin (as the flavoprotein pyridoxamine phosphate oxidase) are important for conversion of vitamin B_6 forms and phosphorylation reactions (Wada and Snell, 1961; Kodentsova et al., 1993). Vitamin B_6 is found in the blood largely as PLP, most of which is derived from the liver after metabolism by hepatic flavoenzymes. Pyridoxal and PLP found in circulation are associated primarily with plasma albumin and red cell hemoglobin (Mehansho and Henderson, 1980). Pyridoxal phosphate accounts for 60% of plasma vitamin B_6.

Pyridoxal crosses the human placenta readily in both directions (Delport et al., 1991; Schenker et al., 1992). Gradients of concentration between maternal and venous cord plasma were 1:5 for PLP (Zempleni et al., 1992). Alcohol inhibited the transport of pyridoxal from the maternal to fetal compartments by 42% (Schenker et al., 1992).

Storage

Only small quantities of vitamin B_6 are stored in the body. The vitamin is widely distributed in various tissues, mainly as PLP or pyridoxamine phosphate. Reports of PLP content of glycogen phosphorylase suggest that 90% or more of the vitamin B_6 present in muscle might be present in this single enzyme (Merrill and Burnhan, 1990). Because the muscle accounts for about 40% of body weight, and because the muscle contains more vitamin B_6 per gram than do other tissues (except kidney), muscle phosphorylase may account for as much as 70 to 80% of the total body store of the vitamin.

Excretion

When B_6 coenzymes are synthesized in excess of the binding capacity of B_6-dependent apoenzymes, they are dephosphorylated by alkaline phosphatase, with the resultant pyridoxal reutilized or oxidized to pyridoxic acid (Fig. 9.1) by aldehyde oxidase and/or NAD-dependent dehydrogenase. Pyridoxic acid is the major route for elimination of vitamin B_6, which is excreted in urine. Also, small quantities of pyridoxol, pyridoxal, and pyridoxamine, as well as their phosphorylated derivatives, are excreted into the urine (Rabinowitz and Snell, 1949; Merrill and Burnhan, 1990). Mahuren et al. (1991) suggested that 5-pyridoxic acid and its lactone account for 10 to 20% of urinary vitamin B_6 metabolites. Biliary excretion and enterohepatic circulation of vitamin B_6 probably play only a minor role in the overall economy of the vitamin (Lui et al.,

1983). Vitamin B$_6$ metabolism is altered in renal failure, as observed in rats exhibiting plasma PLP 43% lower than that of controls (Wei and Young, 1994).

FUNCTIONS

Vitamin B$_6$ in the form of PLP (also named codecarboxylase), and to a lesser degree pyridoxamine phosphate, plays an essential role in the interaction of amino acid, carbohydrate, and fatty acid metabolism and the energy-producing citric acid cycle. More than 60 enzymes are already known to depend on vitamin B$_6$ coenzymes. They typically bind the coenzyme tightly in a Schiff base linkage with the ε-amino group of an active-site lysine, and for most of the enzymes, the incoming substrate displaces the lysine to form a new Schiff base. This results in a strong electron sink adjacent to several of the bonds on the substrate and facilitates a variety of chemical reactions (Merrill and Burnhan, 1990). Pyridoxal phosphate functions in practically all reactions involved in amino acid metabolism, including transamination (aminotransferase), decarboxylation, deamination, and desulfhydration, and in the cleavage or synthesis of amino acids.

The largest group of the vitamin B$_6$-dependent enzymes are the transaminases, most of which use α-ketoglutarates as the amino group acceptor. Aminotransferases are involved in interconversions of a pair of amino acids into their corresponding keto acids; generally, these are α-amino and α-keto acids. For example, amino groups are transferred from glutamate to pyruvate with formation of α-ketoglutarate and alanine, or from aspartate to α-ketoglutarate, forming oxaloacetate and glutamate. Aminotransferases function in both amino acid biosynthesis (nonessential amino acids) and catabolism. Each aminotransferase is specific for a specified pair of amino and keto acids functioning as substrates, but is nonspecific for the other pair. The aminotransferases thus represent an important link between amino acid, carbohydrate, and fatty acid metabolism and the energy-producing citric acid cycle (Fig. 9.2).

Nonoxidative decarboxylation reactions also involve PLP as a coenzyme. Decarboxylases convert amino acids to biogenic amines, such as histamine, hydroxytyramine, serotonin, γ-aminobutyric acid, ethanolamine, and taurine, some of which are substances of high physiological activity (regulation of blood vessel diameter, neurohormonal actions, and essential components of phospholipids and bile acids). In accord with their general importance, these enzymatic reactions take place in

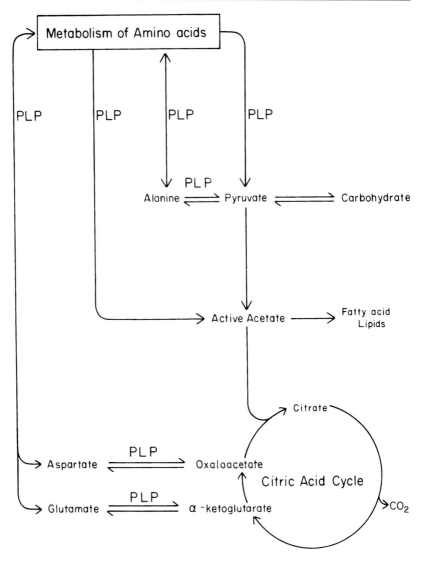

Fig. 9.2 Pyridoxal phosphate (PLP) and amino acid metabolism.

virtually all organs, most intensively in the liver, heart, and brain. Neurological disorders, including states of agitation and convulsions, result from reduction of B_6 enzymes in the brain, including glutamate decarboxylase and γ-aminobutyric acid transaminase. Maternal restriction of B_6 in rats adversely affected synaptogenesis, neurogenesis and neuron longevity, and differentiation of the progeny (Groziak and Kirksey,

1987, 1990). Research in animal models suggests that vitamin B_6 deficiency during gestation and lactation alters the function of N-methyl-D-aspartate receptors, a subtype of receptors of the glutamatergic neurotransmitter system thought to play an important role in learning and memory (Guilarte, 1993).

Vitamin B_6 is involved in many additional reactions, particularly those involving proteins. The vitamin participates in the following functions (Bräunlich, 1974; Marks, 1975; LeKlem, 1991):

1. Deaminases—for serine, threonine, and cystathionine.

2. Desulfhydrases and transulfhyurases—interconversion and metabolism of sulfur-containing amino acids.

3. Synthesis of niacin from tryptophan—hydroxykynurenine is not converted to hydroxyanthranilic acid but rather to xanthurenic acid because of lack of the B_6-dependent enzyme kynureninase (see Chapter 8, Functions).

4. Formation of δ-aminolevulinic acid from succinyl-CoA and glycine, the first step in porphyrin synthesis.

5. Conversion of linoleic to arachidonic acid in the metabolism of essential fatty acids (this function is controversial).

6. Glycogen phosphorylase catalyzes glycogen breakdown to glucose l-phosphate. Pyridoxal phosphate does not appear to be a coenzyme for this enzyme but rather affects the enzyme's conformation.

7. Synthesis of epinephrine and norepinephrine from either phenylalanine or tyrosine—both norepinephrine and epinephrine are involved in carbohydrate metabolism as well as in other body reactions.

8. Racemases—PLP-dependent racemases enable certain microorganisms to utilize D-amino acids. Racemases have not yet been detected in mammalian tissues.

9. Transmethylation by methionine.

10. Incorporation of iron in hemoglobin synthesis.

11. Amino acid transport—all three known amino acid transport systems—(a) neutral amino acids and histidine, (b) basic amino acids, and (c) proline and hydroxyproline—appear to require PLP.

12. Formation of antibodies—B_6 deficiency results in inhibition of the synthesis of globulins, which carry antibodies.

Animal and human studies suggest that vitamin B_6 deficiency affects both humoral and cell-mediated immune responses. In humans, vitamin B_6 depletion significantly decreased percentage and total number of lymphocytes, mitogenic responses of peripheral blood lymphocytes to T-

and B-cell mitogens, and interleukin 2 production (Meydani et al., 1991). Additional human studies indicate that vitamin B_6 status may influence tumor growth and disease processes. Deficiency of the vitamin has been associated with immunological changes observed in the elderly, persons infected with human immunodeficiency virus (HIV), and those with uremia or rheumatoid arthritis (Rall and Meydani, 1993).

Vitamin B_6 has other functions, some of which relate directly or indirectly to overall protein metabolism. The vitamin has been shown to function in blood pressure regulation (Heseker and Kübler, 1992), reduction of edema and inflammation in rats (Lakshmi et al., 1991), carnitine biosynthesis (Cho and LeKlem, 1990), conversion of selenomethionine to glutathione peroxidase and distribution and transport of selenium in the body (Beilstein and Whanger, 1989; Yin et al., 1992), collagen maturation for the connective tissue matrix (Masse et al., 1994), modulate gene expression or transcriptional activation of glycogen phosphorylase in RNA in liver of rats (Oka et al., 1994), detoxification of albizia versicolor poisoning in sheep (Gummow et al., 1992), and rat enterocyte calcium homeostasis—with a 69% reduction in total exchangeable calcium and a 56% reduction in cytosol ionized calcium concentration as a result of vitamin B_6 deficiency (Matyaszczyk et al., 1993).

REQUIREMENTS

Requirement for vitamin B_6 has been found generally to depend on species, age, physiological function, dietary components, the intestinal flora, and other factors that are not yet fully understood. Table 9.1 summarizes the vitamin B_6 requirements for various animal species and humans, with a more complete listing given in the appendix, Table A1. Because of microbial synthesis, ruminants have no dietary requirement for vitamin B_6. Young ruminants that do not have a fully developed rumen, however, require a dietary source. Considerable quantities of vitamin B_6 are synthesized in the relatively large intestinal tract of the horse, but whether this is adequately absorbed to meet requirements is controversial. Vitamin B_6 is also produced by microorganisms of the intestinal tracts of other animals and humans, but whether significant quantities are absorbed and utilized is in doubt. Roth-Maier and Kirchgessner (1993) suggested that adult sows are able to maintain optimal metabolic functions over 8 weeks by utilizing bacterially synthesized vitamin B_6. Cellulose supplement to these pigs increased total vitamin B_6 excretion from 3.4 to 5.2 mg. In rats administered sul-

■ Table 9.1 Vitamin B$_6$ Requirements for Various Animals and Humans

Animal	Purpose or Class	Requirement[a]	Reference
Beef cattle	Adult	Microbial synthesis	NRC (1996)
Dairy cattle	Calf	6.5 ppm milk replacer	NRC (1989a)
	Adult	Microbial synthesis	NRC (1989a)
Chicken	Leghorn, 0–18 weeks	3.0 mg/kg	NRC (1994)
	Laying (100-g intake)	2.5 mg/kg	NRC (1994)
	Broilers, 0–8 weeks	3.0–3.5 mg/kg	NRC (1994)
Duck (Pekin)	All classes	2.5–3.0 mg/kg	NRC (1994)
Japanese quail	All classes	3.0 mg/kg	NRC (1994)
Turkey	All classes	3.0–4.5 mg/kg	NRC (1994)
Sheep	Adult	Microbial synthesis	NRC (1985b)
Swine	Growing-finishing, 3–5 kg	2.0 mg/kg	NRC (1998)
	Growing-finishing, 5–120 kg	1.0–1.5 mg/kg	NRC (1998)
	Adult	1.0 mg/kg	NRC (1998)
Horse	Adult	Microbial synthesis	NRC (1989b)
Goat	Adult	Microbial synthesis	NRC (1981)
Mink	Growing	1.6 mg/kg	NRC (1982a)
Fox	Growing	2.0 mg/kg	NRC (1982a)
Cat	Growing	4.0 mg/kg	NRC (1986)
Dog	Growing	60 µg/kg body wt	NRC (1985a)
Fish	Catfish	3.0 mg/kg	NRC (1993)
	Pacific salmon	5 mg/kg	NRC (1993)
	Rainbow trout	1–10 mg/kg	NRC (1993)
Rat	All classes	6.0 mg/kg	NRC (1995)
Mouse	All classes	8.0 mg/kg	NRC (1995)
Human	Infants	0.3–0.6 mg/day	RDA (1989)
	Children	1.0–1.4 mg/day	RDA (1989)
	Adults	1.7–2.2 mg/day	RDA (1989)

[a]Expressed as per unit of animal feed on either as-fed (approximately 90% dry matter) or dry basis (see Appendix, Tables A1a,b). Human data are expressed as mg/day.

fasalazine, vitamin B$_6$ deficiency was aggravated, suggesting that the intestinal synthesis of the vitamin was affected (Trumbo and Raidi, 1991). Animals practicing coprophagy would obviously be receiving vitamin B$_6$ from this source.

Breed of animal and environmental temperature have been shown to influence vitamin B$_6$ requirements. Lucas et al. (1946) found that crossbred chicks (Rhode Island Red × Barred Plymouth Rock) showed a considerably higher requirement for pyridoxine than had previously been found for White leghorn chicks, and a Japanese strain of chickens was also shown to have a higher B$_6$ requirement (Scott et al., 1982). Two strains of mice have likewise been shown to have greatly different requirements for vitamin B$_6$ (Hoover-Plow and Rice, 1992). Regarding ambient temperature, when rats were housed at 33°C, they needed twice as much vitamin B$_6$ as when they were housed at 19°C (Bräunlich, 1974).

Quantity of dietary protein affects requirement for vitamin B_6 in both animals and humans. Vitamin B_6 requirement is increased when high-protein diets are fed. For example, when feed contained 60% casein instead of 20%, the level of pyridoxine required by mice was three times as high (Miller and Baumann, 1945). Gries and Scott (1972) found a much higher vitamin B_6 requirement in chicks receiving 31% protein than in those receiving a normal 22% protein diet. A number of studies have suggested that amino acid imbalance has an adverse effect on vitamin B_6 status in that weight gain was depressed and survival was decreased when large amounts of a single amino acid were added to rat diets limited in the vitamin. High tryptophan, methionine, and other amino acids increase the need for vitamin B_6 (Scott et al., 1982). Fisher et al. (1984) reported a consistent deleterious effect of a low-quality protein on vitamin B_6 status in rats. Certain feed antagonists (see Chemical Structure, Properties, and Antagonists), bioavailability of B_6 in feeds (see Natural Sources), and nutrients other than protein influence the B_6 requirement. Niacin and riboflavin are needed for interconversions of different forms of vitamin B_6, with an overdose of thiamin reported to produce deficiency of the vitamin in rats (LeKlem, 1991).

In humans, vitamin B_6 requirements are increased with higher dietary protein, pregnancy, lactation, oral contraceptives, alcoholic beverages, liver disease, and certain drugs (see Chemical Structure, Properties, and Antagonists), in the elderly population, and for some individuals with inborn errors of metabolism. The allowance for vitamin B_6 is approximately 2.0 mg/day for adult males and 1.6 mg/day for adult females (RDA, 1989). The RDA for infants begins at 0.3 mg/day, increases to 0.6 mg/day for older infants consuming a mixed diet, and increases from 1 to 2 mg/day from childhood through adolescence. Pregnancy and lactation add 0.6 and 0.5 mg/day, respectively, to the RDA for women. Low milk vitamin B_6 has been associated with long-term use of oral contraceptives (estrogen component). Both the use of oral contraceptives and alcoholism result in lowered plasma PLP levels. Low plasma PLP levels in alcoholics are believed to result from acetaldehyde, which reduces the protein binding of PLP, thereby promoting its dephosphorylation and oxidation to pyridoxic acid. In studies with vitamin B_6-deficient rats, alcohol affected fetal weight and reduced maternal liver PLP by 22% (Lin, 1989). Some individuals have inborn errors of metabolism that greatly increase their B_6 requirement. Fortunately, the number of such individuals appears to be small, but unless they take doses of B_6 starting at birth, they develop convulsions and brain damage, and die (Scriver and Whelan, 1969).

NATURAL SOURCES

Vitamin B$_6$ is widely distributed in foods and feeds (Table 9.2). In general, muscle meats, liver, vegetables, whole-grain cereals and their by-products, and nuts are among best sources; few materials are really poor sources, with the exception of fruits. The vitamin present in cereal grains is concentrated mainly in bran, the rest containing only small amounts. The richest source is royal jelly produced by bees (5,000 µg/g). Most vitamin B$_6$ in animal products is in the form of pyridoxal and pyridoxamine phosphates. In plants and seeds the usual form is pyridoxol. Many analytical figures for vitamin B$_6$, especially older ones, were too low because the assays did not measure all the biologically active forms (Scott et al., 1982).

The level of vitamin B$_6$ contained in all feeds is affected by processing and subsequent storage. Of the several forms, pyridoxine is far more stable than either pyridoxal or pyridoxamine. Therefore, the processing losses of vitamin B$_6$ tend to be highly variable (0 to 40%), with plant-derived foods (which contain mostly pyridoxine) losing little if any of the vitamin and animal products (mostly pyridoxal and pyridoxamine) losing large quantities. Vitamin B$_6$ loss during cooking, processing, refining, and storage has been reported to be as high as 70% (Shideler, 1983) or in the range of 0 to 40% (Birdsall, 1975). Losses may be

■ Table 9.2   Vitamin B$_6$ in Foods and Feedstuffs (mg/kg, dry basis)

Alfalfa leaves, sun cured	4.4	Molasses, sugarcane	5.7
Barley, grain	7.3	Oat, grain	2.8
Bean, navy (seed)	0.3	Oat, grouts	1.2
Blood meal	4.8	Pea, seeds	1.7
Brewer's grains	0.8	Peanut meal, solvent extracted	6.9
Buttermilk (cattle)	2.6	Potato	15.5
Copra meal (coconut)	4.8	Rice, grain	5.0
Corn, gluten meal	8.8	Rice, polished	0.4
Corn, yellow grain	5.3	Rye, grain	2.9
Cottonseed meal, solvent extracted	6.8	Sorghum, grain	5.0
Crab meal	7.2	Soybean meal, solvent extracted	6.7
Fish meal, anchovy	5.0	Spleen, cattle	1.3
Fish meal, menhaden	5.1	Wheat, bran	9.6
Horse meat	0.7	Wheat, grain	5.6
Linseed meal, mechanically extracted	6.1	Whey	3.6
		Yeast, brewer's	39.8
Liver, cattle	18.0	Yeast, torula	38.9
Milk, skim, cattle	4.5		

Source: NRC (1982b).

397

caused by heat, light, and various agents that can promote oxidation. Two-hour sunlight exposure may destroy half the vitamin B_6 in milk. Blanching of rehydrated lima beans resulted in a loss of 20% vitamin B_6, but more significantly, the availability of the vitamin was reduced by almost 50% (Ekanayake and Nelson, 1990). Irradiation as a potential method for microbial control of poultry feed results in a loss of 15% vitamin B_6 potency (Leeson and Marcotte, 1993).

In the early 1950s several infants in the United States were diagnosed as deficient in vitamin B_6 as a result of consuming a commercially sterilized, liquid milk formula. Later studies showed that the vitamin underwent rapid destruction during the autoclaving procedure used in the production of formulas. Also, human milk often does not contain sufficient vitamin B_6 for the newborn (see Deficiency, Effects of Deficiency, Humans). However, human milk could be an adequate source of vitamin B_6 because vitamin levels respond rapidly to dietary intake (Kirksey, 1981; Kang-Yoon et al., 1992). Milk vitamin B_6 concentrations from goats and cows were approximately twice that of human values (Coburn et al., 1992).

Data on vitamin B_6 content of feeds are generally insufficient and information on the vitamin's bioavailability is lacking. Bioavailability of B_6 was found to be greater from beef than from corn meal, spinach, or potatoes (Nguyen and Gregory, 1983). LeKlem et al. (1980) reported that in young adult men, vitamin B_6 bioavailability in whole-wheat bread is lower than that in white bread enriched with pure pyridoxine. Vitamin B_6 in whole-wheat bread and peanut butter was 75 and 63%, respectively, as available as that from canned tuna (Kabir et al., 1983). In studies with young men based upon plasma PLP level or urinary B_6 (i.e., 4-pyridoxic acid) excretion, B_6 bioavailability in the average American diet was estimated to be about 75% (Tarr et al., 1981).

Pyridoxine-5′-β-D-glucoside (PNG), a conjugated form of vitamin B_6, has been shown to be abundant in various plant-derived foods. This form of B_6 may account for up to 50% of the total vitamin B_6 content of oilseeds such as soybeans and sunflower seeds. The utilization of dietary PNG, relative to pyridoxine, has been shown to be 30% in rats (Trumbo et al., 1988) and 50% in humans (Gregory et al., 1991). In suckling rats, the availability of vitamin B_6 derived from PNG is only 25% compared with pyridoxine (Trumbo and Gregory, 1989). Pyridoxine-5′-β-D-glucoside seems to be well absorbed, but the hydrolysis to pyridoxine is poor. The primary site of limited conversion to pyridoxine is the intestinal mucosa, where β-glucosidase activity toward PNG has been demonstrated (Gregory et al., 1991). The glycosylated

PNG can quantitatively alter the metabolism of pyridoxine in vivo; hence, it partially impairs the metabolic utilization of co-ingested non-glycosylated forms of vitamin B$_6$ (Gilbert and Gregory, 1992; Zhang et al., 1993; Nakano and Gregory, 1995; Hansen et al., 1996; Nakano et al., 1997).

DEFICIENCY

Effects of Deficiency

Characteristics of vitamin B$_6$ deficiency are retarded growth, dermatitis, epileptic-like convulsions, anemia, and partial alopecia. Because of the predominant function of the vitamin in protein metabolism, in vitamin B$_6$ deficiency a fall in nitrogen retention is observed, feed protein is not well utilized, nitrogen excretion is excessive, and impaired tryptophan metabolism may result.

Ruminants

Amounts of vitamin B$_6$ that are normally synthesized by microorganisms in the digestive tract of ruminants, when fully developed, are enough to meet needs of these animals. McElroy and Goss (1939) reported vitamin B$_6$ to be 6 to 10 mg/kg of diet in dried rumen contents of mature sheep, even though the diet contained only 1.5 mg/kg. Therefore, no deficiency signs of vitamin B$_6$ have yet been observed in mature ruminants. However, stressed cattle, as a result of long-distance transportation, had very low blood pyridoxine concentrations (Dubeski and Owens, 1993).

Vitamin B$_6$ has been shown to be essential for the young calf when selected experimental diets are used. Calves that were reared on a "milk substitute" lost appetite within 2 to 4 weeks; their growth was impaired; and they progressively showed apathy, diarrhea, loss of appetite, and loss of coordination. In the last stages, convulsions were soon followed by death (Johnson et al., 1947). The convulsions included thrashing of the legs and head and grinding of the teeth (Johnson et al., 1950).

Postmortem examination of vitamin B$_6$ deficient calves revealed hemorrhages in the epicardium and in the kidneys, demyelination of the peripheral nerves, proliferation of Schwann cells, desquamation of the intestinal mucosa, and pneumonia (Johnson et al., 1950). Analyses of the urine from the vitamin B$_6$-deficient calves showed greatly reduced excretion of pyridoxine, pyridoxal, pyridoxamine, and pyridoxic acid (major excretory metabolite).

Swine

In growing pigs, clinical signs of vitamin B_6 deficiency include a poor appetite, slow growth (Fig. 9.3), microcytic hypochromic anemia, epileptic-like seizures or convulsions (Fig. 9.4), fatty infiltration of the liver, diarrhea, rough hair coats, scaly skin, a brown exudate around the eyes, demyelination of peripheral nerves, and subcutaneous edema (Bauernfeind, 1974; Bräunlich, 1974; Cunha, 1977). Like some other vitamins, vitamin B_6 deficiency reduces the immune responses of the pig (Harmon et al., 1963). The first and most conspicuous sign in baby pigs that vitamin B_6 is insufficient is a loss of appetite that, if the deficiency is severe, may appear in less than 2 weeks. This is accompanied by reduced growth, vomiting, diarrhea, and a peculiar compulsion to lick.

When deficiency of vitamin B_6 reaches an advanced stage (probably due to degeneration of the peripheral nerves), disordered movement and ataxia appear. Finally, convulsions develop at irregular intervals, but are, apparently, stimulated by excitement, because they are most often observed at feeding time. Between these convulsions, pigs lie down and are apathetic and unresponsive (Bräunlich, 1974). Bräunlich suggested that a vitamin B_6 deficiency may go unnoticed in swine because of a lack of visible signs associated specifically with the deficiency. Metabolic disor-

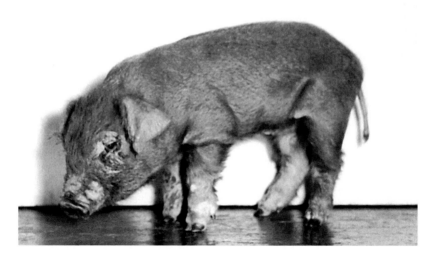

Fig. 9.3 A 6-week-old B_6-deficient pig weighing only 3.6 kg. (Courtesy of R.W. Luecke and E.R. Miller, Michigan Agriculture Experiment Station, and *J. Nutr.* 62 [1957], 405.)

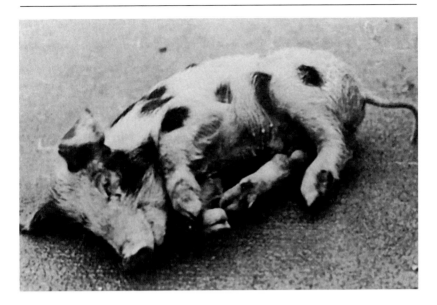

Fig. 9.4 This pig is having an epileptic-like seizure while receiving a diet low in vitamin B$_6$. (Courtesy of E.H. Hughs and H. Heitman, California Agriculture Experiment Station.)

ders may be revealed only by poor appetite, slow growth, and inefficient feed utilization. In some experiments with vitamin B$_6$, protein retention by pigs deficient in the vitamin was reduced to less than half.

During reproduction and lactation, sows fed a corn-sorghum-soybean meal diet responded to vitamin B$_6$ supplementation at a level of 4.4 mg/kg of feed (Adams et al., 1967). Vitamin B$_6$ supplementation of 11 mg/kg of feed produced a slightly superior daily gain in weight, more piglets born alive, and a smaller number of resorbed fetuses compared with control sows that received only 1 mg/kg of vitamin B$_6$ (Ritchie et al., 1960).

Poultry

Chicks fed a vitamin B$_6$-deficient diet have little appetite and grow slowly, with plumage failing to fully develop. Chicks maintained on a B$_6$-deficient diet exhibited general weakness after a few days of deprivation. The birds squat in a characteristic posture, with wings slightly spread and head resting on the ground (Bräunlich, 1974). Miller (1963) observed high proportions of pendulous crops with vitamin B$_6$-deficient chicks.

A more specific sign of B_6 deficiently is the nature of the nervous conditions that develop. Deficient chicks are abnormally excitable. As deprivation continues, nervous disorders become increasingly severe (Bräunlich, 1974). There is a trembling and vibration of the tip of the tail, with movement stiff and jerky. Chicks will run aimlessly about with lowered head and drooping wings. Finally, convulsions develop, during which chicks fall on their side or back, with the legs scrabbling. Violent convulsions cause complete exhaustion and may lead to death. These clinical signs may be distinguished from those of encephalomalacia by the relatively greater intensity of activity during a seizure (Scott et al., 1982).

Blood alterations are also typical of a vitamin B_6 inadequacy in chicks. An extreme deficiency leads to a microcytic, polychromatic hypochromic anemia in conjunction with atrophy of the spleen and thymus (Asmar et al., 1968). Marginal deficiencies provoke a microcytic, normochromic polycythemia (Blalock and Thaxton, 1984), and deficient chicks show decreased immunoglobulin M and immunoglobulin G response to antibody challenge (Blalock et al., 1984).

Similar signs of a vitamin B_6 deficiency have been observed in turkey poults—loss of appetite, poor growth (Fig. 9.5), oversensitivity and cramps, and finally death. Ducklings not receiving enough vitamin B_6 grow slowly, and development of plumage is poor. At 5 days of age, ducklings showed retarded growth (Yang and Jeng, 1989). Clinical signs were first observed at 7 days of age and were characterized by decreased appetite, extreme weakness, hyperexcitability, convulsion, and death. Hematological examination at 3 weeks of age indicated that pyridoxine deficiency in ducklings resulted in microcytic, hypochromic anemia.

Signs of B_6 deficiency in chicks will appear very rapidly after introduction of a B_6-deficient feed. Fuller and Kifer (1959) reported that signs of a deficiency appeared on the eighth day. Chronic, borderline B_6 deficiency produces perosis. Usually one leg is severely crippled, and one or both of the middle toes may be bent inward at the first joint (Gries and Scott, 1972). A marked increase in gizzard erosion was found in vitamin B_6-deficient chicks (Daghir and Haddad, 1981).

In adult poultry, vitamin B_6 deficiency results in reduced egg production and hatchability as well as decreased feed consumption, weight loss, and death. Robel and Christensen (1991) reported that hatchability of pyridoxine-injected white turkey hen eggs was 4.2% higher than non-injected eggs. A severe deficiency (levels of vitamin B_6 below 0.5 mg/kg of diet) causes rapid involution of the ovary, oviduct, comb, and

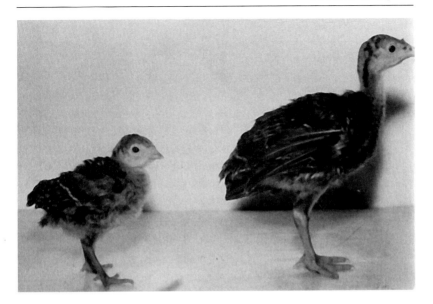

Fig. 9.5 Vitamin B_6-deficient poult (about 4 weeks old) on left and a normal poult on right. (Courtesy of T.W. Sullivan, University of Nebraska.)

wattles in mature laying hens. Involution of testes, comb, and wattle occurs in vitamin B_6-deficient adult cockerels (Scott et al., 1982).

Horses

No experimental information is available on vitamin B_6 requirements or deficiency in the horse. It has been shown that the horse synthesizes vitamin B_6 in the intestinal tract, with the assumption that adequate quantities are absorbed. However, some researchers believe that racehorses need vitamin B_6 supplementation because when these horses undergo intensive training, they need a high proportion of protein in their diets that would increase B_6 requirements (Bräunlich, 1974).

Other Animal Species

DOGS AND CATS

A typical consequence of B_6 deficiency in both young and old dogs is a microcytic, hypochromic anemia. In addition to decreased appetite and body weight loss, pathological changes include ataxia, cardiac dilatation and hypertrophy, congestion of various tissues, and demyelination of peripheral nerves (NRC, 1985a). Acute deficiency of vitamin B_6 in growing puppies may lead to sudden death with clinical signs of only anorexia, slow growth, or body weight loss.

In kittens deficient in B_6, there is growth depression, a mild microcytic, hypochromic anemia, convulsive seizures, and irreversible kidney lesions consisting of areas of tubular atrophy and dilatation (NRC, 1986). Vitamin B_6 deficiency has been reported to produce behavioral, neurophysiological, and neuropathological abnormalities in a variety of species, including cats. Buckmaster et al. (1993) used brainstem auditory evoked potentials and determined that vitamin B_6 deficiency in cats affected peripheral and brainstem auditory pathways. The finding of prolonged interwave intervals in vitamin B_6-deficient cats was consistent with slowed axonal conduction velocity secondary to defective myelination.

FISH

Most fish are sensitive to vitamin B_6 deficiency and show neurological disorders in 3 to 8 weeks (Lovell, 1987). Clinical signs in catfish include hyperirritability, erratic swimming, anorexia, tetany, and greenish-blue coloration. Erratic swimming, hyperirritability, and convulsions have been observed in salmonids, gilthead sea bream, common carp, yellowtail, and Japanese eel (NRC, 1993). Other deficiency signs, such as anorexia and poor growth, usually appear in the fish within 3 to 6 weeks after they have been fed a vitamin B_6-deficient diet. Pyridoxine deficiency has been reported to cause various histopathological changes in rainbow trout liver and kidney and in the intestinal tissue of both rainbow trout and gilthead sea bream.

FOXES AND MINK

Signs of deficiency in growing kits appeared after about 2 weeks on a B_6-deficient diet and included reduced feed intake, weight loss, diarrhea, brown exudate around the nose, excessive lacrimation, swelling and puffiness around the nose and face region, apathy, muscular incoordination, convulsions, and finally death (NRC, 1982a). Reproduction is also affected in mink with testes degeneration and resorption of embryos. Vitamin B_6 deficiency in the fox results in anorexia, growth cessation, and a decrease in hemoglobin.

LABORATORY ANIMALS

Rats fed diets deficient in vitamin B_6 develop symmetrical scaling dermatitis (acrodynia) on the tail, paws, face, and ears; microcytic ane-

mia; hyperexcitability; convulsions; and reduced reproductive performance in both sexes (NRC, 1995). Edema was increased 54% in vitamin
B$_6$-deficient rats (Lakshmi et al., 1991). Subtle abnormalities of gait, consisting of a reduced width of step was detected early in vitamin B$_6$-defi-
cient rats (Schaeffer et al., 1990). Sexual behavior of vitamin B$_6$-deficient
male rats was exhibited as reduced post-ejaculatory intervals and an increased proportion of animals ejaculating (Gorzalka and Moe, 1994).

For mice, vitamin B$_6$ deficiency signs include poor growth, hyperirritability, posterior paralysis, necrotic degeneration of the tail, alopecia,
and progressive hypochromic anemia (NRC, 1995). Loss of appetite is
an early and constant result of B$_6$ deficiency in hamsters. Although acrodynia is characteristic of vitamin B$_6$ deficiency in rats, it is not found in
hamsters. The fur of B$_6$-deprived hamsters has an unkempt appearance,
and crusted lesions are occasionally observed on lips and mouth (NRC,
1995).

Nonhuman Primates

Vitamin B$_6$ deficiency signs in rhesus monkeys consist of weight
loss, hypochromic, microcytic anemia, apathy, and ataxia. There is
widespread arteriosclerosis, fatty metamorphosis of liver, hepatic necrosis and cirrhosis, dental caries, oxaluria, and neuronal degeneration of
the cerebral cortex (NRC, 1978). With cebus monkeys, deficiency consists of weight loss, a profound hypochromic, microcytic anemia, hair
loss, and dermatitis, especially about the hands and toes.

Rabbits

In rabbits, vitamin B$_6$ deficiency signs include a scaly thickening of
the skin of ears and inflammation around eyes and nose. In a few cases
there is a pronounced acrodynia, with severe encrustation and inflammation of nose, eyes, and paws. Alopecia develops most often on
forelegs and is accompanied by skin inflammation and desquamation
(Bräunlich, 1974). Neurological signs observed include convulsions,
partial paralysis, and contracture of extremities. In the advanced stage,
some rabbits are unable to move their hind legs at all, the muscles of the
hind leg having become severely atrophied.

Humans

A high proportion of the human population receives inadequate dietary vitamin B$_6$, particularly young and pregnant or lactating women.
Typical vitamin B$_6$ deficiency symptoms in humans include
hypochromic, microcytic anemia, loss of weight, abdominal distress,

vomiting, hyperirritability, epileptic-type convulsions in infants, depression and confusion followed by convulsions in adults, and electroencephalographic abnormalities (LeKlem, 1991). Seborrhea-like lesions developed about the eyes, nose, and mouth, and some subjects showed cheilosis and glossitis. A depression of the lymphocyte count was a fairly constant finding.

There are a large number of conditions in which vitamin B_6 metabolism is altered. Conditions in which tryptophan metabolism has been altered and in which vitamin B_6 administration was used include asthma, diabetes, certain cancers, pellagra, and rheumatoid arthritis, while diseases and pathological conditions in which plasma PLP levels have been shown to be depressed include asthma, diabetes, renal disorders, alcoholism, heart disease, pregnancy, breast cancer, Hodgkin's disease, and sickle-cell anemia (LeKlem, 1991; Driskell, 1994). Animal and human studies suggest that vitamin B_6 deficiency affects both humoral and cell-mediated immune responses. Lymphocyte differentiation and maturation are altered by deficiency, delayed-type hypersensitivity responses are reduced, and antibody production may be indirectly impaired. Deficiency of the vitamin has been associated with immunological changes observed in the elderly, persons infected with HIV, and those with uremia or rheumatoid arthritis (Rall and Meydani, 1993).

Studies conducted during the 1990s have suggested that in the United States, a large percentage of women of child-bearing age and pregnant and lactating women have vitamin B_6 intakes significantly lower than the recommended dietary allowance (Guilarte, 1993). Vitamin B_6 deficiency has been reported in 83.4% of Turkish children (Wetherilt et al., 1992) and 34% of adolescents in Nigeria (Korede, 1990). In the elderly Greek population, dietary intake of vitamin B_6 was less than 50% of the U.S. RDA (Kafatos et al., 1993).

Convincing evidence of the essential nature of vitamin B_6 in human nutrition was first provided by reports in the United States of infants who developed irritability and convulsive seizures (and sometimes died) when fed autoclaved infant formulas. This autoclaving destroyed much of the vitamin B_6, and infants did not receive adequate quantities of the vitamin. Infants receiving human milk are also sometimes at risk as generally this is a poor source of the vitamin. Other conditions responsive to B_6 first seen in infants are several inborn errors of metabolism resulting in vitamin B_6 dependency.

Reports indicate that unsupplemented mothers have a milk vitamin B_6 level that in some cases is lower than 100 μg/L, a concentration that places infants at risk for development of seizures (Styslinger and Kirksey, 1985; Guilarte, 1993). Although this concentration of vitamin B$_6$ in milk does not always result in clinical signs of apparent vitamin B$_6$ deficiency, it may influence the normal development of the child. Evidence for such an effect was noted in the Egyptian study (McCullough et al., 1990), in which abnormalities in behavior were observed in infants whose mothers had vitamin B$_6$ levels in milk below 85 µg/L. Likewise, these mothers were less responsive to their infants' vocalizations, showed less effective intervention to infant distress, and were more likely to use older siblings as caregivers than were mothers of better vitamin status.

Both pregnancy and use of oral contraceptives increased the vitamin B$_6$ requirement (Miller, 1986). Contractor and Shane (1970) discovered that pregnant women had lower blood levels of PLP than did nonpregnant controls. Brin (1971) reported that pregnant women had increased urinary metabolites of tryptophan. He also found fetal blood levels of B$_6$ two to three times greater than the maternal level, indicating a depletion of the mother's B$_6$ stores. According to Heller et al. (1973), vitamin B$_6$ supplementation is necessary in approximately 50% of pregnant women to maintain normal B$_6$ coenzyme saturation of aspartate aminotransferase.

Alcohol and certain drugs (see Chemical Structure, Properties, and Antagonists) interfere with the metabolic functions of vitamin B$_6$. Vitamin B$_6$ deficiency is viewed as an important nutritional complication in alcoholism, and it has been established that alcoholics absorb less vitamin B$_6$ than do control subjects. Alcoholics have a decreased ability to liberate vitamin B$_6$ from its bound form, and several studies suggest that alcohol interferes with conversion of pyridoxine to PLP (Bonjour, 1980). Certain drugs, including the antituberculosis drug isonicotinic acid hydrazide (INH), have been shown to increase need of vitamin B$_6$. INH forms hydrazone complexes with PLP, which inactivates the coenzyme (Roe, 1973). Studies suggest that vitamin B$_6$ availability is limited in hyperthyroidism, and consequently B$_6$ should be added to antithyroid medication for hyperthyroid patients (Wohl et al., 1960). The use of interleukin-2 for treatment of various cancers depressed vitamin B$_6$ blood concentration to subnormal in 90% of patients (Baker et al., 1992).

Vitamin B$_6$ is affected by uremia and urinary calculi and has been associated with inadequacy of the vitamin. Many symptoms of uremia are quite similar to vitamin B$_6$ deficiency. Convulsions, peripheral neuritis, and depression of the immune response are seen in both conditions. Dobbelstein and coworkers (1974) suggested that uremic toxins exert an inhibitory effect on PLP. The increase in oxalic as well as xanthurenic acid in the urine of B_6-deficient humans has been suggested as a cause for urinary calculi. In a study by Lilum et al. (1981), 85% of 100 rats produced calcium oxalate stones within 6 weeks of being placed on a vitamin B_6-free diet.

Assessment of Status

Several biochemical procedures have been developed and utilized for assessment of vitamin B_6 status of humans and animals. Indices for evaluating vitamin B_6 status and suggested values for adequate status in adult humans have been reported (LeKlem, 1990). Vitamin B_6 deficiency leads to an impairment of protein utilization even before visible signs occur. A widely used approach to assess vitamin B_6 status in humans is measuring urinary metabolites of tryptophan following a tryptophan load test. In a B_6 deficiency, tryptophan is not converted to niacin and is metabolized to other intermediate products at a greater rate than in a nondeficient state. Metabolites most often measured are xanthurenic acid and kynurenic acid. Although the tryptophan load test has been widely used in assessment of vitamin B_6 status, results obtained via this method should be interpreted with care, as several other metabolic and hormonal factors are known to be involved in tryptophan metabolism. The tryptophan load test is a good parameter for the assessment of the vitamin B_6 status of population groups. Some research suggests that this test may be less useful in detecting marginal vitamin B_6 intake.

Direct measurements of one or more forms of vitamin B_6 in plasma, urine, or erythrocytes are relatively reliable indicators of vitamin B_6 status. Urinary 4-pyridoxic acid (4-PA) excretion is considered a short-term indicator of vitamin B_6 status due to the fact that 4-PA reflects recent vitamin B_6 intake rather than the underlying state of tissue reserve (Lui et al., 1985). Often 4-PA is not detectable in the urine of vitamin B_6-deficient subjects. One of the most commonly used measures of vitamin B_6 status is the measurement of erythrocyte alanine and aspartic acid transaminase(s) activity and/or stimulation (LeKlem, 1990). Because of the nature of the life span of the erythrocyte, they are considered long-term measures of vitamin B_6 status. The specific tests employed are the measurement of the basal activity of these transaminases and the activity in the presence of excess PLP.

Over the past 20 years, plasma PLP has been the most frequently used direct measure of vitamin B_6 status. This measure has replaced the tryptophan load test as the method of choice in evaluating status. Plasma PLP is the primary form of circulating vitamin B_6 and comprises 70 to 90% of the total vitamin B_6 in the plasma. Plasma pyridoxal has been suggested as an additional index of vitamin B$_6$ status (LeKlem, 1991).

Other factors may influence plasma PLP and should be considered when using this index as a measure of vitamin B$_6$ status. These include the physiological variables of age, exercise, pregnancy, and dietary components, particularly protein. Plasma PLP has been shown to decrease with advancing age (Löwik et al., 1989), with an age-dependent difference in protein intake related to vitamin B$_6$ requirements. Elderly subjects apparently need less vitamin B$_6$ at higher protein intake based on plasma PLP, pyridoxal, and total vitamin B$_6$ concentrations (Pannemans et al., 1994).

Other vitamin B$_6$ status indicators might include concentrations of the vitamin in milk and eggs. Pyridoxine intakes of breast-fed infants reflected the amount of their mother's supplement (Kang-Yoon et al., 1992). Pyridoxine intake of mothers was a strong indicator of infant pyridoxine status. Concentrations of vitamin B$_6$ in hen egg albumen increased with four incremental dietary pyridoxine levels (Robel, 1992).

SUPPLEMENTATION

Vitamin B$_6$ is one of the B vitamins that is least likely to be deficient in livestock diets, particularly ruminants. However, a supplemental use of vitamin B$_6$ was reported in that 40 to 50 mg pyridoxine hydrochloride/kg body weight administered to sheep was successful in counteracting toxicity of the toxic plant *Albezia versicolor* (Gummow et al., 1992). Only before the rumen is developed should B$_6$ supplementation for ruminants be considered. Young ruminants receiving mother's milk are provided with sufficient quantities of the vitamin. Bräunlich (1974) suggested that the best possible concentration of vitamin B$_6$ in milk substitutes for calves is probably higher than 2.4 mg/kg. Because of its wide dietary distribution, vitamin B$_6$ is seldom deficient in typical swine and poultry diets. Evidence indicates that corn, soybean meal, and other ingredients used to supply energy and protein in practical diets for these species usually also provide sufficient vitamin B$_6$. Consequently, it is not often added in supplemental form. However, the bioavailability of vitamin B$_6$ in corn and soybean meal ranges from only 45 to 65% (Hoffmann-La Roche, 1979).

Under certain conditions vitamin B$_6$ supplementation is warranted for practical growing and breeding diets for poultry and other monogastric or simple-stomached animals. Fuller et al. (1961) believed that although corn-soybean meal practical poultry breeder diets probably contain sufficient vitamin B_6 to support hatchability, there is little margin of safety. The amount of supplemental vitamin B_6 recommended for monogastric species varies from 1 to 10 mg/kg of diet depending on species, age, activity, stress of performance, and field use experience (Bauernfeind, 1974). Reasons for needed supplementation of vitamin B_6 include the following (Perry, 1978): (1) great variations in amounts of B_6 in individual ingredients, (2) variable bioavailability of this vitamin in ingredients, (3) losses reported during processing of ingredients, (4) discrepancies in activity for test organisms versus those for animals, (5) a higher pyridoxine requirement due to a marginal level of methionine in the diet, and (6) high-protein diets.

Variability of vitamin B_6 in feeds depends on the sample origin, conditions of growth, climate, weather conditions, and other local factors (see Natural Sources). For products of animal origin, concentration depends on level of nutrition and environment of original animals. Yen et al. (1976) determined available vitamin B_6 in corn and soybean meal using a chick growth assay. Corn was found to be 38 to 45% available, and B_6 in soybean meal 58 to 62% available. There was little difference in availability between corn samples not heated and those heated to 120°C. However, corn heated at 160°C contained significantly less available B_6. Level of vitamin B_6 contained in feedstuffs is also affected by processing and subsequent storage. In one report a loss of 30% of B_6 contained in alfalfa meal during the coarse-milling and pelleting processes was observed (Bräunlich, 1974). Ink and Henderson (1984) reported that bioavailability can be as low as 40 to 50% after heat processing of foods.

Predominant losses of vitamin B_6 activity in food occur in the pyridoxal and pyridoxamine forms, with pyridoxine being the more stable form. Supplemental vitamin B_6 is reported to have a higher bioavailability and stability than the naturally occurring vitamin, which in retorted milk products exhibited only 50% of the bioavailability of synthetic B_6 or B_6 in formulas that were fortified with the vitamin prior to thermal processing (Tomarelli et al., 1955). Heat sterilization of milk reduced vitamin B_6 activity by irreversible binding to protein, as well as by partial formation of 4-PA (Pingali and Trumbo, 1992).

Commercially, vitamin B_6 is available as crystalline pyridoxine hydrochloride and various dilutions. Pyridoxine hydrochloride contains 82.3% vitamin B_6 activity. The dry dilution is used in feeds, while the crystalline product is used in parenteral and oral pharmaceuticals as well as in feeds. For human nutrition, pyridoxine hydrochloride is used by pharmaceutical companies in the preparation of capsules, tablets, and ampoules. The tablets used for prophylactic purposes usually contain 2 mg per daily dose. For therapeutic purposes, 10- to 150-mg tablets are taken one to three times daily.

The recovery of vitamin B$_6$ as pyridoxine hydrochloride in a multivitamin premix not containing trace minerals was 100%, even after 3 months in storage at 37°C. However, stability in a premix containing trace minerals was poor, with only 45% recovery after 3 months at 37°C (Adams, 1982). Verbeeck (1975) found vitamin B$_6$ to be stable in premixes with minerals as sulfates. However, if minerals in the form of carbonates and oxides are used, 25% of the vitamin can be lost over a 3-month period. Stress agents such as choline chloride help catalyze this destruction. Gadient (1986) considers pyridoxine to be very sensitive to heat, slightly sensitive to moisture and light, and insensitive to oxygen. Retention of B$_6$ activity in pelleted feeds after 3 months at room temperature should be 80 to 100% as a general rule. The retention of pyridoxine in an extruded fish meal fed after 1 month at room temperature was found to be 56%.

Data have accumulated for the need of vitamin B$_6$ supplementation for humans, especially for young and pregnant or lactating women. Requirements for B$_6$ are higher for individuals during pregnancy, use of oral contraceptives, certain drug therapy, radiation sickness, overuse of alcohol, hyperthyroidism, uremia, urinary calculi, and in errors of metabolism (see Deficiency). Vitamin B$_6$ supplements are commonly given when isoniazid is used in tuberculosis treatment and when penicillamine is used in the treatment of Wilson's disease. Vitamin B$_6$ supplements are also frequently given along with most anticonvulsant drugs. Reports indicate that mothers unsupplemented with vitamin B$_6$ produce milk low in the vitamin (Guilarte, 1993). Based on these studies, it is apparent that some degree of vitamin B$_6$ deficiency may be present in infants whose sole source of nutrients is breast milk and whose mothers are not supplemented with the vitamin (see Deficiency). Supplemental vitamin B$_6$ is needed by persons with the "Chinese restaurant syndrome," a condition in which individuals are sensitive to foods heavily seasoned with monosodium glutamate (Folkers et al., 1981). Individuals with carpal tunnel syndrome (pain and/or numbness in hands) require vitamin B$_6$ well in excess of the RDA requirement (LeKlem, 1991). Pyridoxine in pharmacological doses was useful in the management of kidney stones, decreasing urinary oxalate excretion in patients with recurrent oxalate renal calculi (Mitwalli, 1989). In doses of 10 to 25 mg, vitamin B$_6$ increases the conversion of L-dopa to dopamine, which, unlike its precursor, is unable to cross the blood-brain barrier. Thus, vitamin B_6 interferes with L-dopa in the management of Parkinson's disease.

Vitamin B_6 is one of several vitamins currently popular in "orthomolecular" megadose therapy. It has been used for a variety of conditions, including premenstrual syndrome and behavioral disorders. Pyridoxine tablets are available over the counter in dosages of 30 to 500 mg.

TOXICITY

In common with other members of the vitamin B complex, vitamin B_6 has a very low toxicity. Prolonged feeding of pyridoxine-HCl to rats (2.5 mg per day), puppies (20 mg per kilogram body weight per day), and monkeys (10 mg per kilogram body weight per day) produced no toxic signs (Unna and Antopol, 1940).

Large doses of vitamin B_6 can produce detrimental effects in experimental animals and humans. Signs of toxicity occur most obviously in the peripheral nervous system and include changes in gait and peripheral sensation (Krinke and Fitzgerald, 1988). Changes in central nervous system function were detected in rats fed excess vitamin B_6 using techniques of startle behavior measurement (Schaeffer, 1993).

Rats, rabbits, and dogs tolerated 1 g/kg body weight without ill effects; however, larger doses produced adverse manifestations in all three species. Marked impairment of coordination and/or righting reflexes were observed within about 3 days, followed by severe convulsions, paralysis, and death (Unna and Antopal, 1940). Neurohistological examination of rats and dogs that had received 2 to 6 g/kg body weight of the vitamin revealed degeneration of the spinal cord and peripheral nerves (Antopol and Tarlov, 1992). Testicular damage from high doses of vitamin B_6 to rats was reported (Kaido et al., 1991), including retardation in spermiation and Sertoli cell alterations.

Pyridoxal is apparently twice as toxic as pyridoxine or pyridoxamine. Evidence from dog and rat studies suggests that more than 1,000 times the requirement would be needed in diets to produce signs of toxicity (NRC, 1987).

Humans are reported to tolerate daily doses of 20 to 1,000 mg per day of pyridoxine-HCl for prolonged periods without deleterious effects. These doses are 10 to 500 times greater than the recommended daily dietary allowance of vitamin B_6 for adults (Haskell, 1978). Vitamin B_6 is one of several vitamins currently popular in megadose therapy (see Supplementation). Humans have developed a sensory neuropathy as a direct result of taking 2,000 to 6,000 mg of pyridoxine daily (Schaumburg et al., 1983). Subjects developed ataxia and severe sensory nervous system dysfunctions, but substantial improvement occurred with pyridoxine withdrawal.

■ REFERENCES

Adams, C.R. (1982). *In* Vitamins—The Life Essentials. Nutrition Institute, National Feed Ingredient Association, NI-82, 1, Des Moines, Iowa.

Adams, C.R., Richardson, C.E., and Cunha, T.J. (1967). *J. Anim. Sci. 26*, 903 (Abstr.).

Antopol, W., and Tarlov, I.M. (1992). *J. Neuropathol. Exp. Neurol. 1*, 330.

Asmar, J.A., Daghirn, N.J., and Azar, H.A. (1968). *J. Nutr. 95*, 153.

Baker, H., Marcus, S.L., Petrylak, D.P., Frank, O., DeAngelis, B., Baker, E.R., Dutcher, J.P., and Wiernik, P.H. (1992). *J. Am. College Nutr. 11*, 482.

Basu, T.K., and Mann, S. (1997). *J. Nutr. 127*, 117.

Bauernfeind, J.C. (1974). *Feedstuffs, 46*, 30.

Beilstein, M.A., and Whanger, P.D. (1989). *J. Nutr. 119*, 1962.

Birdsall, J.J. (1975). Technology of Fortification of Foods, p. 19. National Academy of Sciences, Washington, D.C.

Blalock, T.L., and Thaxton, J.P. (1984). *Poult. Sci. 63*, 1243.

Blalock, T.L., Thaxton, J.P., and Garlich, J.D. (1984). *J. Nutr. 114*, 312.

Bonjour, J.P. (1980). *Int. J. Vitam. Nutr. Res. 50*, 215.

Bräunlich, K. (1974). Vitamin B$_6$, No. 1451. Hoffmann-La Roche, Basel, Switzerland.

Buckmaster, P.S., Holliday, T.A., Bai, S.C., and Rogers, Q.R. (1993). *J. Nutr. 123*, 20.

Brin, M. (1971). *Am. J. Clin. Nutr. 24*, 704.

Cho, Y.O., and LeKlem, J.E. (1990). *J. Nutr. 120*, 258.

Coburn, S.P., Mahuren, J.D., Pauly, T.A., Ericson, K.L., and Townsend, D.W. (1992). *J. Nutr. 122*, 2348.

Contractor, S., and Shane, B. (1970). *Am. J. Obstet. Gynecol. 107*, 635.

Cunha, T.J. (1977). Swine Feeding and Nutrition. Academic Press, New York.

Daghir, N.J., and Haddad, K.S. (1981). *Poult. Sci. 60*, 988.

Delport, R., Ubbink, J.B., Vermoak, W.J.H., Shaw, A., Bissbort, S., and Becker, P.J. (1991). *Nutr. Burbank 7*, 260.

Dobbelstein, H., Korner, W., Mempel, W., Grosse-Wilde, H., and Edel, H. (1974). *Kidney Int. 5*, 233.

Driskell, J.A. (1994). *Nutr. Res. 14*, 293.

Dubeski, P.L., and Owens, F.N. (1993). *In* Animal Science Res. Rept. No. P-933. Stillwater, Oklahoma.

Durst, L., Kirchgessner, M., and Roth-Maier, D.A. (1989). *J. Anim. Physiol. Anim. Nutr. 62*, 85.

Ekanayake, A., and Nelson, P.E. (1990). *J. Food Sci. 55*, 154.

Fisher, J.H., Willis, R.A., and Haskell, B.E. (1984). *J. Nutr. 114*, 786.

Folkers, K., Shizukuishi, S., Scudder, S.L., Willis, R., Takemura, K., and Longenecker, J.B. (1981). *Biochem. Biophys. Res. Commun. 100,* 972.

Fuller, H.L., and Kifer, P.E. (1959). *Poult. Sci. 38,* 255.

Fuller, H.F., Field, R.C., Roncalli-Amici, A., Dunahoo, W.S., and Edwards, H.M. (1961). *Poult. Sci. 40,* 249.

Gadient, M. (1986). *Proc. Nutr. Conf. Feed Manuf.* College Park, Maryland, p. 73.

Gilbert, J.A., and Gregory, J.F. III. (1992). *J. Nutr. 122,* 1029.

Gorzalka, B.B., and Moe, I.V. (1994). *Nutr. Res. 14,* 279.

Gregory, J.F. III. (1988). *J. Food Comp. Anal. 1,* 105.

Gregory, J.F. III, Trumbo, P.R., Bailey, L.B., Toth, J.P., Baumgartner, T.G., and Cerda, J.J. (1991). *J. Nutr. 121,* 177.

Gries, C.L., and Scott, M.L. (1972). *J. Nutr. 102,* 1269.

Groziak, S.M., and Kirksey, A. (1987). *J. Nutr. 117,* 1045.

Groziak, S.M., and Kirksey, A. (1990). *J. Nutr. 120,* 485.

Guilarte, T.R. (1993). *Nutr. Rev. 51,* 193.

Gummow, B., Bastianello, S.S., Labuschagne, L., and Erasmus, G.L. (1992). *Onderstepoort J. Vet. Res. 59,* 111.

Hansen, C.M., LeKlem, J.E., and Miller, L.T. (1996). *J. Nutr. 126,* 2512.

Harmon, B.G., Miller, E.R., Hoefer, J.A., Ullrey, D.E., and Leucke, R.W. (1963). *J. Nutr. 79,* 263.

Haskell, B.E. (1978). *In* Handbook Series in Nutrition and Food, Section E: Nutritional Disorders (M. Rechcigl Jr., ed.), Vol. 1, p. 43. CRC Press, Boca Raton, Florida.

Heller, S., Salkeld, R.M., and Korner, W.F. (1973). *Am. J. Clin. Nutr. 26,* 1330.

Heseker, H., and Kübler, W. (1992). *In* Nutrition of the Elderly (H.N. Munro and G.J. Schlierf, eds.), Nutrition Workshop Series 29. Raven Press, New York.

Hoffmann-La Roche. (1979). Rationale for Roche Recommended Vitamin Fortification-Poultry Rations. RCD 5692/979. Hoffmann-La Roche, Nutley, New Jersey.

Hoover-Plow, J., and Rice, S. (1992). *Nutr. Res. 12,* 773.

Ink, S.L., and Henderson, L.M. (1984). *Annu. Rev. Nutr. 4,* 455.

Johnson, B.C., Mitchell, H.H., Hamilton, T.S., and Nevens, W.B. (1947). *Fed. Proc. Am. Soc. Exp. Biol. 6,* 410.

Johnson, B.C., Pinkos, J.A., and Burke, K.A. (1950). *J. Nutr. 40,* 309.

Kabir, H., LeKlem, J.E., and Miller, L.T. (1983). *J. Nutr. 113,* 2412.

Kafatos, A., Diacatou, A., Labadarios, D., Kounali, D., Apostolaki, J., Vlachonikolis, J., Mamalakis, G., and Megremis, S. (1993). *J. Am. Coll. Nutr. 12,* 685.

Kaido, M., Mori, K., Ide, Y., Inoue, N., and Koide, O. (1991). *Exp. Mol. Pathol. 55,* 63.

Kang-Yoon, S.A., Kirksey, A., Giacoia, G., and West, K. (1992). *Am. J. Clin. Nutr. 56,* 548.

Kirksey, A. (1981). *In* Vitamin B_6 Methodology and Nutrition Assessment (J.E. LeKlem and R.D. Reynolds, eds.), p. 269. Plenum, New York.

Kodentsova, V.M., Yakushina, L.M., Vrzhesinskaya, O.A., Beketova, N.A., and Spirichev, V.B. (1993). *Voprosy Pitaniya 5,* 32.

Korede, O. (1990). *Ann. Nutr. Metab. 34,* 273.

Krinke, G.J., and Fitzgerald, R.E. (1988). *Toxicology 49,* 171.

Lakshmi, R., Lakshmi, A.V., Divan, P.V., and Bamji, M.S. (1991). *Indian J. Biochem. Biophys. 28,* 481.

Leeson, S., and Marcotte, M. (1993). *World's Poultry Sci. J. 49,* 120.

LeKlem, J.E. (1990). *J. Nutr. 120,* 1503.

LeKlem, J.E. (1991). *In* Handbook of Vitamins (L.J. Machlin, ed.), p. 341. Marcel Dekker, New York.

LeKlem, J.E., Miller, L.T., Perera, A.D., and Peffers, D.E. (1980). *J. Nutr. 110,* 1819.

Lilum, D., Hammond, W., Krauss, D., and Schoonmaker, J. (1981). *Invest. Urol. 18,* 451.

Lin, G.W.J. (1989). *Alcohol. Clin. Exp. Res. 13,* 236.

Loosli, J.K. (1991). *In* Animal Science Handbook (P.A. Putnam, ed.). Academic Press, San Diego, California.

Lovell, R.T. (1987). *Feed Manage. 38,* 28.

Löwik, M.R.H., van den Berg, H., Westenbrink, S., Wedel, M., Schrijver, J., and Ockhuizen, T. (1989). *Am. J. Clin. Nutr. 50,* 391.

Lucas, H.L., Heuser, G.F., and Norris, L.C. (1946). *Poult. Sci. 25,* 137.

Lui, A., Lumeng, L., and Li, T. (1983). *J. Nutr. 113,* 893.

Lui, A., Lumeng, L., Aronoff, G.R., and Li, T. (1985). *J. Lab. Clin. Med. 106,* 491.

Mahuren, J.D., Pauly, T.A., and Coburn, S.P. (1991). *J. Nutr. Biochem. 2,* 449.

Marks, J. (1975). A Guide to the Vitamins, Their Role in Health and Disease, p. 73. Medical and Technical Publ., Lancaster, England.

Masse, P.G., Pritzker, K.P., Mendes, M.G., Boskey, A.L., and Weiser, H. (1994). *Brit. J. Nutr. 71,* 919.

Matyaszczyk, M., Karczmarewicz, E., Czarnowska, E., Reynolds, R.D., and Lorenc, R.S. (1993). *J. Nutr. 123,* 204.

McCullough, A.L., Kirksey, A., and Wacks, T.C. (1990). *Am. J. Clin. Nutr. 51,* 1067.

McCollum, E.V. (1957). *In* A History of Nutrition. The Riverside Press, Cambridge, Massachusetts.

McElroy, L.W., and Goss, H. (1939). *J. Biol. Chem. 130,* 437.

Mehansho, H., and Henderson, L.M. (1980). *J. Biol. Chem. 255,* 11901.

Mehansho, H., Hamm, M.W., and Henderson, L.M. (1979). *J. Nutr. 109,* 1542.

Merrill, A.H., and Burnhan, F.S. (1990). *In* Nutrition Reviews, Present Knowledge in Nutrition (M.L. Brown, ed.), p. 155. The Nutrition Foundation, Washington, D.C.

Meydani, S.N., Ribaya-Mercado, J.D., Russell, R.M., Sahyoun, N., Morrow, F.D., and Gershoff, S.N. (1991). *Am. J. Clin. Nutr. 53,* 1275.

Miller, B.F. (1963). *Poult. Sci. 42,* 795.

Miller, E.E., and Baumann, C.A. (1945). *J. Biol. Chem. 157,* 551.

Miller, L.T. (1986). *J. Nutr. 116,* 1344.

Mitwalli, A. (1989). *Ann. Saudi Med. 6,* 541.

Nakano, H., and Gregory, J.F. III. (1995). *J. Nutr. 125,* 926.

Nakano, H., McMahon, L.G., and Gregory, J.F. III. (1997). *J. Nutr. 127,* 1508.

Nguyen, L.B., and Gregory, J.F. III. (1983). *J. Nutr. 113,* 1550.

NRC. Nutrient Requirements of Domestic Animals. National Academy of Sciences- National Research Council, Washington, D.C.

(1978). Nutrient Requirements of Nonhuman Primates.

(1981). Nutrient Requirements of Goats.

(1982a). Nutrient Requirements of Mink and Foxes.

(1985a). Nutrient Requirements of Dogs, 2nd Ed.

(1985b). Nutrient Requirements of Sheep, 5th Ed.

(1986). Nutrient Requirements of Cats, 3rd Ed.

(1989a). Nutrient Requirements of Dairy Cattle, 6th Ed.

(1989b). Nutrient Requirements of Horses, 5th Ed.

(1993). Nutrient Requirements of Fish.

(1994). Nutrient Requirements of Poultry, 9th Ed.

(1995). Nutrient Requirements of Laboratory Animals.

(1996). Nutrient Requirements of Beef Cattle, 7th Ed.

(1998). Nutrient Requirements of Swine, 10th Ed.

NRC. (1982b). United States-Canadian Tables of Feed Composition, 3rd Ed. National Academy of Sciences-National Research Council, Washington, D.C.

NRC. (1987). Vitamin Tolerance of Animals. National Academy of Sciences-National Research Council, Washington, D.C.

Oka, T., Komori, N., Kuwahata, M., Suzuki, I., Okada, M., and Natori, Y. (1994). *Experientia 50*, 127.

Pannemans, D.L., van den Berg, H., and Westerterp, K.R. (1994). *J. Nutr. 124*, 1207.

Parsons, J.L., and Klostermann, H.J. (1967). *Feedstuffs 39*(45), 74.

Perry, S.C. (1978). *Proc. Roche Vitam. Nutr. Update Meeting*, p. 29. Hot Springs, Arkansas.

Pingali, A.V., and Trumbo, P.R. (1992). *J. Agr. Food. Chem. 40*, 1860.

Price, J.M., Brown, R.R., and Larson, F.C. (1957). *J. Clin. Invest. 36*, 1600.

Rabinowitz, J.C., and Snell, E.E. (1949). *Proc. Soc. Exp. Biol. Med. 70*, 235.

Rall, L.C., and Meydani, S.N. (1993). *Nutr. Rev. 51*, 217.

RDA. (1989). Recommended Dietary Allowances, 10th Ed. National Academy of Sciences-National Research Council, Washington, D.C.

Ritchie, H.D., Miller, E.R., Ullrey, D.E., Hofer, J.A., and Lucke, R.W. (1960). *J. Nutr. 70*, 491.

Robel, E.J. (1992). *Poultry Sci. 71*, 1733.

Robel, E.J., and Christensen, V.L. (1991). *Brit. Poult. Sci. 32*, 509.

Roe, D.A. (1973). *Drug Ther. 3*, 23.

Roth-Maier, D.A., and Kirchgessner, M. (1993). *J. Anim. Physiol. Anim. Nutr. 70*, 6.

Rothschild, B. (1982). *Arch. Intern. Med. 142*, 840 (Abstr.).

Sakurai, T., Asakura, T., Mizuno, A., and Matsuda, M. (1992). *J. Nutr. Sci. Vitaminol. 38*, 227.

Salkeld, R., Knorr, K., and Korner, W. (1973). *Clin. Chim. Acta 49*, 195.

Schaeffer, M.C. (1993). *J. Nutr. 123*, 1444.

Schaeffer, M.C., Cochary, E.F., and Sadowski, J.A. (1990). *J. Am. Coll. Nutr. 9*, 120.

Schaumburg, H., Kaplan, J., Windebank, A., Vick, N., Rasmug, S., Pleasure, D., and Brown, M.J. (1983). *N. Engl. J. Med. 309*, 445.

Schenker, S., Johnson, R.F., Mahuren, J.D., Henderson, G.I., and Coburn, S.P. (1992). *Am. J. Physiol. 262,* R966.

Scott, M.L., Nesheim, M.C., and Young, R.J. (1982). Nutrition of the Chicken, p. 119. Scott, Ithaca, New York.

Scriver, C.R., and Whelan, D.T. (1969). *Ann. N Y Acad. Sci. 166,* 83.

Shideler, C.E. (1983). *Am. J. Med. Technol. 49,* 17.

Snell, E.E. (1986). *In* Pyridoxal Phosphate: Chemical, Biochemical and Medical Aspects, Part A (D. Dolphin, R. Poulson and O. Avramovic, eds.), Vol. 1A, p. 1. John Wiley and Sons, New York.

Styslinger, L., and Kirksey, A. (1985). *Am. J. Clin. Nutr. 41,* 21.

Tarr, J.B., Tamura, T., and Stokstad, E.L.R. (1981). *Am. J. Clin. Nutr. 34,* 1328.

Tomarelli, R.M., Spence, E.R., and Bernhart, F.W. (1955). *J. Agric. Food Chem. 3,* 338.

Trumbo, P.R., and Gregory, J.F. III. (1989). *J. Nutr. 119,* 36.

Trumbo, P.R., and Raidi, M.A. (1991). *Nutr. Res. 11,* 53.

Trumbo, P.R., Gregory, J.F. III, and Sartain, D.B. (1988). *J. Nutr. 118,* 170.

Unna, K., and Antopol, W. (1940). *Proc. Soc. Exp. Biol. Med. 43,* 116.

Vanderslice, J.T., Maire, C.E., Doherty, R.F., and Beecher, G.R. (1980). *J. Agric. Food Chem. 28,* 1145.

Van Schoonhoven, J., Schrijver, J., van den Berg, H., and Haenen, G. (1994). *J. Agr. Food Chem. 42,* 1475.

Verbeeck, J. (1975). *Feedstuffs 47*(36), 4.

Wada, H., and Snell, E.E. (1961). *J. Biol. Chem. 236,* 2089.

Wei, I.L., and Young, T.K. (1994). *Nutr. Res. 14,* 271.

Wetherilt, H., Ackurt, F., Brubacher, G., Okan, B., Aktas, S., and Turdu, S. (1992). *Int. J. Vitam. Nutr. Res. 62,* 21.

Witkowska, D., Sedrowicz, L., and Oledzka, R. (1992). *Bromatologia Chemia Toksykoleziczna 25,* 25.

Wohl, M., Levy, H., Szutha, A., and Maldia, G. (1960). *Proc. Soc. Exp. Biol. Med. 105,* 523.

Yang, C.P., and Jeng, S.L. (1989). *J. Chinese Agr. Chem. Soc. 27,* 450.

Yen, J.T., Jensen, A.H., and Baker, D.H. (1976). *J. Anim. Sci. 42,* 866.

Yin, S., Sato, I., and Yamaguchi, K. (1992). *J. Nutr. Biochem. 3,* 633.

Zempleni, J., Link, G., and Kubler, W. (1992). *Int. J. Vitam. Nutr. Res. 62,* 165.

Zhang, Z., Gregory, J.F. III, and McCormick, D.B. (1993). *J. Nutr. 123,* 85.

PANTOTHENIC ACID

INTRODUCTION

After the discovery of thiamin, riboflavin, and niacin as B-complex vitamins, researchers realized that at least one other unidentified factor remained. Two additional vitamins, pyridoxine (vitamin B_6) and pantothenic acid, were found in the late 1930s as fractions of yeast and liver. Tissue extracts from a variety of biological materials provided a growth factor for yeast that was identified as pantothenic acid, derived from the Greek word *pantos*, meaning "found everywhere."

Pantothenic acid is found in two enzymes, coenzyme A and acyl carrier protein, which are involved in many reactions in carbohydrate, fat, and protein metabolism. Although this vitamin occurs in practically all feedstuffs, the quantity present is generally insufficient for optimum performance of poultry and swine and other monogastric species. There are no reports of deficiency in adult ruminants because of microbial synthesis. Pantothenic acid deficiency occurs only rarely in humans.

HISTORY

Historical aspects of pantothenic acid have been reviewed (Sauberlich, 1973; Fox, 1991; Loosli, 1991). During the 1930s several independent research programs concentrated on either a growth factor for microorganisms or a chick antidermatitis factor. Research to identify pantothenic acid was also closely associated with studies of vitamin B_6 (pyridoxine). Both vitamins were fractions of the "vitamin B_2" complex and were found associated in biological materials. Since pyridoxine was adsorbed on Fuller's earth, from which it could be eluted, and pantothenic acid was not, pantothenic acid was sometimes referred to as

10

"filtrate factor" and pyridoxine as "eluate factor." Pantothenic acid deficiency was first described in the chick as a pellagra-like dermatitis by Norris and Ringrose in 1930. Since the filtrate factor cured dermatitis in chicks, but not rats, one early name of the vitamin was "chick antidermatitis factor."

In independent studies in 1933, Williams and associates fractionated "bios," a growth factor for yeast, particularly *Saccharomyces cerevisiae*. They concentrated the factor, determined many of its properties, and provided the name pantothenic acid. In 1937 Snell and associates independently studied the nature of an essential factor for lactic and propionic acid bacteria. It was soon found that the filtrate factor, the chick antidermatitis factor, and the unknown factor required by yeast and lactic acid bacteria were all pantothenic acid. In 1939 Williams isolated pantothenic acid and determined the structure in 1940. Also in 1940 the vitamin was synthesized independently in three different laboratories. The active form of pantothenic acid, coenzyme A, was discovered as an essential cofactor in acetylation of sulfonamides in the liver by Lipmann and Kaplan in 1947.

CHEMICAL STRUCTURE, PROPERTIES, AND ANTAGONISTS

Pantothenic acid is an amide consisting of pantoic acid (α, γ-dihydroxy-β, β-dimethylbutyric acid) joined to β-alanine. Pantothenic acid and the biologically active coenzyme A, which contains the vitamin as an essential component, are shown in Fig. 10.1. The vitamin is derivatized at its carboxyl end by β-mercaptoethylamine and at its alcohol end by phosphate to form a pseudodinucleotide containing phosphoadenylic acid. Therefore coenzyme A contains the vitamin combined with adenosine 3'-phosphate, pyrophosphate, and β-mercaptoethylamine. Another metabolically active form of pantothenic acid, panthenol, is more easily absorbed and is converted to the acid in vivo.

Analogs of pantothenic acid that have replaced the β-alanine with other amino acids, such as α-alanine, β-aminobutyric acid, aspartic acid, leucine, or lysine, are inactive. The most common antagonist of pantothenic acid is ω-methyl-pantothenic acid, which has been used to produce a deficiency of the vitamin in humans (Hodges et al., 1958). Other antivitamins include pantoyltaurine, phenylpantothenate hydroxycobalamine (c-lactam) (analog of vitamin B_{12}), and antimetabolites of the vitamin containing alkyl or aryl ureido and carbamate components in the amide part of the molecule (Fox, 1991; Brass, 1993). Feeding chickens

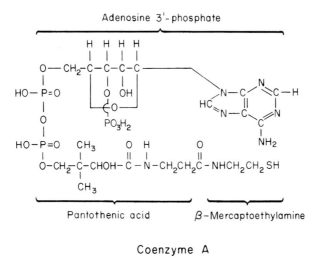

Fig. 10.1 Structures of pantothenic acid and coenzyme A.

on high intakes of copper results in reduced formation of coenzyme A, by increasing the oxidation of cysteine to cystine, and also by the formation of copper-cysteine and copper-glutathione complexes, which render the amino acid unavailable for coenzyme A synthesis (Latymer and Coates, 1981).

The free acid of the vitamin is a viscous, pale yellow oil readily soluble in water and ethyl acetate. The oil is extremely hygroscopic and is easily destroyed by acids, bases, and heat. Maximum heat stability occurs at pH 5.5 to 7.0. Calcium pantothenate, the form used in commerce, crystallizes as white needles from methanol and is reasonably

421

stable to light and air. Pantothenic acid is optically active (characteristic of rotating a polarized light). It may be prepared as either the pure dextrorotatory (*d*-) form or the *dl*-form; the racemic form has approximately one-half the biological activity of *d*-calcium pantothenate. Only the dextrorotatory form, *d*-pantothenic acid, is effective as a vitamin. The *l*-pantothenic acid is inactive for organisms requiring the intact vitamin.

ANALYTICAL PROCEDURES

Pantothenic acid content of various substances has been analyzed by microbiological assay, animal bioassay, radioimmunoassay, and chemical methods (Fox, 1991). The complex nature of natural products has hindered development of chemical methods for assay of the vitamin. Chick growth bioassays have been used extensively and measure bound forms as well as free pantothenic acid.

The rat and chick tests have gradually been replaced by more rapid, simpler, and cheaper microbiological tests. Microbiological procedures for determination of pantothenic acid are widely employed but require that the vitamin be freed from the coenzyme form. Values for pantothenic acid content of feedstuffs obtained by microbiological procedures performed before proper methods were devised for liberating the vitamin from its bound form are much too low. Procedures for cleavage of bound forms to obtain free pantothenic acid can include use of (1) intestinal phosphatase to cleave the phosphate linkage and (2) pigeon or chick liver enzyme preparation to break the linkage between mercaptoethylamine and pantothenic acid. Bound forms cannot be hydrolyzed as this will destroy the vitamin. A number of organisms can be used in the assay method; *Lactobacillus plantarum* (formerly *Lactobacillus arabinosus*) is widely used.

Radioimmunoassay and an automated fluorometric assay technique (Roy and Buccafuri, 1978) have been reported to be successful for pantothenic acid determination. Pantothenic acid levels in blood have been determined by radioimmunoassay (Wyse and Hansen, 1977). After treatment with alkaline phosphatase and liver extract, the pantothenic acid content of whole blood analyzed by radioimmunoassay compared favorably to the microbiological assay with *L. plantarum*. An indirect enzyme-linked immunosorbent assay (ELISA) has been developed for determining pantothenic acid in plasma (Song et al., 1990). The ELISA was based on the competition for the antibody between immobilized pantothenate adsorbed on polystyrene microwells and free pantothenate in samples. This method is easy to use, less expensive, and sensitive.

METABOLISM

Pantothenic acid is found in feeds in both bound and free forms. The bound coenzyme forms are principally coenzyme A and acyl carrier protein (ACP). It is necessary to liberate the pantothenic acid from the bound forms in the digestive process prior to absorption. Coenzyme A and other bound forms are hydrolyzed in the intestinal lumen to 4'-phosphopantetheine. This form is dephosphorylated to yield pantothenate, which is rapidly converted by the intestinal enzyme pantetheinase to pantothenic acid. Pantothenic acid, its salt, and the alcohol are absorbed primarily in the jejunum by a specific transport system that is saturable and sodium ion dependent (Fenstermacher and Rose, 1986). The alcohol form, *panthenol*, which is oxidized to pantothenic acid in vivo, appears to be absorbed somewhat faster than the acid form. After absorption, pantothenic acid is transported to various tissues in the plasma, from which it is taken up by most cells via another active-transport process involving cotransport of pantothenate and sodium in a 1:1 ratio (Olson, 1990).

Within all tissues pantothenic acid is converted to coenzyme A and other compounds in which the vitamin is a functional group (Sauberlich, 1985). Free pantothenate appears to be efficiently absorbed; in the dog, between 81 and 94% of an oral dose of sodium [^{14}C] pantothenate was absorbed (Taylor et al., 1974). Measurement of pantothenic acid bioavailability in adult men consuming a typical United States diet ranged from 40 to 61%, with an average of 50% (Sauberlich, 1985). Urinary excretion represents the major route of body loss of absorbed pantothenic acid, with prompt excretion when taken in excess. Most pantothenic acid is excreted as the free vitamin, but some species (e.g., dog) excrete it as β-glucuronide (Taylor et al., 1972). An appreciable quantity of pantothenic acid (approximately 15% of daily intake) is oxidized completely and is excreted across the lungs as CO_2 (Combs, 1992).

Animals and humans do not appear to have the ability to store appreciable amounts of pantothenic acid, with organs such as the liver and kidney having the highest concentrations. Most pantothenic acid in blood exists in red blood cells as coenzyme A; serum contains no coenzyme A but does contain free pantothenic acid. A number of human studies suggest that stores of pantothenic acid are not great, as tissue levels dropped dramatically and/or clinical signs developed after 7 to 12 weeks on diets low in the vitamin (Fry et al., 1976). Urinary pantothenic acid concentrations dropped from 3 to 8.0 mg in just 63 days in human subjects fed low quantities of the vitamin (Fry et al., 1976). Coenzyme A is synthesized by cells from pantothenic acid, ATP, and cysteine. Pantothenic acid kinase, a cytosolic enzyme, is rate limiting for the overall pathway of coenzyme A biosynthesis (Brass, 1993).

FUNCTIONS

Pantothenic acid functions as a constituent of two important coenzymes—coenzyme A and ACP. Coenzyme A is found in all tissues and is one of the most important coenzymes for tissue metabolism. The important role of coenzyme A is summarized in Fig. 10.2; biochemical reactions catalyzed by coenzyme A are presented in Table 10.1. The coenzymes are known to be involved in more than 100 different metabolic pathways involving the metabolism of carbohydrates, proteins, and lipids, and the synthesis of lipids, neurotransmitters, steroid hormones, porphyrins, and hemoglobin.

The most important function of coenzyme A is to act as a carrier mechanism for carboxylic acids (Marks, 1975). Such acids, when bound to coenzyme A, have a high potential for transfer to other groups and are normally then referred to as "active." The most important of these reactions is the combination of coenzyme A with acetate to form "active acetate" with a high-energy bond that renders acetate capable of further chemical interactions. As an example, it is utilized directly by combination with oxaloacetic acid to form citric acid, which enters the Krebs citric acid cycle. Its combination with two-carbon fragments from fats, carbohydrates, and certain amino acids to form acetyl coenzyme A is an essential step in their complete metabolism, because the coenzyme enables these fragments to enter the citric acid cycle.

Coenzyme A functions as a carrier of acyl groups in enzymatic reactions involved in synthesis of fatty acids, cholesterol, and sterols; in the oxidation of fatty acids, pyruvate, and α-ketoglutarate; and in biological acetylations. In the form of active acetate, acetic acid can also combine with choline to form acetylcholine, the chemical transmitter at the nerve synapse, and can be used for detoxification of drugs including sulfonamides.

Coenzyme A has an essential function in lipid metabolism, fatty acids are activated by formation of the coenzyme derivative, and degra-

424

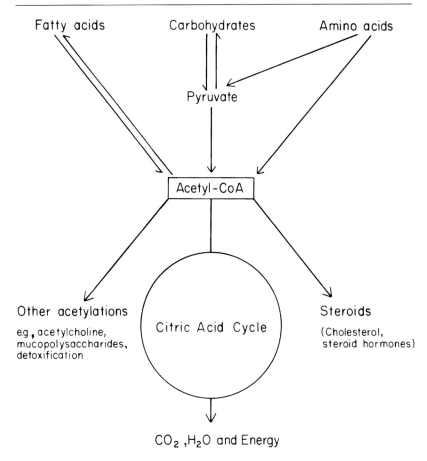

Fig. 10.2 The important role of coenzyme A in metabolism. (Modified from Marks, 1975.)

dation by removal of acetate fragments in beta oxidation also uses another molecule of coenzyme A. These active acetate fragments may directly enter the citric acid cycle or combine to form ketone bodies. A pantothenic acid-dependent enzyme, ACP, that replaces coenzyme A during building of the carbon chain in synthesis of fatty acids, was recognized in 1965 (Pugh and Wakil, 1965). ACP is a protein with a sulfhydryl group covalently attached to acetyl, malonyl, and intermediate-chain acyl groups. The sulfhydryl group at the binding site of the ACP was identified as a cysteine residue, thioethanolamine. Discovery of thioethanolamine and β-alanine residues suggested that both ACP and coenzyme A have similar acyl-binding sites.

425

CHAPTER TEN

■ Table 10.1   Selected Biochemical Reactions Catalyzed by Coenzyme A

Enzyme	Pantothenate Derivative	Reactant	Product	Site
Pyruvic dehydrogenase	CoA	Pyruvate	Acetyl-CoA	Mitochondria
α-Ketoglutarate dehydrogenase	CoA	α-Ketoglutarate	Succinyl-CoA	Mitochondria
Fatty acid oxidase	CoA	Palmitate	Acetyl-CoA	Mitochondria
Fatty acid synthetase	Acyl carrier protein	Acetyl-CoA, Malonyl-CoA	Palmitate	Microsomes
Propionyl-CoA carboxylase	CoA	Propionyl-CoA, carbon dioxide	Methylmalonyl-CoA	Microsomes
Acyl-CoA synthetase	Phosphopanthetheine	Succinyl-CoA, GDP + P_1	Succinate, GTP + CoA	Mitochondria

Source: Modified from Olson (1990).

Decarboxylation of ketoglutaric acid in the citric acid cycle yields succinic acid, which is then converted to the active form by linkage with coenzyme A. Active succinate and glycine are together involved in the first step of heme biosynthesis. Pantothenic acid also stimulates synthesis of antibodies, which increase resistance of animals to pathogens. It appears that when pantothenic acid is deficient, the incorporation of amino acids into the blood albumin fraction is inhibited, which would explain why there is a reduction in the titer of antibodies (Axelrod, 1971). The 4′-phosphopantetheine is the prosthetic group of an enzyme system that synthesizes peptide antibodies, such as gramicidin in bacteria (Olson, 1990).

REQUIREMENTS

Pantothenic acid requirements for selected animals and humans are presented in Table 10.2. For growth and reproduction, the majority of species have a dietary requirement between 5 and 15 mg/kg of diet. For egg production in chickens, the pantothenic acid requirement is very low (2.2 mg/kg) compared to a requirement of 10 mg/kg for growth and reproduction. Requirements are based on typical consumption levels. When energy density of diets is increased, intake is reduced, so higher dietary concentrations of pantothenic acid and other vitamins are required. When the level of energy in the rations of broilers was raised

426

■ Table 10.2   Pantothenic Acid Requirements for Various Animals and Humans

Animal	Purpose or Class	Requirement[a]	Reference
Beef cattle	Adult	Microbial synthesis	NRC (1996)
Dairy cattle	Calf	13 ppm milk replacer	NRC (1989a)
	Adult	Microbial synthesis	NRC (1989a)
Chicken	Leghorn, 0–18 weeks	10.0 mg/kg	NRC (1994)
	Laying (100-g intake)	1.7–2.5 mg/kg	NRC (1994)
	Broilers, 0–8 weeks	10.0 mg/kg	NRC (1994)
Duck (Pekin)	0–7 weeks	11.0 mg/kg	NRC (1994)
Japanese quail	All classes	10.0–15.0 mg/kg	NRC (1994)
Turkey	0–4 weeks	10.0 mg/kg	NRC (1994)
	4–24 weeks	9.0 mg/kg	NRC (1994)
Sheep	Adult	Microbial synthesis	NRC (1985b)
Swine	Growing-finishing, 3–5 kg	12.0 mg/kg	NRC (1998)
	Growing-finishing, 5–110 kg	7.0–10.0 mg/kg	NRC (1998)
	Adult	12.0 mg/kg	NRC (1998)
Horse	Adult	Microbial synthesis	NRC (1989b)
Goat	Adult	Microbial synthesis	NRC (1981b)
Fox	Growing	8.0 mg/kg	NRC (1982a)
Cat	Growing	5.0 mg/kg	NRC (1986)
Dog	Growing	400 µg/kg body wt.	NRC (1985a)
Fish	Catfish	10–15 mg/kg	NRC (1993)
	Pacific salmon	17–50 mg/kg	NRC (1993)
	Rainbow trout	10–20 mg/kg	NRC (1993)
Rat	All classes	8.0 mg/kg	NRC (1995)
Mouse	All classes	16.0 mg/kg	NRC (1995)
Human	Infants	2–3 mg/day	RDA (1989)
	Adults	4–7 mg/day	RDA (1989)

[a]Expressed as per unit of animal feed on either as-fed (approximately 90% dry matter) or dry basis (see Appendix, Tables A1a,b). Human data are expressed as mg/day.

from 2,870 to 3,505 kcal/kg, intake of pantothenic acid fell by 19.1% because appetite is mainly controlled by intake of energy (Friesecke, 1975). For the blue tilapia (*Tilapia aurea*) fish, the growth requirement for pantothenic acid was 6 mg/kg, but based on survival and lack of pathology, a value of 10 mg/kg was recommended (Roem et al., 1991).

Research has shown a wide variation in pantothenic acid requirements, even among animals within a breed. Data from Michigan show that for one-half of growing pigs, 9.13 mg/kg of pantothenic acid was sufficient for growth, whereas the remaining one-half required more than 9.13 but less than 13.5 mg/kg (Luecke et al., 1953).

Antibiotics have a sparing effect on the pantothenic acid requirement. A dietary level of 22 mg/kg aureomycin for weanling pigs (McKigney et al., 1957) and 10 mg/kg of procaine penicillin to turkey poults (Slinger and Pepper, 1954) reduced the pantothenic acid requirement for these species.

If the rumen is functioning normally, ruminal microflora will synthesize enough pantothenic acid to satisfy ruminant needs; however, biosynthesis will depend on the composition of feeds. Vitamin synthesis is reduced with diets high in cellulose but increases with higher quantities of easily soluble carbohydrates (Virtanen, 1966). Certain amounts of B-complex (including pantothenic acid) vitamins are synthesized in the large intestine of monogastric animals. It is doubtful, however, whether much benefit is derived, as only limited pantothenic acid absorption occurs in the large intestine, with greatest benefit found in animals that practice coprophagy (Friesecke, 1975).

Interrelationships with other vitamins (e.g., vitamin B_{12}, vitamin C, and biotin) on pantothenic acid requirements are known (Scott et al., 1982). Pantothenic acid requirement of chicks from B_{12}-depleted hens was found to be greater than that of chicks from normal hens. A five-fold increase in coenzyme A content of liver was found in B_{12}-deficient chicks and rats. There is no evidence of sparing action of B_{12} on pantothenic acid needs for swine as has been observed in poultry (Luecke et al., 1953). There is some evidence that pantothenic acid is involved in ascorbic acid synthesis in plants and animals, with ascorbic acid sparing the pantothenic acid requirement in rats (Barboriak and Krehl, 1957). Also, there have been suggestions of a possible interrelationship between folacin and biotin with pantothenate. Both vitamins were found necessary for pantothenic acid utilization in the rat (Wright and Welch, 1943). The inclusion of biotin in the diet of a pantothenic acid-deficient pig was effective in prolonging the life of the pig, but caused the pantothenic acid deficiency signs to appear in half the time (Colby et al., 1948).

Dietary fat and protein influence the pantothenic acid requirement. Pigs fed a diet deficient in pantothenic acid and high in fat failed to gain weight, exhibited lower feed efficiency, and developed deficiency signs more quickly than those fed diets low in fat (Sewell et al., 1962). Nelson and Evans (1945) found that pantothenic acid-deficient rats fed a high-protein diet excreted more pantothenic acid and had accelerated growth and survival rates compared with rats fed a low-protein diet. The superiority of the high-protein diet may be due to the decreased level of dietary carbohydrate, which would presumably require coenzyme A for metabolism.

The Food and Nutrition Board of the National Research Council (RDA, 1989) has not established a recommended human dietary allowance for pantothenic acid but states that 4 to 7 mg per day for adults and 2 to 3 mg per day for infants are safe and adequate intakes. Women who are pregnant or lactating may have an increased requirement of about 30% (Plaut et al., 1974).

NATURAL SOURCES

Pantothenic acid is widely distributed in foods of animal and plant origin. Alfalfa hay, peanut meal, cane molasses, yeast, rice bran and polishings, green leafy plants, wheat bran, brewer's yeast, and fish solubles are good sources for animals. For human foods, in general, liver, kidney, yeast, egg yolk, and fresh vegetables (e.g., mushrooms, avocados, and broccoli) are the best sources, followed by milk and meat; grains, fruits, and nuts contain the lowest levels. Royal jelly of bees is a rich source (510 ppm), with ovaries of the cod containing more than 2,000 ppm. Analysis of feeds for pantothenic acid are sometimes conflicting depending on whether data were determined by microbiological assays or more recent radio immunoassay procedures. Different methods of sample hydrolysis may also contribute to the variation (see Analytical Procedures). The pantothenic acid content of foods and feedstuffs is shown in Table 10.3.

Many swine and poultry diets are borderline in supplying pantothenic acid requirements, and many are deficient in this vitamin. Diets based on corn and soybean meal are apt to be deficient in pantothenic acid. Milling by-products such as rice bran and wheat bran are good

■ Table 10.3   Pantothenic Acid in Foods and Feedstuffs (mg/kg, dry basis)

Food	Value	Food	Value
Alfalfa hay, sun cured	28.6	Molasses, sugarcane	50.3
Alfalfa leaves, sun cured	32.4	Oat, grain	8.8
Barley, grain	9.1	Pea seeds	21.0
Bean, navy (seed)	2.3	Peanut meal, solvent extracted	50.7
Blood meal	2.6	Potato	22.0
Brewer's grains	8.9	Rice, bran	25.2
Buttermilk (cattle)	40.1	Rice, grain	9.1
Citrus pulp	14.3	Rice, polished	3.9
Clover hay, ladino (sun cured)	1.1	Rye, grain	9.1
Copra meal (coconut)	6.9	Sorghum, grain	12.5
Corn, gluten meal	11.2	Soybean meal, solvent extracted	18.2
Corn, yellow grain	6.6	Soybean seed	17.3
Cottonseed meal, solvent extracted	15.4	Spleen, cattle	8.2
Eggs	27.0	Timothy hay, sun cured	7.9
Fish meal, anchovy	10.9	Wheat, bran	33.5
Fish meal, menhaden	9.4	Wheat, grain	11.4
Fish, sardine	11.8	Whey	49.6
Linseed meal, solvent extracted	16.3	Yeast, brewer's	118.4
Liver, cattle	164.9	Yeast, torula	100.6
Milk, skim, cattle	38.6		

Source: NRC (1982b).

429

sources, being two to three times higher than the respective grains. Biological availability of pantothenic acid is high from corn and soybean meal, but low from barley, wheat, and sorghum (Southern and Baker, 1981). Changing processing methods can greatly alter vitamin feed levels. As an example, with changes in sugar technology, literature values for pantothenic acid content of beet molasses have decreased from 50 to 110 mg/kg in the 1950s to about 1 to 4 mg/kg (Palagina et al., 1990).

Pantothenic acid is reported to be fairly stable in feedstuffs during long periods of storage (Scott et al., 1982). The authors indicate that heating during processing may cause considerable losses, especially if temperatures attain 100 to 150°C for long periods and pH values are above 7 or below 5.

Gadient (1986) considers pantothenic acid to be slightly sensitive to heat, oxygen, or light, but very sensitive to moisture. Pelleting was reported to cause only small losses of the vitamin. As a general guideline, pantothenic acid activity in normal pelleted feed over a period of 3 months at room temperature should be 80 to 100%. Pantothenic acid loss during processing of human foods is significant and can amount to as much as 70% in frozen meat and 80% in canned legumes. Loss of the vitamin in dairy products during processing and storage is about 30 to 35% (Song, 1990).

DEFICIENCY

Effects of Deficiency

On the basis of observations on pantothenic acid-deficient animals and studies in human volunteers, deficiency of the vitamin is shown in the following signs and symptoms:

1. Reduced growth and feed conversion efficiency.
2. Lesions of skin and its appendages.
3. Disorders of the nervous system.
4. Gastrointestinal disturbances.
5. Inhibition of antibody formation and thus decreased resistance to infection.
6. Impairment of adrenal function.

Clinical signs of pantothenic acid deficiency take many forms and differ from one animal species to another. In humans, additional emotional and neurological symptoms include hyperventilation, irritability, insomnia, depression, headache, and dizziness. Since pantothenic acid is so widely distributed in nature, clear-cut deficiency symptoms in humans are rarely found in practice. However, pantothenic acid does occur in animals with certain feeding regimens.

Ruminants

Pantothenic acid is not required in the diet of adult ruminants, because ruminal microorganisms synthesize this vitamin in adequate amounts. Sheppard and Johnson (1957) experimentally produced pantothenic acid deficiencies in calves. Major clinical signs were anorexia, reduced growth, rough hair coat, dermatitis, diarrhea, and eventual death. The most characteristic pantothenic acid deficiency sign in the calf is scaly dermatitis around the eyes and muzzle. Anorexia and diarrhea followed after 11 to 20 weeks on a deficient diet, and calves become weak and unable to stand and may develop convulsions. They are susceptible to mucosal infection, especially in the respiratory tract. Postmortem studies have revealed moderate sciatic and peripheral nerve demyelination. If deficient calves are treated with calcium pantothenate, they respond with increased appetite and weight gains and subsequent reversal of dermatitis.

Swine

Many swine diets are borderline in supplying pantothenic acid, and many are deficient in the vitamin (Cunha, 1977). Nonspecific signs of pantothenic acid deficiency in swine include reduced growth rate, bloody diarrhea, loss of appetite, poor general condition, dermatosis, lowered blood pantothenic acid, and reduced feed conversion.

A characteristic sign of a pantothenic acid deficiency in the pig is locomotor disorder (especially of hindquarters), which has been described by Goodwin (1962). In the early stages of such a deficiency, the movement of back legs becomes stiff and jerky. Standing animals show a slight tremor of the hindquarters. When deficiency persists, this particular action of the back legs grows more exaggerated and resembles a characteristic military gait, or goose step (Fig. 10.3) (Luecke et al., 1953). The condition may be so severe that, as the pig moves forward, the back legs will touch the belly. Finally, increasingly severe paralysis of the hindquarters develops. Affected pigs frequently fall sideways or, with their back legs spread apart, assume a posture that resembles that of a sitting dog (Fig. 10.4). The chief microscopic lesion is a chromatolysis of isolated cells of the dorsal root ganglia, followed by a demyelinating process in brachial and sciatic nerves.

431

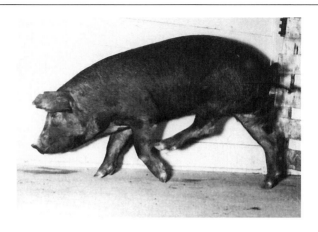

Fig. 10.3 Goose-stepping pig with pantothenic acid deficiency. (Courtesy of R.W. Luecke, Michigan Agriculture Experiment Station.)

Pigs with pantothenic acid deficiency have scurfy skin, thin hair, and brownish secretion around the eyes. The dermatosis associated with deficiency appears principally on the shoulders and behind the ears; the skin appears dirty and scaly. Skin becomes reddened, and the bristles on the rump and along the spine loosen and fall. The dermatosis extends to the mucosa, where it becomes manifest as necrotic enteritis, ulceration, and hemorrhages in the large intestine (Ullrey et al., 1955). As a consequence, the feces contain blood. Goodwin (1962) observed various degrees of gastritis and, occasionally, peritonitis and intestinal fissures.

Ullrey et al. (1955) observed pathological changes in other organs of sows and baby pigs maintained on pantothenic acid-deficient diets. These changes included fatty liver degeneration, enlargement of adrenals, enlargement of heart (with some related flaccidity of the myocardium), and intramuscular hemorrhages. Histopathological studies showed degenerative changes and necroses of the tissue cells.

Pantothenic acid is particularly important in sow fertility, with insufficient quantities of the vitamin resulting in complete reproductive failure. Estrus may occur, but the sows fail to retain the embryos following breeding. Female hogs fed low-pantothenic acid diets exhibited fatty livers, enlarged adrenal glands, intramuscular hemorrhage, heart dilation, small ovaries, and improper uterus development (Ullrey et al., 1955). Ensminger et al. (1951) reported that although gilts on a low-pantothenic acid diet became pregnant, they did not farrow or show any signs of pregnancy. Necropsy of gilts revealed macerating fetuses in the

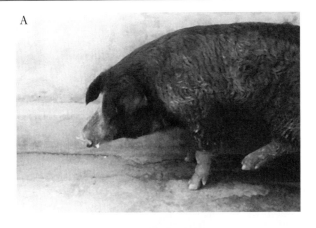

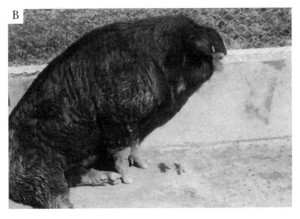

Fig. 10.4 Pantothenic acid deficiency. (A) Locomotor incoordination (goose-stepping). (B) An affected pig often falls sideways or, with its back legs spread apart, assumes a posture that resembles that of a sitting dog. (Courtesy of L.R. McDowell, University of Florida.)

uterine horns in all cases. Minimal pantothenic acid sufficient to result in normal farrowing may still result in an abnormal locomotion in suckling pigs from sows that had received diets low in the vitamin (Teague et al., 1971). Sucking movements in the deficient piglets are impaired, as is the use of the tongue.

Poultry

The major lesions of pantothenic acid deficiency for poultry appear to involve the nervous system, adrenal cortex, and skin (Scott et

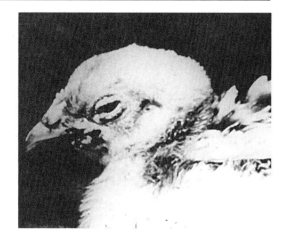

Fig. 10.5 Pantothenic
acid deficiency in a
chick, with dermatitis
around beak. (Courtesy
of G.F. Combs, Univer-
sity of Maryland.)

al., 1982). Pantothenic acid deficiency reduces normal egg production
and hatchability. Subcutaneous hemorrhage and severe edema are
signs of pantothenic acid deficiency in the developing chick embryo.
In chickens, there is first a decline of growth, followed by decline in
feed conversion and retardation of feather growth. Plumage becomes
rough and ruffled, and feathers become brittle and may fall; next, dermatosis rapidly develops in chicks. Corners of the beak and the area
below the beak are the most affected, but the disorder is also observed
in feet. Outer layers of skin between toes and on bottoms of feet peel
off, and small cracks and fissures appear. In some cases, skin layers of
feet thicken and cornify, and wart-like protuberances develop on balls
of the feet. The foot problem is usually exacerbated by bacterial invasion of the lesions. Within 12 to 14 days of receiving a deficient
diet, the margins of the eyelids are sealed closed by a viscous discharge. (Fig. 10.5 illustrates the typical deficiency syndrome in the
chick.)

Pantothenic acid concentrations in liver are reduced during deficiency. Liver is hypertrophied and varies in color from a faint yellow to
a dirty yellow. Nerves and fibers of the spinal cord show myelin degeneration, with these degenerating fibers occurring in all segments of the
cord down to the lumbar region (Scott et al., 1982).

In young chicks, clinical signs of pantothenic acid deficiency are difficult to differentiate from those of biotin deficiency—both cause severe
dermatitis, broken feathers, perosis, poor growth, and mortality (see
Chapter 11, Deficiency). In pantothenic acid deficiency, dermatitis of the

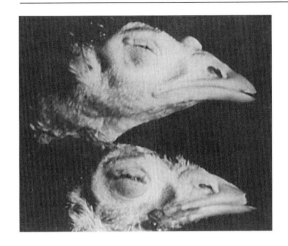

Fig. 10.6 Pantothenic acid deficiency in a turkey with dermatitis on lower beak and at angle of mouth (lower turkey). Sticky exudate that formed on the eyelid resulted in encrustation and caused swollen eyelids to remain stuck together. Normal turkey above is the control. (Courtesy of T.M. Ferguson [deceased] and J.R. Couch, Texas A&M University.)

feet is evident over the toes, in contrast to biotin deficiency, which primarily affects the foot pads and is often more severe than pantothenic acid deficiency.

Signs of pantothenic acid deficiency in young turkeys are similar to those in young chickens and include general weakness, dermatitis, and sticking together of eyelids (Fig. 10.6). Young ducks do not show the usual signs seen in chickens and turkeys, except for retarded growth; however, their mortality rate is very high. Poor feathering is the most prevalent deficiency sign in pheasants and quail (Scott et al., 1964).

Pantothenic acid deficiency does not normally affect egg production but severely depresses hatchability, and chicks that hatch may be too weak to survive. Embryonic mortality in pantothenic acid deficiency occurs usually during the last few days of incubation. A direct linear relationship exists between diet pantothenic acid and hatchability. Beer et al. (1963) fed a purified diet to White Leghorn hens that contained 0.9 mg of pantothenic acid per kilogram of diet. They found that the hens required addition of 1.0 mg/kg for optimum egg production, at least 4.0 mg/kg for maximum hatchability, and 8.0 mg/kg for optimum hatchability and viability of offspring. Dawson et al. (1962) reported that turkey breeder hens fed a diet deficient in pantothenic acid demonstrated a high embryonic mortality during the first week of development. After 17 days, the surviving embryos were small and poorly feathered, and showed signs of edema, hemorrhaging, fatty livers, and pale dilated hearts.

Horses

Pantothenic acid deficiency has not been reported in the horse (NRC, 1989b). Likewise, no requirement for the vitamin has been reported. Pantothenic acid is synthesized in the intestinal tract of adult horses. Carroll et al. (1949) fed a diet containing 0.8 mg of pantothenic acid per kilogram of dry matter and found the following pantothenic acid concentrations (ppm dry matter) in ingesta: duodenum, 11.7; ileum, 9.2; cecum, 39.2; anterior large colon, 34.4; and anterior small colon, 20.5. No signs of pantothenic acid deficiency were observed in horses on this diet or on a second diet containing less than 0.2 mg/kg.

Other Animal Species

Experimental pantothenic acid deficiencies have been induced in most animal species studied. However, the deficiency is not present in animals with sufficient microbial fermentation (e.g., ruminants and horses) or animals that practice sufficient coprophagy (e.g., rabbits).

DOGS AND CATS

Pantothenic acid-deficient dogs exhibit erratic appetites, reduced rates of growth, lowered antibody response, and reduced blood concentrations of cholesterol and total lipids. Diarrhea becomes severe and bloody just prior to death. Vomiting is frequent. Animals become quiet and very weak prior to death. Schaeffer et al. (1942) reported that vomiting was sometimes so severe in pantothenic acid-deficient dogs that feces occurred in the vomit. In terminal stages of deficiency, dogs exhibited spasticity of the hindquarters, sudden prostration, or coma, usually accompanied by rapid respiratory and cardiac rates and possibly convulsions (NRC, 1985a). Deficient dogs have reduced pantothenate concentrations in urine, blood, liver, muscle, and brain.

In kittens, pantothenic acid deficiency is characterized chiefly by emaciation (NRC, 1986). Moderate to marked fatty metamorphosis of the liver occurs, with both fine and coarse vacuolar formation. Giant, blunted villi are seen in some areas of the jejunum and upper ileum, with the tops of the villi in some animals necrotic.

FISH

In rapidly growing fish (e.g., fingerling yellowtail), pantothenic acid deficiency has been found to appear within 10 to 14 days. Gill lamellar hyperplasia, or clubbed gills, is a characteristic sign of pantothenic acid deficiency in most fish (Lovell, 1987; NRC, 1993). In addition to clubbed gills, anemia and high mortality have been observed in pantothenic acid-deficient salmonids. In blue tilapia and rainbow trout, deficiency signs included exudated gills, fusion of gill filaments and lamellae, severe fin erosion, and abnormal swimming (Roem et al., 1991; Masumoto et al., 1994). Pantothenic acid-deficient Japanese parrot fish exhibited anorexia, convulsions, cessation of growth, and a high mortality rate (Ikeda et al., 1988). Poor growth, hemorrhage, skin lesions, and abnormal swimming were found in Japanese eels receiving pantothenic acid-deficient diets (NRC, 1993).

FOXES AND MINK

Deficiency signs in pantothenic acid-deprived mink include severe emaciation, enlarged adrenals, and general gastric ulceration, with petechial (minute) hemorrhages in the jejunum (NRC, 1982a). No definitive pantothenic acid studies in foxes have been completed.

LABORATORY ANIMALS

Pantothenic acid deficiency retards the development of weight in all laboratory animals. Feed consumption is reduced because of appetite loss. Animals become apathetic and noticeably less active (Friesecke, 1975). In mild pantothenic acid deficiency, serum triglyceride and free fatty acid levels are elevated prior to weight loss and more severe signs of the deficiency (Wittwer et al., 1990).

In rats, lack of pantothenic acid results in premature graying of hair (achromotrichia). For this reason pantothenic acid has been called the "anti-gray-hair factor." Another term applied to rats on a deficient diet is "bloody whiskers." Porphyrin from the lachrymal glands of the pantothenic acid-deficient rat accumulates on the whiskers and gives the appearance of blood. The same condition can be produced when water intake is reduced to 50% of normal, so it may be due to adrenal degeneration. Pantothenic acid deficiency also induces exfoliative dermatitis, oral hyperkeratosis, necrosis, and ulceration of the gastrointestinal tract. Focal or generalized hemorrhagic necrosis of the adrenals may occur, and death results after 4 to 6 weeks of deficiency (NRC, 1995). Pantothenic acid-deficient rats have impaired antibody synthesis, decreased serum globulins, and decreased antibody-forming cells in response to antigen. Reproduction is affected, with litter size and birth weight reduced. Newborn rats exhibit neurological defects in the form of locomotor disturbances, incoordination of movements, and motor spasms.

437

Signs of pantothenic acid deficiency in growing mice are reported to be weight loss, hair loss (particularly on the ventral surface, flanks, and legs), dermatosis, partial posterior paralysis, other neurological abnormalities, and achromotrichia. Young guinea pigs fed a purified, pantothenic acid-deficient diet developed signs of deficiency such as decreased growth rate, anorexia, weight loss, rough hair coat, diarrhea, weakness, and death. Adult guinea pigs fed a pantothenic acid-deficient diet died within 10 to 41 days. Many of them had adrenal and gastrointestinal hemorrhages (NRC, 1995).

NONHUMAN PRIMATES

Pantothenic acid deficiency in rhesus monkeys results in reduced growth, anemia, hair loss, and ataxia (NRC, 1978).

Humans

In humans, pantothenic acid deficiency has not been observed under natural conditions except when associated with severe malnutrition. The main reason is that pantothenic acid deficiency is rare because of the vitamin's widespread distribution in foods. Deficiency has been produced in volunteers consuming a pantothenic acid-deficient diet, but more rapidly by also including the antagonist ω-methylpantothenic acid (see Chemical Structure, Properties, and Antagonists) in the diet. The deficient diet alone may require about 12 weeks to produce recognizable symptoms (Hodges et al., 1958). Symptoms most commonly present were persistent and annoying fatigue, headache, muscle weakness, and cramps. Some subjects demonstrated impaired motor coordination and peculiar gait. The neuromotor disorders included paresthesia of the hands and feet with hyperactive deep tendon reflexes. Neuromotor disorders could be explained by the role of acetyl coenzyme A in the synthesis of the neurotransmitter acetylcholine.

Other signs of pantothenic acid deficiency are gastrointestinal disturbances, apathy, depression, cardiovascular instability, increased susceptibility to infections, and impaired adrenal function. Increased susceptibility to upper respiratory tract infections presumably reflects the impairment of immune response.

Deficiency of the vitamin was reported to cause "burning feet syndrome" during World War II among prisoners in Japan and the Philippines (Gopalan, 1946). This syndrome is occasionally described in malnourished people in developing countries. Symptoms include abnormal skin sensations of the feet and lower legs, which were increased by warmth and lessened by cold. Supplementation with large quantities of pantothenic acid increased the ability of subjects to withstand stress.

Assessment of Status

Urinary excretion has been used in humans to estimate status of pantothenic acid as well as the vitamin content of the diet. Urinary excretions of less than 1 mg/day are considered to be in the deficiency zone corresponding to intakes of possibly less than 4 mg/day (Olson, 1990). Like urine, the pantothenic acid content of human milk reflects the pantothenic acid content of the diet. Johnston et al. (1981) reported a correlation of 0.62 between dietary and milk content of pantothenic acid. Total pantothenic acid levels in whole blood below 100 µg/dL would be suggestive of deficiency (Fox, 1991).

Studies of pantothenic acid deficiency in various animal species indicate lowered tissue levels and decreased urinary excretion of the vitamin, and decreased tissue coenzyme A (Nelson, 1978). However, data are insufficient to establish pantothenic acid status for animals based on critical concentrations. There is a close relationship between the amounts of dietary pantothenic acid in hen diets, egg production, egg concentrations, and newly hatched chicks and poults (Pearson et al., 1945; Robel, 1993), indicating potential for status determination.

SUPPLEMENTATION

Monogastric animal diets based on grains, particularly corn, are routinely supplemented with pantothenic acid. Scott et al. (1982) concludes that practical diets usually contain sufficient pantothenic acid for all classes of chickens, but a number of factors may influence the requirement for this vitamin. Because of this, supplemental calcium pantothenate is usually added to diets for chicks and breeding hens. Increasing supplemental pantothenic acid to turkey breeding hens increased the transfer of pantothenic acid in eggs (Robel, 1993). Scott (1966) indicated that the pantothenic acid requirement for poultry may have to be increased 60 to 80% because of a lack of availability from bound forms in feeds. Southern and Baker (1981) estimated that pantothenic acid present in both corn and dehulled soybean meal was 100% bioavailable. The bioavailability of pantothenic acid in barley, wheat, and sorghum, however, was estimated to be only 60% available based upon chick growth bioassay. Nevertheless, corn and sorghum contained less bioavailable total pantothenic acid than barley and wheat because of less total content of the vitamin. Clinical pantothenic acid deficiency signs appear to be completely reversible, if not too far advanced, by oral treatment or injection with the vitamin followed by restoration of an adequate level of pantothenic acid in the diet.

Type of diet will influence need for pantothenic acid supplementation. High-protein diets would reduce pantothenic acid needs due to the decreased level of dietary carbohydrate, which would presumably require coenzyme A for metabolism. Pigs fed a pantothenic acid-deficient, high-fat diet failed to gain weight, exhibited a lower feed-efficiency ratio, and developed deficiency signs more quickly than pigs fed a diet low in fat (Sewell et al., 1962). Biotin and folacin have been found necessary for pantothenic acid utilization, and vitamin B_{12} and antibiotics (see Requirements) have a sparing effect for chicks (Latymer and Coates, 1981) and pigs (Latymer et al., 1985).

Pantothenic acid is available as a commercially synthesized product for addition to feed. It is available as d- or dl-calcium pantothenate. One gram of d-calcium pantothenate is equivalent to 0.92 g of d-pantothenic acid activity, while the combination of 1 g of the dl-form has 0.46 g of d-pantothenic acid activity. A racemic mixture (equal parts of d- and l-calcium pantothenate) is generally sold to the feed industry. Because livestock and poultry can biologically utilize only the d-isomer of pantothenic acid, nutrient requirements for the vitamin are routinely expressed in the d-form.

Feed-grade pantothenic acid products are available in a number of potencies. Products that are sold on the basis of racemic mixture content can be misleading and confusing to a buyer who is not fully aware of the biological activity supplied by d-pantothenic acid. To avoid confusion, the label should clearly state the grams of d-calcium pantothenate or its equivalent per unit weight and the grams of d-pantothenic acid.

A straight racemic mixture (90%) is available to people in the feed industry, but its hygroscopic and electrostatic properties contribute to handling problems. Because it readily picks up moisture, it sticks to bags, cans, and scoops and can become hard after prolonged exposure to air. Its electrostatic properties cause it to cling to metallic and other objects, and losses can be significant. Through complexing procedures, several companies now market free-flowing and essentially nonhygroscopic and nonelectrostatic products.

Verbeeck (1975) reported calcium pantothenate to be stable in premixes with or without minerals and regardless of the mineral form. Losses of calcium pantothenate may occur in premixes that are extremely acidic in nature, however. If a calcium pantothenate–calcium chloride complex is used instead of the plain calcium pantothenate, this problem should be alleviated.

In the United States, estimates of pantothenic acid dietary intakes in the human adult population range between 5 and 20 mg/day (Chung et al., 1961). These levels are higher than estimated requirements of 4 to 7 mg/day for children and adults (RDA, 1989). Therefore, supplementation would not normally be recommended unless associated with general malnutrition. Humans at greatest risk and needing supplementation include alcoholics and diabetics; adrenal and digestive dysfunctions also influence need for the vitamin (Fox, 1991).

TOXICITY

Pantothenic acid toxicity has not been reported in humans. The LD_{50} in milligrams per kilogram of body weight for mice and rats has been reported to range from 0.83 to 10.0 for calcium pantothenate (Unna and Greslin, 1941). In rats, 100 times the dietary requirement resulted in nonfatal liver damage (NRC, 1987).

Pantothenic acid has only limited pharmacological effects when administered to animals or humans. Dexpanthenol, the alcohol synthetically derived from d-pantothenic acid, has been administered to increase gastrointestinal peristalsis and applied topically to alleviate itching and improve minor skin irritations (Fox, 1991). Pantothenic acid has been reported to have a protective effect against radiation sickness (Egarova and Perepelkin, 1979). Some work suggests that pantothenic acid may accelerate wound healing in rabbits by increasing the fibroblast content of scar tissue (Aprahamian et al., 1985).

■ REFERENCES

Aprahamian, M., Dentinger, A., Stock-Damge, C., Kouassi, J.C., and Grenier, J.F. (1985). *Am. J. Clin. Nutr. 41, 578.*
Axelrod, A.E. (1971). *Am. J. Clin. Nutr. 24, 265.*
Barboriak, J.J., and Krehl, W.A. (1957). *J. Nutr. 63, 601.*
Beer, A.E., Scott, M.L., and Neshein, M.C. (1963). *Br. Poult. Sci. 4, 243.*
Brass, E.P. (1993) *J. Nutr. 123, 1801.*
Carroll, F.D., Gross, H., and Howell, C.E. (1949). *J. Anim. Sci. 8, 290.*
Chung, A.S.M., Pearson, W.N., Darby, W.J., Miller, O.N., and Goldsmith, G.A. (1961). *Am. J. Clin. Nutr. 9, 573.*
Colby, R.W., Cunha, T.J., Lindley, C.E., Cordy, D.R., and Ensminger, M.E. (1948). *J. Am. Vet. Med. Assoc. 113, 589.*
Combs, G.F. Jr. (1992). The Vitamins. Academic Press, San Diego, California.

Cunha, T. J. (1977). Swine Feeding and Nutrition. Academic Press, Inc., New York. *7,* 1074.

Dawson, E., Ferguson, T.M., Deyoe, C.W., and Couch, J.R. (1962). *Poult. Sci. 41,* 1639.

Egarova, N.D., and Perepelkin, S.R. (1979). *Gig. Sanit. 10, 25.*

Ensminger, M. E., Colby, R. W., and Cunha, T. J. (1951). Wash. Agric. Exp. Stn. Circ. 134, Pullman, Washington.

Fenstermacher, D.K., and Rose, R.C. (1986). *Am. J. Physiol. 250,* G155.

Fox, H.M. (1991). *In* Handbook of Vitamins (L.J. Machlin, ed.), p. 437. Marcel Dekker, New York.

Friesecke, H. (1975). *In* Pantothenic Acid, No. 1533. Hoffmann-La Roche, Basel, Switzerland.

Fry, P.C., Fox, H.M., and Tao, H.G. (1976). *J. Nutr. Sci. Vitaminol. 22,* 339.

Gadient, M. (1986). *In* Proc. Maryland Nutrition Conference for Feed Manufacturers, p. 73. College Park, Maryland.

Goodwin, R.F.W. (1962). *J. Comp. Pathol. 72,* 214.

Gopalan, C. (1946). *Indian Med. Gaz. 81,* 23.

Hodges, R.E., Ohison, M.A., and Bean, W.B. (1958). *J. Clin. Invest. 37,* 1642.

Ikeda, M., Ishibashi, Y., Murata, O., Nasu, T., and Harada, T. (1988). *Bull. Jpn. Soc. Sci. Fish 54,* 2029.

Johnston, L., Vaughan, L., and Fox, H.M. (1981). *Am. J. Clin. Nutr. 34,* 2205.

Latymer, E.A., and Coates, M.E. (1981). *Br. J. Nutr. 45,* 431.

Latymer, E.A., Mitchell, G., Coates, M.E., Keol, H.D., Thomas, J., and Woodley, S.C. (1985). *Livest. Prod. Sci. 12,* 265.

Loosli, J. K. (1991). *In* Handbook of Animal Science (P. A. Putnam, ed.). Academic Press, San Diego, California.

Lovell, R.T. (1987). *Feed Manage. 38,* 28.

Luecke, R. W., Hoefler, J.A., and Thorpe, F. Jr. (1953). *J. Anim. Sci. 12,* 605.

Marks, J. (1975). A Guide to the Vitamins. Their Role in Health and Disease, p. 73. Medical and Technical Publ., Lancaster, England.

Masumoto, T., Hardy, R.W., and Stickney, R.R. (1994). *J. Nutr. 124,* 430.

McKigney, J.I., Wallace, H.D., and Cunha, T.J. (1957). *J. Anim. Sci. 16,* 35.

Nelson, M.M., and Evans, H.M. (1945). *Proc. Soc. Exp. Biol. Med. 60,* 319.

Nelson, R.A. (1978). *In* Handbook Series in Nutrition and Food. Section E: Nutritional Disorders (M. Rechcigl Jr., ed.), Vol. 3, p. 33. CRC Press, Boca Raton, Florida.

NRC. Nutrient Requirements of Domestic Animals. National Academy of Sciences-National Research Council, Washington, D.C.
(1978). Nutrient Requirements of Nonhuman Primates.
(1981). Nutrient Requirements of Goats.
(1982a). Nutrient Requirements of Mink and Foxes.
(1985a). Nutrient Requirements of Dogs, 2nd Ed.
(1985b). Nutrient Requirements of Sheep, 5th Ed.
(1986). Nutrient Requirements of Cats, 3rd Ed.
(1989a). Nutrient Requirements of Dairy Cattle, 6th Ed.
(1989b). Nutrient Requirements of Horses, 5th Ed.
(1993). Nutrient Requirements of Fish.
(1994). Nutrient Requirements of Poultry, 9th Ed.

(1995). Nutrient Requirements of Laboratory Animals.

(1996). Nutrient Requirements of Beef Cattle, 7th Ed.

(1998). Nutrient Requirements of Swine, 10th Ed.

NRC. (1982b). United States-Canadian Tables of Feed Composition, 3rd Ed. National Academy of Sciences-National Research Council, Washington, D.C.

NRC. (1987). Vitamin Tolerance of Animals. National Academy of Sciences-National Research Council, Washington, D.C.

Olson, R.E. (1990). *In* Nutrition Reviews, Present Knowledge in Nutrition (R.E. Olson, ed.), p. 208. Nutrition Foundation, Washington, DC.

Palagina, N.K., Meledina, T.V., and Karpisheva, I.A. (1990). *Appl. Biochem. Microbiol. 26,* 688.

Pearson, P.B., Melass, V.H., and Sherwood, R.M. (1945). *Arch. Biochem. 7,* 353.

Plaut, G.W.E., Smith, C.M., and Alworth, W.L. (1974). *Annu. Rev. Biochem. 43,* 899.

Pugh, E.L., and Wakil, S.J. (1965). *J. Biol. Chem. 240,* 4727.

RDA. (1989). Recommended Dietary Allowances, 10th Ed., National Academy of Sciences-National Research Council, Washington, D.C.

Robel, E.J. (1993). *Poult. Sci. 72,* 1740.

Roem, A.J., Stickney, R.R., and Kohler, C.C. (1991). *Prog. Fish Culturist 53,* 216.

Roy, R.B., and Buccafuri, A. (1978). *J. Assoc. Off. Anal. Chem. 61,* 720.

Sauberlich, H.E. (1973). *In* Modern Nutrition in Health and Disease, 5th ed. (R.S. Goodhart and M.E. Shils, eds.), p. 203. Lea and Febiger, New York.

Sauberlich, H.E. (1985). *Prog. Food Nutr. 9,* 1.

Schaefer, A.E., McKibben, J.M., and Elvehjem, C.A. (1942). *J. Biol. Chem. 143,* 321.

Scott, M.L. (1966). *Proc. Cornell Nutr. Conf.* p. 35.

Scott, M.L., Holm, E.R., and Reynolds, R.E. (1964). *Poult. Sci. 43,* 1543.

Scott, M.L., Nesheim, M.C., and Young, R.J. (1982). Nutrition of the Chicken. Scott & Associates, Ithaca, New York.

Sewell, R.F., Price, D.G., and Thomas, M.C. (1962). *Fed. Proc. Fed. Am. Soc. Exp. Biol. 21,* 468(Abstr.).

Sheppard, A.J., and Johnson, B.C. (1957). *J. Nutr. 61,* 195.

Slinger, S.J., and Pepper, W.F. (1954). *Poult. Sci. 33,* 633.

Song, W.O. (1990). *Nutr. Today, March-April,* 19.

Song, W.O., Smith, A.,Wittwer, C.,Wyse, B., and Hansen, G. (1990). *Nutr. Res. 10,* 439.

Southern, L.L., and Baker, D.H. (1981). *J. Anim. Sci. 53,* 403.

Taylor, T., Hawkins, D.R., Hathway, D.E., and Partington, H. (1972). *Br. Vet. J. 128,* 500.

Taylor, T., Cameron, B.D., Hathway, D.E., and Partington, H. (1974). *Res. Vet. Sci. 16,* 271.

Teague, H.S., Grifo, A.P. Jr., and Palmer, W.M. (1971). *J. Anim. Sci. 33,* 239(Abstr.).

Ullrey, D.E., Becker, D.E., Terrill, S.W., and Notzold, R.A. (1955). *J. Nutr. 57,* 40.

Unna, K., and Greslin, J.C. (1941). *J. Pharmacol. Exp. Ther. 73,* 85.

Verbeeck, J. (1975). *Feedstuffs 47* (36), 4.

Virtanen, A.I. (1966). *Science 153*, 1603.

Wittwer, C.T., Beck, S., Peterson, M., Davidson, R., Wilson, D.E., and Hansen, R.G. (1990). *J. Nutr. 120*, 719.

Wright, L.D., and Welch, A.D. (1943). *Science 97*, 426.

Wyse, B.W., and Hansen, R.G. (1977). *Fed. Proc. 36*, 1169.

BIOTIN

INTRODUCTION

For many years it was believed that supplemental biotin was not required in swine and poultry diets because of its wide distribution in feedstuffs and because of known biotin synthesis by the intestinal microflora. However, in the mid-1970s, field cases in these species were found under modern production systems. These conditions, characterized by specific clinical signs, responded to supplemental biotin. On the basis of these findings, nutritionists have had to reexamine the role of biotin in livestock and poultry diets. In many different animal species, biotin deficiency is usually associated with epidermal lesions.

Incidence of biotin deficiency has been found occasionally when humans and animals have consumed excessive quantities of raw eggs, which contain a biotin complexing factor (avidin). Likewise, biotin deficiency is reported in children with inborn errors of metabolism when there are insufficient biotin-dependent enzymes. Such cases in children respond dramatically to high-level dietary supplementations with biotin.

HISTORY

Discovery of the physiological significance of biotin is the history of the merging of different lines of investigation that appeared to be unrelated (Scott et al., 1982; Bonjour, 1991; Loosli, 1991). Biotin was the name given to a substance isolated from egg yolk by Kögl and Tönnis in 1936 that was necessary for yeast growth. This substance was discovered to be identical to a growth factor named coenzyme R that was required by legume nodule bacteria.

The toxic properties of feeding raw egg white to animals were first observed by Bateman in 1916. Clinical signs of dermatitis and hair loss due to egg-white injury were prevented by several researchers by feeding certain foods, notably liver and kidney. György studied the chemistry of this protective factor in certain foods, which he named factor H in 1937. The term vitamin H was chosen by György because the factor protected the *haut*, the German word for skin.

In 1940 György and associates found that biotin, vitamin H, and coenzyme R were the same substance. Other names given to this factor were protective factor X, egg-white injury protection factor, factor S, and factor W (or vitamin B_w). Egg-white injury resulted from its inactivating dietary biotin because of a specific constituent, avidin. Heat was found to destroy avidin, therefore revealing that this biotin antagonistic factor was heat labile. Avidin is a protein that is a secretory product of the mucosa of the oviduct and therefore is found in the albuminous part of eggs.

The structure and properties of biotin were established by U.S. and European investigators between 1940 and 1943. The first chemical synthesis was completed by Harris and associates of the Merck Company in 1943. In 1949 Goldberg and Sternbach developed a technique for industrial production of biotin.

CHEMICAL STRUCTURE, PROPERTIES, AND ANTAGONISTS

The chemical structure of biotin in metabolism includes a sulfur atom in its ring (like thiamin) and a transverse bond across the ring (Fig. 11.1). The empirical formula for biotin is $C_{11}H_{18}O_3N_2S$. Biotin is a fusion of an imidazolidone ring with a tetrahydrothiophene ring bearing a valeric acid side chain. It is a monocarboxylic acid with sulfur as a thioether linkage. Biotin, with its rather unique structure, contains three asymmetric carbonations, and therefore eight different isomers are possible. Of these isomers only one contains vitamin activity, *d*-biotin. The stereoisomer *l*-biotin is inactive.

Biotin crystallizes from water solution as long, white needles. Its melting point is 232 to 233°C. Free biotin is soluble in dilute alkali and hot water and practically insoluble in fats and organic solvents. Biotin is quite stable under ordinary conditions. It is destroyed by nitrous acid, other strong acids, strong bases, and formaldehyde and is inactivated by rancid fats and choline (Scott et al., 1982). It is gradually destroyed by ultraviolet radiation.

446

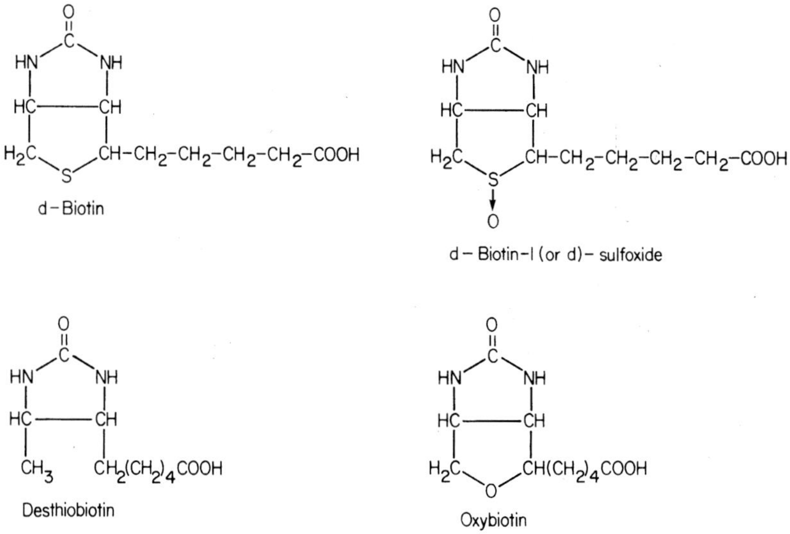

Fig. 11.1 Structures of biotin and some derivatives.

Structurally related analogs of biotin (Fig. 11.1) can vary from no activity to partial replacement value and to antibiotin activity. Mild oxidation converts biotin to sulfoxide, and strong oxidation converts it to sulfone. Strong agents result in sulfur replacement by oxygen, resulting in oxybiotin and desthiobiotin. Oxybiotin has some biotin activity for chicks (one-third) but less for rats (one-tenth). Both desthiobiotin and biotin sulfone are active for yeast but are inhibitory to bacteria. Biocytin, a bound form of biotin, is also biologically active in several species, including animals. This naturally occurring compound has been shown to be ε-N-biotinyl-L-lysine. Besides these biotin analogs, other compounds exist that can bind biotin to form a stable complex, thus preventing the utilization of the vitamin by animals and/or microorganisms. The microorganism *Saccharomyces avidinii* produces a biotin-binding protein streptavidin and other compounds that can inactivate free biotin and apparently inhibit biotin synthesis in susceptible microorganisms. Oleic acid and related compounds, in the presence of aspartic acid, satisfy the biotin requirement of many microorganisms, but are inactive for some and actually toxic for others.

ANALYTICAL PROCEDURES

A number of methods are available for estimating biotin content of feeds and supplements. An enzyme-linked immunosorbent assay has been used to determine biotin in blood and other fluids (Wellenberg and Banks, 1993). This assay utilizes the strong binding property of streptavidin. Bioassay procedures with animals (rats and chicks) and microorganisms are employed because of the difficulty of establishing chemical or physical methods suitable for natural materials. However, Achuta Murthy and Mistry (1977) reported progress in the use of colorimetric, gas chromatographic, and polarographic methods of analyses. Isotope dilution and radiotracers have been used for biotin analysis and are sensitive, yielding results comparable to the *Lactobacillus plantarum* assay (Bonjour, 1991). Nevertheless, such analytical methods are not capable of identifying amounts of this vitamin that are biologically available to the animal.

In the biological estimation, rats and chicks are made biotin deficient by the use of special diets. Rats are made deficient by resorting to the use of sulfonamides, preventing coprophagy, feeding egg white (avidin), or combinations of these techniques. However, deficiency in the chick can be produced by a diet low in biotin alone. For both species, biotin content of the test sample can be calculated from growth-response curves. The healing of skin lesions in avidin-fed rats is a sensitive indicator of biotin availability. An additional test to evaluate feeds is based on the pyruvate carboxylase activity in poultry or rat blood, either directly or by assaying the in vitro activity before and after addition of biotin (Whitehead et al., 1982; Bonjour, 1991). Most studies of biotin content of feedstuffs have been conducted by microbiological assay. *Lactobacillus plantarum* is often employed with other suitable organisms, including *L. casei* and *Saccharomyces cerevisiae*. The procedure with microorganisms includes heating with H_2SO_4 to liberate bound forms and removing unsaturated fatty acids that interfere with the assay. A simple, rapid, and economic method for assessing biotin availability of feedstuffs was developed using egg yolk and plasma biotin concentrations after hens were fed specific feeds (Buenrostro and Kratzer, 1984).

METABOLISM

Biotin exists in natural materials in both bound and free forms, with much of the bound biotin apparently not available to animal species. For poultry, often less than one-half of the microbiologically determined biotin in a feedstuff is biologically available (Scott, 1981). Naturally occurring biotin is found partly in the free state (fruit, milk, vegetables) and partly in a form bound to protein in animal tissues, plant seeds, and yeast. Variation in availability appears to be due to differential susceptibilities to digestion of the biotin-protein linkages in which the vitamin is found in natural products. Those linkages involve the formation of covalent bonds between the carboxyl group of the biotin side-chain with the amino acid lysine or to protein.

Biotinidase, present in pancreatic juice and intestinal mucosa, releases biotin from biocytin during the luminal phase of proteolysis. In most species that have been investigated, physiological concentrations of biotin are absorbed from the intestinal tract by a sodium-dependent active transport process, which is inhibited by desthiobiotin and biocytin (Said and Derweesh, 1991). Absorption of biotin by a Na^+-dependent process was noted to be higher in the duodenum than the jejunum, which was in turn higher than that in the ileum, and it was concluded that the proximal part of the human small intestine was the site of maximum transport of biotin (Said et al., 1988).

The few studies conducted in animals on biotin metabolism revealed that biotin is absorbed as the intact molecule in the first third to half of the small intestine (Bonjour, 1991). There is also absorption of biotin from the hind gut of the pig, with disappearance of between 50 and 61% of infused biotin between the cecum and feces that was accompanied by more than a fourfold increase of plasma biotin concentration and more than a sixfold increase of urinary biotin excretion (Barth et al., 1986). Kopinski and Leibholz (1985) reported that postileal absorption was 10 to 15% of that from the small intestine after oral ingestion. Eighty percent of a labeled biotin dose infused into the cecum of minipigs appeared in portal blood (Drouchner and Volker, 1984) with the largest proportion appearing in feces. Using ^{14}C-labeled biotin, Kopinski et al. (1989a,b) reported similar findings in that absorption of free biotin in the postileal digestive tract was about 8% as efficient as that from a similar labeled dose of orally administered biotin. Kopinski et al. (1989c) observed that even with extensive microbial synthesis of biotin in the postileal tract, low concentrations of biotin in plasma and tissue, and the presence of deficiency signs indicated that postileal synthesized biotin is of limited benefit to the pig. Scholtissek et al. (1990) suggested that under basal conditions, 1.7 to 17% of the requirement for biotin is provided by colonic bacteria.

Biotin appears to circulate in the bloodstream both free and bound

449

to a serum glycoprotein, which also has biotinidase activity, catalyzing the hydrolysis of biocytin. In humans, 81% of biotin in plasma was free and the remainder bound (Mock and Malik, 1992). Information is very limited on biotin transport, tissue deposition, and storage in animals and humans. Mock (1990) reported that biotin is transported as a free water-soluble component of plasma, is taken up by cells via active transport, and is attached to its apoenzymes. Said et al. (1992) reported that biotin is transported into human liver via a specialized carrier-mediated transport system. This system is Na^+-gradient dependent and transports biotin via an electroneutral process.

Disappearance of an intravenous dose of radioactive biotin from blood of biotin-deficient rats was more rapid than for controls (Petrelli et al., 1979). Also, rate and extent of deposition into deficient liver, particularly mitochondrial and cytosolic fractions, were favored. This research supports the concept of homeostatic mechanisms responding to provide biotin in relation to needs. All cells contain some biotin, with larger quantities in the liver and kidneys. Intracellular distribution of biotin corresponds to known localization of biotin-dependent enzymes (carboxylases).

Investigations into biotin metabolism in animals and humans are difficult to interpret, as biotin-producing microorganisms exist in the intestinal tract distal to the cecum. Often, the amount of biotin excreted in urine and feces together exceeds total dietary intake, whereas urinary biotin excretion is usually less than intake. ^{14}C-labeled biotin showed that the major portion of intraperitoneally injected radioactivity was excreted in the urine and none in the feces or expired as CO_2 (Lee et al., 1973). In rats and pigs, biliary excretion of biotin and metabolites was negligible (Zempleni et al., 1997).

The brush border of the kidney cortex has a sodium-biotin transport system similar to that in the intestinal mucosa, thus providing for resorption of free biotin filtered into the urine. It is only when this resorption mechanism is saturated that there will be significant excretion of biotin. Efficient conservation of biotin, together with the recycling of biocytin released from the catabolism of biotin-containing enzymes, may be as important as intestinal bacterial synthesis of the vitamin in meeting biotin requirements (Bender, 1992).

FUNCTIONS

Biotin is an essential coenzyme in carbohydrate, fat, and protein metabolism. It is involved in conversion of carbohydrate to protein and vice versa as well as conversion of protein and carbohydrate to fat. Biotin also plays an important role in maintaining normal blood glucose levels from metabolism of protein and fat when dietary intake of carbohydrate is low. Biotin functions as a carboxyl carrier in four carboxylase enzymes: pyruvate carboxylase, acetyl CoA carboxylase, propionyl CoA carboxylase, and 3-methylcrotonyl CoA carboxylase. As a component of these carboxylating enzymes, there is the capacity to transport carboxyl units and to fix carbon dioxide (as bicarbonate) in tissue. Biotin serves as a prosthetic group in a number of enzymes in which the biotin moiety functions as a mobile carboxyl carrier. The biotin prosthetic group is linked covalently to the ε-amino group of a lysyl residue of the biotin-dependent enzyme.

In carbohydrate metabolism, biotin functions in both carbon dioxide fixation and decarboxylation, with the energy-producing citric acid cycle dependent on the presence of this vitamin. It is suggested that part of the effect of biotin on energy production is through stimulation of phosphorylation pathways (Moretti et al., 1990). Glucokinase activity is affected by biotin, with activity of the enzyme decreasing with biotin deficiency (Li-Hsieh and Mistry, 1992). Specific biotin-dependent reactions in carbohydrate metabolism are the following:

- Carboxylation of pyruvic acid to oxaloacetic acid.
- Conversion of malic acid to pyruvic acid.
- Interconversion of succinic acid and propionic acid.
- Conversion of oxalosuccinic acid to α-ketoglutaric acid.

In protein metabolism, biotin enzymes are important in protein synthesis, amino acid deamination, purine synthesis, and nucleic acid metabolism. Biotin is required for transcarboxylation in degradation of various amino acids. Deficiency of the vitamin in mammals hinders the normal conversion of the deaminated chain of leucine to acetyl-CoA. Depletion of hepatic biotin results in reduction of hepatic activity of methylcrotonyl-CoA carboxylase, which is needed for leucine degradation (Mock and Mock, 1992). Ability of liver homogenates to incorporate labeled CO_2 was directly related to biotin level of the animal (Terroine, 1960). Likewise, ability to synthesize citrulline from ornithine was reduced in liver homogenates from biotin-deficient rats. The urea cycle enzyme ornithine transcarbamylase was significantly lower in livers of biotin deficient rats (Maeda et al., 1996).

Acetyl-CoA carboxylase catalyzes addition of CO_2 to acetyl-CoA to form malonyl-CoA. This is the first reaction in the synthesis of fatty

451

acids. A cytosolic multienzyme complex, fatty acid synthetase, then accomplishes synthesis of palmitate from malonyl-CoA. Biotin is required for normal long-chain unsaturated fatty acid synthesis and is important for essential fatty acid metabolism (Kramer et al., 1984). Deficiency in rats inhibited arachidonic acid (20:4 ω-6) synthesis from linoleic acid (18:2 ω-6) while increasing linolenic acid (18:3 ω-3) and its metabolite (22:6 ω-3) (Kramer et al., 1984; Watkins and Kratzer, 1987a). Biotin deficiency resulted in reduced arachidonic acid (20:4) in chicks, and therefore reduced plasma prostaglandin E_2 (PGE_2) as a result of having less of the prostaglandin precursor (20:4) (Watkins and Kratzer, 1987b; Watkins, 1989).

REQUIREMENTS

Estimates of biotin requirements for various animals and humans are presented in Table 11.1. Biotin requirements are difficult to establish because of variability in feed content and bioavailability. Likewise, it is difficult to obtain a quantitative requirement for biotin because the vitamin is synthesized by many different microorganisms and certain fungi. These microorganisms are found in the lower part of the intestinal tract, a region in which absorption of nutrients is generally reduced. However, it is believed that intestinal microflora make a significant contribution to the body pool of available biotin. In general, combined urinary and fecal excretion of biotin exceeds the dietary intake. What is not known for the various species is the extent of microbial synthesis or the biotin availability to the host.

It is concluded that microorganisms contribute to animal and human requirements because the use of some sulfa drugs, such as Sulfathalidine, can induce deficiency under some circumstances. Microorganisms that provide significant quantities of biotin to most species apparently supply a variable and undependable amount of biotin for poultry (Scott, 1981). Biotin deficiency was less severe in cecectomized than normal chickens, indicating that cecal microorganisms do not supply chickens with significant amounts of biotin but instead compete with the host animal for dietary biotin, thus increasing the requirement (Sunde et al., 1950).

Rate and extent of biotin synthesis may be dependent on the level of other dietary components. In poultry and rats, it has been shown that polyunsaturated fats, ascorbic acid, and other B vitamins may influence the demand for biotin. Addition of polyunsaturated fatty acids to fat-

■ Table 11.1 Biotin Requirements for Various Animals and Humans

Animal	Purpose or Class	Requirement[a]	Reference
Beef cattle	Adult	Microbial synthesis	NRC (1996)
Dairy cattle	Calf	0.1 ppm milk replacer	NRC (1989a)
	Adult	Microbial synthesis	NRC (1989a)
Chicken	Leghorn, 0–6 weeks	0.15 mg/kg	NRC (1994)
	Leghorn, 6–18 weeks	0.10 mg/kg	NRC (1994)
	Laying (100-g intake)	0.10 mg/kg	NRC (1994)
	Broilers, 0–6 weeks	0.15 mg/kg	NRC (1994)
Japanese quail	Starting and growing	0.3 mg/kg	NRC (1994)
	Breeding	0.15 mg/kg	NRC (1994)
Turkey	0–4 weeks	0.25 mg/kg	NRC (1994)
	4–8 weeks	0.20 mg/kg	NRC (1994)
	Breeding hens	0.10 mg/kg	NRC (1994)
Sheep	Adult	Microbial synthesis	NRC (1985b)
Swine	Growing-finishing	0.05 mg/kg	NRC (1998)
	Breeding-lactating	0.20 mg/kg	NRC (1998)
Horse	Adult	Microbial synthesis (?)	NRC (1989b)
Goat	Adult	Microbial synthesis	NRC(1981b)
Cat	All classes	0.07 mg/kg	NRC (1986)
Mink	Growing	0.12 mg/kg	NRC (1982a)
Hamster	All classes	0.6 mg/kg	NRC (1978a)
Fish	Common carp	1 mg/kg	NRC (1993)
	Pacific salmon	1–1.5 mg/kg	NRC (1993)
	Rainbow trout	0.05–0.14 mg/kg	NRC (1993)
Human	Infants	10–15 µg/day	RDA (1989)
	Adults	30–100 µg/day	RDA (1989)

[a]Expressed as per unit of animal feed on either as-fed (approximately 90% dry matter) or dry basis (see Appendix, Tables A1a,b). Human data are expressed as µg/day. Often requirements are unknown, so the best recommendation is used.

free, biotin-deficient diets increased severity of dermal lesions (Roland and Edwards, 1971). Biotin is rapidly destroyed as feeds become rancid. Pure biotin was inactivated to the extent of 96% in 12 hours when linoleic acid of a high peroxide number was added to the diet (Pavcek and Shull, 1942). In the presence of α-tocopherol, this destruction amounted to only 40% after 48 hours.

Verification that humans require biotin was documented in two situations: prolonged consumption of raw egg white and parenteral nutrition without biotin supplementation in patients with short-gut syndrome and other causes of malabsorption (Mock, 1990). General recommendations for human biotin requirements vary from 10 to 100 µg/day; uncertainty of requirements is due to lack of information on the nutritional significance of biotin synthesis and utilization of biotin by enteric bacteria (RDA, 1989).

NATURAL SOURCES

Biotin is present in many foods and feedstuffs (Table 11.2). The richest sources of biotin are royal jelly, liver, kidney, yeast, blackstrap molasses, peanuts, and eggs. Most fresh vegetables and some fruits are fairly good sources. Corn, wheat, other cereals, meat, and fish are relatively poor sources. In comparison to cereal grains, oilseed meals are better sources of total biotin. Soybean meal, for instance, contains a mean biotin content of 270 ppb, with a range of 200 to 387 ppb (Frigg and Volker, 1994).

Animal proteins, on the other hand, are rather unreliable sources of biotin. For instance, highly variable levels are found in fish meals (135 ppb on average, ranging from 11 to 421 ppb) and meat meals (88 ppb on average, ranging from 17 to 322 ppb).

The biotin content of cereal grains appears to be influenced by variety, season, and yield (in particular, the endosperm-pericarp ratio) (Brooks, 1982). Harvest conditions, origin of sample, year of collection, postharvest treatment, and storage conditions all appear to play a part in determining biotin content and may also affect the availability. There is considerable variation in biotin content within individual sources. For example, 65 samples of corn analyzed for biotin varied between 0.012 and 0.072 ppm, and 20 samples of meat meal varied between 0.008 and 0.20 ppm (Brooks, 1982).

Less than one-half of the biotin in various feedstuffs is biologically available (Table 11.2) as determined by microbiological assay (Frigg, 1976, 1984; Frigg and Volker, 1994). Thus, it is important to know the chemical form of biotin (e.g., bound or unbound) as well as its overall content in feed. Oilseed meals, alfalfa meals, and dried yeast are excellent sources of biologically available biotin. Meat meal and fish meals contain biotin of relatively poor biological availability. Sauer et al. (1988) determined that an apparent biotin digestibility of soybean meal was 55.4%, while that of meat and bone meal was only 2.7%, and canola meal was 3.9%. Grains are poor sources of biotin, with corn and oats more available than wheat, hull-less barley, or regular barley. Frigg (1976) reported that the biotin content of wheat and barley may be totally unavailable. The excretion of biotin in feces of pigs given wheat was 10 times greater than from corn, indicating greater utilization of corn biotin (Bryden, 1989).

Biotin in feedstuffs may be destroyed by heat curing, solvent extraction, and improper storage conditions, while pelleting has little ef-

■ Table 11.2   Typical Biotin Contents and Bioavailability in Various Foods and Feedstuffs (as-fed basis)

Food or Feedstuff	Biotin Levels (μg/g)	Biotin Availability (%)
Alfalfa meal, dehydrated	0.33	75–100
Barley	0.14	10
Beef, steak	0.04	—
Cabbage	0.02	—
Carrots	0.03	—
Chicken	0.10	—
Corn, yellow	0.08	100
Corn gluten meal	0.19	100
Cottonseed meal, solvent extracted	0.08–0.47	100
Distiller's solubles, dried	0.44–1.1	90
Eggs, whole	0.25	—
Fish meal	0.14	100
Liver, beef	1.00	—
Meat and bone meal	0.08	100
Milk, cow's	0.05	—
Molasses, blackstrap	0.70	—
Oats	0.25	35
Peanut meal	1.63	53
Rice bran	0.42	—
Rice polishings	0.37	20
Skim milk, dried	0.25	65
Sorghum	0.29	20
Soybean meal	0.27	100
Wheat	0.10	—
Wheat bran	0.36	20
Yeast, brewer's	0.63	100

Sources: Modified from NRC (1982b) and Frigg and Volker (1994).

fect on biotin content of feed (McGinnis, 1986a,b). Milling of wheat or
corn and canning of corn, carrots, spinach, or tomatoes reduced biotin
concentrations (Bonjour, 1991). Biotin is unstable to oxidizing conditions and therefore is destroyed by heat, especially under conditions that
support simultaneous lipid peroxidation. These losses can be reduced by
the use of an antioxidant (e.g., vitamin C, vitamin E). After baby foods
were stored for 6 months, an approximate 15% reduction in biotin content was found (Karlin and Foisy, 1972).

DEFICIENCY

Effects of Deficiency

Biotin is important for normal function of the thyroid and adrenal
glands, the reproductive tract, and the nervous system. However, the ef-

455

fect of biotin deficiency on the cutaneous system is most dramatic since a severe dermatitis is the major obvious clinical sign of deficiency in livestock and poultry.

Ruminants

Biotin deficiency, identified by hindquarter paralysis, decreased urinary excretion of biotin, and correction of the problem with biotin injections was reported in calves (Wiese et al., 1946). Flipse et al. (1948) reported a potassium-biotin interrelationship in calves, with the result that calves fed purified diets low in potassium and biotin developed progressive paralysis of the hind legs that spread to the forelegs, neck, and respiratory system. Death may result within 12 to 24 hours of the first signs; however, the condition can be cured by injections of potassium salts or biotin.

Due to ruminal and intestinal synthesis of biotin, a need for supplemental sources was at one time not expected for ruminants. Nevertheless, promising preliminary results in preventing lameness in dairy cattle with biotin supplementation were reported (Frigg et al., 1993). Successful biotin treatment of dairy cows with claw problems was reported by Nietlis-Bash and Triebel (1988). In biotin-deficient dairy cows, the hoof horn is of poor quality, soft, and crumbling, with no distinct separation of keratinizing and cornified cells. This results in the omission of the granular layer at the epidermis of the bulb of the heel. Decreased stabilizing filaments in the upper spiny layer of the hoof corium in biotin-deficient cows reveals the depressed hormone-like activity of biotin in the synthesis of protein (Budras et al., 1997).

Increased plasma biotin levels have been associated with hardness and conformational changes in the bovine hoof. Dairy cows supplemented with 20 mg of biotin per cow over an 11-month period expressed a steepened angle of the dorsal border and height of the heel; length of the diagonal and size of the ground surface increased (Distl and Schmid, 1994). The hardness of the hoof was also significantly greater in the biotin-treated group. Greenough et al. (1999) reported that biotin supplementation (20 mg/day) to dairy cows not only reduced hoof lesions, but significantly increased milk production.

Beef cattle suffer from a common hoof defect known as sandcracks, which are vertical fissures in the hoof. These tend to be more prevalent in older, heavier cows and often result in chronic lameness problems in beef cattle. Biotin supplementation in 15 beef cow herds in which 37.2% of the cows were affected with sandcracks dramatically reduced the proportion of affected cows (Campbell et al., 1995). This study indicates that biotin supplementation appears to improve hoof quality by lowering the number of sandcracks per cow and decreases occurrence of other hoof defects, such as broken toes and abnormal coronary bands. Feeding dairy and beef cows 20 mg/day of supplemental biotin resulted in reduced incidence of hoof lesions and increased milk production (Seymour, 1999).

Swine

Biotin deficiency was produced in 1946 in swine by feeding a purified diet containing Sulfathalidine or raw egg white (Cunha et al., 1946; Lindley and Cunha, 1946). For many years it was concluded that biotin supplementation was not needed since it is synthesized by intestinal microorganisms and is widely distributed in feed. Nevertheless, clinical signs of deficiency were observed by feed company personnel and scientists under field conditions. However, it wasn't until the 1970s that a greater awareness of the problem of biotin field deficiency became apparent (Cunha, 1984).

Biotin deficiency results in reduced growth rate and impaired feed conversion as well as a wide variety of clinical signs. These include alopecia (hair loss); dermatitis characterized by dryness, roughness, and a brownish exudate; ulceration of the skin; inflammation of the mouth mucosa; hind-leg spasticity; and transverse cracking of the soles and tops of hooves (Cunha, 1977). Clinical signs of biotin deficiency in swine are shown in Figs. 11.2 and 11.3.

Growth depression may become evident in biotin-deficient swine before clinical signs are seen. The first clinical signs are generally excessive hair loss and dermatitis, with complete hair loss in severe cases. Dermatitis first appears as scaly skin, often starting on the ears, neck, shoulder, and tail and eventually spreading over the entire body. In later stages, crust and cracks appear on the face and extremities.

After 5 to 7 weeks on a biotin-deficient diet, swine may show claw defects. Foot lesions may be the most characteristic sign of biotin deficiency. The hoof horn becomes soft and rubbery and is poorly resistant to abrasions. The slow growth-and-repair process in the hoof tissue and the considerable weight on the feet add to the problem. Depending on the floor type on which the animal is kept, this may have little effect or may lead to the development of cracks and necrotic lesions, resulting in extreme lameness (Glättli, 1975). Secondary infections may gain entry through claw cracks and result in infected joints, which may lead to premature removal from the herd. Feeding and breeding activities are also adversely affected; in particular, the sow becomes unable to support the

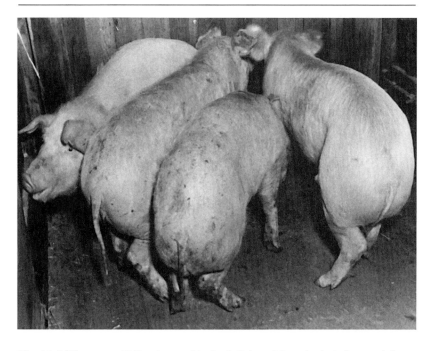

Fig. 11.2 The two middle pigs are biotin deficient. Note the hair loss and dermatitis. (Courtesy of T.J. Cunha and Washington State University.)

weight of the boar. Also, because the hog's ability to eat may be impaired, these problems will obviously lead to economic losses.

Biotin supplementation improved the strength of the pig claw horn (Kempson et al., 1989). Supplementary biotin affected the structure of the coronary epidermis; there was an increase in the density of the horn tubules in the stratum medium, the horny squames in the stratum medium were more tightly packed, and the tubules were more clearly defined in the pigs receiving biotin. The body condition of sows during lactation, and in the period from weaning to remating, was improved by biotin supplementation (Greer et al., 1991). Twelve months after the experiment commenced, the percentage of sows with foot lesions was lower in the biotin-supplemented than the unsupplemented group (42 versus 55). Investigations of lameness in sows showed that pigmented claws were less liable to develop lesions than unpigmented claws, that claws with high moisture content were relatively weak, that feeding biotin increased claw hardness under certain conditions, and that the frequency of claw lesions increased during pregnancy (Kroneman et al., 1992).

458

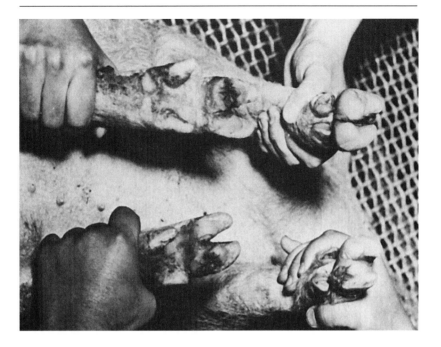

Fig. 11.3 Biotin-deficient pigs. Note transverse cracking of the soles and the tops of the hooves. (Courtesy of T.J. Cunha and Washington State University.)

Supplementation of the diet of breeding sows with biotin from an early stage of development made a significant contribution to the maintenance of hoof-horn integrity (Simmins and Brooks, 1988). Tagwerker (1983) noted that foot lesions were responsible for 4 to 8% of all sows culled in Europe. Also, he noted a Denmark study that reported 8.5% of hoof lesions in biotin-supplemented sows compared to 25% for controls. After biotin supplementation, in Holland, culling rate due to lameness was decreased from 25 to 14% (de Jong and Sytsema, 1983).

Cunha (1984) noted that in most of the 40 countries he visited during the past 30 years, biotin deficiency signs were observed in swine operations. These signs, observed under field conditions, occurred in only 10 to 20% of sows or less. Baby pigs nursing these sows usually showed no biotin deficiency signs but responded to biotin supplementation. Unfortunately, many swine producers are of the opinion that it is natural for a swine herd to have a few animals with hair loss, dermatitis, and cracked feet and therefore are not overly concerned when a small percentage of sows exhibit these clinical signs (Cunha, 1984).

459

Biotin supplementation of sow diets has significantly improved reproductive performance, including the number of pigs farrowed and weaned, litter weaning weight, and number of days from weaning to estrus (Brooks et al., 1977; Simmins and Brooks, 1983; Misir and Blair, 1984; Kornegay, 1986).

In a field study, sows had severe lameness and impaired reproduction (Fonge, 1977). After these sows received supplemental biotin, normal foot health and normal reproductive performance were restored. Researchers also found that sows housed in total confinement showed a positive response to conception rate and interval from weaning to first estrus and a trend to larger litters when supplemented with biotin (Bryant et al., 1985). In an earlier study (Brooks et al., 1977), sows fed supplemental biotin had more pigs born alive (9.8 versus 8.1), more pigs weaned (7.8 versus 6.8), increased litter weight at weaning (71.0 versus 64.5 kg), and reduced time interval from weaning to first estrus after weaning (6.2 versus 15.3 days) compared to unsupplemented controls.

Poultry

Biotin requirement in the turkey is higher than that of the chick, so more field problems with biotin deficiency have arisen in turkeys. Biotin deficiency in chicks and poults results in a wide range of clinical signs (Figs. 11.4 through 11.7), with considerable variation in time of appearance of individual signs (NRC, 1994). The principal effects in both species are reduced growth rate and feed efficiency, disturbed and broken feathering, dermatitis, and leg and beak deformities. First signs of deficiency are usually growth depression and loose feathering; signs of dermatitis then appear and, finally, disorders of the leg (perosis) and beak become apparent. With dermal lesions, bottoms of feet become rough and calloused and contain deep fissures that show some hemorrhaging. Feet problems are usually exacerbated by bacterial invasion of lesions. Toes may become necrotic and slough off. Tops of feet and legs usually show only a dry scaliness. Lesions appear in the corner of the mouth and slowly spread to the whole area around the beak. Eyelids eventually swell and stick together.

Dermal lesions have a characteristic order of appearance, although speed of onset depends on deficiency severity. For chicks fed severely deficient diets, dryness and flakiness of the feet first become noticeable at about 14 days of age, and slight encrustations and superficial fissures develop in the undersurfaces of the feet at about 18 days (Whitehead, 1978). These increase in severity until, by about 25 days, the fissures be-

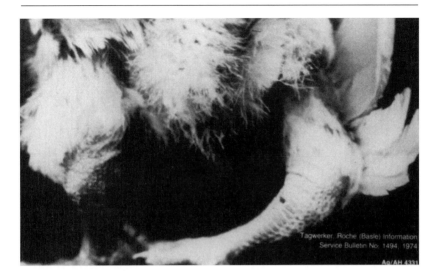

Fig. 11.4 Perosis (bone deformities) as a result of biotin deficiency. Chicks showed perosis as early as 17 days of age, with rigid limb joints that resulted in a stilted walk. (Courtesy of Hoffmann-La Roche Inc., Nutley, New Jersey.)

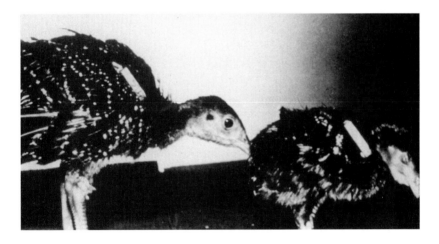

Fig. 11.5 Normal (left) and biotin-deficient (right) Broad-Breasted Bronze male turkeys at 3 weeks of age. (Courtesy of D.C. Dobson, Utah State University.)

461

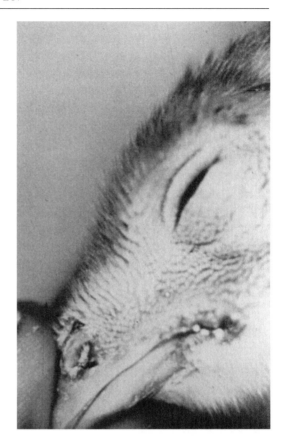

Fig. 11.6 Biotin deficiency in a poult. Note lesion at apex of mouth. (Courtesy of L.S. Jensen and Washington State University).

come hemorrhagic. Between 3 and 4 weeks, dermatitis may also appear on the eyelids and, as this develops, the bird becomes unable to keep the lids apart and they eventually become stuck together.

Dermal lesions are similar to those of pantothenic acid deficiency (see Chapter 10). However, with biotin deficiency, lesions occur first in the feet and later around the beak and eyes, whereas in pantothenic acid deficiency, the signs occur first in the corners of the mouth and eyes and only in prolonged cases appear in the feet. Because of the difficulty of making a differential diagnosis between the two vitamins, it is often necessary to examine the diet composition and decide which is most likely to be deficient.

Biotin deficiency is a cause of hock disorders in both poults and chicks. The major deficiency sign affecting market turkeys is severe leg weakness. Lesions caused by biotin deficiency are brought about by

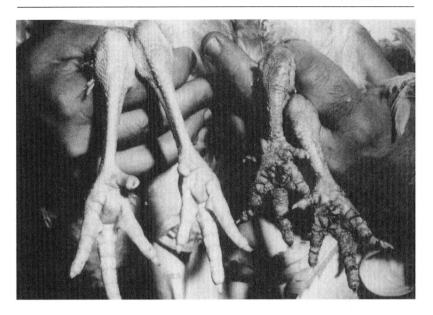

Fig. 11.7 Severe foot-pad lesions in the growing turkey as a result of biotin deficiency. Less severe lesions are more common. (Courtesy of Richard Miles, University of Florida.)

chondrodystrophy, a condition in which bone mineralization is normal, but linear growth of long bones is impaired. Chondrodystrophy caused by biotin deficiency can result in shortening of metatarsal bones and perosis. Perosis occurs when irregular bone development results in enlargement and deformity of the hock joint. Crippling in turkeys can occur as early as 3 to 4 weeks of age and often seems to disappear at 6 to 7 weeks. Then it reappears with great severity between 13 and 16 weeks (Scott, 1981). At this stage, the birds are unable to walk and thus can be trampled by other turkeys. Perosis can occur at any stage in the growth of the turkey from 3 to 24 weeks of age. In general, young chickens are less susceptible than poults to leg disorders, although biotin deficiency does cause problems of the same type in chicks as in poults (Whitehead, 1978). Once the deformities of perosis occur, biotin administration is not curative.

Bain et al. (1988) report that "twisted leg" is the most common limb disorder in broiler chickens and that biotin deficiency adversely affected tibiotarsal bone growth. Tibiotarsal bones are frequently longitudinally distorted in biotin-deficient poultry. Presumably, reduced biotin prevents

463

ready formation of prostaglandins from essential fatty acids, and bone growth fails to respond to stresses during development (Watkins et al., 1989).

Low dietary fat and the necessity for fatty acid synthesis lead to an abnormal array of fatty acids that predisposes poultry to a fatty liver and kidney syndrome (FLKS) (Whitehead, 1988). This condition, which has caused heavy economic losses in commercial broiler flocks, was found to be due to a suboptimal dietary biotin coupled with certain nutritional and environmental stress factors. Situations increasing the metabolic rate of biotin-dependent enzymes (pyruvate, acetyl-CoA carboxylase), such as low fat or protein levels, aggravate the condition. Although the signs of FLKS are not those of classic biotin deficiency, they can virtually be eliminated by supplementing chick starter or breeder diets with biotin.

In turkeys, dry and brittle feathers usually accompany the other signs of clinical biotin deficiency. Bronze poults can exhibit white barring of the feathers, usually affecting just tom turkeys. Likewise, deficient chicks have rough and broken feathering, with head and breast feathers often having a spiky, matted appearance.

Poor egg production and hatchability will result from clinical biotin deficiency (Robel, 1991; NRC, 1994). In breeder chickens, biotin deficiency will reduce hatchability but is less likely to affect egg production. Clinical signs and conditions associated with biotin deficiency in chick embryos and/or newly hatched chicks include bone deformities (perosis), impaired muscle coordination (ataxia), skeletal deformities (e.g., crooked legs), extensive foot webbing, abnormal cartilage development (chondrodystrophy), embryonic mortality, twisted and malformed beak ("parrot beak"), and reduced size. In turkeys, Ferguson et al. (1961) reported that biotin deficiency resulted in a marked decrease in hatchability and a high rate of embryonic mortality during the first week of incubation. At the end of the second week, hatchability decreased from 83 to 14%. At the end of the third week, hatchability was zero. Embryonic mortality because of inadequate biotin occurs largely during the last 3 days of incubation. Feeding the biotin-deficient diet resulted in an abrupt decrease in egg production after 13 weeks.

Horses

Biotin is synthesized in the lower digestive tract of the horse, but information on dietary requirement is lacking (NRC, 1989b). Hoof integrity for a number of cases has been reported to improve as a result of biotin supplementation (Fig. 11.8). Such cases were characterized by

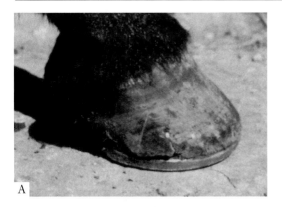

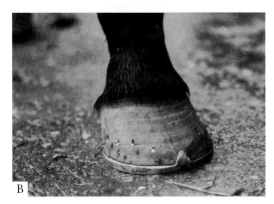

Fig. 11.8 Hoof condition of a 7-year-old 18-hands heavyweight show hunter resulting from biotin supplementation. The horse had a history of tender feet. (A) The walls of the hooves were very weak, crumbling at the lower edges, with large areas breaking out and detaching when shoes were nailed. (B) Five months after supplementation with 15 mg of biotin per day, the walls of the hooves were thicker and harder, so nailing was achieved. (Courtesy of N. Comben, R.J. Clark, and D.J.B. Sutherland and permission of *Veterinary Record* 115 [1984], 642–645.)

horn that tended to crumble at the lower edges of the hoof walls and that was generally prone to poor conformation and damage to the walls, soles, and the white line junction (Comben et al., 1984).

Biotin supplementation was given to 38 horses at 5 mg/150 kg body weight once daily for at least 9 months (Schulze and Scherf, 1989). Initially, all horses had hoof horn of poor quality. By the end of treatment the hoof defects were regarded as cured in 24 horses and improved in the remainder. In a 19-month experiment with Lipizzaner stallions, biotin supplementation decreased incidence and severity of horn defects, increased tensile strength (4.5 versus 3.7 kp/mm^2), and improved condition of the white line (Linden et al., 1993).

Other Animal Species

For a number of species, including guinea pigs, rats, hamsters, cats, and rabbits, no deficiency signs have been observed when animals were fed purified diets and/or natural diets containing low biotin concentrations. However, with these same species, feeding a biotin-deficient diet containing raw egg white (Fig. 11.9) produced typical deficiency signs, often including weight loss and alopecia.

DOGS AND CATS

Biotin-responsive disease conditions in dogs include dull coat, brittle hair, loss of hair, scaly skin pruritis, and dermatitis (NRC, 1985a; Frigg et al., 1989). In a study with small animal practitioners, 60% of clinical signs in dogs were cured, and another 31% improved (119 cases) in dogs with hair and skin conditions (Frigg et al., 1989).

In cats, severe, experimental biotin deficiency may be marked by bloody diarrhea, anorexia, and emaciation. Scaly dermatitis about the nose and mouth, generalized alopecia, and hypersalivation have been noted (NRC, 1986; Pastoor et al., 1991). Most cats with the deficiency develop signs of alopecia; dried secretion around the eyes, nose, mouth, and feet; focal dermatitis of the lips near the eyeteeth; and a brownish appearance of the skin (Pastoor et al., 1991).

FISH

Biotin is synthesized in many species of fish by intestinal microflora, but supplemental biotin may be required for maximum growth and to prevent clinical deficiency signs (NRC, 1993; Shiau and Chin, 1998). Signs of biotin deficiency in trout and salmon include anorexia, slow growth, increased mortality, and poor feed conversion. The "blue slime" disease of trout can be prevented with dietary biotin. Biotin-deficient catfish develop light skin pigmentation and anemia. Japanese eels fed a biotin-deficient diet exhibited reduced growth, abnormal swimming behavior, and dark coloration.

Common carp and channel catfish required from 8 to 12 weeks, and rainbow trout from 4 to 8 weeks, to show growth depression when fed biotin-deficient diets (NRC, 1993). Signs of biotin deficiency were not detected in rainbow trout or channel catfish fed natural ingredient diets without supplemented biotin for 24 and 17 weeks, respectively (NRC, 1993). These studies concluded that adequate biotin was available in the natural feed ingredients.

FOXES AND MINK

Biotin deficiencies have been produced by feeding purified diets or diets containing egg products to growing mink. Apparently, the short intestinal tract of the mink and rapid feed passage make it impossible for

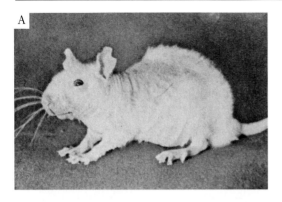

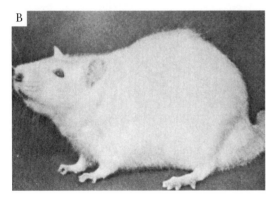

Fig. 11.9 (A) Egg-white injury as a result of feeding a rat raw egg white, which contains a biotin antagonist, avidin. The resulting dermatitis progressed to generalized alopecia. (B) After 3 months of treatment, the animal returned to normal. (Courtesy of Alan T. Forrester, *Scope Manual on Nutrition*, The Upjohn Company, Kalamazoo, Michigan.)

the animal to obtain adequate biotin from that synthesized by its intestinal flora. Stout et al. (1966) reported biotin deficiency in mink when diets contained 40% or more offal from breeder hen turkeys. Presence of raw eggs in the offal was presumed responsible for the deficiency. Later studies in Oregon showed that inclusion of spray-dried egg in the diet can have a similar effect (Wehr et al., 1980). In both mink and foxes, biotin deficiency resulted in graying or discoloration of hair (Fig. 11.10) and, in extreme cases, hair loss (NRC, 1982a).

LABORATORY ANIMALS

Signs of biotin deficiency (Fig. 11.9) in avidin-fed rats are weight loss, exfoliative dermatitis, alopecia, achromotrichia, and an abnormal, spastic gait (NRC, 1995). Heard et al. (1989) reported that biotin deficiency causes impaired auditory brainstem function in young biotin-deficient rats. Skin from biotin deficient rats contained a different pattern

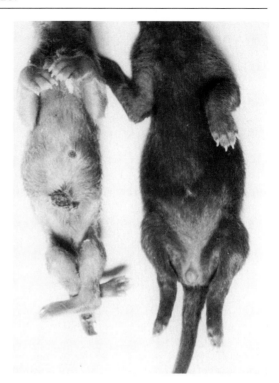

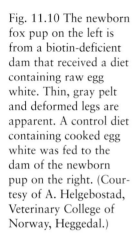

Fig. 11.10 The newborn fox pup on the left is from a biotin-deficient dam that received a diet containing raw egg white. Thin, gray pelt and deformed legs are apparent. A control diet containing cooked egg white was fed to the dam of the newborn pup on the right. (Courtesy of A. Helgebostad, Veterinary College of Norway, Heggedal.)

of fatty acids than that of controls (Proud et al., 1990). Biotin deficiency in rats and mice can result in a hind limb paralysis referred to as kangaroo gait.

Clinical signs for biotin deficiency in mice, hamsters, and guinea pigs included alopecia, achromotrichia, and growth failure (NRC, 1995). Biotin supplementation improved reproduction and lactation in mice when added to a purified diet devoid of egg white (NRC, 1995). Biotin deficiency interfered with synthesis of specific proteins, which resulted in congenital malformations (e.g., cleft palate) (Watanabe, 1995). On day 10 of gestation in hamsters, biotin deficiency resulted in a high incidence of resorbed and dead embryos, and by day 14, for the remaining embryos, there were growth retardation, morphological abnormalities, and skeletal defects (Watanabe, 1993).

NONHUMAN PRIMATES

Biotin deficiency was produced in adolescent rhesus monkeys with thinning of hair and loss of hair color as a result of a low-biotin diet for

468

long periods (15 to 28 months) (Waisman et al., 1945). Use of diets with egg white and/or sulfonamides greatly hastened and intensified biotin-deficiency signs.

RABBITS

Deficiency of biotin, characterized by loss of hair and dermatitis, occurred in rabbits that were fed raw egg white over a period of time (Lease et al., 1937).

Humans

Except in infants, there is no evidence of spontaneous biotin deficiency in humans. This is probably due to the ubiquitous nature of the vitamin in diets plus benefits derived from microbial synthesis. Biotin deficiency occurs in individuals consuming a large number of raw eggs daily because of the antagonistic effect of the egg-white protein avidin (see History). Adult volunteers fed 200 g of dehydrated egg white daily for 5 weeks displayed symptoms of mild depression, lassitude, somnolence, hallucination, anxiety with muscle pain, and hyperesthesia (Sydenstricker et al., 1942). After 8 weeks, anorexia and a striking grayish pallor with dermatitis and desquamation occurred. The experiment was terminated because of a marked fall in food intake.

Biotin deficiency has also been demonstrated in biotinidase deficiency, with many clinical findings and biochemical abnormalities similar to those associated with biotin deficiency (Mock, 1990). Patients with biotinidase deficiency cannot utilize biocytin, which is excreted in their urine, and must depend solely upon free biotin from food to maintain normal biotin levels. Two conditions in infants—seborrheic dermatitis and desquamative erythroderma (Leiner's disease)—are apparently connected with biotin deficiency, since children with these diseases have subnormal biotin in blood and urine and respond to supplementation with the vitamin. Some children have an inborn error of metabolism resulting from lack of biotin-dependent carboxylases. Children with this disorder can be divided into two groups, namely, those affected by an isolated defect in only one and those with a combined deficiency of the four biotin-dependent enzymes. The multiple carboxylase deficiency apparently results from a deficiency in biotinidase activity.

Biotin deficiency can result when insufficient biotin is added to infant milk formulations or to total parenteral nutrition solutions. Infants with short bowel syndrome receiving total parenteral nutrition lacking in biotin showed an increase in serum odd-chain saturated fatty acids and a decrease in linoleic acid compared with controls (Anonymous,

1989). Although the evidence is circumstantial, some researchers have suggested that sudden infant death syndrome (SIDS) may be related to low biotin intakes of bottle-fed infants (Bonjour, 1991). The median biotin levels in the livers of infants who died from SIDS between 1 and 52 weeks of life were significantly lower than those of infants who died from explicable causes (Heard et al., 1983). Anticonvulsant drugs (e.g., carbamazepine and primidone) are competitive inhibitors of biotin transport in the intestine and would relate to inadequate biotin status for long-term therapy of these drugs (Said et al., 1989). Cases of low circulating plasma biotin have also been reported for alcoholics, elderly persons, epileptics, and burn victims.

Assessment of Status

Detection of subclinical or marginal biotin deficiency, which is most likely to occur under field conditions, is difficult. Field observations are important, but it is essential to realize that there may be no clinical signs in spite of deficiency. If clinical signs are seen, they may not all be present, and only a small percentage of animals may exhibit such clinical signs. Chemical, chick, or microbiological assays often give different results for feed biotin concentrations. Likewise, there is great variability in feed biotin concentrations and availability in various feeds (see Natural Sources).

Whitehead et al. (1980) and Misir and Blair (1984) suggested that plasma biotin concentration and plasma pyruvate carboxylase activity are methods of assessing the biotin status of pigs. However, blood biotin concentrations often lack dependability as a good indicator of biotin status of pigs (Cunha, 1984). This is particularly true with borderline deficiency, in which plasma biotin varies with dietary intake and shows considerable individual variation among pigs. In chickens, several reports have indicated that plasma biotin concentration below 100 ng/100 ml is indicative of biotin deficiency (Scott et al., 1982). In three experiments using chickens and turkeys, plasma pyruvic carboxylase activity was positively related to supplemental biotin in both species (Whitehead and Bannister, 1978). Robinson and Lovell (1978) reported that biotin status in fish may be assessed by measuring pyruvate carboxylase activity in the liver. Hepatic pyruvate carboxylase activity in rainbow trout fed a lipid-free and biotin-deficient diet decreased to 3.3% of normal (Walton et al., 1984). Biotin concentration in egg yolk is an additional method of evaluating the status of the vitamin (see Analytical Procedures). In both poultry and swine, the ratio of the blood fatty acids is likewise indicative of biotin status, with palmitoleic acid particularly increasing in relation to stearic acid (Edwards, 1974).

Mock and Mock (1992) reported abnormal catabolism of leucine as a basis for early detection of biotin deficiency in rats. 3-Methylcrotonyl-CoA originates from catabolism of leucine and is normally metabolized to acetyl-CoA. However, in biotin deficiency, reduced hepatic activity of the biotin-dependent enzyme methylcrotonyl-CoA carboxylase causes the enzyme's substrate 3-methylcrotonyl-CoA to be shunted via an alternate pathway to 3-hydroxyisovaleric acid (3-HIA), which is excreted at increased rates in the urine. Elevated concentrations of 3-HIA would be an early indication of biotin inadequacy.

Evaluation of human biotin status employs blood and urinary biotin and biotin metabolites (Mock et al., 1997). As with animals, there are considerable differences and variations among humans that are difficult to explain. From the available data, a biotin level in urine of approximately 70 nmol/L and a circulating level in plasma of around 1,500 nmol/L seem to indicate an adequate supply of biotin for humans (Bonjour, 1991).

SUPPLEMENTATION

For supplementation in livestock, consideration must be given to cost, as biotin is one of the more expensive vitamins. However, based on the requirements and recommended industry levels for biotin supplementation, it costs less than other vitamins, such as choline and vitamin E, in monogastric diets. In view of the considerable cost of synthetically produced biotin, the question of biotin supplementation of practical diets is economically significant.

Although clinical signs were found for poultry and swine under experimental conditions in the 1940s, for many years it was believed that supplemental biotin was not needed in swine and poultry diets because of the production of biotin by the animal's intestinal microflora. In 1967 for poultry and in the mid-1970s for swine, interest was rekindled when more field cases occurred than in the past. Interference with the biosynthesis of biotin by intestinal bacteria can individually or collectively lead to biotin deficiency. These interferences can be in the form of therapeutic administration of antibacterial agents and modern housing systems, which limit animals' access to feces. Additionally, biotin deficiency is now more prevalent because of limited bioavailability of biotin found in some grains (e.g., wheat, barley, sorghum) and in some animal protein sources (e.g., meat meal, poultry by-product meal), biotin antagonists including molds, feed rancidity, and improved genetic characteristics for greater production. Cunha (1984) summarized the possible reasons for more frequent occurrence of biotin deficiency in swine (Table 11.3); the majority of these reasons are likewise applicable to the poultry industry. Biotin deficiency in fur-bearing animals caused by feeding of egg products is economically disastrous because of interference with fur coloration, and supplementation is mandated.

Some reports conclude that foot lesions in adult sows healed in a matter of weeks (Tagwerker, 1974) when sows were supplemented with high levels of biotin, while Brooks et al. (1977) found that biotin supplementation resulted in a 28% reduction in lesions after 6 months. Pigs housed on badly designed floors have little opportunity for recovery, as traumatic injury exceeds the capacity of the hoof for growth and repair. Brooks (1982) summarized data from Great Britain, Denmark, and Switzerland and concluded that where foot lesions already existed, dietary supplements of 2,000 to 3,000 µg of biotin per kilogram of diet were beneficial.

For many species receiving typical diets, supplementation is not needed because of adequate sources in feed ingredients and/or intestinal microflora synthesis. As an example of dietary adequacy, practical diets for channel catfish made from the commonly used ingredients—soybean meal, corn, and menhaden fish meal—did not need supplemental biotin (Lovell and Buston, 1984). There may be less need for biotin supplementation for swine fed a high-quality corn-soybean diet that has no mold (short-term storage) and for swine raised under favorable environmental and nutritional conditions (Watkins et al., 1991).

For some species, including equines, the need for supplemental biotin is controversial. If hoof problems exist, daily biotin supplementation has been suggested (Comben et al., 1984) for each animal as follows: donkeys and ponies, 5 to 10 mg; riding horses, 15 mg; and heavy horses, up to 30 mg. The recommendation is to continue supplementation as increased hoof horn strength may be anticipated within 3 to 5 months. Using scanning electron microscope observations, Kempson (1987, 1994) concluded that biotin-related improvements in hoof quality are limited to the stratum externum and not the stratum medium or stratum internum. He suggested that structural defects in the stratum externum of the hoof horn could be remedied by biotin supplementation alone, but poor attachment of the horn squames required biotin plus supplemental calcium and protein.

Young ruminants not receiving their mother's milk and before the

■ Table 11.3   Possible Explanations Why Biotin Deficiencies Have Become More
Prevalent in Swine and Poultry Operations in Recent Years

Increased use of confinement, which lessens opportunity for coprophagy (feces eating);
feces containing biotin synthesized in the intestines.
Increased use of grain–soybean meal diets, with less utilization of biotin-rich feeds including whey, fermentation by-products, yeast, dehydrated alfalfa, and pasture.
Biotin antagonists in feeds such as streptavidin, certain antimicrobial drugs, and dieldrin
(a pesticide). *Streptomyces* are molds affecting biotin availability that are found in
soil, moldy feeds, manure, and litter.
Rancidity in feeds causes biotin to be readily destroyed. Biotin in feedstuffs may be destroyed by heat curing, solvent extraction, pelleting, and improper storage conditions.
Length of storage, temperature, and humidity result in biotin loss.
Reduced intestinal synthesis and/or absorption of biotin may result from diseases and
other conditions affecting the gastrointestinal tract.
Improved genetic characteristics (breed, type, and strain) and intensified production for
faster weight gains and better feed conversion. Increased reproductive performance
with more farrowings per sow yearly or increased egg production in poultry operations.
Decreased level of biotin or its availability in feeds because of new plant varieties, new
feed production practices, and processing methods.
For swine, reduced feed consumption (thus reduced biotin intake) by sows to avoid excess weight, which is detrimental to reproduction. Sows now receive 1.4–2.3 kg feed
per day during gestation whereas previously they had received 2.7–3.2 kg.
Interrelationships between biotin and other nutrients affect requirements. Dietary fats,
pantothenic acid, vitamin B_6, vitamin B_{12}, folacin, thiamin, riboflavin, *myo*-inositol,
and ascorbic acid are related to biotin requirements and metabolism.
Lower levels and availability of biotin in feeds. Different batches of the same feed may
vary considerably in biotin content. Biotin in feeds exists in both free and bound
forms. Certain feeds have a low availability (i.e., wheat, barley, sorghum). A shift
from use of corn, soybean meal, and cottonseed meal often results in diets with less
available biotin.

Source: Adapted from Cunha (1984).

rumen is developed are recommended to receive supplemental biotin.
Milk replacers for calves are recommended to contain 0.1 mg/kg of biotin (NRC, 1989a). In acute cases of biotin deficiency in calves, single
injections of 100 µg of biotin subcutaneously or 1 mg of biotin intravenously reversed the deficiency (Wiese et al., 1946). Dietary biotin supplementation (e.g., 20 mg/day) for adult ruminants would be recommended where field conditions suggest a need (Seymour, 1999). Ruminal
bacteria involved in the synthesis of biotin appear to be sensitive to low
pH; therefore, high grain diets reduce rumen synthesis (Seymour, 1999).

Supplementation of human diets is generally considered unnecessary
because of adequate dietary intakes as well as intestinal microbial synthesis. Exceptions would be for individuals consuming raw eggs and infants with inborn errors of metabolism. Eggs are a good source of biotin;
however, the biotin contained in egg yolk is inadequate to counteract the

473

deficiency of the vitamin caused by the avidin in egg white, so unheated dried whole egg is deficient in this vitamin (Kratzer et al., 1988). In addition, since the advent of total parenteral nutrition, biotin deficiency has resulted in some cases in which biotin was omitted from intravenous fluids (Bonjour, 1991). In humans, biotin supplements in the form of injections of 150 to 300 µg/day can clear up symptoms of deficiency in a matter of a few days.

Biotin is commercially available as a 100% crystalline product or as dilutions (45.5 mg/kg and as a 1% premix). The form containing vitamin activity is d-biotin, which occurs in nature and is the commercially available form. A 2% spray-dried biotin product is also available for use in either feed or drinking water. An example of supplemental biotin provided in water for biotin-deficient young turkeys is 0.25 mg of biotin per gallon of drinking water for 3 to 4 weeks, and for older birds 0.50 mg per gallon (Bauernfeind, 1969).

Losses of biotin during storage can be considerable. Biotin is readily destroyed by feed rancidity (Pavcek and Shull, 1942). Preparing fresh feeds, storing them for only short periods, and keeping them dry and in a well-ventilated storage area will minimize rancidity problems. Hamilton and Veum (1984) have suggested that overdrying, poor storage conditions, and presence of mold may reduce the availability of biotin in corn. Also, the diet should be low in feeds that are high in prooxidants and/or properly protected by an effective antioxidant to avoid destruction of biotin, vitamin E, selenium, and other nutrients.

Biotin is relatively stable in multivitamin premixes, unless combined with choline or trace minerals. Coelho (1991) reported only 57% retention of biotin when the vitamin supplement contained choline and trace minerals. Biotin is generally stable in feeds, but losses of the vitamin during processing do occur. Processing losses of biotin in extruded pet food have been reported at about 15% (Anonymous, 1981).

TOXICITY

For both humans and animals, biotin is apparently not toxic even in large doses. However, Paul et al. (1973) reported that an acute dose of biotin (5 mg/100 g of body weight) caused irregularities of the estrus cycle, with heavy infiltration of leukocytes in the vagina of the rat up to 14 days after treatment. In additional rat studies, a dose of biotin at least 5,000 or 10,000 times the daily requirement had no deleterious effects (Mittelholzer, 1976). Studies with poultry and swine indicate a safety tolerance of 4 to 10 times their requirement, with maximum tolerable level probably much higher (NRC, 1987). Likewise with humans, no adverse effects have resulted from oral or intravenous administration of high doses over prolonged periods.

■ REFERENCES

Achuta Murthy, P.N., and Mistry, S.P. (1977). *Prog. Food Nutr. Sci. 2,* 450.
Anonymous (1981). Rationale for Roche Recommended Vitamin Fortification, RCD 5963/1280. Hoffmann-La Roche, Nutley, New Jersey.
Anonymous (1989). *Nutr. Rev. 47,* 121.
Bain, S.D., Newbrey, J.W., and Watkins, B.A. (1988). *Poult. Sci. 67,* 590.
Barth, C.A., Frigg, M., and Hagemeister, H. (1986). *J. Anim. Phys. Anim. Nutr. 55,* 128.
Bauernfeind, J.C. (1969). *World Rev. Anim. Prod. 5,* 20.
Bender, D.A. (1992). Nutritional biochemistry of the vitamins, Cambridge University Press, Cambridge, England.
Bonjour, J.P. (1991). *In* Handbook of Vitamins 2nd Ed. (L.J. Machlin, ed.), p. 403. Marcel Dekker, New York.
Brooks, P.H. (1982). *Pig News Inf. 3,* 1.
Brooks, P.H., Smith, D.A., and Irwin, V.C.R. (1977). *Vet. Res. 101,* 46.
Bryant, K.L., Kornegay, E.T., Knight, J.W., Webb, K.E. Jr., and Notter, D.R. (1985). *J. Anim. Sci. 60,* 145.
Bryden, W.L. (1989). *Br. J. Nutr. 62,* 389.
Budras, K.D., Hochstetter, T., Muelling, Ch., and Natterman, W. (1997). *J. Dairy Sci. 80*(Suppl. 1), 192.
Buenrostro, J.L., and Kratzer, F.H. (1984). *Poult. Sci. 63,* 1563.
Campbell, J., Greenough, P.R., and Petrice, L. (1995). Western College of Vet. Med. University of Saskatchewan, Saskatoon, Canada.
Coelho, M.B. (1991). Vitamin Stability in Premixes and Feeds: A Practical Approach, p. 56. BASF Technical Symposium, Bloomington, Minnesota.
Comben, N., Clark, R.J., and Sutherland, D.J.B. (1984). *Vet. Rec. 115,* 642.
Cunha, T.J. (1977). Swine Feeding and Nutrition, Academic Press, New York.
Cunha, T.J. (1984). *Feed Manage. 35,* 14.
Cunha, T.J., Lindley, D.C., and Ensminger, M.E. (1946). *J. Anim. Sci. 5,* 219.
de Jong, M.F., and Sytsema, J.R. (1983). *Vet. Q. 5,* 58.
Distl, O., and Schmid, D. (1994). *Tierarzliche Umschauy 49,* 581.
Drouchner, W., and Völker, L. (1984). Proc. TAD Symposium, Cattle and Pig Diseases. *Cuxhaveny 1,* 105.
Edwards, H.M. (1974). *In* Proc. Nutr. Conf., p. 1. Atlanta.
Ferguson, T.M., Whiteside, C.H., Creger, C.R., Jones, M.L., Atkinson, R.L., and Couch, J.R. (1961). *Poult. Sci. 40,* 1151.
Flipse, R.J., Huffman, C.F., Duncan, G.W., and Thorp, F. (1948). *J. Anim. Sci. 7,* 525.
Fonge, J. (1977). *Pig Farm. 25*(6), 61.
Frigg, M. (1976). *Poult. Sci. 55,* 2310.
Frigg, M. (1984). *Poult. Sci. 63,* 750.

Frigg, M., and Volker, L. (1994). *Feedstuffs* 66(1), 12.

Frigg, M., Schulze, J., and Volker, L. (1989). *Schweizer-Archiv-fur-Tierheilkunde* *131*, 621.

Frigg, M., Straub, O.C., and Harmann, D. (1993). *Int. J. Vit. Nutr. Res.* 63, 122.

Glättli, H.R. (1975). *Zentralbl. Veterinaermed. A* 22, 102.

Greenough, P.R., Gay, J.M., Dobson, R.C., and Gay, C.C. (1999). *J. Dairy Sci.* 82(Suppl. 1.), 34 (Abstr.)

Greer, E.B., Leibholz, J.M., Pickering, D.I., Macoun, R.E., and Bryden, W.L. (1991). *Aust. J. Agr. Res.* 42, 1013.

Hamilton, C.R., and Veum, T.L. (1984). *J. Anim. Sci.* 59, 151.

Heard, G.S., Hood, R.L., and Johnson, A.R. (1983). *Med. J. Aust.* 2, 305.

Heard, G.S., Lenhardt, M.I., Bowie, R.M., Clarke, A.M., Harkins, S.W., and Wolf, B. (1989). *FASEB J.* 3, A1242.

Karlin, R., and Foisy, C. (1972). *Int. J. Vit. Nutr. Res.* 42, 545.

Kempson, S.A. (1987). *Vet. Rec.* 120, 568.

Kempson, S.A. (1994). *In* Ninth Annual Bluegrass Laminitis Symposium. Louisville, Kentucky.

Kempson, S.A., Currie, R.J.W., and Johnston, A.M. (1989). *Vet. Rec.* 124, 37.

Kopinski, J.S., and Leibholz, J. (1985). *Proc. Nutr. Soc. Aust.* 10, 170.

Kopinski, J.S., Leibholz, J., and Love, R.J. (1989a). *Brit. J. Nutr.* 62, 767.

Kopinski, J.S., Leibholz, J., and Love, R.J. (1989b). *Brit. J. Nutr.* 62, 781.

Kopinski, J.S., Leibholz, J., Bryden, W.L., and Fogarty, A.C. (1989c). *Brit. J. Nutr.* 62, 751.

Kornegay, E.T. (1986). *Livestock Prod.* 14, 65.

Kramer, T.R., Briske-Anderson, M., Johnson, S.B., and Holman, R.T. (1984). *J. Nutr.* 114, 2047.

Kratzer, F.H., Knollman, K., Earl, L., and Buenrostro, J.L. (1988). *J. Nutr.* 118, 604.

Kroneman, A., Vellenga, L., Vermeer, H.M., and Van-der Wilt, F.J. (1992). *Proefverslag-Proefstation-Voor-de-Varkenshouderij*, pp. 1, 78.

Lease, J.G., Parsons, H.T., and Kelly, E. (1937). *Biochem. J.* 31, 433.

Lee, H.M., McCall, N.E., Wright, L.D., and McCormick, D.B. (1973). *Proc. Soc. Exp. Biol. Med.* 142, 642.

Li-Hsieh, Y.T., and Mistry, S.P. (1992). *Nutr. Res.* 12(6), 787.

Linden, J., Josseck, H., Zenker, W., Geyer, H., and Schulze, J. (1993). *In* Proc. 13th Equine Nutrition and Physiology Symposium, p. 58. University of Florida, Gainesville.

Lindley, D.C., and Cunha, T.J. (1946). *J. Nutr.* 32, 47.

Loosli, J.K. (1991). *In* Animal Science Handbook (P.A. Putnam, ed.). Academic Press, San Diego.

Lovell, R.T., and Buston, J.C. (1984). *J. Nutr.* 114, 1092.

Maeda, Y., Kawata, S., Inui, Y., Fukuda, K., Igura, T., and Matsuzawa, Y. (1996). *J. Nutr.* 126, 61.

McGinnis, C.H. (1986a). Water Soluble Vitamins. Rhone Poulenc, Atlanta.

McGinnis, C.H. (1986b). Bioavailability of Nutrients in Feed Ingredients, p. 1. National Feed Ingredient Association (NFIA), Des Moines, Iowa.

Misir, R., and Blair, R. (1984). *J. Anim. Sci.* 59(Suppl. 1), 254.

Mittelholzer, E. (1976). *Int. J. Vit. Res.* 46, 33.

Mock, D.M. (1990). *In* Nutrition Reviews, Present Knowledge in Nutrition (R.E. Olson, ed.), p. 189. Nutritional Foundation, Washington, D.C.

Mock, D.M., and Malik, M.I. (1992). *Am. J. Clin. Nutr. 56*, 427.

Mock, D.M., Stadler, D.D., Stratton, S.L., and Mock, N.I. (1997). *J. Nutr. 127*, 710.

Mock, N.I., and Mock, D.M. (1992). *J. Nutr. 122*, 1493.

Moretti, P., Petrelli, C., Petrelli, F., and Sciarresi, P. (1990). *Med. Sci. Res. 18*, 73.

Nietlis-Bash, C., and Triebel, D.F. (1988). *Die Gruene 116*, 28.

NRC. Nutrient Requirements of Domestic Animals. National Academy of Sciences-National Research Council, Washington, D.C.

   (1981). Nutrient Requirements of Goats.

   (1982a). Nutrient Requirements of Mink and Foxes.

   (1985a). Nutrient Requirements of Dogs, 2nd Ed.

   (1985b). Nutrient Requirements of Sheep, 5th Ed.

   (1986). Nutrient Requirements of Cats, 3rd Ed.

   (1989a). Nutrient Requirements of Dairy Cattle, 6th Ed.

   (1989b). Nutrient Requirements of Horses, 5th Ed.

   (1993). Nutrient Requirements of Fish.

   (1994). Nutrient Requirements of Poultry, 9th Ed.

   (1995). Nutrient Requirements of Laboratory Animals.

   (1996). Nutrient Requirements of Beef Cattle, 7th Ed.

   (1998). Nutrient Requirements of Swine, 10th Ed.

NRC. (1982b). United States-Canadian Tables of Feed Composition, 3rd Ed. National Academy of Sciences-National Research Council, Washington, D.C.

NRC. (1987). Vitamin Tolerance of Animals. National Academy of Sciences-National Research Council, Washington, D.C.

Pastoor, F.J.H., Van Herick, H., Van't Klooster, A., and Beynen, A.C. (1991). *J. Nutr. 121*, 573.

Paul, P.K., Duttagupta, P.N., and Agarwal, H.C. (1973). *Curr. Sci. 42*, 613.

Pavcek, P.L., and Shull, G.M. (1942). *J. Biol. Chem. 146*, 351.

Petrelli, F., Moretti, P., and Paparelli, M. (1979). *Mol. Biol. Rep. 4*, 247.

Proud, V.K., Rizzo, W.B., Patterson, J.W., Heard, G.S., and Wolf, B. (1990). *Am. J. Clin. Nutr. 51*, 853.

RDA. (1989). Recommended Dietary Allowances, 10th Ed. National Academy of Sciences-National Research Council, Washington, D.C.

Robel, E.J. (1991). *Poult. Sci. 70*, 1716.

Robinson, E.H., and Lovell, R.T. (1978). *J. Nutr. 108*, 1600.

Roland, D.A., and Edwards, H.M. (1971). *J. Nutr. 101*, 811.

Said, H.M., and Derweesh, I. (1991). *Am. J. Phys. 261*, R94.

Said, H.M., Redha, R., and Nylander, W. (1988). *Gastroenterology 95*, 1312.

Said, H.M., Redha, R., and Nylander, W. (1989). *Am. J. Clin. Nutr. 49*, 127.

Said, H.M., Hoefs, J., Mohammadkhani, R., and Horne, D.W. (1992). *Gastroenterology 102*, 2120.

Sauer, W.C., Mosenthin, R., and Ozimek, L. (1988). *J. Anim. Sci. 66*, 2583.

Scholtissek, J., Barth, C.A., Hagemeister, H., and Frigg, M. (1990). *Br. J. Nutr. 64*, 715.

Schulze, J., and Scherf, H. (1989). *Tierarztliche-Umschau 44*, 187.

Scott, M.L. (1981). *Feedstuffs 53*(8), 59.

Scott, M.L., Nesheim, M.C., and Young, R.J. (1982). Nutrition of the Chicken, p. 119. Scott, Ithaca, New York.

Seymour, W.M. (1999). *In* Proc. "Tri-state Dairy Nutrition Conference," p. 43, Grand Wayne Center, Fort Wayne, Indiana.

Shiau, S., and Chin, Y. (1998). *J. Nutr. 128*, 2494.

Simmins, P.H., and Brooks, P.H. (1983). *Vet. Rec. 112*, 425.

Simmins, P.H., and Brooks, P.H. (1988). *Vet. Rec. 122*, 431.

Stout, F.M., Adair, J., and Oldfield, J.E. (1966). *Nutr. Fur. News 38*, 13.

Sunde, M.L., Cravens, W.W., Elvehjem, C.A., and Halpin, J.G. (1950). *Poult. Sci. 29*, 10.

Sydenstricker, V.P., Singal, S.A., Briggs, A.P., DeVaughn, N.M., and Isbell, H. (1942). *JAMA 118*, 1199.

Tagwerker, F. (1974). Roche Information Service Bulletin No. 1494. Hoffmann-La Roche & Co., Ltd., Basel, Switzerland.

Tagwerker, R.J. (1983). *Feed Int. 4*, 22.

Terroine, T. (1960). *Vitam. Horm. 18*, 1.

Waisman, H.A., McCall, K.B., and Elvehjem, C.A. (1945). *J. Nutr. 29*, 1.

Walton, M.J., Cowey, C.B., and Andron, J.W. (1984). *Aquaculture 37*, 21.

Watanabe, T. (1993). *J. Nutr. 123*, 2101.

Watanabe, T., Dakshinamurti, K., and Persaud, T.V.N. (1995). *J. Nutr. 125*, 2114.

Watkins, B.A. (1989). *Brit. J. Nutr. 61*, 99.

Watkins, B.A., and Kratzer, F.H. (1987a). *Poult. Sci. 66*, 1818.

Watkins, B.A., and Kratzer, F.H. (1987b). *Poult. Sci. 66*, 306.

Watkins, B.A., Bain, S.D., and Newbrey, J.W. (1989). *Calcif. Tissue Int. 46*, 41.

Watkins, K.L., Southern, L.L., and Miller, J.E. (1991). *J. Anim. Sci. 69*, 201.

Wehr, N.B., Adair, J., and Oldfield, J.E. (1980). *J. Anim. Sci. 50*, 877.

Wellenberg, G.J., and Banks, J.N. (1993). *J. Sci. Food Agric. 63*, 1.

Whitehead, C.C. (1978). *In* Handbook Series in Nutrition and Food, Section E: Nutritional Disorders (M. Rechcigl Jr., ed.),Vol. 2, p. 65. CRC Press, Boca Raton, Florida.

Whitehead, C.C. (1988). *Broiler Industry 51*(9), 60.

Whitehead, C.C., and Bannister, D.W. (1978). *Br. J. Nutr. 39*, 547.

Whitehead, C.C., Armstrong, J.A., and Waddington, D. (1982). *Br. J. Nutr. 48*, 81.

Whitehead, C.C., Bannister, D.W., and D'Mello, J.P.F. (1980). *Res. Vet. Sci. 29*, 126.

Wiese, A.C., Johnson, B.C., and Nevens, W.B. (1946). *Proc. Soc. Exp. Biol. Med. 63*, 521.

Zempleni, J., Green, G.M., Spannagel, A.W., and Mock, D.M. (1997). *J. Nutr. 127*, 1496.

FOLACIN

INTRODUCTION

Folacin and folate are generic terms used to describe folic acid and related compounds that exhibit the biological activity of folic acid. The terms folacin, folate, and folic acid will be used interchangeably. A number of researchers in both developed and developing countries have reported a high incidence of folacin deficiency in pregnant women. It has been estimated that up to one-third of all pregnant women in the world may experience folacin deficiency of varying severity (Rothman, 1970). Because of their rapid growth rate, cancer cells have an exceptionally high folacin requirement. Therefore, drugs that inhibit folacin-requiring enzymes are widely used in medicine for cancer chemotherapy. Megaloblastic anemia of pregnancy, resulting from low folacin intakes, is associated with poverty and poor diet selection. While folacin deficiency is extremely common in women 16 to 40 years of age because of the effects of pregnancy and lactation, it is rare in men younger than 60 years of age. After age 60, folacin deficiency is equally high in both men and women.

Recent research has shown that adequate serum folacin not only corrects megaloblastic anemia but prevents a number of life threatening diseases, including cardiovascular disease, neural tube defects (e.g., spina bifida and anencephaly), and risk of colorectal and other forms of cancer (Glynn and Albanes, 1994; Bower, 1995; Brattström, 1996). In relation to cardiovascular disease, moderate hyperhomocysteinemia is a risk factor. Supplementation with folacin and vitamin B_{12} reduces elevated plasma homocysteine (Brattström, 1996).

For animals, folacin needs are met principally by dietary sources and to some extent by intestinal bacterial synthesis. Different species vary in ability to utilize microbial intestinal synthesis as a source of folacin. Poultry and swine need supplemental folacin under certain conditions. Folacin supplementation is most important when poultry and swine receive diets containing sulfa drugs and grains contaminated with toxin-producing molds. To maximize reproductive efficiency, gestating swine often receive supplemental folacin.

HISTORY

In the 1930s and early 1940s, a number of active substances were described that were effective against nutritional deficiencies in humans, certain animals, and bacteria. Factors that later were found to be folacin-related include vitamin M, factor U, vitamin Bc, Bc conjugate, *Lactobacillus casei* factor, *Streptococcus lactis* R. (SLR) factor, folic acid, citrovorum factor, and others. The early history of folacin is discussed by Scott et al. (1982), Blakely and Benkovic (1984), and Loosli (1991). Willis in 1931 demonstrated a factor from yeast that was active in treating a tropical macrocytic anemia seen in women of India. An anemia-preventive factor for monkeys was found in yeast or liver extracts and designated vitamin M in 1935 by Day and associates. In 1939 Hogan and Parrot prevented anemia in chicks with a factor in liver called Bc. In the late 1930s, factors needed for growth and anemia prevention in poultry were referred to as Bc, factor U, or factor R. In 1940 Snell and coworkers found a growth factor for *L. casei*, and in the same year, a growth factor for *S. lacti* was found in spinach. The growth factor had been isolated from 4 tons of spinach leaves. The isolated factor was called folic acid from *folium,* the Latin word for leaf.

Folic acid was isolated from the liver with the structure and synthesis accomplished by the Lederly group, who named it pteroylglutamic acid on the basis of chemical structure. Active forms were found to contain a formyl group or a methyl group attached to the number 5 nitrogen of the pteridine nucleus.

Confusion existed in the 1940s concerning the identity of these various factors because both *L. casei* factor and folic acid were active for both microorganisms and animals, whereas vitamin M, factor R, and vitamin Bc were active for monkeys and chicks but not microorganisms. This was resolved when studies showed that folacin exists in nature in both free and bound (additional glutamic acid molecules) forms. Incubating vitamin M with rat or chick liver enzymes markedly increased activity for *L. casei* and *S. faecalis*. Folacin conjugases (enzymes that hydrolyze polyglutamates to monoglytamyl forms) were also shown to occur in hog kidney and chick pancreas. These studies, therefore, showed that most species except microorganisms are able to utilize bound forms.

Taking advantage of the high folacin requirement of cancer cells, during the 1950s, two drugs, methotrexate and 5-fluorouracil, were found to be useful in cancer chemotherapy. Both of these drugs are powerful inhibitors of folacin-requiring enzymes and are widely used in medicine. In the 1960s Herbert, of Boston College, clarified biochemical and hematological changes associated with a low folacin diet on himself and established progressive abnormalities as the deficiency intensified. In the 1970s the widespread world incidence of megaloblastic anemia was established, and in the 1980s and 1990s, the importance of folacin for reducing the incidence of neural tube defects, cardiovascular disease, and cancer began to emerge.

CHEMICAL STRUCTURE, PROPERTIES, AND ANTAGONISTS

Folacin is the group name used to distinguish naturally occurring compounds of this class; the pure substance is designated pteroyl-monoglutamic acid. The chemical structure of folacin (pteroylglutamic acid) is shown in Fig. 12.1. Its chemical structure contains three distinct parts. Reading from right to left, this compound consists of glutamic acid, ρ-aminobenzoic acid (PABA), and a pteridine nucleus, the last two making up pteroic acid. Thus the name pteroylglutamic acid was suggested. The PABA portion of the vitamin structure was once thought to be a vitamin. If the folacin requirement is met, there is no need to add PABA to the diet (see Chapter 17).

Much of the folacin in natural feedstuffs is conjugated with a varying number of extra glutamic acid molecules. Folacin as pteroyloligo-γ-L-glutamates (PteGlu$_n$) is generally from one to nine glutamates long, with n indicating the number of glutamyl residues. Polyglutamate forms—usually of 3 to 7 glutamyl residues linked by peptide bonds—of folacin are the natural coenzymes that are most abundant in every tissue examined (Wagner, 1984). The conjugated forms with two or more glutamic acid residues are joined by γ-glutamyl linkages to the single glutamic acid moiety of the vitamin. Synthetic folacin, however, is in the monoglutamate form.

It has been concluded that there are more biologically active forms of folacin than any other known vitamin. Naturally occurring pteroylpolyglutamates constitute a large family of closely related com-

481

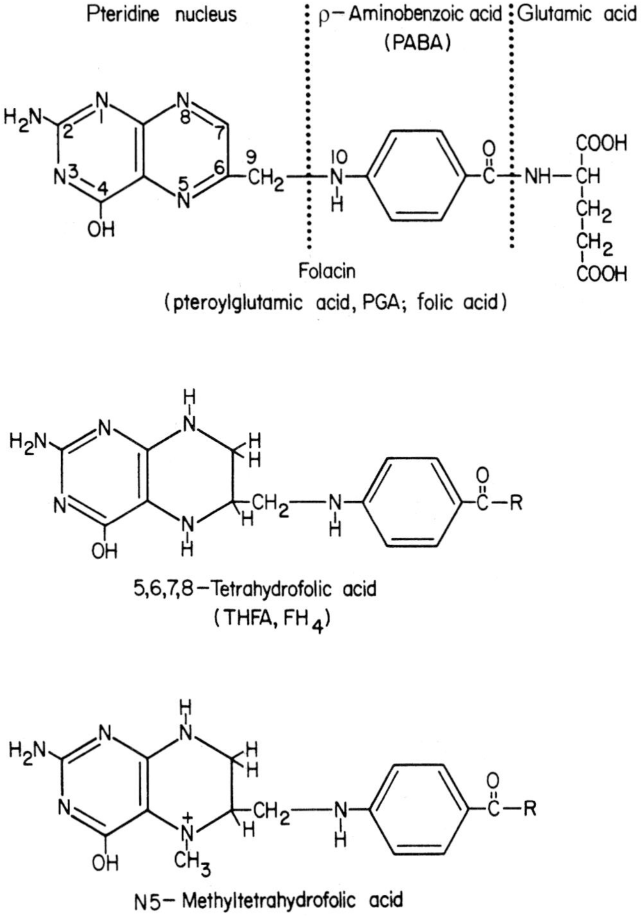

Fig. 12.1 Structures of folacin compounds. (R is one or more glutamic acid molecules.)

pounds arising from modifications of the three parts of the parent compound pteroylglutamic acid. Changes in the state of reduction of the pteridine moiety, addition of various kinds of one-carbon substituents, and addition of glutamic acid residues lead to a wide array of compounds. Baugh and Krumdieck (1971), on the basis of the three known states of reduction of the pyrazine ring, the six different one-carbon substituents that may occur at N-5 and/or N-10, and assuming that the polyglutamyl chain would have no more than seven glutamyl residues, calculated that the theoretical number of folacins approached 150. However, this figure includes compounds that have never been identified in natural materials. Since it is clear now that the polyglutamyl chain reaches at least 8 or 9 residues in animal tissues (and as many as 12 in bacterial cells), the number of folacin compounds that might be expected to occur in animal tissues still approaches 100 compounds. The active forms of folacin contain a formyl group or a methyl group attached to the number 5 or number 10 nitrogens of the compound, or a methylene group between nitrogens 5 and 10. Tetrahydrofolic acid is the principal coenzyme form, while the main storage form is 5-methyltetrahydrofolic acid (Fig. 12.1).

Folacin is a yellowish-orange crystalline powder, tasteless and odorless, and insoluble in alcohol, ether, and other organic solvents. It is slightly soluble in hot water in the acid form but quite soluble in the salt form. It is fairly stable to air and heat in neutral and alkaline solution, but unstable in acid solution. From 70 to 100% of folacin activity is destroyed on autoclaving at pH 1 (O'Dell and Hogan, 1943). Large losses in food folate can occur during food preparation such as heating, particularly under oxidative conditions (Gregory, 1989). Oxidation of reduced folates usually results in cleavage products lacking vitamin activity. Folacin is readily degraded by light and ultraviolet radiation. Cooking can considerably reduce folacin food content (see Natural Sources).

A great variety of folate analogs have been prepared, mainly for the purposes of anticancer (e.g., methotrexate and 5-fluorouracil) and antitumoral therapy (Brody, 1991). Since folacin deficiency is more detrimental to cells that are rapidly growing, these antagonists are used as potent antibacterial and antitumoral agents. Folacin antagonists can act by (1) blocking conversion of pteroylmonoglutamic acid to tetrahydrofolic acid by binding to dihydrofolic acid reductase or (2) blocking the transfer of single-carbon units from tetrahydrofolic acid to acceptors, such as in synthesis of methionine or purines (Scott et al., 1982). The folacin enzyme dihydrofolate reductase is the usual target of these antifolacin drugs. Methotrexate binds extremely tightly to dihydrofolate reductase. This drug is used both as an anticancer agent and (in low doses) as a treatment for a number of nonmalignant disorders, such as psoriasis and rheumatoid arthritis.

Sulfonamides, though not folacin analogs, are analogs of the folacin biosynthetic intermediate PABA and are widely used as antibacterial agents (Brown, 1962). By competing with PABA, sulfonamides prevent folacin synthesis so the microorganisms cannot multiply, with the result that an important source of folacin to the animal is reduced or eliminated. The anticonvulsant phenytoin is antagonistic to folacin, inhibiting the formation of polyglutamyl folates in rat liver (Carl et al., 1997).

ANALYTICAL PROCEDURES

Determination of folacin in biological materials is a difficult analytical problem because of the existence of a number of folacin complexes that exhibit the vitamin activity. High sensitivity is essential in methods of analysis because of the low concentration of folacin in foods and feedstuffs. Both microbiological and chemical methods have been employed to identify folacin and its derivatives. Because folacin in natural feedstuffs is conjugated with varying numbers of extra glutamic acid molecules, the bound forms must be freed to be active for the assay microorganisms. Conjugase enzymes, widely distributed in animal tissues, are capable of releasing free folacin. Typically, conjugases from the pancreas, liver, or kidney are used to reduce the conjugate to the monoglutamate form.

Folacin can be detected by microbiological assays (O'Broin and Kelleher, 1992). The microbiological assay can use *L. casei,* which responds to all the common monoglutamate forms of folacin, and a differential assay using *Enterococcus hirae* (formerly known as *S. faecalis*) and *L. citrovorum.* A radiometric microbiological method has also been reported, as well as a fluorometric procedure (Cruces-Blanco et al., 1994). For a biological assay of feeds, the chick is the preferred animal. Although growth may not be a specific indicator of available dietary folacin, plasma and liver folacin are highly sensitive criteria.

Various methods have been developed for separation of folacins by high-pressure liquid chromatography (HPLC). Separations of monoglutamyl folacins have been accomplished by anion-exchange, paired-ion reverse-phase, and conventional reverse-phase HPLC methods (Gregory et al., 1984; Selhub, 1989). Quantitation of the major folacin compounds in biological materials has been reported by Gregory et al. (1984) to combine fluorometric determination with HPLC. Methods have been developed for simultaneous measurement of one-carbon and polyglutamate derivatives of folacin using enzymatic interconversions of folates and ternary complexes separated by isoelectric focusing (Carl and Smith, 1995).

METABOLISM

Digestion, Absorption, and Transport

Polyglutamate forms are digested via hydrolysis to pteroylmonoglutamate prior to transport across the intestinal mucosa. Intraluminal polyglutamate hydrolysis is catalyzed by a conjugase intestinal enzyme found in the brush border. This brush border pteroylpolyglutamate hydrolase (γ-carboxy peptidase) is an exopeptidase that cleaves the polyglutamyl chain one residue at a time starting from the carboxyl end. It has a pH optimum near neutrality and is activated by zinc (Chandler et al., 1986). In humans, a zinc deficiency resulted in a decreased intestinal hydrolysis of pteroylpolyglutamate (Tamura et al., 1978). Conjugase activity is widely distributed in the mucosa of the proximal small intestine, both intracellularly and in association with the brush border. Conjugase activities have also been found in bile, pancreatic juice, kidney, and liver. Conjugase activity is reduced by nutritional zinc deficiency, chronic consumption of alcohol, and exposure to naturally occurring inhibitors in foods.

Pteroylmonoglutamate is absorbed predominantly in the jejunum, with lesser amounts in the duodenum, by a Na^+-coupled carrier-mediated process. Folacin is also absorbed passively, presumably by diffusion; this mechanism accounts for 20 to 30% of folacin absorption, regardless of folate concentration.

Dietary folates, after hydrolysis and absorption from the intestine, are transported in plasma as monoglutamate derivatives, with only limited methylation (5-methyltetrahydrofolate). Folacin taken up by the liver is converted primarily to 5-methyltetrahydrofolate and 10-formyltetrahydrofolate and then transported to the peripheral tissues. The monoglutamate derivatives are then taken up by cells in tissues by specific transport systems. There, the pteroylpolyglutamates—the major folacin form in cells—are built up again in stepwise fashion by the enzyme folate polyglutamate synthetase. Polyglutamation traps folates inside cells at concentrations one to two orders of magnitude greater than those of extracellular fluids. Polyglutamates serve to keep folacin within the cells since only the monoglutamate forms are transported across membranes, and only the monoglutamates are found in plasma and urine (Wagner, 1995). Folacin enzymes are compartmentalized between the cytosol and the mitochondria. Almost all the folate in the cell is distributed equally between the two compartments. There are also mitochondrial and cytosolic isoforms of the same enzymes (Wagner, 1996).

Studies showed that about 79 to 88% of labeled folacin is absorbed, and that absorption is rapid since serum concentrations usually peak about 2 hours after ingestion. Using in vitro studies, Wagonfeld et al. (1975) showed that the rate-limiting step in folacin absorption is transport of the monoglutamyl folacin into the mesenteric circulation rather than hydrolysis of polyglutamyl folacins, which is very rapid. However, in cases where the conjugase is strongly inhibited, absorption of polyglutamyl folacins may be reduced. Low availability in orange juice is due to the inhibition of conjugase activity by the low pH. Therefore, drugs that drastically alter intraluminal pH and/or inhibit conjugase activity will also decrease folacin absorption.

Specific folate-binding proteins (FBPs) that bind folacin monoglutamates and polyglutamates are known to exist in many tissues and body fluids, including liver, kidney, small intestinal brush border membranes, leukemic granulocytes, blood serum, allantoic fluid, and milk (Tani and Iwai, 1984; Shoda et al., 1990; Muldoon et al., 1996; Vallet et al., 1999). The physiological roles of these FBPs are not completely known, but it has been suggested that they play a role in folacin transport analogous to the intrinsic factor in the absorption of vitamin B_{12}. The FBPs may play a role in tissue storage of folacin by protecting the polyglutamate derivatives from the action of degradative or hydrolytic enzymes (Brody, 1991). The FBPs (also referred to as folate receptors) are abundant in the kidney proximal tubule and are involved with reabsorption of 5-methyl THF_4 (Muldoon et al., 1996). Tani and Iwai (1984) reported that FBPs of bovine milk affected bioavailability of folacin in vivo by resulting in a more uniform absorption throughout the small intestine and reduced loss of 5-methyltetrahydrofolacin in the urine.

Storage

Folacin is widely distributed in tissues largely in the conjugated polyglutamate forms. Normal body stores in humans have been estimated at 5 to 10 mg, with approximately half in the liver (Brody, 1991). Well-nourished adults may have stores that can meet normal body requirements for up to 4 or 5 months (Baker and DeMaeyer, 1979). Body folacin stores are small at birth and are rapidly depleted, particularly in small premature infants. In vitamin B_{12} deficiency, there are defects in the conversion of pteroylmonoglutamates to polyglutamate forms that lead to a decreased tissue ability to retain intracellular folacin. Vitamin B_{12} deficiency has been shown to lead to functional folacin deficiency even when folacin intake and absorption are normal. Giugliani et al.

(1985) reported a significantly higher serum folacin concentration for patients receiving vitamin B_{12} supplementation during pregnancy.

Excretion

Urinary excretion of folacin represents a small fraction of total excretion (e.g., < 1% of total body stores). Fecal folacin concentrations are quite high, often higher than intake, representing not only undigested folacin but, more important, the considerable bacterial synthesis of the vitamin in the intestine. In tracer studies for the first 24 hours after the dose, much of the dose in urine is as intact folacins. After longer time periods, all the excreted label was in degradative products, primarily pteridines and acetaminobenzoylglutamate (Murphy et al., 1976). Over half of labeled dietary folacin is excreted in feces. This is expected, as bile contains high levels of folacin due to enterohepatic circulation, with most of bile folacin reabsorbed in the intestine.

FUNCTIONS

Folacin, in the form 5,6,7,8-tetrahydrofolic acid, is indispensable in transfer of single-carbon units in various reactions, such as those occurring in the biosynthesis of lipids, proteins, nucleic acid derivatives, hormones, and neurotransmitters—a role analogous to that of pantothenic acid in the transfer of two-carbon units. The one-carbon units can be formyl, formimino, methylene, or methyl groups. The major in vivo pathway providing methyl groups involves transfer of a one-carbon unit from serine to tetrahydrofolate to form 5,10-methylenetetrahydrofolate, which is subsequently reduced to 5-methyltetrahydrofolate. Methyltetrahydrofolate then supplies methyl groups to remethylate homocysteine in the activated methyl cycle, providing methionine for synthesis of the important methyl donor agent S-adenosylmethionine (Krumdieck, 1990; Jacob et al., 1994). Some biosynthetic relationships of one-carbon units are shown in Fig. 12.2. These one-carbon units are generated primarily during amino acid metabolism and are used in the metabolic interconversions of amino acids and in the biosynthesis of the purine and pyrimidine components of nucleic acids that are needed for cell division. The important physiological function of tetrahydrofolate (THF) consists of binding the C_1 units to the vitamin molecule and thus transforming them to "active formic acid" or "active formaldehyde," so that these are interconvertible by reduction or oxidation and transferable to appropriate acceptors.

Ability of the vitamin as a coenzyme is governed by three factors: (1)

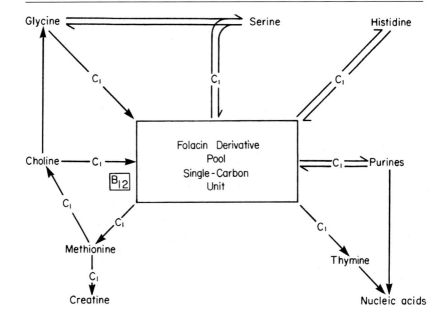

Fig. 12.2 Folacin metabolism requiring one-carbon units. (Modified from Scott et al., 1982.)

the nature of the carbon-containing substituent attached at either the N-5 or the N-10 position, or bridging them; (2) the state of oxidation or reduction of the pyrazine ring; and (3) the number of glutamic acid units attached in gamma linkage to the glutamate of pteroylglutamic acid. Certain polyglutamates may serve as cofactors for one enzyme while inhibiting another (White et al., 1976).

Folacin polyglutamates work at least as well as or better than the corresponding monoglutamate forms in every enzyme system examined (Wagner, 1995). It is now accepted that the pteroylpolyglutamates are the acceptors and donors of one-carbon units in amino acid and nucleotide metabolism, while the monoglutamate is merely a transport form.

Glutamate chain length of folacin polyglutamate may affect metabolism of one-carbon units (Foo and Shane, 1982). In hamster ovary cells with normal extracellular methionine, polyglutamate chain lengths were longer, with high levels of octaglutamates, nonaglutamates, and even decaglutamates occurring, while with suboptimal levels of methionine, shorter chain lengths were found. This observed phenomenon of a profound effect of extracellular methionine concentration on glutamate chain elongation may be interpreted to mean that there is a regulatory action of polyglutamate chain length on one-carbon metabolism.

Specific reactions involving single-carbon transfer by folacin compounds are (1) purine and pyrimidine synthesis, (2) interconversion of serine and glycine, (3) glycine-α-carbon as a source of C_1 units for many syntheses, (4) histidine degradation, and (5) synthesis of methyl groups for such compounds as methionine, choline, and thymine.

Purine bases (adenine and guanine) as well as thymine are constituents of nucleic acids, and with folacin deficiency, there is a reduction in the biosynthesis of nucleic acids essential for cell formation and function. Hence, deficiency of the vitamin leads to impaired cell division and alterations of protein synthesis; these effects are most noticeable in rapidly growing tissues. In absence of adequate nucleoproteins, normal maturation of primordial red blood cells does not take place, and hematopoiesis is inhibited at the megaloblast stage. As a result of this megaloblastic arrest of normal red blood cell maturation in bone marrow, a typical peripheral blood picture results that is characterized by macrocytic anemia. White blood cell formation is also affected, resulting in thrombopenia, leukopenia, and old, multilobed neutrophils.

In folacin deficiency, formiminoglutamic acid (FIGLU), formed as an intermediate in degradation of histidine, can no longer be transformed completely into glutamate and formiminotetrahydrofolic acid, and is therefore excreted in urine. This excretion is suitable as a biochemical criterion for diagnosis of folacin deficiency, appearing at an early stage of deficiency.

Vitamin B_{12} is also closely associated with the progress of the folacin-dependent reactions of intermediary metabolism (Savage and Lindenbaum, 1995). Vitamin B_{12} has two main effects in facilitating folacin: (1) Vitamin B_{12} regulates the proportion of methyl to nonmethyl tetrahydrofolates according to the methyl trap theory, and (2) vitamin B_{12} is necessary for transport of methyl-THF across the cell membrane and promotes folacin retention by tissues. According to the methyl trap concept (Herbert and Zalusky, 1962), vitamin B_{12} deficiency decreases the formation of methionine from homocysteine and methyl-THF by the B_{12}-dependent methionine synthetase (see Chapter 13, Functions). This results in an increase in methyl-THF and a decrease in THF, which is the active coenzyme form that functions in the degradation of FIGLU and formate.

Vitamin B_{12} is necessary in the reduction of one-carbon compounds of the oxidation stage of formate and formaldehyde, and in this way, it participates, with folacin, in biosynthesis of labile methyl groups. Folacin is also essentially involved in all these reactions of labile methyl groups. The metabolism of labile methyl groups plays an important role for the body in the biosynthesis of methionine from homocysteine and of choline from ethanolamine. Folacin has a sparing effect on requirements of choline (the importance of both folacin and vitamin B_{12} on synthesis of choline is discussed in Chapter 14).

Folacin is needed to maintain the immune system; the blastogenic response of T lymphocytes to certain mitogens is decreased in folacin-deficient humans and animals, and the thymus is preferentially altered (Dhur et al., 1991). The effects of folacin deficiency upon humoral immunity have been more thoroughly investigated in animals than in humans, and the antibody responses to several antigens have been shown to decrease. As de novo synthesis of methyl groups requires the participation of folacin coenzymes, the effect of folacin deficiency on pancreatic exocrine function was examined in rats (Balaghi and Wagner, 1992; Balaghi et al., 1993). Pancreatic secretion was significantly reduced in the deficient group compared with the pair-fed control groups after 5 weeks. The results indicate that severe folacin deficiency impairs pancreatic exocrine function. The ratio of S-adenosylmethionine to S-adenosylhomocysteine was rapidly reduced in the deficient pancreas. The pancreas of deficient rats had more immature secretory granules, and the ducts were devoid of secreted material.

REQUIREMENTS

Various animal species differ markedly in their requirements for folacin. Because of microbial synthesis in their digestive tracts, ruminants have no dietary requirement for folacin. Only young ruminants that do not have a fully developed rumen would be expected to require a dietary source. Folacin requirements for monogastric species would be dependent on degree of intestinal folacin synthesis and utilization by the animal (Rong et al., 1991). Animals that practice coprophagy would also have a lower dietary need for folacin, as feces is a rich source of the vitamin (Abad and Gregory, 1987). Many species apparently do not require dietary folacin because of their ability to utilize microbial intestinal synthesis (Rong et al., 1991).

Poultry, swine, guinea pigs, and primates (including humans) do develop deficiencies on low dietary folacin. Even though deficiencies can be produced with special diets, corn, soybean meal, and other common feedstuffs in a practical poultry diet usually provide ample folacin under most conditions (Scott et al., 1982). However, marginal inadequacies have been produced in chicks fed corn-soybean meal diets (Pesti et al., 1991).

Self-synthesis of folacin is dependent on dietary composition. For poultry, some research has indicated higher folacin requirements for very high protein diets, or when sucrose was the only source of carbohydrates (Scott et al., 1982). Keagy and Oace (1984) reported that dietary fiber had an effect on folacin utilization; xylan, wheat bran, and beans stimulated folacin synthesis in the rat, reflected as higher fecal and liver folacin. For humans it was concluded that milk type differentially affects intestinal folacin biosynthesis and the superior folacin availability from human (versus cow and goat) milk-containing diets is due in part to enhanced intestinal biosynthesis of folacin (Semchuk et al., 1994).

The levels of antibacterials added to the feed will affect microbial synthesis of folacin. Sulfa drugs, which are commonly added to livestock diets, are folacin antagonists (see Deficiency). In the chicken, sulfa drugs have been shown to increase the requirement (Scott et al., 1982). Moldy feeds (e.g., aflatoxins) have also been shown to contain antagonists that inhibit microbial intestinal synthesis in swine (Purser, 1981).

Folacin requirements are dependent on the form in which it is fed and concentrations and interrelationships of other nutrients. Deficiencies of choline, vitamin B_{12}, iron, and vitamin C all have an effect on folacin needs. Although most folacin in poultry feedstuffs is present in conjugated form, the young chick is fully capable of utilizing it. On the contrary, Baker et al. (1978) reported that human patients over 60 years of age utilized conjugated forms of folacin much less efficiently than monoglutamates.

Folacin requirements are related to type and level of production. Growth rate, age, and pregnancy influence folacin requirements. The requirement decreases with age because diminished growth rate reduces the need for DNA synthesis. Increased catabolism of folacin is a feature of pregnancy. Studies with both rats (McNulty et al., 1993) and humans (McPartlin et al., 1993) demonstrated an enhanced folacin catabolism that was a feature of pregnancy per se and not simply due to increased weight. In poultry the folacin requirement for egg hatchability is higher than that for production (NRC, 1994). Taylor (1947) reported that 0.12 mg of folacin per kilogram of diet was satisfactory for egg production, but higher levels were required for good hatchability. Table 12.1 summarizes the folacin requirements for various livestock species and humans; a more complete listing is given in the appendix, Table A1.

The current Recommended Dietary Allowances (RDAs) for folates

■ Table 12.1   Folacin Requirements for Various Animals and Humans

Animal	Purpose or Class	Requirement[a]	Reference
Beef cattle	Adult	Microbial synthesis	NRC (1984)
	Calf	0.1 ppm milk replacer	NRC (1984a)
Dairy cattle	Adult	Microbial synthesis	NRC (1989a)
Chicken	Leghorn, 0–6 weeks	0.55 mg/kg	NRC (1994)
	Leghorn, 6–18 weeks	0.25 mg/kg	NRC (1994)
	Laying (100-g intake)	0.25 mg/kg	NRC (1994)
	Broilers, 0–6 weeks	0.55 mg/kg	NRC (1994)
	Broilers, 6–8 weeks	0.50 mg/kg	NRC (1994)
Japanese quail	All classes	1.0 mg/kg	NRC (1994)
Turkey	Growing, 0–8 weeks	1.0 mg/kg	NRC (1994)
	Growing, 8–16 weeks	0.8 mg/kg	NRC (1994)
	Breeding hens	1.0 mg/kg	NRC (1994)
Sheep	Adult	Microbial synthesis	NRC (1985b)
Swine	Growing-finishing	0.3 mg/kg	NRC (1998)
	Gestating-lactating	1.30 mg/kg	NRC (1998)
Horse	Adult	Microbial synthesis	NRC (1989b)
Goat	Adult	Microbial synthesis	NRC (1981b)
Cat	Adult	0.8 mg/kg	NRC (1986)
Mink	Growing	0.5 mg/kg	NRC (1982a)
Fox	Growing	0.2 mg/kg	NRC (1982a)
Dog	Growing	0.2 mg/kg	NRC (1985a)
Hamster	All classes	0.6 mg/kg	NRC (1978a)
Fish	Catfish	1.5 mg/kg	NRC (1993)
	Pacific salmon	2–10 mg/kg	NRC (1993)
	Rainbow trout	1 mg/kg	NRC (1993)
Rat	All classes	1.0 mg/kg	NRC (1978a)
Human[b]	Infants	25–30 µg/day	RDA (1989)
	Children	50–100 µg/day	RDA (1989)
	Adults	150–400 µg/day	RDA (1989)

[a]Expressed as per unit of animal feed on either as-fed (approximately 90% dry matter) or dry basis (see Appendix, Tables A1a,b). Requirements established for some species, while only suggested for others. Human data are expressed as µg/day.

[b]A number of nutritionists believe the RDA (1989) was ultraconservative in recommending folacin allowances. Research findings would suggest the 1980 RDA to have more realistic recommendations as follows: Infants (30–45 µg/day), children (100–300 µg/day), and adults (400–800 µg/day).

are set at 200 µg/day for adult males and 180 µg/day for adult females (RDA, 1989). This represents a significant reduction from the previously recommended (RDA, 1980) amount of 400 µg/day for adult males and females (Bailey, 1995). The later RDA also reduced the recommended requirement for children and infants (Table 12.1). Many nutritionists feel that the 1989 RDA committee was ultraconservative in suggesting folacin recommendations and prefer the 1980 RDA values. Also, research associating folacin deficiency with hyperhomocysteinemia and increased heart disease risk (Kang et al., 1992), cervical dysplasia (Butterworth et al., 1992), bronchial metaplasia (Heimburger et al., 1988), and neural tube defects (Centers for Disease Control, 1992), and the wide use of folate-antagonist medications, clearly demonstrate an increased need for higher levels of dietary folacin (see Supplementation). As an example, the U.S. Public Health Service issued a recommendation that all U.S. women of childbearing age capable of becoming pregnant should consume 0.4 mg (400 µg) of folacin per day for the purpose of reducing their risk of a pregnancy affected with spina bifida or other neural tube defects (Centers for Disease Control, 1992).

In pregnancy and lactation, folate requirements clearly increase. The burden of lactation on maternal folacin reserves is estimated to be 20 to 50 µg/day, varying with the folacin content and volume of milk (Matoth et al., 1965). This estimate, based on production of 850 cc of average milk folacin content, should be doubled to meet the needs of mothers producing milk with high folate content. An additional 100 µg of dietary folacin should provide for the absorption of the excess need. The recommended daily allowance (RDA, 1980) for folacin is necessarily in excess of the minimum daily requirement to provide a margin of safety and allow for losses in preparation of foods as well as the decreased availability of food folacin as compared to folacin in the monoglutamate form. The newer RDA (1989) has set 400 µg/day during pregnancy and 280 µg/day during the first 6 months of lactation as a folacin recommendation. This likewise is low compared with the earlier RDA (1980) recommendation. It should be noted that a study of 10 nonpregnant women followed for 92 days in a metabolic unit arrived at a higher recommended intake of 300 µg/day to meet requirements and provide an allowance for storage (Sauberlich et al., 1987).

Smoking, alcohol consumption, antifolacin drugs (e.g., methotrexate), anticonvulsant drugs, oral contraceptives, and certain antibiotics (e.g., sulfasalazine) interfere with folacin activity and therefore increase the body's folacin requirements (Brody, 1991). Tobacco smoking is believed to represent a second model of localized folacin deficiency often associated with preneoplastic changes of the affected tissues (Krumdieck, 1990). Methotrexate lowers folacin status, whether used as an anticancer agent or in low doses as a treatment for psoriasis and rheumatoid arthritis (Green and Jacobsen, 1995). Anticonvulsant drugs have been found to reduce blood folacin and lead to problems such as megaloblastic anemia (Porras-Tejero and Lluch-Fernandez, 1993). As many as 19% of the users of oral contraceptive agents showed cytological abnormalities that, although not associated with systemic evidence of folacin or vitamin B_{12} deficiency, were corrected by the administration of oral folic acid (Krumdieck, 1990).

493

NATURAL SOURCES

Folacin is widely distributed in nature, almost exclusively as THF acid derivatives; the stable ones have a methyl or formyl group in the 5-γ position and generally possess three or more glutamic acid residues in glutamyl linkages. Only limited amounts of free folacin occur in natural products, with most feed sources containing predominantly polyglutamyl folacin. However, in seeds or fruit, which presumably store the vitamin, a considerable amount is present as a monoglutamate. More than a third of the folates in orange juice are present as monoglutamates and nearly half as pentaglutamates. A high proportion of monoglutamate forms of folacin are found in milk and soybeans. Much of the folacin in milk is available in the monoglutamate form, which is necessary for absorption by the newborn (Wagner, 1984). The predominant form of folacin in vegetables such as spinach, asparagus, broccoli, lettuce, yeast, rice, and peas is the N-10 formyl derivative. Folates in tissues such as liver, kidney, and red blood cells are predominantly pentaglutamates.

Folacin is abundant in green leafy materials and organ meats. Soybeans, other beans, nuts, some animal products, and citrus fruits are good sources. Cereal grains, milk, and eggs are generally poor sources of the vitamin. Any animal or human diet without green leafy materials or animal protein, especially organ meats, is likely to be low in folacin. Human diets may be particularly low during the winter season, when green vegetables and citrus fruits are less plentiful. The folacin content of typical foods and feedstuffs is shown in Table 12.2.

Folacin bioavailability of beef liver, lima beans, peas, spinach, mushrooms, collards, and wheat germ was found to generally exceed 70% (Clifford et al., 1990). Bioavailability of monoglutamate folacin was substantially greater than polyglutamyl forms (Clifford et al., 1991 Gregory et al., 1991). The availability of food folacins may range from 30 to 80% that of the monoglutamate form, being generally less well utilized from plant-derived foods than from animal products. Deficiencies of both iron and vitamin C in humans is associated with impaired utilization of dietary folacin (see Deficiency, Assessment of Status). Bioavailability of orally administered 5-methyl folacin and 5-formyl folacin compared to folacin were found to be equal for rats (Bhandari and Gregory, 1992).

A considerable loss of folacin (50 to 90%) occurs during cooking or processing of foods. Folacin is sensitive to light and heating, particularly in acid solution. Under aerobic conditions, destruction of most folacin

■ Table 12.2   Typical Folacin Concentrations in Foods and Feedstuffs (ppm, dry basis)

Alfalfa meal, dehydrated	5.5	Milk, skim, cow's	0.7
Asparagus, fresh	1.4	Orange juice, fresh	1.4
Bananas, fresh	0.28	Peanut meal, solvent extracted	0.7
Barley, grain	0.6	Rice, bran	2.4
Blood meal, dehydrated	0.1	Rice, grain	0.4
Brewer's grains	7.7	Rice, polished	0.2
Broccoli, fresh	1.69	Rye, grain	0.7
Broccoli (boiled), fresh	0.65	Sorghum, grain	0.2
Cabbage, fresh	0.3	Soybean meal	0.7
Cabbage (boiled), fresh	0.16	Soybean, seeds	3.9
Carrot, roots	1.2	Spinach, fresh	1.93
Coconut meal	1.5	Spinach (boiled), fresh	0.91
Corn (maize), grain	0.3	Sugarcane molasses	0.1
Corn (maize), gluten meal	0.3	Timothy hay, sun cured	2.3
Cottonseed meal, solvent extracted	2.8	Wheat, bran	1.6
Fish meal, anchovy	0.2	Wheat, grain	0.5
Fish meal, menhaden	0.2	Whey, cattle	0.9
Linseed meal, solvent extracted	1.4	Yeast, brewer's	10.3
Liver, cattle	8.4		

Sources: Concentrations from NRC (1982a) and Brody (1991).

forms is significant with heating, with reduced folacins more stable in foods due to relatively anaerobic conditions and because folacin is protected from light (Brody 1991). Fresh cabbage and broccoli are good sources of folacin and contain (wet-weight basis) 0.30 and 1.69 ppm, respectively. However, when these vegetables are boiled and the water is discarded, losses are considerable, reducing concentrations to 0.16 and 0.65 ppm, respectively (Leichter et al., 1978). Although the cooking losses of folacin in vegetables may be great, the bioavailability of the remaining folacin is quite high (Clifford et al., 1990): broccoli 80 to 90% and cabbage 79%.

DEFICIENCY

Folacin deficiency has been produced experimentally in many animal species, with macrocytic anemia (megaloblastic anemia) and leukopenia (reduced number of white cells) being consistent findings. Tissues that have a rapid rate of cell growth or tissue regeneration, such as epithelial lining of the gastrointestinal tract, the epidermis, and bone marrow, are principally affected (Hoffbrand, 1978).

For some animals, such as the chick, guinea pig, monkey, and pig, the presence of adequate amounts of folacin in the diet is essential, and deficiency signs can readily be induced by feeding a diet deficient in the

495

vitamin. In other animals, such as the rat and dog, folacin produced by the intestinal microflora is usually adequate to meet requirements. Consequently, deficiency signs do not develop unless an intestinal antiseptic is also included in the diet to depress bacterial growth.

Effects of Deficiency

Ruminants

Folacin synthesis occurs in the rumen. However, young animals that do not have a fully developed rumen would be expected to be folacin deficient. Draper and Johnson (1952) reported folacin deficiency in lambs fed synthetic diets. The disease was characterized by leukopenia followed by diarrhea, pneumonia, and death. Folacin therapy promoted regeneration of white blood cells, and 0.39 mg/L of milk in control animal diets prevented the deficiency. There was no indication of folacin deficiency in calves fed synthetic milk containing 52 mg of folacin per kilogram of liquid feed fed at 10% of live weight (Wiese et al., 1947). In later studies, dairy veal calves were fed daily 0, 4, or 16 mg of folacin in milk (Lévesque et al., 1993). Supplemental folacin increased serum and red blood cell folacin concentrations and reduced the rearing period to reach 180 kg without increasing feed intake.

Girard et al. (1994) studied whether ruminal folacin is affected by dietary folacin and if this response is modified by the diet. Concentrations of folacin in rumen contents were increased by supplemental folacin and by ingestion of concentrate compared with hay-based diets.

The efficiency of folacin and synthesis by rumen microflora and whether this is adequate at weaning and later is not yet established. For example, in an experiment in which supplemental folacin was administered to dairy heifers intramuscularly weekly during the first 4 months of life, average daily gain increased by 8% during the 5 weeks following weaning (Dumoulin et al., 1991). This supplementation also increased serum and hepatic folates, as well as blood hemoglobin and packed cell volume. Girard et al. (1989a) observed that concentration of serum folacin of calves at 2 weeks of age is half that of 4-month-old heifers. Girard et al. (1992) fed supplemental folacin to both preruminant and ruminant calves in an attempt to maintain high serum folacin concentrations. Serum folacin was increased in both groups receiving dietary folacin, but the amount needed to reach similar concentrations was higher in ruminant than in preruminant calves. These observations seem to confirm that during the weeks before and after weaning, the supply of folates by the diet and the rumen microorganisms might not be optimum for dairy heifers and possibly other preruminants and ruminant livestock.

Girard et al. (1989b) evaluated serum folates in gestating and lactating dairy cows and found that serum folacin decreased by 40% from 2 months postpartum (around mating) to parturition. The synthesis of folacin by rumen microorganisms was not sufficient to prevent fluctuations of serum folacin during gestation and lactation in dairy cows. Moreover, serum folacin can be increased by an intramuscular injection of folacin at the end of gestation, but in cows during early lactation, this did not markedly affect serum and milk folacin concentrations. Girard et al. (1995) injected folacin (160 mg) weekly to dairy cows 45 days after mating to 6 weeks after parturition. The supply of folates by the diet and the synthesis by ruminal microflora were found to be sufficient to prevent folacin deficiency in dairy cows and to maintain normal gestation and lactation, but not to achieve maximal production of milk and protein in multiparous, but not primiparous, dairy cows during gestation and lactation (Girard et al., 1995; Girard and Matte, 1998).

Swine

Earlier, folacin deficiency in swine had only been produced by the simultaneous feeding of sulfa drugs, indicating that intestinal synthesis was adequate to meet needs. Deficiencies were not observed when young pigs were fed only purified diets or low natural diets alone (Johnson et al., 1948), indicating that intestinal synthesis was adequate to meet needs. Feeding a purified diet containing 2% sulfasuxidine to weanling pigs resulted in reduced gains and alopecia (Cartwright and Wintrobe, 1949). The pigs also developed a milk normochromic, normocytic anemia; in bone marrow there was a decrease in the ratio of leukocytes to erythrocytes and an increase in the number of immature nucleated red blood cells. Positive response was obtained after supplementation with folacin. Cunha et al. (1948) found that folacin was needed for normal hematopoiesis with 8-week-old pigs fed a purified diet with sulfasuxidine for 21 weeks. A normocytic anemia resulted that was prevented by folacin, whereas a more severe anemia was produced by using a crude folacin antagonist. A combination of folacin and biotin was more effective than folacin alone in counteracting the anemia. Lindemann and Kornegay (1986) reported that combination of the antibiotic mixture ASP 250 (which includes chlortetracycline, sulfamethazine, and penicillin) and folacin to a corn-soybean meal diet increased gains and feed consumption, with no effect of either used alone.

More severe deficiency signs that responded to folacin supplementation were induced by feeding diets containing a sulfonamide and a folacin antagonist (Welch et al., 1947). Under such circumstances, pigs became listless, had a reduced growth rate, and developed diarrhea. Hematological manifestations were severe macrocytic anemia, leukopenia with a more marked reduction in the number of polymorphonucleocytes, and mild thrombocytopenia. Cartwright et al. (1952) reported a combined folacin and vitamin B_{12} deficiency in pigs receiving a purified soybean protein diet that included a folacin antagonist. Growth rate was reduced, and macrocytic anemia, leukopenia, and neutropenia developed, with erythroid hyperplasia of the bone marrow. Folacin supplementation immediately resulted in a normal blood and bone marrow picture, but growth was decreased, and the blood picture subsequently relapsed.

In addition to sulfa drugs and other folacin antagonists, moldy feeds can increase the need for the vitamin. In seven swine-feeding trials involving more than 1,000 pigs fed corn with mold infestation, additional folacin increased growth rate up to 15% and improved feed efficiency up to 9% (Purser, 1981). Folacin supplementation was of no value when normal corn was fed. Improvements in growth rate for pigs receiving 840 ppb aflatoxin were obtained with addition of 2 ppm folacin (Lindemann et al., 1993).

Inadequate folacin has been associated with suboptimal reproductive performance of sows in some studies (Matte et al., 1984b; Lindemann and Kornegay, 1989; Tremblay et al., 1989; Lindemann, 1993; Matte and Girard, 1999) but without affect in others (Matte et al., 1993; Harper et al., 1994). In sows a dramatic decrease in serum folacin concentrations was observed during early and mid-gestation (Matte et al., 1984a; Harper et al., 1994). Low folacin during gestation may be associated in part with embryonic mortality. In one trial, folacin was administered intramuscularly according to a schedule that maintained serum folacin concentrations at approximately the same level between weaning and 60 days of gestation (Matte et al., 1984b). Average live litter size was 12 piglets per litter for sows receiving folacin and flushing treatments compared with 10.5 for sows without any treatment. In another study, addition of 5.0 mg of folacin per kilogram of diet improved survival rate of fetuses during early gestation (62.2 versus 55.1%) compared with those not receiving folacin (Tremblay et al., 1989). Lindemann and Kornegay (1989) found the number of matings required per female farrowing was lower with folacin supplements (1.07 versus 1.16 for controls). Matte et al. (1992) reported that growth of piglets and total litter weight from birth to 8 weeks of age increased linearly from the level of folacin that had been provided to sows during the gestation diet.

There seems to be no major benefits to lactational supplementation, although it is effective in elevating sow serum folacin, milk folacin, and nursing pig serum folacin. The response in gestation of increased litter size seems to be a result of improved embryo or fetal survival rather than increased ovulation, although the mechanism whereby survival rate is improved is not yet understood (Lindemann, 1993). Gilts fed 4 mg of folacin per kilogram of feed 17 days before and 7 days after insemination had an average embryo survival rate (based on ovulation rate) of 88.5 versus 62.9% for controls and 4.4 versus 22.4% degenerated embryos for the treatments, respectively (Stancic et al., 1993). Additional research is required to determine if supplemental dietary folacin will reduce embryonic death loss under differing management systems to improve overall efficiency of production (i.e., to optimize pig survival and litter size).

Poultry

Poultry are more susceptible to lack of folacin than other farm livestock, as deficiency can readily be produced by feeding a folacin-deficient diet. Folacin deficiency, as indicated by retarded growth and feed efficiency, was produced in 15-day-old chicks fed corn-soybean meal diets (Pesti et al., 1991).

In folacin deficiency, megaloblastic arrest of erythrocyte formation in bone marrow causes severe macrocytic anemia as one of the first signs. Folacin deficiency in chicks is also characterized by poor growth, very poor feathering, anemic appearance, and perosis (Figs. 12.3 and 12.4). The chicks become lethargic and feed intake declines. As anemia develops, the comb becomes waxy white, and mucous membrane of the mouth becomes pale (Siddons, 1978). Turkey poults fed a folacin-deficient diet show reduced growth rate and increased mortality (Fig. 12.5). The birds develop a spastic type of cervical paralysis in which the neck is stiff and extended, but with only a moderate degree of anemia. Poults with cervical paralysis will die within 2 days after the onset of these signs unless folacin is administered immediately (Scott et al., 1982). Erythrocytes of deficient birds tend to be larger in diameter, and their nuclei are less dense than those of birds receiving supplementary folacin (Schweigert et al., 1948).

In chicks and turkeys, folacin deficiency also results in poor feather development, with the shafts weak and brittle. Folacin, along with lysine and iron, is required for feather pigmentation, as depigmentation occurs in colored feathers during folacin deficiency.

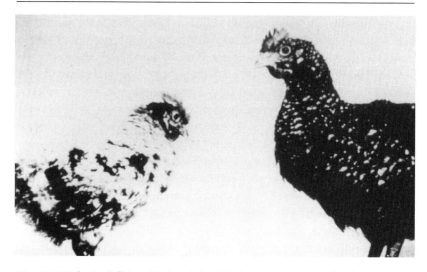

Fig. 12.3 Folacin-deficient bird on left with depigmentation and reduction in growth (compare with normal bird on the right). (Courtesy of G.F. Combs, Department of Poultry Science, University of Maryland.)

Fig. 12.4 Folacin-deficient chick, with cervical paralysis, at 5 weeks of age. Note the weakened condition of legs and the way the bird holds the left wing. Folacin-deficient bird will shake the end of the wing, and the whole bird will quiver at times. (Courtesy of M.L. Sunde, University of Wisconsin.)

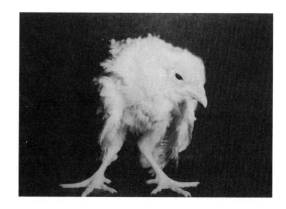

It appears that egg production is less affected by folacin deficiency than the development of the chick or poult. Egg and poult weights were significantly increased when turkey hens received higher dietary folacin and when eggs were injected with folacin (Robel, 1993). Inadequate folacin provided to the hen impairs the oviduct's response to estrogen and the ability to form albumen (NRC, 1994). Inadequate intake of folacin by breeding hens results in poor hatchability and a marked increase in

500

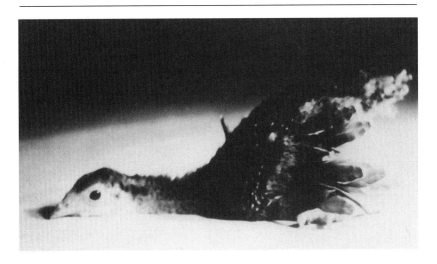

Fig. 12.5 Folacin-deficient poult was hatched from a hen fed a diet low in fo-lacin. (Courtesy of M.L. Sunde, University of Wisconsin.)

embryonic mortality (Fig. 12.6), which occurs during the last days of in-cubation. A deformed beak and bending of the tibiotarsus are signs of the embryonic deficiency. Chicks that successfully emerge are stunted and have feathers that are poorly developed and abnormally pigmented (NRC, 1994).

Folacin deficiency has sometimes been associated with perosis, or slipped tendon. Pollard and Creek (1964) demonstrated histologically that the lesions of folacin-deficient bones and cartilage are different from those produced by choline or manganese deficiencies. Abnormal structure of the hyaline cartilage is found in folacin-deficient chicks, and ossification is retarded. These disorders are not found in chicks deficient in choline or manganese, although bone deformities and slipped tendons are found in both types of disorders. However, Bechtel (1964) claimed that choline is effective in preventing perosis only when sufficient folacin is present in the diet. Dietary choline content has been shown to affect the chick's requirement for folacin. When the diet contained adequate choline, the folacin requirement was 0.46 mg/kg diet, but this increased to 0.96 mg/kg diet when the diet was choline deficient (Young et al., 1955). Increasing the protein content of the diet has also been shown to increase the incidence and severity of perosis in chicks receiving low lev-els of dietary folacin. It is suggested that this increased requirement for folacin in high protein diets for poultry is a consequence of greater de-

501

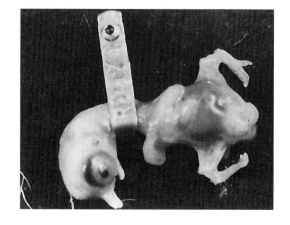

Fig. 12.6 Folic acid deficiency. Abnormal embryo from an egg laid by a hen on a low-folacin diet. (Courtesy of M.L. Sunde, University of Wisconsin.)

mand for folacin in uric acid formation (Creek and Vasaitis, 1963).

Folacin appears to be necessary for cell mitosis. In the absence of folacin, oviduct growth is not increased in estrogen-treated chicks. The production of water-soluble proteins (particularly the albumin fraction) in the hormone-stimulated oviduct is also greatly reduced, and the amino acid composition of these proteins is altered. The percentages of arginine, leucine, serine, and tryptophan are decreased and those of glycine and methionine increased (Siddons, 1978).

Horses

It has been shown that the horse synthesizes folacin in the intestinal tract. Carroll et al. (1949) fed a diet containing less than 0.1 mg of folacin per kilogram of dry matter and found the following folacin concentrations in ingesta (mg/kg dry matter): duodenum, 0.9; ileum, 0.5; cecum, 3.0; anterior large colon, 4.7; and anterior small colon, 2.7. Folacin synthesis may not be sufficient; Seckington et al. (1967) reported a case of folacin deficiency in a 7-year-old gelding that had been receiving a diet lacking in fresh grass for many months. The folacin-deficient animal had poor performance associated with low serum folacin. Administration of 20 mg of folacin dramatically increased performance and elevated blood folacin. Roberts (1983) examined serum and erythrocyte folacin levels in Australian horses and found higher concentrations in those on pasture than in permanently stabled horses.

Other Animal Species

Folacin deficiency has been reported using only purified feed ingredients or only diets naturally low in the vitamin for a number of species,

502

including the dog, fox, guinea pig, hamster, mink, monkey, salmon, and trout. For other species, including the rat, cat, carp, and catfish, folate deficiencies are difficult to establish unless use is made of an intestinal antiseptic (sulfa drug) or folate antagonist. For mice and certain other species, care must be taken to prevent coprophagy if folacin deficiency is to be produced on a diet without the aid of an antagonist or sulfa drug.

DOGS AND CATS

Folacin deficiency was produced in cats by adding sulfonamides to semipurified diets; the deficiency was characterized by weight loss, anemia (macrocytic tendencies), and leukopenia. Blood-clotting time was increased, and plasma iron concentrations were elevated (Carvalho da Silva et al., 1955).

Folacin deficiency resulted in erratic appetite, decreased gain, water exudate from eyes, glossitis, leukopenia, hypochromic anemia, and decreased antibody response to infectious canine hepatitis and canine distemper virus (NRC, 1985a). A positive response was obtained by subcutaneous injections of folacin. Serum folacin was increased in various breeds of dogs that received dietary folacin (Davenport et al., 1994). A fox terrier bitch with chronic ehrlichiosis exhibited a regenerative anemia and thrombopenia associated with marrow hypercellularity. Dyserythropoiesis and dysthrombopoiesis were attributed to folacin and vitamin B_{12} deficiency, which was thought to have been the result of medullary hyperconsumption during the subclinical phase of the disease (Caprelli et al., 1994). Sheffy (1964) illustrated the importance of folacin in the immune response of folacin-deficient puppies inoculated with distemper and hepatitis antigens. Half the dogs were also given 27.5 µg of folacin per kilogram of body weight. Depleted dogs had delayed antibody production responses against both distemper and infectious hepatitis antigens. Antibodies were detected in depleted dogs supplemented with folacin 8 days after challenge with antigen, whereas depleted dogs without folacin did not show antibodies until 17 days.

FISH

Signs of folacin deficiency in trout and salmon include anorexia, reduced growth, poor feed conversion, and macrocytic, normochromic, megaloblastic anemia characterized by pale gills and poikilocytosis (increased numbers of hemocytoblasts) (Cowey and Woodward, 1993; NRC, 1993). Anorexia, poor growth, and dark skin coloration were noted in Japanese eels fed a folacin-deficient diet for 10 weeks (Arai et

al., 1972). Folacin-deficient yellowtail fingerlings also showed congestion in fins and bronchial mantle, dark skin coloration, and anemia
(Hosokawa, 1989). Folacin deficiency signs in channel catfish included
reduced growth, anemia, and increased sensitivity to bacterial infection
(Duncan and Lovell, 1991). Anemia in folate-deficient channel catfish
was characterized by pale livers, spleens, gills, and kidneys and by poikilocytosis (Duncan et al., 1993).

An anemic disease in catfish known as "no blood disease" or "white
lip disease" was reported to result in catfish fed sulfonamide-degrading
Pseudomonas bacteria (Plumb et al., 1991). The researchers were able
to isolate two strains of folacin-degrading enzymes from feed, environment, and catfish tissue samples. Catfish fed sulfonamide showed higher
mortality, lower weight gain, lower thrombocyte counts, higher hemo-
cytoblast and neutrophil counts, and lower liver folacin values compared with controls (no folacin), indicating that significant intestinal
bacterial synthesis of folacin occurs in channel catfish (Duncan et al.,
1993).

Foxes and Mink

Both adult and growing foxes receiving a folacin-deficient diet exhibit anorexia; body weight loss; and a decrease in hemoglobin, erythrocyte, and leukocyte concentrations (NRC, 1982a; Pölönen et al.,
1997). Folacin deficiency in mink results in anorexia, growth depression, diarrhea, and ulcerative hemorrhagic gastritis (NRC, 1982a; Siddons, 1978).

Laboratory Animals

Rodent species have generally similar folacin-deficiency signs, including reduced growth, anemia, leukopenia, evidence of reduced protein synthesis, reduced folacin tissue levels, and impaired antibody response (Siddons, 1978; NRC, 1995; Achón et al., 1999). An increase in
urinary excretion of FIGLU occurs with folacin deficiency in the rat and
mouse. In rats, severe folacin deficiency caused secondary hepatic
choline deficiency (Kim et al., 1994). Folacin deficiency has been shown
to have a teratogenic effect on the rat, with congenital abnormalities in
offspring, including hydrocephalus. Hamsters resemble guinea pigs
rather than rats in their ability to develop folacin deficiency without the
use of intestinal antiseptic or folacin antagonist (Cohen et al., 1971). For
the rat, folacin biosynthesis by intestinal bacteria may meet much of the
requirement for the vitamin (Rong et al., 1991).

Deficiency of folacin in the pregnant mouse has an adverse effect on reproduction and lactation. Shaw et al. (1973) observed decreased growth, especially of brain and liver, in young mice deprived of folate both prenatally and postnatally. Cerecedo and Mirone (1947) reported that folacin increased survival to weaning of suckling mice from 34% (basal diet) to 69%.

NONHUMAN PRIMATES

After 3 to 9 months, monkeys on a low-folacin diet lost weight, became inactive, and between 3 and 18 months, developed a megaloblastic macrocytic anemia (NRC, 1978; Siddons, 1978; Thenen et al., 1991). In rhesus monkeys a variety of clinical and hematological signs arise as a result of the deficiency, including weight loss, anorexia, listlessness, mucoid to bloody diarrhea, gingivitis and oral ulceration, increased susceptibility to infection (especially dysentery), macrocytic anemia, leukopenia, and increased excretion of FIGLU. Leukopenia is the most characteristic hematological sign, and in some monkeys, it may prove fatal without the development of anemia.

Humans

For humans, folacin deficiency is probably the most common vitamin deficiency in the world. Infants, adolescents, elderly persons, and pregnant women seem particularly vulnerable. Studies involving the World Health Organization in various countries suggest that up to one-third of all pregnant women in the world have folacin deficiency (Herbert, 1981). In a clinic in New York City, 16% of pregnant women were deficient, with erythrocyte folacin below 150 ng/ml. A further 14% had erythrocyte folacin concentrations suggestive of a deficiency. In a study in Paris, 18% of immigrant pregnant women were deficient in folacin (Hercberg et al., 1987). Black South African women had a high incidence of megaloblastic anemia of pregnancy, and 40% of apparently otherwise healthy pregnant women had morphological and biochemical evidence of folate deficiency (Colman, 1982).

Adolescent girls have a greater nutritional requirement for folacin in relation to body size than do adult women (Heald, 1975). Additional folacin demand of pregnancy and poor dietary habits may compromise their growth potential and increase risk in pregnancy. Folacin deficiency in the older population is due in part to an impairment of dietary folate utilization (Baker et al., 1978). Elderly subjects (older than 60 years) were unable to utilize polyglutamate forms of folacin effectively compared to younger subjects, indicating a lack of conjugase enzymes. In Italy (Maiani et al., 1992), 15% of free living elderly were deficient in folacin, while in Holland (Lowik et al., 1992), 28% of elderly women living in a nursing home were deficient in the vitamin. In Spain 80% of free living elderly subjects were deficient in folacin on the basis of low serum and red blood cell folacin values (Ortega et al., 1993).

Infants have a high requirement for folacin, with preterm infants reported to have significantly lower erythrocyte folacin than those born at term (Ek, 1980). These data would suggest a heightened maternofetal transfer of folacin during the last few weeks of pregnancy. One study evaluated the folacin status of 31- to 210-day-old Brazilian infants from low-income families (Trugo et al., 1991). Some of the babies were exclusively breast-fed, and some were partially weaned. Low serum folacin was found in 33% of exclusively breast-fed infants and in 27% of partially weaned infants.

Typical reaction to folacin deficiency in the human is megaloblastic red cell maturation in the bone marrow with resulting macrocytic anemia (Fig. 12.7), which is accompanied by leukopenia. The macrocytic anemia that occurs resembles pernicious anemia without the nervous system involvement. Glossitis, gastrointestinal lesions, diarrhea, and intestinal malabsorption may accompany macrocytic anemia. Likewise, clinical findings of folacin deficiency include pallor, weakness, forgetfulness, sleeplessness, and bouts of euphoria (Herbert, 1962). The most rapidly proliferating tissues of the body, such as the bone marrow for blood cell production, have the greatest requirement for DNA synthesis and thus are principally affected when severe deficiency occurs.

The sequence of signs in the development of human folacin deficiency was reported by Herbert (1967), who examined biochemical and hematological changes in himself as he consumed a low-folacin diet over time (Table 12.3). After only 3 weeks of dietary folacin deprivation, his serum folacin dropped from 7 to less than 3 ng/ml. However, low erythrocyte folacin did not appear until 4 months after initiation of folacin deprivation. At about 4.5 months, his bone marrow became megaloblastic and anemia developed.

Apart from features due to megaloblastic anemia or to abnormalities of the epithelial cell surfaces, sterility and gastrointestinal abnormalities are established effects of folacin deficiency (Hoffbrand, 1978). Sterility in both men and women and, in a small percentage of cases, widespread reversible melanin pigmentation of the skin, mainly affecting the skin creases and nail-beds, have been reported (Fleming and Dawson, 1972). Folacin deficiency may be related to abnormalities of pregnancy, including postpartum hemorrhage, antepartum hemorrhage, congenital malformation, and prematurity. Clinical signs related to the

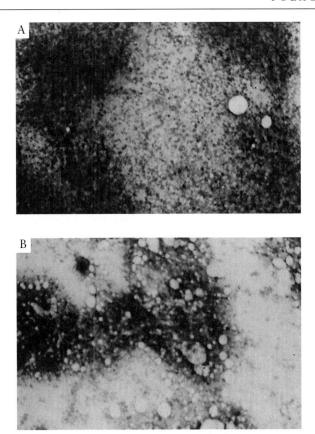

Fig. 12.7 Pernicious anemia in a human, characterized by (A) marked hyperplasia in bone marrow compared to (B) normal. Deficiency of either folacin or vitamin B_{12} results in ineffective erythropoiesis. (Courtesy of R.R. Streiff, Veterans Administration, University of Florida.)

gastrointestinal tract include sore tongue, angular cheilosis, loss of appetite, and diarrhea (Rose, 1971). The tongue may appear red and shiny or smooth, pale, and atrophic. Some researchers have shown structural and functional jejunal changes in nutritional folacin deficiency that can be reversed by supplemental folacin (Hoffbrand, 1978). There is a complicated relationship between tropical sprue and folacin deficiency. Nutritional folacin deficiency may predispose to the disease, and that deficiency, due to reduced diet and to malabsorption, may aggravate the small intestinal lesion.

Numerous studies have shown that supplemental folacin (0.4 to 4

507

■ Table 12.3   Progressive Folacin Deficiency Sequence of Events in a 35-
Year-Old Human Male

Time (weeks)	Biochemical and Hematological Events
3	Low serum folacin (< 3 ng/ml)
7	Hypersegmentation of neutrophils (leukocytes)
13	High urine formiminoglutamic acid (FIGLU)
17	Low RBC folacin (< 20 ng/ml)
19–20	Megaloblastic anemia

Source: Modified from Herbert (1967).

mg) can prevent serious birth defects, known as neural tube defects, in developing fetuses (Rush, 1992; Bower, 1995; Scott et al., 1995). In the United States and around the world, neural tube defects—anencephaly, spina bifida, and encephalocoele—contribute significantly to infant mortality and morbidity. According to the Centers for Disease Control report (1992), 4,000 infants with neural tube defects are born annually in the United States; worldwide, nearly 400,000 are born with these conditions (Rush, 1992). Neural defects occur when the neural tube, which will develop into the spinal cord, fails to close 18 to 26 days after actual conception. If the neural tube defect occurs toward the top of the tube, the child is born with anencephaly (without a brain) and will die soon after birth. If the defect occurs further down the tube, the child will be born with spina bifida (an open spine) and will be crippled for life (Bower, 1995).

The exact mechanism by which folacin prevents these birth defects is not known. There is substantial geographical and ethnic variation in the prevalence of neural tube defects; the etiology is unknown but is believed to be multifactorial, involving both genetic and environmental determinants. Evidence indicates that vitamin B_{12} is also an independent risk factor, which makes it very probable that, either directly or indirectly, the primary cause of neural tube defects is a defective enzyme. This enzyme is most probably in the affected fetus as well as in the mother, namely methionine synthase, since this is the only point in metabolism at which both folacin and vitamin B_{12} interact (Scott et al., 1995; see also Chapter 13, Deficiency, Humans).

Data have accumulated indicating that low folacin status may promote cancer. Low folacin levels are associated with cytogenetic abnormalities in vivo and in vitro. Epidemiological studies examined the association between folacin and cancer of the cervix, colorectum, lung, esophagus, and brain and suggested that low folacin status may play an important role early in the neoplastic process (Glynn and Albanes, 1994). Butterworth (1993) suggested that a significant reduction in early cervical cancer could be achieved in up to two-thirds of high-risk populations through improved nutritional intake of folacin before exposure to an oncogenic strain of papilloma virus.

In a prospective analysis of over 25,000 men and women, Giovannucci et al. (1993) found an inverse association between dietary folacin and the incidence of adenomatous polyps in the distal colon and rectum. They also found an inverse association with another dietary source of methyl groups (methionine), as well as a direct association with moderate alcohol consumption, which is known to adversely affect folacin metabolism. This suggests that diminished folacin status and excessive alcohol intake, which may decrease S-adenosyl-methionine levels, may induce hypomethylation of DNA, thereby promoting colorectal cancer.

Studies suggest that folacin deficiency may be an important cause of a moderate hyperhomocysteinemia, which is an independent risk factor for cardiovascular disease (Boushey et al., 1995; Selhub et al., 1996). All but a few of over 75 studies, including a total of more than 15,000 investigated patients and controls, support this issue (Brattström, 1996). Basal hyperhomocysteinemia unmasked by a methionine load test is a marker for increased cardiovascular risk (Ueland et al., 1992).

Some studies suggest that folacin deficiency may be responsible for up to 40% of the heart attacks and strokes suffered by American men every year (Raeburn, 1995). Studies have consistently found that men with elevated homocysteine levels in the blood are three times more likely to have a heart attack over the next 5 years than men with normal homocysteine levels. Elevated homocysteine levels can be caused by genetic defects in homocysteine metabolism, or by lack of vitamin B_6 or folacin, and vitamin B_{12}. Supplementation with folacin has been shown to markedly reduce elevated plasma homocysteine concentrations and reduce normal homocysteine concentrations (Brattström, 1996). Folacin doses of less than 1 mg/day may be effective. Supplementation with a combination of folacin and vitamin B_{12} will secure the full homocysteine-lowering effect and prevent occurrence of a vitamin B_{12} deficiency during the course of therapy.

Folacin deficiency is often associated with chronic alcoholism. Between 40 and 87% of alcoholics admitted to municipal hospitals in the United States have low serum folacin, and between 40 and 61% have megaloblastic anemia (Halsted and Tamura, 1979). Folacin deficiency appears to be a result of a complex interaction between nutritional deprivation and chronic alcohol ingestion. Alcohol specifically inhibits hematopoiesis, and Halsted et al. (1973) reported that the jejunal uptake of folacin was significantly greater in subjects who remained sober. Hidiroglou et al. (1994) suggested that alcohol exerts its effect through (1) inhibition of B_{12}-dependent methyl transfer from methyltetrahydrofolate to homocysteine; (2) diversion of formylated tetrahydrofolates toward serine synthesis; and (3) interaction of acetaldehyde with tetrahydrofolates, which thereby interferes with folacin coenzyme metabolism.

Both poor folacin status and moderate to excessive alcohol consumption have been associated with increased risk of colorectal cancer, although the mechanisms through which these effects occur have not been established. Reports suggest that diminished folacin status and excessive alcohol intake—which may decrease S-adenosylmethionine levels, thereby depleting methionine—may induce hypomethylation of DNA, thus promoting colorectal cancer (Giovannucci et al., 1993).

Folacin has been shown to have a role in neuropsychiatry. In many countries there is a high incidence of folacin deficiency in psychiatric and psychogeriatric patients, especially inpatients (Bottiglieri et al., 1995). The deficiency can be associated with any diagnostic category but is more common in patients with depression and dementia. There is some evidence that even a borderline deficiency can be harmful to the mental state (Godfrey et al., 1990). There is growing evidence that whether the deficiency is primary or secondary to the psychiatric disorder, folacin replacement may improve mental function when added to standard psychotropic medication.

Assessment of Status

Assessment of nutritional status of folacin can involve dietary evaluation, clinical signs, response to supplementation, and laboratory analysis. Regarding dietary history, humans or animals (particularly poultry) that have not received green leafy plant sources or organ meats would suggest reduced folacin intake. Because liver contains a high percentage of stored folacin, concentration in this organ would serve as a folacin status indicator. On low-folacin diets, liver concentrations are depleted in a few months. Clinical signs of folacin deficiency are extremely variable and are less precise than laboratory analysis to confirm deficiency. Using a protocol of folacin depletion-repletion of rats, followed by assessment of growth and liver, serum, and erythrocyte folacin concentrations, has been successful in evaluating bioavailability of food folacin sources (Clifford et al., 1990, 1991).

In humans, a positive diagnosis of folacin deficiency is usually made by the finding of subnormal serum and erythrocyte levels. Cutoff values of less than 0.3 ng/ml for serum folacin and less than 140 ng/ml for erythrocyte folacin are the basis for estimation of the prevalence of low values of the vitamin (Senti and Pilch, 1985). Patients with vitamin B_{12} deficiency exhibit all the clinical and hematological features and many of the biochemical features of folacin deficiency. Thus, erythrocyte folacin assay is better used in conjunction with the values for serum vitamin B_{12}.

Measurement of tissue content of several forms of folacin and urinary excretion of FIGLU, a histidine catabolite that cannot be normally metabolized in folacin deficiency, is utilized to assess folacin nutrition. It has been shown that the amount of FIGLU excreted in urine roughly parallels the erythrocyte folate and hepatic folacin levels in both anemic and nonanemic folacin-deficient patients and thus, like the erythrocyte folate and hepatic folacin levels, appears to be a satisfactory index of tissue folacin stores (Herbert, 1967). A 24-hour urinary excretion level after a single oral dose of isotopically labeled folacin is a functional indicator of folacin status (Gregory et al., 1998).

Deficiencies of iron and vitamin C can be related to folacin status, but it has not yet been proven that folacin requirement is increased in either iron deficiency anemia or scurvy. The frequent occurrence of combined iron and folacin deficiencies has led to the suggestion that iron deficiency may be responsible for the development of secondary folacin deficiency. Iron deficiency has been reported to influence folacin metabolism in pregnant women. The stress of lactation in rats superimposed on iron deficiency was found to alter milk folacin concentration, resulting in folacin depletion in rat pups (Kochanowski et al., 1983). Both iron and folacin are required for normal hematopoiesis, with anemia resulting from lack of either nutrient. Iron deficiency may mask the changes in the developing erythroblasts but does not affect the white cell abnormalities. Anemia in humans is often assumed to be the result of iron deficiency; however, Bailey et al. (1980) reported that folacin deficiency was much more prevalent than iron deficiency in a lower-income pregnant Florida population. Whether the association of scurvy and megaloblastic anemia is due to increased folacin requirements secondary to lack of vitamin C or is merely the result of a double nutritional deficiency is unresolved. However, it is interesting to speculate that many cases of vitamin C deficiency could likewise be folacin deficiencies, since both vitamins are rich in green plants and citrus fruits and lacking in most other food sources.

The measurement of serum homocysteine was shown to be a good indicator of folacin and vitamn B_{12} nutritional status (Krumdieck, 1990;

Jacob, 1998). The folate-vitamin B_{12}-requiring remethylation of homocysteine to methionine normally converts approximately 50% of available homocysteine back to methionine.

In most human patients with folacin deficiency, a combination of factors leads to negative folacin balance. Poor diet is usually the major cause, since few diseases cause malabsorption or poor folacin utilization to become so severe that good intake of the vitamin cannot overcome losses. It is likely that severe folacin deficiency may occur in tropical sprue and congenital specific malabsorption of folacin, despite a normal dietary folacin content (Hoffbrand, 1978).

SUPPLEMENTATION

Folacin needs for livestock are often met by good practical diets, and for most species, substantial quantities of folacin are provided through microbial synthesis. Nevertheless, field observations have been made on folacin-insufficient diets. Green forage is an excellent source of folacin. Supplementation of folacin would be most needed when animals are in confinement without access to green grazing or preserved green forages. The successful treatment of field cases of folacin deficiency with supplemental folacin has demonstrated that commercial feeds do not always supply adequate quantities of the vitamin to poultry (Pesti et al., 1991).

Of farm livestock, poultry would most likely need supplemental folacin and then only under certain conditions. Newly weaned pigs may also need additional folacin in their diets for optimum growth and feed efficiency. The supplementation of gestating swine diets with folacin to maximize sow productivity is indicated by research (Matte et al., 1984b; Tremblay et al., 1989; Lindemann, 1993). There was consistent increase in total and live pigs born when reproducing females received supplemental folacin during gestation. The increase has occurred at dietary supplementation levels from 0.2 mg/kg (Easter et al., 1983) to 15 mg/kg (Matte et al., 1990) as well as with folacin injections throughout the first 12 weeks of gestation (Matte et al., 1984b, 1992). Matte et al. (1992) observed that dietary supplementation of 15 mg/kg was necessary to avoid the drop in concentrations of serum folates of sows in gestation and seemed to influence some traits of the reproductive performance. It seems apparent and logical that supplementation must occur in early gestation. The response appears to be greater in conditions of increased ovulation (e.g., sows versus gilts, flushed versus nonflushed), which suggests that there may be breed differences in response to folacin supplementation (Lindemann, 1988).

Only young ruminants that do not have a fully developed rumen would be expected to require a dietary source. Fluctuations in the concentration of serum folacin observed during the first months of life of young ruminants may be an indication that synthesis of folacin by ruminal microflora is not sufficient to meet requirements during weaning (Girard et al., 1989a). The age effect on development of the rumen was observed, in which parenterally administered folacin markedly increased serum folacin in 2-week-old heifers, while in 4-month-old heifers, the increase was less marked. For adult dairy cows, Girard et al. (1989b) reported that serum folacin can be increased by intramuscular injection of folacin, but in cows during early lactation, this does not markedly affect serum and milk folacin. Girard et al. (1995) injected folacin (160 mg) weekly into dairy cows from mating to 6 weeks postparturition; the supplementation achieved maximal production of milk and protein in multiparous cows.

Folacin may be of little benefit when poultry and swine receive only low levels of sulfa drugs and consume grains relatively free of toxin-producing molds. However, since a large percentage of the U.S. corn crop has some mold contamination, folacin supplementation should have a positive effect in many commercial poultry and hog operations as well as in other livestock enterprises (Purser, 1981). This would likely be an even more important consideration in developing tropical countries, where conditions favoring mold growth are optimized. Individual responses to folacin supplementation to counteract mold effect will obviously vary with the class of livestock being fed, species of mold present, and the levels of toxin encountered (Bhavanishankar et al., 1986). Purser (1981) fed supplemental folacin to pigs weaned at 3, 4, or 5 weeks of age. At the end of the 4-week feeding period, the younger pigs showed the greatest response to diets providing the supplemental vitamin.

Gadient (1986) found folacin to be very sensitive to heat and light, slightly sensitive to moisture, and insensitive to oxygen. Frye (1978) found that folacin can be lost during storage of premixes, particularly at elevated temperatures. After 3 months of room-temperature storage, 43% of the original folacin activity was lost. Verbeeck (1975) found folacin to be stable in premixes without minerals, but there may be as much as 50% loss in a premix with minerals kept at room temperature for 3 months. Adams (1982) reported only 38% retention of folacin activity in a premix without minerals after 3 weeks at 45°C. However, he reported 57% retention of activity after 3 months at room temperature. One suggestion would be to almost double the amount of folacin in a premix at the time of manufacture to ensure that poultry or swine receive the desired amount from that premix, since a 3- to 4-month period is not an unreasonable amount of time from premix manufacture to customer purchase to (ultimately) diet mixing and feeding.

Slinger et al. (1979) reported processing and storage losses of folacin in fish feeds of 5 to 10% for steam-pelleted crumbles and 3 to 7% for extruded crumbles, depending on dietary level. Scott (1966) indicated that an adjustment of 10 to 20% in the folacin level in poultry feed may be necessary because of pelleting losses. Coelho (1994) reported a 21% loss of folacin in feeds as a result of pelleting and 2 weeks of storage.

It is important that women begin supplementation of folacin before they plan to become pregnant, or at least to consume adequate folacin if there is a chance of pregnancy occurring. They should not wait until pregnancy is confirmed, because supplementation at that time is too late to provide protection from birth defects. Neural tube defects develop very early in pregnancy (18 to 26 days); therefore supplemental folacin must be provided in the preconception period before a woman knows she is pregnant.

Humans obtain folacin primarily from fruits and vegetables, and an average western diet supplies 0.15 to 0.2 mg/day (Metz, 1995). Women of childbearing age would need to increase their folacin intake threefold to reach the level of 0.4 mg/day, the amount of folacin known to be effective against neural tube defects and which does not mask the diagnosis of pernicious anemia and/or vitamin B_{12} deficiency.

Supplementation with large doses of folacin will cure the macrocytic anemia in human patients with the vitamin B_{12} deficiency, pernicious anemia. However, folacin will not prevent the often irreversible neurological lesions of vitamin B_{12} deficiency or pernicious anemia. Therefore, large quantities (more than 1 mg/day) of supplemental folacin should not be taken indiscriminately as they may obscure a diagnosis of vitamin B_{12} deficiency. The U.S. Public Health Service cautioned against recommending daily intakes above 1 mg/day, except under physician supervision (Anonymous, 1996).

To reduce the risk of neural tube defects, the U.S. Food and Drug Administration (FDA) has required (since January 1, 1998) that folacin be added to most enriched flour, breads, corn meals, rice, noodles, macaroni, and other grain products (Anonymous, 1996). These foods were chosen for folacin fortification because they are staple products for most of the U.S. population, and because they have a long history of being successful vehicles for improving nutrition by reducing the risk of classic nutrient deficiency diseases. The FDA is requiring that the above-noted food products be fortified with folacin at a level of 140 mg/100 g. This supplementation level will likely provide at least 0.4 mg folacin daily. The purpose of mandatory folacin supplementation in the United States is to reduce neural tube defects; however, benefits will surely be derived in providing protection against megaloblastic anemia, cardio-vascular disease, and various forms of cancer (e.g., colorectal), and in preventing other conditions that result from folacin deficiency. As an example, assuming that correction of the homocysteinemia diminishes the risk of vascular disease and given the apparent high prevalence of the trait, a vast opportunity for prevention of coronary disease by giving these patients supplemental folacin may exist. Likewise, folacin deficiency enhances tumor development in rats, which is preventable with folacin supplementation (Henning et al., 1997).

Crystalline folacin, produced by chemical synthesis, is available for feeds, foods, and pharmaceuticals. Although folacin is only sparingly soluble in water, the sodium salt is quite soluble and is used in injections as well as feed supplements (McGinnis, 1986; Tremblay et al., 1986). For humans, folacin supplements (monoglutamate form) ranging from 100 to 1,000 µg/day have been recommended by different investigators. Oral supplementation appears to be desirable to maintain maternal stores and to keep pace with the increased folacin turnover that is seen in rapidly growing tissue. Synthetic folacin supplements are convenient to take and highly available; natural forms are approximately 50% less available than synthetic forms.

TOXICITY

Folacin generally has been regarded as a nontoxic vitamin (NRC, 1987). Acute intravenous toxicity is very low, with the LD_{50} as follows (in milligrams per kilogram of body weight): mice, 600; rats, 500; rabbits, 410; and guinea pigs, 120. In rats, most of the deaths occurred within 30 minutes of injection (Anonymous, 1961). Rabbits given 50 mg/kg/day intraperitoneally for 10 weeks were possibly retarded in growth and did not differ in blood picture, number of deaths, or general appearance, but did show signs of renal injury at autopsy. Folacin has a low acute and chronic toxicity for humans. In adults, no adverse effects were noted after 400 mg/day for 5 months or after 10 mg/day for 5 years (Brody, 1991). The danger of excess folacin is indirect in that the folacin supplements can obscure the diagnosis of vitamin B_{12} deficiency; they can prevent anemia while permitting neurological damage.

■ REFERENCES

Abad, A.R., and Gregory, J.F. (1987). *J. Nutr.* 117, 866.
Achón, M., Reyes, L., Alonso-Aperte, E., Ubeda, N., and Varela-Moreiras, G. (1999). *J. Nutr.* 129, 1204.
Adams, C.R. (1982). *In* Vitamins—The Life Essentials. Nutrition Institute, National Feed Ingredients Association, NI-82, 1, Des Moines, Iowa.
Anonymous (1961). Vitamin Manual, p. 53. Upjohn, Kalamazoo, Michigan.
Anonymous (1996). *Nutr. Rev.* 54(3), 94.
Arai, S., Nose, T., and Hashimoto, Y. (1972). *Bull Freshwater Res. Lab. Tokyo* 22, 69.
Bailey, L.B. (1995). *In* Folate in Health and Disease (L.B. Bailey, ed.), p. 123. Marcel Dekker, New York.
Bailey, L.B., Manan, C.S., and Dimpeno, D. (1980). *Am. J. Clin. Nutr.* 33, 1997.
Baker, H., Jaslow, S.P., and Frank, O. (1978). *J. Am. Geriatr. Soc.* 26, 218.
Baker, S.J., and DeMaeyer, E.M. (1979). *Am. J. Clin. Nutr.* 32, 368.
Balaghi, M., and Wagner, C. (1992). *J. Nutr.* 122, 1391.
Balaghi, M., Horne, D.W., Woodward, S.C., and Wagner, C. (1993). *Am. J. Clin. Nutr.* 58, 198.
Baugh, C.M., and Krumdieck, C.L. (1971). *Ann. N. Y. Acad. Sci.* 186, 7.
Bechtel, H.E. (1964). *Feedstuffs* 36(45), 18.
Bhandari, S.D., and Gregory, J.F. (1992). *J. Nutr.* 122, 1847.
Bhavanishanker, T.N., Shantha, T., and Ramesh, H.P. (1986). *Nutr. Rep. Int.* 33, 603.
Blakley, R.L., and Benkovic, S.J. (1984). Folates and Pterins. Wiley, New York.
Bottiglieri, T., Crellin, R.F., and Reynolds, E.H. (1995). *In* Folate in Health and Disease (L.B. Bailey, ed.), p. 435. Marcel Dekker, New York.
Boushey, C.J., Beresford, S.A.A., Omenn, G.S., and Motulsky, A.G. (1995). *JAMA* 274, 1049.
Bower, C. (1995). *Nutr. Rev.* 53, S33.
Brattström, L. (1996). *J. Nutr.* 126, 1276S.
Brody, T. (1991) *In* Handbook of Vitamins (L.J. Machlin, ed.), 2nd Ed., p. 453. Marcel Dekker, New York.
Brown, G.M. (1962). *J. Biol. Chem.* 237, 536.
Butterworth, C.E. (1993). *Pennington Cent. Nutr. Ser.* 3, 196.
Butterworth, C.E. Jr., Hatch, K.D., Macaluso, M., Cole, P., Sauberlich, H.E., Soong, S.J., Borst, M., and Baker, V.V. (1992). *JAMA* 267, 528.
Caprelli, J.L., Bohlay, P., and Barre, D. (1994). *Pratique-Medicale-et-Chirurgicale-de-l'Animal-de-Compagnie* 29, 395.
Carl, G.F., and Smith, M.L. (1995). *J. Nutr.* 125, 1245.
Carl, G.F., Hudson, F.Z., and McGuire, B.S. (1997). *J. Nutr.* 127, 2231.

Carroll, F.D., Gross, H., and Howell, C.E. (1949). *J. Anim. Sci. 8*, 290.

Cartwright, G.E., and Wintrobe, M.M. (1949). *Proc. Soc. Exp. Biol. Med. 71*, 54.

Cartwright, G.E., Tatting, B., Kurth, D., and Wintrobe, M.M. (1952). *Blood 7*, 992.

Carvalho da Silva, A., deAngelis, R.C., Pontes, M.A., and Mansurguerios, M.F. (1955). *J. Nutr. 56*, 199.

Centers for Disease Control (1992). *Morb. Mortal. Wkly. Rep. 41*, RR-14 (September 11, 1992).

Cerecedo, L.R., and Mirone, L. (1947). *Arch. Biochem. 12*, 154.

Chandler, C.J., Wang, T.T.Y., and Halsted, C.H. (1986). *J. Biol. Chem. 261*, 928.

Clifford, A.J., Jones, A.D., and Bills, N.D. (1990). *J. Nutr. 120*, 1640.

Clifford, A.J., Heid, M.K., Peerson, J.M., and Bills, N.D. (1991). *J. Nutr. 121*, 445.

Coelho, M.B. (1994). *In* BASF Technical Symposium, p. 60. Clarion, Arkansas.

Cohen, N.L., Reyes, P.S., and Briggs, G.M. (1971). *Lab. Anim. Sci. 21*, 350.

Colman, N. (1982). *Nutr. Rev. 49*, 225.

Cowey, C.B., and Woodward, B. (1993). *J. Nutr. 123*, 1594.

Cravo, M.L., Mason, J.B., and Dayal, Y. (1992). *Cancer Res. 52*, 5002.

Creek, R.D., and Vasaitis, V. (1963). *Poult. Sci. 42*, 1136.

Cruces-Blanco, C., Segura-Carretero, A., Fernandez-Guitierrez, A., and Roman-Ceba, M. (1994). *Anal. Lett. 27*, 1339.

Cunha, T.J., Colby, R.W., Bustad, L.K., and Bone, J.F. (1948). *J. Nutr. 36*, 215.

Davenport, D.J., Ching, R.J.W., Hunt, J.H., Bruyette, D.S., and Gross, K.L. (1994). *J. Nutr. 124*, 2559S.

Dhur, A., Galan, P., and Hereberg, S. (1991). *Prog. Food Nutr. Sci. 15*, 43.

Draper, H.H., and Johnson, B.C. (1952). *J. Nutr. 46*, 123.

Dumoulin, P.G., Girard, C.L., Matte, J.J., and St-Laurent, G.J. (1991). *J. Anim. Sci. 69*, 1657.

Duncan, P.L., and Lovell, R.T. (1991). Twenty-second Ann. Confer. World Aquacul. Soc. San Juan, Puerto Rico, June 16–20, 1991.

Duncan, P.L., Lovell, R.T., Butterworth, C.E., Jr., Freeberg, L.E., and Tamura, T. (1993). *J. Nutr. 123*, 1888.

Easter, R.A., Anderson, P.A., Michel, E.J., and Corley, J.R. (1983). *Nutr. Rep. Int. 28*, 945.

Ek, J. (1980). *J. Pediatr. 97*, 288.

Fleming, A.F., and Dawson, I. (1972). *Br. Med. J. 4*, 236.

Foo, S.K., and Shane, B. (1982). *J. Biol. Chem. 257*, 13587.

Frye, T.M. (1978). *Proc. Roche Vitam. Nutr. Update Meet.* Arkansas Nutr. Conf. p. 54.

Gadient, M. (1986). *Proc. Nutr. Conf. Feed Manuf.*, College Park, Maryland, p. 73.

Giovannucci, E., Stampfer, M.J., and Colditz, G.A. (1993). *J. Natl. Cancer Inst. 85*, 875.

Girard, C.L., and Matte, J.J. (1998). *J. Dairy Sci. 81*, 1412.

Girard, C.L., Matte, J.J., and Roy, G.L. (1989a). *Br. J. Nutr. 61*, 595.

Girard, C.L., Matte, J.J., and Tremblay, G.F. (1989b). *J. Dairy Sci. 72*, 3240.

Girard, C.L., Matte, J.J., and Lévesque, J. (1992). *J. Anim. Sci. 70*, 2847.

Girard, C.L., Chiquett, J., and Matte, J.J. (1994). *J. Anim. Sci. 72*, 1023.

Girard, C.L., Matte, J.J., and Tremblay, G.F. (1995). *J. Dairy Sci. 78*, 404.

Giugliani, E.R.J., Jorge, S.M., and Goncalves, A.L. (1985). *Am. J. Clin. Nutr. 41*, 330.

Glynn, S.A., and Albanes, D. (1994). *Nutr. Cancer, 22*, 101.

Godfrey, P.S.A., Toone, B.K., and Carney, M.W.P. (1990). *Lancet 336*, 392.

Green, R., and Jacobsen, D.W. (1995). *In* Folate in Health and Disease (L.B. Bailey, ed.), p. 75. Marcel Dekker, New York.

Gregory, J.F. (1989). *Adv. Food Nutr. Res. 33*, 1.

Gregory, J.F., Sartain, D.B., and Day, B.P.F. (1984). *J. Nutr. 114*, 341.

Gregory, J.F., Bhandari, S.D., Bailey, L.B., Toth, J.P., Baumgartner, T.G., and Cerda, J.J. (1991). *Am. J. Clin. Nutr. 53*, 736.

Gregory, J.F., Williamson, J., Bailey, L.B., and Toth, J.P. (1998). *J. Nutr. 128*, 1907.

Halsted, C.H., and Tamura, R. (1979). Problems in Liver Disease (C.S. Davidson, ed), p. 91. Stratton, New York.

Halsted, C.H., Robles, E.A., and Mezey, E. (1973). *Gasteroenterology 64*, 526.

Harper, A.F., Lindemann, M.D., Chiba, L.I., Combs, G.E., Handlin, D.L., Kornegay, E.T., and Southern, L.L. (1994). *J. Anim. Sci. 72*, 2338.

Heald, F.P. (1975). *Med. Clin. North Am. 59*, 1329.

Heimburger, D.C., Alexander, C.B., Birch, R., Butterworth, C.E. Jr., Bailey, W.C., and Krumdieck, C.L. (1988). *JAMA 259*, 1525.

Henning, S.M., Swendseid, M.E., and Coulson, W.F. (1997). *J. Nutr. 127*, 30.

Herbert, V. (1962). *Trans. Assoc. Am. Physicians 75*, 307.

Herbert, V. (1967). *Am J. Clin. Nutr. 20*, 562.

Herbert, V. (1981). *Proc. Fla. Symp. Micronutr. Hum. Nutr.* Univ. Fla., Gainesville, p. 121.

Herbert, V., and Zalusky, R. (1962). *J. Clin. Invest. 41*, 1263.

Hercberg, S., Bichon, L., Galan, P., Christides, J.P., Carroget, C., and Potier de Courcey, G. (1987). *Nutr. Rep. Int. 35*, 915.

Hidiroglou, N., Camilo, M.E., Beckenhauer, H.C., Tuma, D.L., Barak, A.J., Nixon, P.F., and Selhub, J. (1994). *Biochem. Pharm. 47*, 1561.

Hoffbrand, A.V. (1978). Handbook Series in Nutrition and Food, Section E: Nutritional Disorders (M. Rechcigl, ed.), Vol. 2, p. 55. CRC Press, Boca Raton, Florida.

Hosokawa, H. (1989). The vitamin requirements of fingerling yellowtail, *Seriola quinqueradiata*, Ph.D. dissertation. Kochi University, Japan.

Jacob, R.A. (1998). *Nutr. Rev. 56*, 212.

Jacob, R.A., Wu, M., Henning, S.M., and Swendseid, M.E. (1994). *J. Nutr. 124*, 1072.

Johnson, B.C., James, M.F., and Krider, J.L. (1948). *J. Anim. Sci. 7*, 486.

Kang, S.S., Wong, P.W.K., and Malinow, M.R. (1992). *Ann. Rev. Nutr. 12*, 279.

Keagy, P.M., and Oace, S.M. (1984). *J. Nutr. 114*, 1252.

Kim, Y., Miller, J.W., DaCosta, K.A., Nadeau, M., Smith, D., Selhub, J. Zeisel, S.H., and Mason, J.B. (1994). *J. Nutr. 124*, 2197.

Kochanowski, B.A., Smith, A.M., Picciano, M.F., and Sherman, A.R. (1983). *J. Nutr. 113*, 2471.

Krumdieck, C.L. (1990). *In* Present Knowledge in Nutrition (M.L. Brown, ed.), 6th Ed., p. 179. International Life Sciences Institute/Nutrition Foundation, Washington, D.C.

Leichter, J., Switzer, V.P., and Landymore, A.F. (1978). *Nutr. Rep. Int. 18*, 475.

Lévesque, J., Girard, C.L., Matte, J.J., and Brisson, G.J. (1993). *Livestock Prod. Sci. 34*, 71.

Lindemann, M.D. (1988). *Feedstuffs 60*(46), 15.

Lindemann, M.D. (1993). *J. Anim. Sci. 71*, 239.

Lindemann, M.D., and Kornegay, E.T. (1986). *J. Anim. Sci. 63*(Suppl. 1), 35(Abstr).

Lindemann, M.D., and Kornegay, E.T. (1989). *J. Anim. Sci. 67*, 459.

Lindemann, M.D., Blodgett, D.J., Kornegay, E.T., and Schurig, G.G. (1993). *J. Anim. Sci. 71*, 171.

Loosli, J.K. (1991). *In* Handbook of Animal Science (P.A. Putnam, ed.), p. 25. Academic Press, San Diego, California.

Lowik, M.R.H., Berg, H., Schrijver, J., Odink, J., Wedel, M., and Van Houten, P. (1992). *J. Am. Coll. Nutr. 11*, 673.

Maiani, G., Polito, A., Ranaldi, L., Azzini, E., Raguzzini, A., Mobarhan, S., and Ferro-Luzzi, A. (1992). *Age Nutr. 3*, 48.

Matoth, Y., Pinkas, A., and Sroka, C. (1965). *Am. J. Clin. Nutr. 16*, 356.

Matte, J.J., and Girard, C.L. (1999). *J. Anim. Sci. 77*, 159.

Matte, J.J., Girard, C.L., and Brisson, G.J. (1984a). *J. Anim. Sci. 59*, 158.

Matte, J.J., Girard, C.L., and Brisson, G.J. (1984b). *J. Anim. Sci. 59*, 1020.

Matte, J.J., Girard, C.L., and Brisson, G.J. (1990). *J. Anim. Sci. 68*(Suppl. 1), 370(Abstr.).

Matte, J.J., Girard, C.L., and Brisson, G.J. (1992). *Livestock Prod. Sci. 32*, 131.

Matte, J.J., Girard, C.L., and Tremblay, G.F. (1993). *J. Anim. Sci. 71*, 151.

McGinnis, C.H. (1986). Bioavailability of Nutrients in Feed Ingredients, p. 1. National Feed Ingredient Association (NFIA), Des Moines, Iowa.

McNulty, H., McPartlin, J.M., and Weir, D.G. (1993). *J. Nutr. 123*, 1089.

McPartlin, J., Scott, J.M., Halligan, A., Darling, M., and Weir, D.G. (1993). *Lancet 341*(8838), 148.

Metz, J. (1995). *Med. J. Aust. 163*, 231.

Muldoon, R.T., Ross, D.M., and McMartin, K.E. (1996). *J. Nutr. 126*, 242.

Murphy, M., Keating, M., Boyle, P., Weir, D.G., and Scott, J.M. (1976). *Biochem. Biophys. Res. Commun. 71*, 1017.

NRC. Nutrient Requirements of Domestic Animals. National Academy of Sciences-National Research Council, Washington, D.C.
(1978). Nutrient Requirements of Nonhuman Primates.
(1981). Nutrient Requirements of Goats.
(1982a). Nutrient Requirements of Mink and Foxes.
(1985a). Nutrient Requirements of Dogs, 2nd Ed.
(1985b). Nutrient Requirements of Sheep, 5th Ed.
(1986). Nutrient Requirements of Cats, 3rd Ed.
(1989a). Nutrient Requirements of Dairy Cattle, 6th Ed.
(1989b). Nutrient Requirements of Horses, 5th Ed.
(1993). Nutrient Requirements of Fish.
(1994). Nutrient Requirements of Poultry, 9th Ed.

(1995). Nutrient Requirements of Laboratory Animals, 4th Ed.

(1996). Nutrient Requirements of Beef Cattle, 7th Ed.

(1998). Nutrient Requirements of Swine, 10th Ed.

NRC. (1982b). United States-Canadian Tables of Feed Composition, 3rd Ed. National Academy of Sciences-National Research Council, Washington, D.C.

NRC. (1987). Vitamin Tolerance of Animals. National Academy of Sciences-National Research Council, Washington, D.C.

O'Broin, S., and Kelleher, B. (1992). *J. Clin. Pathol. 45,* 344.

O'Dell, B.L., and Hogan, A.G. (1943). *J. Biol. Chem. 149,* 323.

Ortega, R.M., Redondo, R., Andres, P., and Equileor, I. (1993). *Int. J. Vit. Nutr. Res. 63,* 17.

Pesti, G.M., Rowland, G.N., and Ryu, K.S. (1991). *Poult. Sci. 70,* 600.

Plumb, J.A., Liu, P.R., and Butterworth, C.E., Jr. (1991). *J. Appl. Aquacult. 1,* 33.

Pollard, W.O., and Creek, R.D. (1964). *Poult. Sci. 43,* 1415.

Pölönen, I.J., Vahteristo, L.T., and Tanhuanpää, E.J. (1997). *J. Anim. Sci. 75,* 1569.

Porras-Tejero, E., and Lluch-Fernandez, M.D. (1993). *Anales Espanoles de Pediatria 38,* 113.

Purser, K. (1981). *Anim. Nutr. Health April,* 38.

Raeburn, P. (1995). Vitamin Deficiency Tied to Heart Attacks, *San Francisco Examiner, July 25.*

RDA. (1980). Recommended Dietary Allowances, 9th Ed. National Academy of Sciences-National Research Council, Washington, D.C.

RDA. (1989). Recommended Dietary Allowances, 10th Ed. National Academy of Sciences-National Research Council, Washington, D.C.

Robel, E.J. (1993). *Poult. Sci. 72,* 546.

Roberts, M.C. (1983). *Aust. Vet. J. 60,* 106.

Rong, N., Selhub, J., Goldin, B.R., and Rosenberg, I.A. (1991). *J. Nutr. 121,* 1955.

Rose, J.A. (1971). *Lancet 2,* 453.

Rothman, D. (1970). *Am. J. Obstet. Gynecol. 108,* 149.

Rush, D. (1992). *Nutr. Rev. 50(1),* 25.

Sauberlich, H.E., Kretsch, M.J., Skala, J.H., Johnson, H.L., and Taylor, P.O. (1987). *Am. J. Clin. Nutr. 46,* 1016.

Savage, D.G., and Lindenbaum, J. (1995). *In* Folate in Health and Disease (L.B. Bailey, ed.), p. 237. Marcel Dekker, New York.

Schweigert, B.S., German, H.L., Pearson, P.B., and Sherwood, R.M. (1948). *J. Nutr. 35,* 89.

Scott, J.M., Weir, D.G., and Kirtie, P.N. (1995). *In* Folate in Health and Disease (L.B. Bailey, ed.), p. 329. Marcel Dekker, New York.

Scott, M.L. (1966). *Proc. Cornell Nutr. Conf.,* p. 35. Ithaca, New York.

Scott, M.L., Nesheim, M.C., and Young, R.J. (1982). Nutrition of the Chicken, p. 119. Scott, Ithaca, New York.

Seckington, I.M., Huntsman, R.G.,and Jenkins, G.C. (1967). *Vet. Rec. 81,* 158.

Selhub, J. (1989). *Anal. Biochem. 182,* 84.

Selhub, J., Jacques, P.F., Bostom, A.G., D'Agostino, R.B., Wilson, P.W.F., Belanger, J., O'Leary, D.H., Wolf, P.A., Rush, D., Schaefer, E.J., and Rosenberg, I.H. (1996). *J. Nutr. 126*, 1258S.

Semchuk, G.M., Allen, O.B., and O'Connor, D.L. (1994). *J. Nutr. 124*, 1118.

Senti, F.R., and Pilch, S.M. (1985). *J. Nutr. 115*, 1398.

Shaw, W., Schreiber, R.A., and Zemp, J.W. (1973). *Nutr. Rep. Int. 8*, 219.

Sheffy, B.E. (1964). *In* Cornell Nutr. Conf., p. 159. Cornell University, Ithaca, New York.

Shoda, R., Mason, J.B., Selhub, J., and Rosenberg, I.H. (1990). *J. Nutr. Biochem. 1*(5), 257.

Siddons, R.C. (1978). Handbook Series in Nutrition and Food: Section E: Nutritional Disorders (M. Rechcigl Jr., ed.), Vol. 2, p. 123. CRC Press, Boca Raton, Florida.

Slinger, S.J., Razzaque, A., and Cho, C.Y. (1979). *Proc. World Symp. Finfish Nutr. Fishfeed Technol. 2*, 425.

Stancic, B., Piuko, J., Grafenau, P., Sijacic, L., Laurincik, J., Oberfranc, M., and Sahinovic, R. (1993). *J. Farm Anim. Sci. 26*, 13.

Tamura, T., Shane, B., Baer, M.T., King, J.C., Margen, S., and Stokstad, E.L.R. (1978). *Am. J. Clin. Nutr. 31*, 1984.

Tani, M., and Iwai, K. (1984). *J. Nutr. 114*, 778.

Taylor, L.W. (1947). *Poult. Sci. 26*, 372.

Thenen, S.W., Hwang, S.M., Blocker, D.E., and Meadows, C.A. (1991). *Int. J. Vitam. Nutr. Res. 61*, 310.

Tremblay, G.F., Matte, J.J., Lemieux, L., and Brisson, G.J. (1986). *J. Anim. Sci. 63*, 1173.

Tremblay, G.F., Matte, J.J., Dufour, J.J., and Brisson, G.J. (1989). *J. Anim. Sci. 67*, 724.

Trugo, N.M.F., Donangelo, C.M., Koury, J.C., Freitas, L.A., and Feldheim, W. (1991). *Ecol. Food Nutr. 25*, 333.

Ueland, P.M., Refsum, H., and Brattström, L. (1992). *In* Cardiovascular Disease, Hemostasis, and Endothelial Function (R.B. Francis Jr., ed.), p. 183. Marcel Dekker, New York.

Vallet, J.L., Christenson, R.K., and Klemcke, H.G. (1999). *J. Anim. Sci. 77*, 1236.

Verbeeck, J. (1975). *Feedstuffs 47*(36), 4, 45.

Wagner, C. (1984). Nutrition Reviews: Present Knowledge in Nutrition (R.E. Olson, H.P. Broquist, C.O. Chichester, W.J. Darby, A.C. Kolbye, and R.M. Stalvey, eds.), 5th Ed. Nutrition Foundation, Washington, D.C.

Wagner, C. (1995). *In* Folate in Health and Disease (L.B. Bailey, ed.), p. 23. Marcel Dekker, New York.

Wagner, C. (1996). *J. Nutr. 126*, 1228S.

Wagonfeld, J.B., Dudzinsky, D., and Rosenberg, I.H. (1975). *Clin. Res. 23*, 259(Abstr.).

Welch, A.D., Heinle, R.W., Sharpe, G., George, W.L., and Epstein, M. (1947). *Proc. Soc. Exp. Biol. Med. 65*, 364.

White, W.E., Yielding, K.L., and Krumdieck, C.L. (1976). *Biochem. Biophys. Acta. 429*, 689.

Wiese, A.C., Johnson, B.C., Mitchell, H.H., and Nevens, W.B. (1947). *J. Dairy Sci. 30*, 87.

Young, R.J., Norris, L.C., and Heuser, G.F. (1955). *J. Nutr. 55*, 353.

VITAMIN B$_{12}$

INTRODUCTION

Vitamin B$_{12}$ was the last vitamin to be discovered (1948) and the most potent of the vitamins, with the lowest concentrations required to meet daily requirements. Vitamin B$_{12}$ is unique in that it is synthesized in nature only by microorganisms; therefore, it is usually not found in plant feedstuffs. Consequently, humans and other monogastric species who subsist entirely on plant foods would be susceptible to vitamin B$_{12}$ deficiency. It is also unique in that the trace element cobalt is an integral part of the molecule.

The discovery of this vitamin was dramatic and made possible by the combined efforts of microbiologists, biochemists, nutrition scientists, and physicians working in various laboratories. Three seemingly unrelated conditions attributed to lack of the vitamin or its precursor were identified: (1) a fatal anemia in humans, (2) a potent growth factor for monogastric species, and (3) a relationship to cobalt, the lack of which resulted in wasting diseases in ruminants.

HISTORY

The history of vitamin B$_{12}$ in human and animal nutrition is both exciting and stimulating and has been reviewed (Sebrell and Harris, 1968; Folkers, 1982; Loosli, 1991). In 1824 Combe described a fatal anemia, pernicious anemia, and suggested that it could be related to a disorder of the digestive tract. The existence of an unknown factor in liver, effective in treatment of pernicious anemia, was recognized in 1926 when Minot and Murphy showed that large amounts (120 to 240 g/day) of raw liver given by mouth daily would alleviate this previously

13

fatal disease. In 1920 Whipple provided liver in diets to dogs and showed regenerated blood and a specific liver protein that was needed for the formation of hemoglobin. Minot, Murphy, and Whipple received the Nobel Prize in 1934 for liver therapy of pernicious anemia. Two years after the Nobel Prize was awarded it became apparent that the reason the dogs responded to liver was the iron content of the liver and not the vitamin B_{12} content.

During the next 20 years following the Minot and Murphy discovery, research resulted in concentrating the activity of 400 g of liver to 1 mg of active substance. From 1929 onward, Castle postulated that pernicious anemia was due to the interaction of a dietary (extrinsic) factor and an intrinsic factor produced by the stomach. Mixing beef muscle and gastric juice prevented anemia; thus a factor in gastric juice was the intrinsic factor, while a different substance in beef muscle was the extrinsic factor. Castle took the extraordinary step of using his own stomach to process food for his anemic patients, then regurgitated his partially digested meals to supplement their diets.

For many years following the discovery that liver contained a substance that could cause remission of pernicious anemia, scientists tried unsuccessfully to isolate from liver the antipernicious anemia (APA) factor. Progress was slow because no experimental animal for laboratory trials exhibited this condition, thus human patients with pernicious anemia were required for experimental studies. In 1947 Shorb of the University of Maryland reported that a factor (LLD factor) in liver extract required by the bacterium *Lactobacillus lacatis* Dorner was in concentrations bearing an almost linear relationship to the APA activity of the extract. Making use of this organism, Rickes and coworkers in the United States in 1948, isolated, in crystalline form, a factor from the liver that cured pernicious anemia. They named this factor vitamin B_{12}. Three weeks after the Rickes and coworkers publication, a similar article from Smith of Great Britain also indicated isolation of the APA factor. West (1948) confirmed the clinical activity of the vitamin, which prevented pernicious anemia with a single dose of 3 to 6 µg. During these early years of isolating the APA factor, the production of 15 mg of crystalline vitamin B_{12} required 1,000 kg of fresh liver.

Although isolated by the two laboratories in 1948, it was not until 1956 that the complicated vitamin B_{12} structure was ascertained. In 1961 Lenhert and Hodgkin reported the structure of the enzyme form of vitamin B_{12}. In 1964 another Nobel Prize was awarded to Hodgkin for her part in the elucidation of the chemical structure of vitamin B$_{12}$ by x-ray crystallography.

Attempts to raise pigs and chickens by feeding all vegetable diets resulted in poor performance. In 1926 it was recognized that liver extracts and other concentrates of animal origin stimulated growth of rats, chicks, and pigs. Because the true nature of the active principle of such animal products was unknown, it was called animal protein factor (APF). It was also referred to as the chick growth factor, and the same factor was found essential for hatchability. Manure from cattle (cow manure factor) was also found to contain the factor. The APF found in animal excrement was particularly potent in the summer, when feces were rich in bacteria. This led to the isolation of a microorganism from chicken feces and its cultivation in a simple fermentation medium. The discovery of microbial production of vitamin B$_{12}$ opened the way to economical industrial production of vitamin B$_{12}$, which is based entirely on bacterial fermentation.

Vitamin B$_{12}$ became available for animal experiments in 1948 as the crystalline vitamin B$_{12}$ was isolated from liver and crude fermentation products, which contained considerable concentrations of the vitamin. To the surprise of researchers, the growth effect of pure vitamin B$_{12}$ in animals was not quite as good as that observed from APF supplements. Eventually, it was found that crude vitamin B$_{12}$ concentrates contained more than one active principle, namely, vitamin B$_{12}$, some essential amino acids, and small concentrations of compounds with antibiotic activity. The growth-promoting effects of antibiotics were discovered practically as a by-product of research on vitamin B$_{12}$ in animal nutrition. These discoveries were important considerations to providing complete confinement for certain classes of livestock.

The significance of vitamin B$_{12}$ for ruminants was discovered to be the requirement of cobalt by rumen microorganisms in order to synthesize the vitamin (McDowell, 1985, 1992). Cobalt, the central ion in vitamin B$_{12}$, was shown to be a dietary essential for sheep in 1935 by Underwood and others in Australia (Underwood, 1977). The Australians showed that the deficiency caused debilitating diseases of sheep known as "coast disease" and "wasting disease." In Florida in 1937, cobalt deficiency was reported by Becker and coworkers (1965) to be responsible in part for "salt sick" cattle, describing a severe wasting disease. In 1951, Smith and coworkers at Cornell discovered that injections of vitamin B$_{12}$ prevented all signs of cobalt deficiency.

CHEMICAL STRUCTURE, PROPERTIES, AND ANTAGONISTS

Vitamin B_{12} is now considered by nutritionists as the generic name for a group of compounds having B_{12} activity. These compounds have very complex structures. The empirical formula of B_{12} is $C_{63}H_{88}O_{14}N_{14}PCo$, and among its unusual features is the content of 4.5% cobalt. The structure of one B_{12} compound, cyanocobalamin, is shown in Fig. 13.1. Vitamin B_{12} resembles a porphyrin structure consisting of four pyrrole nuclei coupled directly to each other, with the inner nitrogen atom of each pyrrole coordinated with a single atom of cobalt. The basic tetrapyrrole structure is the corrin nucleus, which positionally is a planar structure coupled below to the nucleotide 5,6-dimethylbenzimidazole and above to cyanide or some other derivative. The large ring formed by the four reduced rings is called "corrin" because it is the core of the vitamin. The vitamin belongs to the corrinoid group of compounds that have a corrin nucleus; however, numerous other corrinoids do not possess vitamin B_{12} activity. The name "cobalamin" is used for compounds in which the cobalt atom is in the center of the corrin nucleus.

In vitamin B_{12} the base is coupled directly to the cobalt atom, and an ester linkage from the phosphate group of the nucleotide to the propionic acid group of the D ring of the corrin nucleus adds further stability to the molecule. Cyanide, which lies above the planar ring, is attached to the cobalt atom—thus the name cyanocobalamin. The cyanide can be replaced by other groups, including OH (hydroxycobalamin), H_2O (aquacobalamin), NO_2 (nitrocobalamin), and CH_3 (methylcobalamin). All these compounds are referred to as cobalamins and have activity. In addition, several other compounds, referred to as "pseudo" vitamin B_{12} complexes or vitamin B_{12}-like factors that have some activity, have been isolated or synthesized. Their structure differs regarding the nucleotide moiety. These pseudovitamins are probably intermediates of the biosynthesis of vitamin B_{12} and are found in sewage, manure, rumen contents, and residues from fermentation. Some of these pseudovitamin B_{12} compounds are analogs without a nucleotide, while others contain a nucleotide other than 5,6-dimethylbenzimidazole. Some analogs have incorporated other metals (e.g., Cu, Ni, Mn, Fe) into them, but without corrinoids have no biological activity. Some of the corrinoid pseudovitamins that are growth factors for microorganisms not only have no vitamin B_{12} activity, but may be antagonists or antimetabolites of the vitamin.

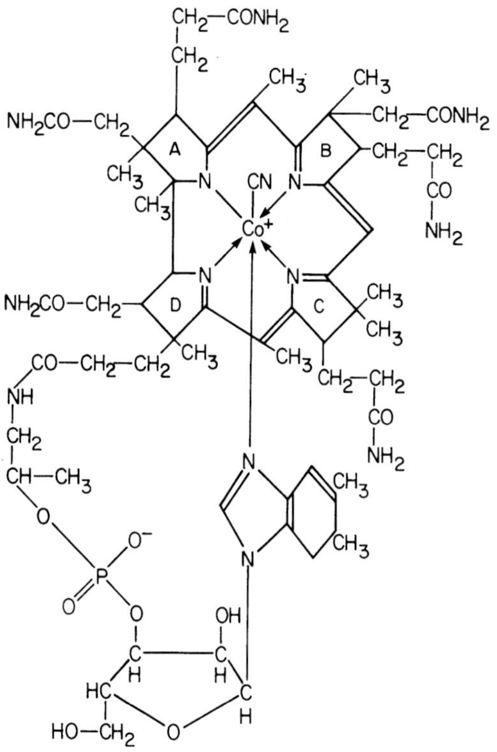

Fig. 13.1 Structure of vitamin B$_{12}$ (cyanocobalamin).

The isolation of coenzyme forms of vitamin B$_{12}$ led to the recognition that cyanocobalamin is not the naturally occurring form of the vitamin but is rather an artifact that arises from the original isolation procedure, which absorbed the vitamin by activated charcoal. Adenosylcobalamin, hydroxocobalamin, methylcobalamin, cyanocobalamin, and sulfitocobalamin have been determined in feedstuffs, with the first three being the most predominant forms in animal tissue (Farquharson and Adams, 1976).

The two coenzyme forms of cobalamin found in animals are adenosylcobalamin and methylcobalamin. Cyanocobalamin, however, is the most widely used form of cobalamin in clinical practice because of its relative availability and stability (particularly to light). Most metabolic studies utilize cyanocobalamin. Hydroxocobalamin is also used in pharmaceutical preparations, and is better retained after parenteral administration than is cyanocobalamin.

Vitamin B_{12} is a dark red, crystalline, hygroscopic substance, freely soluble in water and alcohol but insoluble in acetone, chloroform, or ether. Cyanocobalamin has a molecular weight of 1354 and is the most complex structure and heaviest compound of all the vitamins. Oxidizing and reducing agents and exposure to sunlight tend to destroy its activity. Losses of vitamin B_{12} during cooking are usually not excessive.

ANALYTICAL PROCEDURES

Several techniques are employed for analyses of vitamin B_{12}. Chemical assays, including spectrophotometric and colorimetric procedures, have been developed for pharmaceutical preparations but are not sensitive enough for determination of the vitamin in natural materials (Scott et al., 1982). Colorimetric procedures rely on measurement of cyanide released or a color complex with 5,6-dimethyl-benzimidazole.

Microbiological assays for vitamin B_{12} are sensitive and can be applied to crude materials. Microbiological methods using *L. leichmannii* can determine quantities less than 0.01 µg of the vitamin per milliliter of assay solution. The organism responds, however, to deoxyribonucleosides and to several B_{12} pseudovitamins. Treatment of the sample with alkali destroys vitamin B_{12}, leaving the deoxyribonucleosides intact; thus the vitamin B_{12} plus pseudo forms can be determined by difference. Also, response to deoxyribonucleosides is less serious, since *L. leichmannii* requires about 1,000 times more deoxyribonucleosides than vitamin B_{12} for growth.

The protozoans *Euglena gracilis* and *Ochromonas malhamensis* are also successfully used for vitamin B_{12} determination. Vitamin B_{12} assays involving animals are somewhat more difficult and time-consuming than microbiological assays. Large stores of vitamin B_{12} found in young, growing animals reared from normal mothers present the biggest problem (Ellenbogen and Cooper, 1991). A biological assay for vitamin B_{12} uses growth of chicks hatched from eggs of vitamin B_{12}-deficient hens, and assays have been conducted with young rats born from depleted dams. Thyroid-stimulating material often is added to assay diets to increase the B_{12} requirement in the young animal.

The radioisotope dilution methods for the assay of cobalamins have been replacing the microbiological methods and are used more widely than most other methods. These assays measure the extent to which cobalamin, after first being liberated from bound materials, competes with radioactively labeled cyanocobalamin for binding sites on a protein (Ellenbogen and Cooper, 1991).

Ramoz et al. (1994) reported that the radioassay method was as reliable as the microbiological method for measuring vitamin B_{12} in ovine milk, except for very low levels. A radioimmunoassay was found not to detect vitamin B_{12} concentration in plasma samples containing elevated concentrations of methylmalonic acid (Kennedy et al., 1992b). Muhammad et al. (1993) compared a competitive binding assay with a microbiological assay and found a high correlation between methods for estimating B_{12} concentrations in foods.

METABOLISM

Digestion, Absorption, and Transport

Passage of vitamin B_{12} through the intestinal wall requires intervention of certain carrier compounds able to bind the vitamin molecule. Vitamin B_{12} in the diet is bound to food proteins. In the stomach, the combined effect of gastric acid and peptic digestion releases the vitamin, which is then bound to a nonintrinsic factor–cobalamin complex (Toskes et al., 1973). The nonintrinsic protein that is secreted in the saliva has been named cobalophilin, formerly known as R-proteins, because of their rapid electrophoretic mobility compared with other cobalamin-binding proteins.

Vitamin B_{12} is bound preferentially to cobalophilin in the acid medium of the stomach rather than to intrinsic factor. The B_{12} remains bound to cobalophilin in the slightly alkaline environment of intestine until pancreatic proteases (e.g., trypsin) partially degrade the cobalophilin protein and thereby enable B_{12} to become bound exclusively to intrinsic factor. Therefore, patients with pancreatic insufficiency absorb B_{12} poorly (Jorgensen et al., 1991), and this malabsorption is completely corrected by administration of pancreatic enzymes or purified trypsin.

A prerequisite for intestinal absorption of physiological amounts of cobalamin is binding to intrinsic factor. Intrinsic factor is a glycoprotein (mucoprotein) synthesized and secreted by parietal cells of the gastric mucosa. Atrophy of the fundus, where intrinsic factor is produced, and lack of free HCl (achlorhydria) are usually associated with pernicious anemia (Behrns et al., 1994). Gastric juice defects are responsible for most cases of food-vitamin B_{12} malabsorption (Carmel, 1994). The formation of this intrinsic factor complex protects the vitamin from bacterial utilization and/or degradation as it traverses the lumen of the small intestine to the terminal ileum, where absorption occurs (Ellenbogen and Highley, 1970). The intrinsic factor–B_{12} complex is transiently attached to an ileal receptor. The proximal small intestine does not have the ability to enhance absorption of the vitamin—only the ileum has this property. In the ileum, the intrinsic factor moiety of the intrinsic factor–B_{12} complex binds to a specific receptor protein on the microvillus membrane of brush borders of intestinal epithelial cells. Next there is transport of vitamin B_{12} from the receptor intrinsic factor–B_{12} complex through the epithelial cell to portal blood.

The absorption of vitamin B_{12} is limited by the number of intrinsic factor–vitamin B_{12} binding sites in the ileal mucosa, so that not more than about 1 to 1.5 μg of a single oral dose of the vitamin in humans can be absorbed (Bender, 1992). The absorption is also slow; peak blood concentrations of the vitamin are not achieved for some 6 to 8 hours after an oral dose.

When B_{12} enters the portal blood, it is no longer bound to intrinsic factor but to specific transport proteins called transcobalamins. Three binding proteins have been identified in normal human serum and are designated as transcobalamin I, II, and III. The transcobalamins are synthesized by several tissues, including intestinal mucosa and liver, and have been shown to deliver B_{12} to various tissues, such as liver, kidney, spleen, heart, lung, and small intestine (Rothenberg and Cotter, 1978). Transcobalamin II appears to be primarily concerned with transport of vitamin B_{12}, whereas transcobalamin I is involved in storage of the vitamin.

The function of transcobalamin III is to provide a mechanism for returning vitamin B_{12} from peripheral tissues to the liver, as well as for clearance of other corrinoids without vitamin activity (e.g., undesired analogs of B_{12}), which may arise either from foods or from the products of intestinal bacterial action and be absorbed passively across the lower gut (Bender, 1992). These corrinoids are then secreted into the bile, bound to cobalophilins. Like dietary vitamin B_{12} bound to salivary cobalophilin, the biliary cobalophilins are hydrolyzed in the duodenum, and the released vitamin B_{12} binds to intrinsic factor, permitting reabsorption into the ileum.

To summarize, B_{12} absorption for most species studied requires the following: (1) adequate quantities of dietary B_{12}, (2) normal stomach for breakdown of food proteins for release of B_{12}, (3) normal production of cobalophilin (nonintrinsic factor) secreted in saliva, (4) normal stomach for production of intrinsic factor for absorption of B_{12} through the ileum, (5) normal pancrease (trypsin) required for release of bound B_{12}

prior to combining the vitamin with the intrinsic factor, and (6) normal ileum with receptor and absorption sites. Additional factors that diminish vitamin B$_{12}$ absorption include deficiencies of protein, iron, and vitamin B$_6$; thyroid removal; and dietary tannic acid (Anonymous, 1984).

Intrinsic-factor concentrates prepared from one animal's stomach do not in all cases increase B$_{12}$ absorption in other species or in humans. There are structural differences in the B$_{12}$ intrinsic factor among species. Likewise, species differences exist for B$_{12}$ transport proteins (Polak et al., 1979). Intrinsic factor has been demonstrated in the human, monkey, dog, pig, rat, cow, ferret, rabbit, hamster, fox, lion, tiger, and leopard. It has not been detected in the guinea pig, horse, sheep, chicken, or a number of other species. The dog stomach produces only small amounts of intrinsic factor, with larger amounts produced by the pancreas (Simpson et al., 1989).

Absorption of vitamin B$_{12}$ does not completely depend on active intervention of the intrinsic factor. Both active and passive mechanisms exist for absorption of B$_{12}$ (Herbert, 1990). The passive mechanism, simple diffusion, has low efficiency (approximately 1%) and is operative throughout the digestive tract; it becomes practically important only in the presence of large quantities of the vitamin, in excess of those present in most foods.

About 3% of ingested cobalt is converted to vitamin B$_{12}$ in the rumen. Of the vitamin B$_{12}$ produced, only 1 to 3% is absorbed. In the rumen, iron interacts with cobalt so that iron deficiency enhances cobalt absorption (Keen and Graham, 1989). As in most species, the absorptive site for ruminants is the lower portion of the small intestine. Substantial amounts of B$_{12}$ are secreted into the duodenum and then reabsorbed in the ileum.

Tissue Distribution and Storage

In normal human subjects, vitamin B$_{12}$ is found principally in the liver; the average amount is 1.5 mg. Kidneys, heart, spleen, and brain each contain about 20 to 30 μg (Ellenbogen and Cooper, 1991). Vitamin B$_{12}$ is stored in the liver in the largest quantities for most animals that have been studied, but it is stored in the kidney of the bat. Vitamin B$_{12}$ storage in humans can exceed the daily requirement by about 1,000-fold.

Henderickx et al. (1964) reported a total retention of 20 to 23% of an oral dose of vitamin B$_{12}$ in pigs, about two-thirds of which was present in the liver. Even though vitamin B$_{12}$ is a water-soluble vitamin, there is a considerable degree of tissue storage. The great storage and long biological half-life (350 to 400 days in humans) of the vitamin provides substantial protection against periods of deprivation.

To become metabolically active, vitamin B_{12} must be converted into one of its various coenzyme forms. This transformation takes place mainly in liver but also in kidneys. Most of the cobalamins in humans occur as two coenzymatically active forms, adenosylcobalamin and methylcobalamin. In humans, methylcobalamin constitutes 60 to 80% of total plasma cobalamin, while adenosylcobalamin is the major cobalamin in all cellular tissues, constituting about 60 to 70% in the liver and about 50% in other organs (Ellenbogen and Cooper, 1991). In subjects with pernicious anemia, methylcobalamin is disproportionately reduced in relation to the other major components. Cyanocobalamin is converted within cells to either methylcobalamin, a coenzyme for methyltransferase, or adenosylcobalamin, the coenzyme for mutase.

Excretion

The main excretion of absorbed vitamin B_{12} is via urinary, biliary, and fecal routes. Total body loss ranges from 2 to 5 µg daily in humans (Shinton, 1972). Urinary excretion of the intact vitamin B_{12} by kidney glomerular filtration is minimal. Biliary excretion via feces is the major excretory route. Approximately 0.5 to 5 µg of cobalamin is secreted into the alimentary tract daily, mainly in bile (Ellenbogen and Cooper, 1991). Most of the cobalamin excreted in bile is reabsorbed; at least 65 to 75% is reabsorbed in the ileum by means of the intrinsic factor, active transport mechanism.

FUNCTIONS

Vitamin B_{12} is an essential part of several enzyme systems that carry out a number of very basic metabolic functions. Specific biochemical reactions in which cobalamin coenzymes participate are of two types: (1) those that contain 5′-deoxyadenosine linked covalently to the cobalt atom (adenosylcobalamin) and (2) those that have a methyl group attached to the central cobalt atom (methylcobalamin). A number of vitamin B_{12}-dependent metabolic reactions have been identified in microorganisms; however, only three vitamin B_{12}-dependent enzymes have been discovered in animals: methylmalonyl CoA mutase and leucine mutase, which each require adenosylcobalamin, and methionine synthetase, which requires methylcobalamin. Most reactions requiring adenosylcobalamin can be classified as rearrangement reactions of the carbon skeleton of several metabolic intermediates; a hydrogen atom moves from one carbon atom to an adjacent one in exchange for an alkyl, acyl, or electronegative group, which migrates in the opposite direction (Ellenbogen and Cooper, 1991). In all these rearrangement reactions, adenosylcobalamin is an intermediate hydrogen carrier. The reactions requiring methylcobalamin involve transfer or synthesis of one-carbon units, for example, methyl groups.

Vitamin B$_{12}$ is metabolically related to other essential nutrients, such as choline, methionine, and folacin (Savage and Lindenbaum, 1995). Interrelationships of these nutrients with vitamin B$_{12}$ (and in particular to transmethylation and biosynthesis of labile methyl groups) are discussed in Chapters 12 and 14. Though the most important tasks of vitamin B$_{12}$ concern metabolism of nucleic acids and proteins, it also functions in metabolism of fats and carbohydrates. A summary of B$_{12}$ functions would include (1) purine and pyrimidine synthesis, (2) transfer of methyl groups, (3) formation of proteins from amino acids, and (4) carbohydrate and fat metabolism. A general function of B$_{12}$ is to promote red blood cell synthesis and to maintain nervous system integrity, which are functions noticeably affected in the deficient state.

Vitamin B$_{12}$ is necessary in reduction of one-carbon compounds of formate and formaldehyde, and in this way it participates with folacin in biosynthesis of labile methyl groups. Formation of labile methyl groups is necessary for biosynthesis of purine and pyrimidine bases, which represent essential constituents of nucleic acids. Disorders of nucleic acid synthesis in vitamin B$_{12}$ deficiency are connected with this. The purine bases (adenine and guanine) as well as thymine are constituents of nucleic acids, and with folacin deficiency there is a reduction in biosynthesis of nucleic acids essential for cell formation and function. Hence, deficiency of either folacin or B$_{12}$ leads to impaired cell division and alterations of protein synthesis; these effects are most noticeable in rapidly growing tissues.

Deficiency of B$_{12}$ will induce folacin deficiency by blocking utilization of folacin derivatives. A vitamin B$_{12}$-containing enzyme removes the methyl group from methylfolate, thereby regenerating tetrahydrofolate (THF), from which is made the 5,20-methylene-THF required for thymidylate synthesis. Because methylfolate returns to the body's folacin pool only via the vitamin B$_{12}$-dependent step, vitamin B$_{12}$ deficiency results in folacin being "trapped" as methylfolate, and thus becoming metabolically useless. The "folate trap" concept explains why hematological damage of vitamin B$_{12}$ deficiency is indistinguishable from that of folacin deficiency by alleging that in both instances the defective synthesis of DNA results from the same final common pathway defect, namely, an inadequate quantity of 5,10-methylene-THF to participate adequately in DNA synthesis (Herbert and Zalusky, 1962).

Metabolism of labile methyl groups plays a significant part in biosynthesis of methionine from homocysteine. A vitamin B_{12}-requiring enzyme, 5-methyl-tetrahydrofolate-homocysteine methyltransferase, catalyzes reformation of methionine from homocysteine according to the following reaction:

5-Methyltetrahydrofolate + homocysteine $\rightleftarrows$ methionine + tetrahydrofolate

The mechanism of converting homocysteine to methionine has utilized a methyl group from folacin, the mechanism for maintaining folacin in a reduced form. Activity of this enzyme is depressed in liver of vitamin B_{12}-deficient sheep (MacPherson, 1982), which could lead to a deficiency of available methionine that may account for impairment of nitrogen metabolism in vitamin B_{12}-deficient sheep.

Overall synthesis of protein is impaired in vitamin B_{12}-deficient animals. Wagle et al. (1958) demonstrated that rats and baby pigs deprived of vitamin B_{12} were less able to incorporate serine, methionine, phenylalanine, and glucose into liver proteins. There is good reason to believe that impairment of protein synthesis is the principal reason for the growth depression that is frequently observed in animals deficient in vitamin B_{12} (Friesecke, 1980).

In the metabolism of animals, propionate of dietary or metabolic origin is converted into succinate, which then enters the tricarboxylic acid (Krebs) cycle. Because propionate is a three-carbon and succinate a four-carbon compound, this process requires the introduction of a one-carbon unit. Methylmalonyl-CoA isomerase (mutase) is a vitamin B_{12}-requiring enzyme (5'-deoxyadenosylcobalamin) that catalyzes the conversion of methylmalonyl-CoA to succinyl-CoA. Flavin and Ochoa (1957) established that for succinate production, the following steps are involved:

Propionate + ATP + CoA $\rightleftarrows$ propionyl-CoA
Propionyl-CoA + CO_2 + ATP $\rightleftarrows$ methylmalonyl-CoA (a)
Methylmalonyl-CoA (a) $\rightleftarrows$ methylmalonyl-CoA (b)
Methylmalonyl-CoA (b) $\rightleftarrows$ succinyl-CoA

Methylmalonyl-CoA (a) is an inactive isomer. Its active form (b) is converted into succinyl-CoA by a methylmalonyl isomerase, or methyl-malonyl mutase (fourth reaction).

Vitamin B$_{12}$ is a metabolic essential for all animal species studied, and vitamin B$_{12}$ deficiency can be induced with the addition of high dietary levels of propionic acid. However, metabolism of propionic acid is of special interest in ruminant nutrition because large quantities are produced during carbohydrate fermentation in the rumen. Propionate production proceeds normally, but in cobalt or vitamin B$_{12}$ deficiency, its rate of clearance from blood is depressed, and methylmalonyl-CoA accumulates. This results in increased urinary excretion of methylmalonic acid and in loss of appetite because impaired propionate metabolism leads to higher blood propionate levels, which are inversely correlated to voluntary feed intake (MacPherson, 1982). Injection of cobalt-deficient animals with vitamin B$_{12}$ produces overnight improvement in appetite, whereas oral dosing with cobalt takes 7 to 10 days to produce the same effect.

A further important function of vitamin B$_{12}$ in intermediary metabolism consists of maintaining glutathione and sulfydryl groups of enzymes in the reduced state (Marks, 1975). The reduced activity of glyceraldehyde-3-phosphate dehydrogenase, which needs glutathione as a coenzyme, is possibly responsible for carbohydrate metabolism being impaired in vitamin B$_{12}$ deficiency. Vitamin B$_{12}$ also influences lipid metabolism via its effect on the thiols.

REQUIREMENTS

Vitamin B$_{12}$ requirements are exceedingly small; an adequate allowance is only a few micrograms per kilogram of feed, making B$_{12}$ the most potent of vitamins. Estimated requirements of vitamin B$_{12}$ for various animals and humans are presented in Table 13.1.

The vitamin B$_{12}$ requirements of various species depend on the levels of several other nutrients in the diet. Excess protein increases the need for B$_{12}$ as does performance level (NRC, 1994). The B$_{12}$ requirement depends on levels of choline, methionine, and folacin in the diet and is interrelated with ascorbic acid metabolism (Scott et al., 1982). The requirements for both vitamin B$_{12}$ and folacin are reduced when the diet contains an abundance of compounds that can supply methyl groups. Sewell et al. (1952) showed that B$_{12}$ has a sparing effect on the methionine needs of the pig. A reciprocal relationship occurs between B$_{12}$ and pantothenic acid in chick nutrition, with pantothenic acid sparing the B$_{12}$ requirement. Dietary ingredients may also affect the require-

535

■ Table 13.1   Vitamin B$_{12}$ Requirements for Various Animals and Humans

Animal	Purpose or Class	Requirement[a]	Reference
Beef cattle	Adult	Microbial synthesis[b]	NRC (1996)
Dairy cattle	Calf (milk replacer)	0.07 ppm	NRC (1989a)
	Adult	Microbial synthesis[b]	NRC (1989a)
Chicken	Leghorn, 0–6 weeks	9 µg/kg	NRC (1994)
	Leghorn, 6–18 weeks	3 µg/kg	NRC (1994)
	Laying (100-g intake)	4 µg/kg	NRC (1994)
	Broilers, 0–6 weeks	10 µg/kg	NRC (1994)
	Broilers, 6–8 weeks	7 µg/kg	NRC (1994)
Japanese quail	All classes	3 µg/kg	NRC (1994)
Turkey	All classes	3 µg/kg	NRC (1994)
Sheep	Adult	Microbial synthesis[b]	NRC (1985b)
Swine	Growing-finishing	5–20 µg/kg	NRC (1998)
	Breeding-lactating	15 µg/kg	NRC (1998)
Horse	Adult	Microbial synthesis	NRC (1989b)
Goat	Adult	Microbial synthesis[b]	NRC (1981)
Dog	Growing	26 µg/kg	NRC (1985a)
Cat	Growing	20 µg/kg	NRC (1986)
Mink	All classes	30 µg/kg	NRC (1982a)
Rabbit	All classes	Microbial synthesis	NRC (1977)
Fish	Pacific salmon	15–20 µg/kg	NRC (1993)
	Yellowtail	53 µg/kg	NRC (1993)
Rat	Growing	50 µg/kg	NRC (1995)
Hamster	Growing	10 µg/kg	NRC (1995)
Human	Infants	0.3–0.5 µg/day	RDA (1989)
	Children	0.7–1.4 µg/day	RDA (1989)
	Adults	2 µg/day	RDA (1989)
	Pregnancy-lactation	2.2–2.6 µg/day	RDA (1989)

[a]Expressed as per unit of animal feed on either as-fed (approximately 90% dry matter) or dry basis (see Appendix, Tables A1a,b). Human data are expressed as µg/day.

[b]Only young ruminants have a dietary need for B$_{12}$ prior to ruminal development. Practical vitamin B$_{12}$ deficiency is a secondary result of cobalt deficiency. Suggested cobalt requirements for ruminants range from 0.07 to 0.2 mg/kg of diet.

ment, as wheat bran has been known to reduce availability of vitamin B$_{12}$ in humans (Lewis et al., 1986).

Dietary need depends on intestinal synthesis and tissue reserves at birth. Intestinal synthesis probably explains frequent failures to produce B$_{12}$ deficiency in pigs and rats on diets designed to be B$_{12}$ free. The deficiency can be readily produced in rats, however, when coprophagy is completely prevented (Barnes and Fiala, 1958). Coprophagous animals and poultry on deep litter receive excellent supplies of B$_{12}$ from microbial fermentation. Litter would be a less valuable source of vitamin B$_{12}$ under cold conditions, in which bacterial numbers are greatly reduced. Poultry obtain some vitamin B$_{12}$ by direct absorption of the vitamin produced by bacterial synthesis in the intestine (NRC, 1994), however, the amount from this source is not reliable.

Intestinal microfloral synthesis of vitamin B$_{12}$ has been demonstrated in common carp, channel catfish, Nile tilapia, rainbow trout, ayu, and goldfish (NRC, 1993). Sugita et al. (1991) found a close relationship between the amount of vitamin B$_{12}$ and the viable counts of *Bacteroides* type A in the intestinal contents of the various fish studied. They found that this bacterium was present in the intestinal contents of fish that do not require vitamin B$_{12}$ and was absent in fish that do require the vitamin.

Requirement for vitamin B$_{12}$ in ruminant diets is closely associated with the requirement for cobalt since this trace mineral is a component of the B$_{12}$ molecule. Ruminant animals have the ability to synthesize vitamin B$_{12}$ provided they are supplied with an adequate dietary supply of cobalt (0.07 to 0.2 ppm) and have a normally functioning rumen. Under typical conditions a rumen would be functional for synthesis of all B vitamins at 6 to 8 weeks of age. Therefore, only young ruminants that do not have a fully developed rumen would be expected to require a dietary source of B$_{12}$.

Cobalt content of the diet is the primary limiting factor for synthesis of vitamin B$_{12}$ by ruminal microflora. However, studies indicate that synthesis of vitamin B$_{12}$ could be restricted even when the diet is adequate in cobalt, as several factors can influence synthesis and perhaps utilization. For animals on high-concentrate diets, there is a decrease in vitamin B$_{12}$ synthesis, and more analogs are produced than the vitamin itself (Sutton and Elliot, 1972). These natural analogs have little or no vitamin B$_{12}$ activity. Lopez-Guisa and Satter (1992) suggested that cobalt and copper requirements higher than NRC recommendations may aid in digestibility of low-quality forages (i.e., corn crop residues), but cobalt was without effect for digestibility of high-quality forages (Hussein et al., 1994).

The established dietary cobalt requirements for ruminants are 0.1 to 0.2 mg/kg of diet (NRC, 1985b, 1989a, 1996). It has been suggested that the requirement for vitamin B$_{12}$ in dairy cattle is between 0.34 and 0.68 µg/kg of live weight (NRC, 1989a). Precise estimates of minimum cobalt requirements are difficult because of the influence of many variables, such as seasonal changes in herbage cobalt concentrations, selective grazing habits, and soil contamination. Under grazing conditions, lambs are the most sensitive to cobalt deficiency, followed by mature sheep, calves, and mature cattle (Andrews, 1956).

Ruminants have higher vitamin B$_{12}$ requirements than nonruminants, presumably because of its involvement in the metabolism of propionic acid. Vitamin B$_{12}$ is essential as a cofactor for methyl-malonyl-

CoA isomerase, an enzyme necessary for propionic acid utilization that is produced in much greater quantities in ruminants. Experiments with sheep suggest an oral requirement for growing lambs of some 200 μg/day, about 10 times the reported oral requirement of other species per unit of food intake (Marston, 1970). The surprisingly high requirement of ruminants for cobalt arises partly from the low efficiency of production of vitamin B_{12} from cobalt by the rumen microorganisms and partly from the low efficiency of absorption of vitamin B_{12}.

It has been reported that grass in healthy areas contains around 0.1 mg of cobalt per kg (dry basis) of cobalt or more, on the average, as compared with 0.05 to 0.07 mg/kg for deficient areas. As little as 0.1 mg/kg has restored sick animals to health. Further evidence of 0.1 mg/kg as the dietary requirement for sheep was provided by Mohammed (1983), who fed various levels of cobalt and found that vitamin B_{12} and propionic acid in rumen concentrations were maximal at 0.1 mg of cobalt per kg.

Vitamin B_{12} requirements for humans have been estimated from three different types of studies (Ellenbogen and Cooper, 1991): (1) determination of the amount necessary to treat megaloblastic anemia from vitamin B_{12} deficiency, (2) comparison of blood and liver concentration in normal and cobalamin-deficient subjects, and (3) body stores and turnover rates of the vitamin. Obviously, the requirement for B_{12} will be substantially higher for humans lacking intrinsic factor or other conditions that affect absorption and metabolism of the vitamin (see Metabolism).

For adults, recommendations vary from 1 to 2 μg of vitamin B_{12} daily. Higher vitamin B_{12} requirements would be for pregnancy; during the last half, the fetus removes 0.2 μg daily from maternal stores, and during lactation, 0.3 μg is lost daily in breast milk (Herbert, 1990).

NATURAL SOURCES

The origin of vitamin B_{12} in nature appears to be microbial synthesis. It is synthesized by many bacteria but apparently not by yeasts or by most fungi. There is little evidence that the vitamin is produced in tissues of higher plants or animals. A few reports have suggested limited B_{12} synthesis by a few plants, but in insignificant quantities in relation to animal requirements. Synthesis of this vitamin in the alimentary tract is of considerable importance for animals; if sufficient cobalt is available, ruminants are independent of external sources of vitamin B_{12}.

Foods of animal origin are reasonably good sources, including meat,

■ Table 13.2 Vitamin B$_{12}$ Concentrations of Various
Foods and Feedstuffs (ppb, dry basis)

Blood meal	49
Corn, grain	0
Crab meal	475
Distiller's solubles	3
Fish solubles	1007
Fish meal, anchovy	233
Fish meal, herring	467
Fish meal, menhaden	133
Fish meal, tuna	324
Horse meat	142
Liver meal	542
Meat meal	72
Milk, skim, cow's	54
Poultry by-product meal	322
Soybean meal	0
Spleen, cow	247
Wheat, grain	1
Whey, cow	20
Yeast	1

Source: NRC (1982b).

liver, kidney, milk, eggs, and fish (Table 13.2). Milk and milk products are good sources of vitamin B$_{12}$, but the vitamin content is reduced considerably in whey (Sato et al., 1997). Kidney and liver are excellent sources, and these organs are richer in vitamin B$_{12}$ from ruminants than from most nonruminants. In one study, goat milk was found to contain significantly less vitamin B$_{12}$ than cow milk (Dostalova, 1994). Vitamin B$_{12}$ presence in tissues of animals is due to the ingestion of vitamin B$_{12}$ in animal foods or from intestinal or ruminal synthesis. Among the richest sources are fermentation residues, activated sewage sludge, and manure.

Plant products are practically devoid of vitamin B$_{12}$. The vitamin B$_{12}$ reported in higher plants in small amounts may result from synthesis by soil microorganisms and excretion of the vitamin into soil, with subsequent absorption by the plant. Root nodules of certain legumes contain small quantities of B$_{12}$. Certain species of seaweed (algae) have been reported to contain appreciable quantities of vitamin B$_{12}$ (up to 1 μg/g of solids). Seaweed does not synthesize vitamin B$_{12}$, but it is synthesized by the bacteria associated with seaweed and then concentrated by the seaweed (Scott et al., 1982).

Little is known about the bioavailability of orally ingested B$_{12}$ in foods and feeds. Dagnelie et al. (1991) reported that vitamin B$_{12}$ from algae is largely unavailable. Providing algae to B_{12}-deficient children was ineffective in elevating blood parameters compared to B_{12} from fish sources. Vitamin B_{12} was found to be more available in pasteurized milk (1.91 pmol/ml) than in raw milk (1.54 pmol/ml), sterilized milk (1.25 pmol/ml), and dried milk (1.27 pmol/ml), indicating that heat treatment probably affects the bioavailability (Fie et al., 1994).

To supply the ruminant with vitamin B_{12}, the important consideration is dietary sources of cobalt. Although most feeds are adequate in cobalt, the element is deficient in forages for the grazing ruminant in many parts of the world (McDowell, 1985, 1992). Concentration of cobalt in crops and forages is dependent on soil factors, plant species, stage of maturity, yield, pasture management, climate, and soil pH. Soil containing less than 2 mg/kg of cobalt is generally considered deficient for ruminants (Corrêa, 1957). Raising the pH by liming reduces the cobalt uptake by the plant and may increase the severity of the deficiency. Plants grown on 15-ppm cobalt soil that is neutral or slightly acid may contain more cobalt than those grown on 40-ppm cobalt alkaline soil (Latteur, 1962). High rainfall tends to leach cobalt from the topsoil. This problem is often aggravated by rapid growth of forage during the rainy season, which dilutes the cobalt content. Plants have varying degrees of affinity for cobalt, some being able to concentrate the element much more than others. Legumes, for example, generally have greater ability to concentrate cobalt than do grasses (Underwood, 1977). Cobalt is needed by the N-fixing bacteria in the root nodules of legumes.

DEFICIENCY

The result of vitamin B_{12} deficiency in humans is megaloblastic anemia (pernicious anemia) and neurological lesions. Vitamin B_{12} deficiency in humans usually is conditioned by a deficiency of intrinsic factor necessary for its absorption or is found in humans consuming strict vegetarian diets. In animals, pernicious anemia—or in fact any anemia—is not characteristic of vitamin B_{12} shortage. In rats, guinea pigs, swine, and poultry, vitamin B_{12} functions as a growth factor, although mild anemia does occur in a small percentage of deficient swine. In ruminants, vitamin B_{12} deficiency is closely associated with their requirement for cobalt, since the trace mineral is a component of the B_{12} molecule. In all species, as vitamin B_{12} deficiency progresses, depletion of vitamin B_{12} (and cobalt) occurs concurrently in serum and tissue reserves.

Effects of Deficiency

Ruminants

Vitamin B$_{12}$ deficiency can occur in young ruminants as long as the microflora of the forestomachs is not yet far enough developed and hence unable to furnish sufficient amounts of the vitamin. Lassiter et al. (1953) demonstrated vitamin B$_{12}$ deficiency in calves less than 6 weeks old that received no dietary animal protein. Clinical signs characterizing the deficiency included poor appetite and growth, muscular weakness, demyelination of peripheral nerves, and poor general condition. Young lambs (up to 2 months of age), if weaned early, likewise had a need for dietary vitamin B$_{12}$ (NRC, 1985b). In vitamin B$_{12}$-deficient lambs, there was a sharp decrease of vitamin B$_{12}$ concentrations in blood and liver before signs like anorexia, loss of body weight, and a decrease in hemoglobin concentration were observed. Sheep were more sensitive to cobalt deficiency than cattle, and Mburu et al. (1993) suggested that sheep are likewise less resistant to low dietary cobalt than goats, based on blood parameters.

As cobalt is required for biosynthesis of vitamin B$_{12}$, lack of cobalt may cause deficiency of the vitamin in adult ruminants. Cobalt-deficient soils occur in large areas of many countries, therefore grazing ruminants may be particularly affected by the deficiency. With the exception of phosphorus and copper, cobalt deficiency is the most extensive mineral limitation to grazing livestock in tropical countries (McDowell, 1997).

Cobalt deficiency signs are not specific, and it is often difficult to distinguish between an animal with cobalt deficiency and malnutrition due to low intake of energy and protein and an animal that is diseased or parasitized. Acute clinical signs of cobalt deficiency include lack of appetite, rough hair coat, thickening of the skin, anemia (normocytic and normochromic), wasting away (Fig. 13.2), and eventually death, if the animals are not moved to "healthy" pastures or if cobalt supplements are not made available.

Cobalt deficiency has been reported to reduce lamb survival and increase susceptibility to parasitic infection in cattle and sheep (Ferguson et al., 1988; Suttle and Jones, 1989). Cobalt deficiency was associated with photosensitization of lambs, characterized by a swollen head (Hesselink and Vellema, 1990). The condition responded to two injections of vitamin B$_{12}$ 3 weeks apart. Cobalt-deficient ewes produced fewer lambs and had more stillbirths and neonatal mortality than cobalt-sufficient

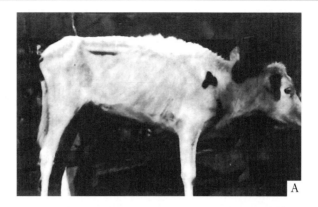

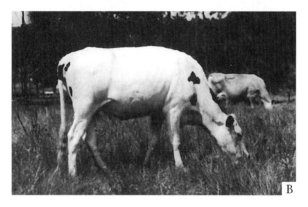

Fig. 13.2 (A) A cobalt-deficient heifer that had access to an iron-copper salt supplement. Note severe emaciation, which resulted from failure to synthesize B_{12}. Her blood contained 6.6 g of hemoglobin per 100 ml on February 25, 1937. (B) The same heifer fully recovered with an iron-copper-cobalt salt supplement while on the same pasture. (Courtesy of R.B. Becker, University of Florida.)

controls (Fisher and MacPherson, 1991). Lambs from deficient ewes were also slower to start suckling. Auricular myocardial necrosis was reported in cobalt-deficient sheep (Mohammed and Lamand, 1986).

At necropsy, the body of a severely affected cobalt-deficient animal presents a picture of extreme emaciation, often with a total absence of body fat. The liver is fatty, the spleen hemosiderized, and in some animals there is hypoplasia of the erythrogenic tissue in the bone marrow (Filmer, 1933). The anemia in lambs is normocytic and normochromic, but the mild anemia is not responsible for the main signs of cobalt deficiency. Inappetence and marasmus invariably precede any considerable degree of anemia. Clinical signs of cobalt deficiency are identical to those of simple starvation, and may indicate that the signs observed with adequate cobalt may be simply due to the inappetence caused by the lack of cobalt. The first discernible response to cobalt feeding or parenteral vitamin B$_{12}$ is rapid improvement in appetite and body weight.

Two other conditions attributed to cobalt deficiency are ovine white liver disease and Phalaris staggers (Graham, 1991; McDowell, 1992; Kennedy et al., 1994b). Ovine white liver disease is characterized by hepatic lipidosis and emaciation. At necropsy, affected lambs had pale, swollen, and friable fatty livers and showed accumulation of lipofuscin (Kennedy et al., 1994b). Alteration in choline synthesis presumably leads to impaired lipid mobilization, but white liver disease may be complicated by other factors. Similarly, the persistent neural effects of *Phalaris* spp., inducing Phalaris staggers, have been shown to be preventable with oral cobalt supplementation, but not with B$_{12}$.

Prior to the recognition of cobalt deficiency in livestock in many parts of the world, cattle could be maintained on deficient pastures only if they periodically were relocated to so-called healthy ground. Cobalt deficiency can be prevented by moving animals for a few months every year to a healthy region, preferably during the rainy season. An example of the necessity of periodically moving animals was illustrated in a disease condition known as "togue" in Espirito Santo, Brazil (Tokarnia et al., 1971). The disease was observed when animals stayed for longer than 60 to 180 days on certain pastures. Sick animals isolated themselves from the rest of the herd; were apathetic; showed loss of appetite, rough hair coat, and dry feces; and lost body condition. If the animals were not moved from the pasture, they died, but if they were taken to a pasture where the disease did not occur, the animals recovered quickly.

Cobalt subclinical deficiencies or borderline states are extremely common and are characterized by low production rates unaccompanied by clinical manifestations or visible signs (McDowell, 1985). Subclinical deficiencies often go unnoticed, thereby resulting in great economic losses to the livestock industry. No estimate can be made of the effect of cobalt subdeficiency on animal performance in general, but in many areas of the world, it is one of the major causes of poor production.

Swine

The general signs of vitamin B$_{12}$ deficiency in pigs are comparable to those observed in other species, principally a loss of appetite, variable feed intake, and a dramatic growth decline (Fig. 13.3). In addition,

543

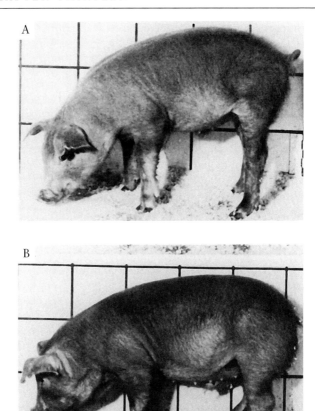

Fig. 13.3 (A) Vitamin B_{12}-deficient pig. Note rough hair coat and dermatitis. (B) Control pig. (Courtesy of the late D.V. Catron and Iowa State University.)

sometimes there is rough skin and hair coat, vomiting and diarrhea, voice failure, and slight anemia (Catron et al., 1952). Microcytic to normocytic anemia is typical; however, observations on anemia are not unanimous and are sometimes contradictory. Nervous disorders occur in the pig, including increased excitability, and unsteady gait (i.e., hind leg incoordination). The thymus and spleen become atrophied, while liver and tongue are frequently enlarged as a result of proliferation of granulomatous tissue.

In the reproducing animal, litter size and pig survival are reduced. Abortions, small litters and birth weights, some deformities, and inability to rear young occur in breeding sows. Later estrus, fewer corpora lutea, and fewer embryos are produced in B$_{12}$-deficient animals. During reproduction and lactation, vitamin B$_{12}$ supplementation was shown to increase birth weight and survival of young pigs (Vestal et al., 1950). Frederick and Brisson (1961) found that sows deficient in vitamin B$_{12}$ had fewer pigs, and these had a lower viability than the pigs born from sows that were supplemented with vitamin B$_{12}$. Successive litters from deficient sows became progressively weaker. In a study of sows supplemented with 80 to 100 μg of vitamin B$_{12}$ daily during pregnancy, there were improved piglet and litter weights and a decreased percentage of stillbirths (Reinisch and Gebhardt, 1987). Under some conditions, reproductive performance of sows were improved by inclusion of higher than recommended levels of dietary vitamin B$_{12}$ (Cunha, 1977). The response was evidenced by an increase in litter size and birth weight of pigs.

Poultry

In growing chicks, turkey poults, and quail, vitamin B$_{12}$ deficiency reduces body weight gain, feed intake, and feed conversion. Vitamin B$_{12}$ deficiency in growing chicks and turkeys may result in a nervous disorder and defective feathering. It has also been related to leg weakness and perosis; however, this appears to be a secondary effect. Perosis may occur in vitamin B$_{12}$-deficient chicks or poults when the diet lacks choline, methionine, or betaine as sources of methyl groups. Addition of B$_{12}$ may prevent perosis under these conditions because of its effect on synthesis of methyl groups. Additional clinical signs in B$_{12}$ deficiency include anemia, gizzard erosion, and fattiness of heart, liver, and kidneys. Poor feathering and mortality are the most obvious signs of vitamin B$_{12}$ deficiency, and gizzard erosions may also appear (NRC, 1994).

In hens, body weight and egg production are maintained despite deficiency, but B$_{12}$ has an important influence on egg size (Scott et al., 1982). However, Squires and Naber (1992) reported that both egg production and hen weight increased with vitamin B$_{12}$ supplementation, as well as increased hatchability and egg weight.

Hatchability of incubated eggs may be severely reduced if the breeder diet contains inadequate vitamin B$_{12}$. Changes that manifest themselves in vitamin B$_{12}$-deficient chick embryos (Olcese et al., 1950) may be summarized as (1) general hemorrhagic condition; (2) fatty liver in varying degrees; (3) heart often enlarged and irregular in shape; (4) kidneys pale or yellow, sometimes hemorrhagic, incidence of perosis; (5) myoatrophy of the leg; (6) fewer myelinated fibers in the spinal cord; and (7) high incidence of embryonic malpositions. Hypertrophy of the thyroid gland has also been repeatedly observed (Ferguson and Couch, 1954).

The most obvious change in B_{12}-deficient embryos is myoatrophy of the leg, a condition characterized by atrophy of thigh muscles (Olcese et al., 1950). Two to 5 months may be needed to deplete hens of vitamin B_{12} stores to such an extent that progeny will hatch with low vitamin B_{12} reserves. The rate of depletion is most rapid when hens are fed high-protein diets (Scott et al., 1982). Chicks that hatch without adequate carryover of vitamin B_{12} from the dam have a high rate of mortality. Vitamin B_{12}-deficient embryos die at about day 17.

Horses

Vitamin B_{12} deficiency has not been described in the horse. It has been concluded that for mature horses, supplemental vitamin B_{12} is not necessary, as the vitamin can be synthesized in the large intestine, where it is absorbed (NRC, 1989b). Davies (1971) subsequently demonstrated increased vitamin B_{12} concentration in gut contents from stomach to rectum. Values (ng/ml) were as follows: stomach, 4; small intestine, 5; cecum, 30; ventral colon, 84; dorsal colon, 197; and small colon, 301. These increasing concentrations were presumably the consequence of synthesis by intestinal anaerobes. Of 97 gut microbe isolates, 47% were found to produce vitamin B_{12} in vitro.

Even with low dietary cobalt intake, B_{12} deficiency would not be expected because dietary cobalt levels greatly exceed the theoretical need for vitamin B_{12} synthesis. In addition, horses have remained in good health while grazing pastures so low in cobalt that cattle and sheep confined to them have died (Filmer, 1933).

Other Animal Species

BATS

Neurological impairment associated with experimentally induced vitamin B_{12} deficiency was produced in bats (Vieira-Makings et al., 1990). Methionine, valine, and isoleucine have been shown to delay onset of the deficiency.

DOGS AND CATS

Vitamin B_{12}-deficient kittens exhibited poor growth, lethargy, emaciation and a high level of methylmalonic acid excretion (Keesling and Morris, 1975; Vaden et al., 1992). Morris (1977) reported that kittens given a vitamin B_{12}-deficient diet at first grew normally for 3 to 4 months, after which growth ceased. Subsequently, body weight was lost at an accelerating rate until supplementation was initiated with parenteral vitamin B$_{12}$, which restored weight gain.

Vitamin B$_{12}$ deficiency has been described in the dog (NRC, 1985a). Earlier reports noted reduced growth (Arnrich et al., 1952) and impaired reproduction (Campbell and Phillipps, 1952) with B$_{12}$ deficiency. An inherited intestinal vitamin B$_{12}$ malabsorption disorder was reported in dogs as a result of a defective brush-border expression of intrinsic factor–vitamin B$_{12}$ receptor (Fyfe et al., 1989, 1991). Vitamin B$_{12}$-deficient dogs developed chronic inappetence, lethargy, chronic nonregenerative anemia, and failure to thrive at 12 weeks of age. Vitamin B$_{12}$ deficiency has been identified in 50% of German shepherds with degenerative myelopathy; however, the clinical signs were not responsive to vitamin B$_{12}$ treatment (Toenniessen and Morin, 1995).

FISH

Salmon and trout fed low dietary B$_{12}$ showed high variability in numbers of fragmented erythrocytes and in hemoglobin values, with a propensity for microcytic, hypochromic anemia (NRC, 1993). Channel catfish and grass shrimp fed a vitamin B$_{12}$-deficient diet exhibited reduced growth rates (NRC, 1993; Shiau and Lung, 1993a). John and Mahajan (1979) observed reduced growth and lower hematocrit in rohu fed a vitamin B$_{12}$-deficient diet. Japanese eel were found to require vitamin B$_{12}$ for normal appetite and growth (Arai et al., 1972). Intestinal microflora synthesis of vitamin B$_{12}$ was shown to be sufficient to meet the requirements for carp, tilapia, rainbow trout, ayu, and goldfish (NRC, 1993; Shiau and Lung, 1993b). Of 746 bacteria strains tested in carp, 8% of the bacteria consumed vitamin B$_{12}$ and the remaining 92% produced it (Sugita et al., 1994). More than 50% of the obligate anaerobes, especially the genus *Clostridium,* produced large amounts of vitamin B$_{12}$.

LABORATORY ANIMALS

In practically all laboratory animals, growth is retarded in vitamin B$_{12}$ deficiency (NRC, 1995), and there are changes in relative weights of certain organs. In B$_{12}$-deficient rats, there are kidney lesions and mucoid structures in the urinary bladders, with reduced muscle mass and fibrotic degeneration of heart. In rats, deficiency in the diet of the mother can result in hydrocephalus, eye defects, and bone defects in the newborn, and mothers may eat the offspring. In mice deficient in B$_{12}$, there is death of young, retarded growth, and renal atrophy. Hamsters receiving low dietary vitamin B_{12} exhibited reduced feed efficiency, but there was no apparent effect on body weight or blood parameters (Scheid et al., 1950). Under practical conditions, vitamin B_{12} deficiency would not be expected in most laboratory animals because of intestinal synthesis and the significant amounts of the vitamin obtained by coprophagy.

MINK

Mink kits deficient in vitamin B_{12} exhibit anorexia, loss of body weight, and severe fatty degeneration of liver (NRC, 1982a). Such deficiency is unlikely in these animals, which are commonly fed diets rich in animal protein. Oral vitamin B_{12} supplementation, but not injections, had some effect in preventing iron-deficiency anemia, indicating an influence on intestinal iron absorption (Pezacka et al., 1992).

NONHUMAN PRIMATES

Megaloblastic anemia reminiscent of pernicious anemia in humans has not been reported in vitamin B_{12}-deficient monkeys. However, abnormalities of the central and peripheral nervous systems in several species of monkeys have been attributed to B_{12} deficiency as a result of vegetarian diets (NRC, 1978). Agamanolis et al. (1976) described demyelination and axon loss in the papillomacular bundle and optic nerve, degeneration within the optic chiasm, and loss of nuclei in all six layers of the lateral geniculate body of rhesus monkeys fed a B_{12}-deficient diet for 4 years.

RABBITS

High urinary and fecal excretion rates of B_{12} have been reported in rabbits receiving diets practically devoid of the vitamin (NRC, 1977). As a result of coprophagy, rabbits should not be deficient in vitamin B_{12}, assuming adequate cobalt is available.

Humans

In humans, pernicious anemia, a fatal megaloblastic anemia with neurological involvement, is the result of vitamin B_{12} deficiency. This megaloblastic anemia is not found in animals. This finding by itself does not elucidate whether the condition is due to deficiency of B_{12} or folacin. Either vitamin B_{12} or folacin supplementation will cure the megaloblastic anemia; however, folacin is ineffective in preventing degenerative changes in the nervous system. In macrocytic anemia, erythrocytes are larger than normal and show great variation in size and normal hemoglobin saturation. The bone marrow shows a megaloblastic pattern of red cell maturation as opposed to the usual normoblast pattern.

In addition to megaloblastic anemia, the most prominent signs and symptoms of vitamin B$_{12}$ deficiency are weakness, tiredness, lightheadedness, pale and smooth tongue with inflammation (Fig. 13.4), dyspnea, splenomegaly, leukopenia, thrombocytopenia, achlorhydria, paresthesia, neurological changes, loss of appetite, loss of weight, and low serum cobalamin levels. The condition results in stiffness of limbs, progressive paralysis, mental disorders, diarrhea, and finally death.

The basic pathological lesion is demyelination of nervous system tissue, seen mainly in the posterolateral columns of the spinal cord but occurring also as foci of demyelination in the cerebral white matter (Metz, 1993). Neurological B$_{12}$ deficiency results in axon degeneration of nerves in the spinal cord. The deficiency produces patchy, diffuse, and progressive demyelination. The clinical picture of the diffuse, uneven demyelination is one of an insidiously progressive neuropathy, often beginning in the peripheral nerves and progressing centrally to involve the posterior and lateral columns of the spinal cord (Herbert, 1990). In addition to subacute combined degeneration of the cord, hypovitaminosis B$_{12}$ may give rise to a severe psychosis with extensive mental deterioration.

The function of B$_{12}$ and folacin in DNA synthesis accounts for some of the pathological findings when deficiency of either of these vitamins occurs. The most rapidly proliferating tissues of the body, such as bone marrow for blood cell production, have the greatest requirement for DNA synthesis and thus are principally affected by megaloblastic anemia when severe deficiency of either B$_{12}$ or folacin occurs. Disturbed division and nuclear maturation of proliferating epithelial cells can be observed in buccal mucosal scrapings and intestinal biopsies of B$_{12}$-deficient patients. The proliferating epithelial cells, as is true for bone marrow, have a high B$_{12}$ and folacin requirement for DNA synthesis.

At the biochemical level the lesion responsible for neuropathy was often attributed to defective functioning of the adenosylcobalamin-dependent folacin-independent methylmalonyl CoA mutase reaction, rather than of the cobalamin-dependent folacin-dependent methionine synthetase reaction (Metz, 1992). However, it is postulated that in vitamin B$_{12}$ deficiency, impaired methionine synthetase activity leads in turn to deficiencies of methionine and S-adenosylmethionine (SAM). Low levels of cerebrospinal SAM are related to abnormal myelination in inherited disorders that affect vitamin B$_{12}$ and folacin metabolism (Metz, 1993). Because SAM is a key intermediary in methylation reactions, de-

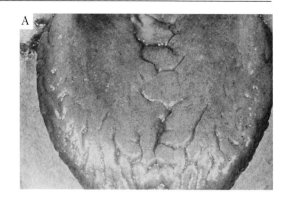

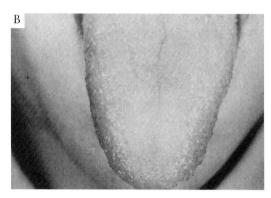

Fig. 13.4 Pernicious anemia. In addition to megaloblastic anemia, an additional sign with vitamin B$_{12}$ deficiency is a pale, smooth tongue with inflammation (A), which is found in one-third to one-half of pernicious anemia patients. The normal tongue (B) has papilla. (Courtesy of R.R. Streiff, Veterans Administration, University of Florida.)

ficiency of SAM could be expected to impair methylation reactions in myelin; thus, methyl group deficiency could result in demyelination and clinical neuropathy (Metz, 1993). A report of studies on infants and children with inborn errors of the methyl-transfer pathway provided further evidence of an association between reduced cerebrospinal fluid SAM levels and abnormal myelination in the nervous system (Surtees et al., 1991).

Vitamin B$_{12}$ deficiency in humans is influenced by one or more of the following considerations:

1. Dietary intake—Inadequate vitamin B$_{12}$ intake is occasionally seen in geriatric patients and in vegetarians. A completely vegetarian diet (one devoid of meat, eggs, and dairy products) can produce B$_{12}$ deficiency if consumed for several years. In some areas of India, religion and poverty result in a basic diet of polished rice, cereals, some vegetables, and fruit, with an inadequate intake of milk and eggs (Rothenberg and Cotter, 1978). Inci-

dence of serum vitamin B$_{12}$ deficiencies were great in Thailand in women practicing vegetarianism for 6 to 10 years (Tungtrongchitr et al., 1993). In Mexico, 62% of breast milk samples from women consuming high-vegetable diets were deficient in vitamin B$_{12}$ (Black et al., 1994). Vitamin B$_{12}$ deficiency was very prevalent in lactating Guatemalan women and their infants at 3 months postpartum (Casterline et al., 1997). There have also been reports of cobalamin deficiency in infants breast-fed by strictly vegetarian mothers (Higginbottom et al., 1978). Breast-fed babies of mothers who are vitamin B$_{12}$ deficient may develop megaloblastic anemia and neurologic symptoms in the first few months of life. Graham et al. (1992) described vitamin B$_{12}$ deficiency in six infants 8 to 15 months old. Consistent clinical signs were irritability, anorexia, and failure to thrive, associated with marked developmental regression and poor brain growth. After follow-up for several years, two of four children tested had mild to borderline intellectual retardation.

2. Failure of absorption or transport—Pernicious anemia is most commonly acquired because of a failure to secrete intrinsic factor. This may be due to deranged stomach activity or may follow total gastrectomy. Total gastrectomy in humans always produces cobalamin deficiency, since it completely removes the site and source of intrinsic factor secretion.

Patients with certain small intestine defects have failure of B$_{12}$ absorption. Impaired absorption of cobalamin is a regular manifestation of tropical sprue. Patients with lesions such as blind loops or small bowel diverticula have demonstrated that an inappropriate bacterial overgrowth in stagnant areas may introduce into the intestinal stream sufficient organisms to absorb all or adsorb much of the dietary cobalamin. Fish tapeworm (*Diphyllobothrium latum*) infestation is a well-recognized cause of impaired B$_{12}$ absorption, as the worm sequesters the vitamin as it progresses through the small intestine. Other conditions that result in reduced B$_{12}$ absorption or transport include excessive intake of alcohol or certain drugs, chronic pancreatitis, diseased B$_{12}$ ileal receptors, and abnormalities related to B$_{12}$ transport proteins.

3. Storage—Vitamin B$_{12}$ stores in the human body exceed the daily requirement by about 1,000-fold (Ellenbogen and Cooper, 1991), which helps explain why clinical B$_{12}$ deficiency due to dietary insufficiency is not more common. It may take as long as 5 to 7 years after cessation of intrinsic-factor secretion before any outward signs of pernicious anemia are evident. Moreover, the small intestine contains microflora that can synthesize significant amounts of cobalamin.

4. Heredity—Pernicious anemia, inherited as an autosomal dominant trait, chiefly affects persons past middle age and results in lack of intrinsic-

factor production. The incidence of pernicious anemia in the general population is one to two per 1,000 and about 25 per 1,000 among relatives of pernicious anemia patients (Ellenbogen and Cooper, 1991).

Neural tube defects (NTDs) are associated with inadequate dietary folacin (see Chapter 12, Deficiency, Humans). Evidence indicates that vitamin B_{12} is also an independent risk factor for NTDs, and the enzyme methionine synthase is involved either directly or indirectly, as this is the only enzyme in metabolism that requires both folate and vitamin B_{12} to function. Further evidence that methionine synthase is defective in mothers who have NTD-affected pregnancies has been reported (Scott et al., 1995). Methionine synthase is required to demethylate 5-CH_3THF with the methyl group used to remethylate homocysteine to produce methionine and SAM, the latter being required for methylation reactions. Low levels of the active form of folacin could impair synthesis of DNA and SAM. Alternatively, impaired activity of methionine synthase might in itself decrease DNA or SAM biosynthesis. Any of the above events could lead to an NTD (Scott et al., 1995).

Carriers of the defective enzyme methionine synthase may also be at risk of other diseases in later life. Homocysteine, the substrate of the enzyme may be inadequately metabolized, leading to hyperhomocysteinemia, a condition that is known to predispose to cardiovascular and cerebrovascular diseases (Clark et al., 1991; Herzlich et al., 1996). Such a defect would be exacerbated by low plasma folate and/or plasma vitamin B_{12} levels (see Chapter 12, Deficiency, Humans).

Assessment of Status

A positive diagnosis of vitamin B_{12} deficiency is usually made by finding subnormal serum and tissue B_{12} concentrations. Low serum levels are associated with low body content of the vitamin. Microbiological assay methods or radioisotopic dilution techniques may be used for this purpose. The normal range for vitamin B_{12} in human serum (or plasma) is 200 to 900 pg/ml. Values between 150 and 200 pg/ml strongly suggest B_{12} deficiency (Rothenberg and Cotter, 1978). A serum concentration of vitamin B_{12} below 110 pmol/L is associated with megaloblastic bone marrow, incipient anemia, and myelin damage, and below 150 pmol/L, there are early bone marrow changes (Bender, 1992).

Analysis of serum levels of both B_{12} and folate can sometimes differentiate which nutrient is deficient for a given megaloblastic anemia (see Chapter 12). However, serum vitamin B_{12} concentration has been shown to have limitations in specificity and sensitivity in diagnosing vitamin B$_{12}$ deficiency and predicting response to therapy in subjects with clinical deficiency syndromes. Frequently, both serum folacin and vitamin B$_{12}$ concentrations are found to be low or low normal in a patient with megaloblastic anemia, making distinction between the two syndromes difficult (Lindenbaum et al., 1994; Savage et al., 1994). In addition to problems with diagnosis, the serum B$_{12}$ concentration cannot be used to monitor response to therapy because it increases in all subjects who receive parenteral B$_{12}$ regardless of whether they were deficient or not.

Contrary to serum vitamin B$_{12}$, elevations of methylmalonic acid and total homocysteine are very sensitive and specific in diagnosing vitamin B$_{12}$ deficiency and can be used to help differentiate vitamin B$_{12}$ deficiency from folacin deficiency (Stabler et al., 1996). Elevated total homocysteine concentrations that may have been attributed to folacin deficiency in elderly subjects may in many instances be the result of vitamin B$_{12}$ deficiency even though serum vitamin B$_{12}$ concentrations are within normal limits. Vitamin B$_{12}$ deficiency is confirmed by determining serum levels of homocysteine and methylmalonic acid. Urinary methylmalonic acid is a sensitive, convenient, and noninvasive indicator for vitamin B$_{12}$ versus folacin deficiency and has been used as a screening procedure in elderly populations (Norman and Morrison, 1993).

Different methods involving various radioactive isotopes of cobalt are available for determining the absorption of an oral dose of radioactive B$_{12}$ in humans. The Schilling urinary excretion test is one of the simplest and most generally used. The basis of this test is giving large doses of unlabeled B$_{12}$ to saturate blood binding protein so any absorbed radioactive B$_{12}$ will be excreted by the kidney. Other procedures include direct determination of fecal radioactivity after a test dose of B$_{12}$-labeled cobalt (i.e., ^{58}Co or ^{56}Co) or measurement of hepatic uptake of B$_{12}$.

Biochemical detection of B$_{12}$ deficiency in both humans and animals includes increased urinary excretion of formiminoglutamic acid (FIGLU) following loading with histidine and a greater percentage of serum folate as 5-methyl-THF rather than THF. Since vitamin B$_{12}$ participates in demethylation of methylfolate, patients with pernicious anemia show an accumulation of the methylfolate and an increased excretion of FIGLU. For deamination of histidine, THF is required rather than methyl-THF.

In laying poultry, vitamin B$_{12}$ concentrations in egg yolk can be used as a status indicator. Squires and Naber (1992) reported that egg yolk vitamin B$_{12}$ concentrations respond rapidly to dietary changes in the level of this vitamin and are indicative of the vitamin B_{12} status of the hen. At four times the dietary requirement, efficiency of transfer to eggs remained nearly constant for vitamin B_{12} (Naber and Squires, 1993). Hence, vitamin B_{12} fortification of eggs is easily accomplished.

In ruminants, the best indicators of cobalt deficiency are low levels of cobalt and B_{12} in tissues, loss of appetite, elevated blood pyruvate, and elevated urinary methylmalonic acid. A vitamin B_{12} enzyme (methylmalonyl-CoA mutase) is required for conversion of propionate to succinate and, with the vitamin deficiency, methylmalonic acid is excreted. Methylmalonic acid concentrations would be higher in all species with B_{12} deficiency but particularly high in ruminants because of the large quantities of propionic acid metabolized. Other indicators of low vitamin B_{12} status have been increased plasma homocysteine (Kennedy et al., 1994b) and low liver methionine synthase activity in sheep (Kennedy et al., 1992a).

In sheep consuming low dietary vitamin B_{12}, plasma vitamin B_{12} concentration decreased below the lower limit of normal after 6 weeks, and plasma methylmalonic acid concentration increased above the upper limit after 10 weeks (Kennedy et al., 1994a). However, Fisher and MacPherson (1990) suggested that serum methylmalonic acid concentrations are less variable and provide a more accurate diagnosis of cobalt deficiency than serum vitamin B_{12}. Normal concentrations of serum methylmalonic acid were tentatively suggested as being less than 2 µmol/L; subclinically cobalt deficient, 2 to 4 µmol/L; and cobalt deficient greater than 4 µmol/L (Paterson and MacPherson, 1990). Graham (1991) suggested that in ruminants, plasma B_{12} is marginally deficient at 380 to 760 pmol/L and deficient when under 380 pmol/L. In goats, serum vitamin B_{12} concentrations below 200 pg/ml were indicative of cobalt deficiency (Mburu et al., 1994).

The levels of cobalt in the livers of sheep and cattle are sufficiently responsive to changes in cobalt intake to have value in the detection of cobalt deficiency, with liver vitamin B_{12} an even more reliable criterion. Values of 0.10 µg or less of vitamin B_{12} per gram wet weight are "clearly diagnostic of cobalt deficiency disease" (Underwood, 1979). Liver cobalt concentrations in the range of 0.05 to 0.07 ppm (dry basis) or below are critical levels indicating deficiency (McDowell, 1985). While herbage and tissue analyses are helpful in diagnosing the deficiency, the definite proof is the prompt improvement in feed intake following injection of vitamin B_{12}.

SUPPLEMENTATION

Vitamin B$_{12}$ is produced by fermentation and is available commercially as cyanocobalamin for addition to feed. Vitamin B$_{12}$ is only slightly sensitive to heat, oxygen, moisture, and light (Gadient, 1986; Coelho, 1994). Verbeeck (1975) reported vitamin B$_{12}$ to have good stability in premixes with or without minerals regardless of mineral source. Scott (1966) indicated that there is apparently little effect of pelleting on vitamin B$_{12}$ content of feed. Vitamin leaching is a problem when feed is administered in water for fish. Pannevis and Earle (1994) reported a 90% loss of vitamin B$_{12}$ after only 30 seconds through water leaching of the feed.

Results of a large number of animal experiments are about equally divided between those reporting a positive response to dietary cyanocobalamin and those reporting little or no response. Variable responses may be due to several factors: initial body stores, environmental sources of the vitamin (such as molds, soil, and animal excreta), microbial synthesis in the intestinal tract, and adequacy or deficiency of other nutrients that influence B$_{12}$ requirements.

Vitamin B$_{12}$ is normally added to diets of all classes of swine and poultry. Swine and poultry raised in confinement, in management systems where there is less access to feces for coprophagy, should have a greater dietary requirement for the vitamin. Although dietary supplements would be recommended, injections of vitamin B$_{12}$ are often given to animals with a poor health appearance. Animals coming into a feedlot are sometimes given B$_{12}$ injections, along with other vitamins, as insurance against not quickly adapting to new feeding regimes. This use of B$_{12}$ may be warranted under certain conditions in which stress, disease, or parasites lower feed intake, impair ruminal function, and/or reduce intestinal absorption.

Intramuscular administration of vitamin B$_{12}$ at the rate of 100 μg each week or of 150 μg every second week were shown to produce a rapid remission of all signs of deficiency in lambs and are just as effective as cobalt administered orally at the rate of 7 mg per week (Andrews and Anderson, 1954). For rapid correction of cobalt deficiency in cattle, intramuscular administration of vitamin B$_{12}$ at 500 to 3,000 μg per head is recommended, which may be repeated weekly (Graham, 1991). Intramuscular administration of vitamin B$_{12}$ to cobalt-deficient animals produced overnight improvement in appetite, whereas oral dosing with cobalt required 7 to 10 days to produce the same effect (MacPherson, 1982). Although parenteral vitamin B_{12} injections prevent cobalt deficiency in ruminants, it is more convenient and economical to supplement the diet with cobalt, allowing the microorganisms to synthesize the vitamin for subsequent absorption by the host.

Since many forages and some concentrate feeds do not supply 0.10 ppm cobalt, an adequate dietary allowance, cobalt supplementation is needed. Ruminants that consume concentrates are more likely to receive adequate dietary cobalt than grazing livestock; however, growth responses to supplemental cobalt were demonstrated in steers fed finishing diets based on barley grain (Raun et al., 1968), sorghum grain, and silage (Morris and Gartner, 1967).

Available cobalt must be present in the animal diet for ruminal and intestinal synthesis to occur. Cobalt deficiency in ruminants can be cured or prevented through treatment of soils or pastures with cobalt-containing fertilizers or by direct oral administration of cobalt to the animals through free-choice mineral supplements (McDowell, 1985, 1992). In deficient areas, where the pastures require regular fertilizer applications, adequate cobalt intakes can usually be ensured by including cobalt salts or oxide ores. Often, use of fertilizer cobalt is impractical and uneconomical for extensive range conditions in developing countries (McDowell et al., 1984).

Cobalt deficiency in grazing ruminants can best be prevented by direct oral administration of cobalt through free-choice mineral supplements. During critical periods cobalt supplementation must be continuous. Cobalt supplementation in either the first or second half of pregnancy only did not fully alleviate adverse effects on ewe reproductive performance and lamb viability (Fisher and MacPherson, 1991). Cobalt-deficient livestock respond quickly to cobalt treatment and recover appetite, vigor, and weight; this serves as an easy practical test to determine whether cobalt deficiency exists. Large, frequent injections of vitamin B_{12} can effectively prevent or cure cobalt deficiency but are much more expensive. Oral dosing or drenching with dilute cobalt solutions are satisfactory if the doses are regular and frequent. Dosing sheep twice weekly with 2 mg of cobalt or once weekly with 7 mg of cobalt, or dosing cattle with 5 to 10 times those amounts, depending on their size and age, is fully adequate for severely deficient regions (Underwood, 1981).

An additional method of providing cobalt, developed in Australia, is the use of an orally administered, heavy pellet (bullet), made of cobalt oxide plus finely divided iron, that remains in the reticulorumen for an extended period. Pellets may be lost through regurgitation or become ineffective because of formation of a surface coating of calcium phosphate. The addition of a steel grinder, which provides an abrasive action, reduces the surface coating and extends the usefulness of the pellet. A multiple slow-release trace element (including cobalt) rumen bolus is available (Judson et al., 1988; Ritchie et al., 1991).

The need for continual cobalt supplementation is difficult to assess, as the incidence of cobalt deficiency can vary greatly from year to year, from undetectable mild deficiency to an acute stage. Lee (1963) illustrated this variation in a 14-year experiment with sheep in southern Australia. Half the ewes, replacements, and progeny were dosed with cobalt and remained healthy. The undosed half had the following performance for the 14 years: in 2 years, lambs were unthrifty, but there were no deaths; in 3 years, growth rate of the lambs was slightly retarded; in 4 years, 30 to 100% of the lamb crop was lost; in 5 years, the performance of the remaining stock was as good as that of dosed animals.

The most important cobalt supplements produced for feed use are cobalt carbonate, a fine powder containing over 46% cobalt; cobalt sulfate crystal, a fine granular crystal containing 21% cobalt; and cobalt sulfate monohydrate, a powder containing 33% cobalt. Carbonate, chloride, sulfate, and oxide forms of cobalt were proposed as satisfactory dietary sources of the mineral (Ammerman and Miller, 1972). However, observations by Ammerman et al. (1982) suggested that the oxide form may be considerably less available than either the carbonate or sulfate form.

For human therapy, during the stage of relapse of pernicious anemia, intramuscular doses of vitamin B$_{12}$ at the rate of 15 to 30 µg/day should be given (Marks, 1975). A single injection of 100 µg or more will produce complete remission in any patient whose vitamin B$_{12}$ deficiency is not complicated by unrelated systemic disease or other factors. When pernicious anemia is due to inadequate absorption, 1 µg of the vitamin by injection daily is adequate therapy. Remission is sustained for life by monthly injections of 100 µg of vitamin B$_{12}$ (Herbert, 1990). In patients treated successfully with intramuscular vitamin B$_{12}$, the first response occurs within about 2 days of the start of treatment and consists of an intense feeling of well-being and an increase in appetite.

Single, large oral doses (1,000 µg) of vitamin B$_{12}$ without intrinsic factor have proven effective in treatment of pernicious anemia. Absorption of a small amount of B$_{12}$ from massive doses is independent of the action of intrinsic factor and is believed to occur by a "mass-action" effect, resulting in diffusion of some of the vitamin. An oral dose of at least 150 µg/day is deemed necessary to maintain the pernicious anemia patient. Single weekly oral doses of 1,000 µg satisfactorily maintain some pernicious anemia patients (Ellenbogen and Cooper, 1991). For vegetarian patients who have a normal secretion of intrinsic factor, 1.0 to 1.5 µg/day of vitamin B_{12} orally is sufficient to prevent pernicious anemia.

Vitamin B_{12} supplementation is particularly important for individuals consuming all-vegetable diets. Supplementation of B_{12} should be considered by vegetarians, particularly for lactating mothers to provide vitamin B_{12} to their offspring. If malabsorption and chronic diarrhea are combined with low dietary intake of vitamin B_{12}, as is the case for many children in the Third World, depletion of vitamin B_{12} stores may result (Paerregaard et al., 1990). Premature infants require additional folacin and vitamin B_{12} to reduce the severity of the anemia of prematurity (Worthington-White et al., 1994). When high amounts of supplemental folacin are administered (e.g., to prevent NTDs), the risk of undiagnosed vitamin B_{12} deficiency could be reduced by simultaneous supplementation with generous doses (1 mg/day) of vitamin B_{12}. A 20% prevalence of abnormal vitamin B_{12} metabolism was found in 64 patients with human immunodeficiency virus (HIV) who were referred for neurological evaluation (Kieburtz et al., 1991). Vitamin B_{12} deficiency may be a frequent and treatable cause of neurological dysfunction in patients with HIV infection.

Supplementation with large doses of vitamin B_{12} has falsely been advocated for various disorders in humans. The red color of the vitamin, along with its almost total lack of known toxicity, makes it an almost ideal placebo. It is, unfortunately, used in large quantities to defraud unsuspecting buyers.

TOXICITY

Addition of vitamin B_{12} to food in amounts far in excess of need or absorbability appears to be without hazard. Dietary levels of at least several thousand times the requirement are safe (NRC, 1987; Ellenbogen and Cooper, 1991). However, the maximum tolerable amount of dietary cobalt for ruminants is estimated at 5 ppm. Cobalt toxicosis in cattle is characterized by mild polycythemia; excessive urination, defecation, and salivation; shortness of breath; and increased hemoglobin, red cell count, and packed cell volume. Although most researchers consider the margin between safe and toxic doses wide enough to make toxicity under natural conditions unlikely, several reports have appeared in the literature concerning cobalt toxicity. These reports almost invariably have involved management mistakes in formulating mineral mixtures.

■ REFERENCES

Agamanolis, D.P., Chester, E.M., Victor, M., Kark, J.A., Hines, J.S., and Harris, J.W. (1976). *Neurology 26*, 905.
Ammerman, C.B., and Miller, S.M. (1972). *J. Anim. Sci. 35*, 681.
Ammerman, C.B., Henry, P.R., and Loggins, P.R. (1982). *J. Anim. Sci. 55*(Suppl. 1), 403.
Andrews, E.D. (1956). *N. Z. J. Agric. 92*, 239.
Andrews, E.D., and Anderson, J.P. (1954). *N. J. Z. Sci. Tech. A35*, 483.
Anonymous (1984). Vitamin B$_{12}$. *Roche Tech. Bull.* Hoffmann-LaRoche, Nutley, New Jersey.
Arai, S., Nose, T., and Hashimoto, Y. (1972). *Bull. Freshwater Res. Lab.* Tokyo 22, 69.
Arnrich, L., Lewis, E.M., and Morgan, A.F. (1952). *Proc. Soc. Exp. Biol. Med. 80*, 401.
Barnes, R.H., and Fiala, G. (1958). *J. Nutr. 65*, 103.
Becker, R.B., Henderson, J.R., and Leighty, R.B. (1965). *Fla. Univ. Agric. Exp. Stn. Tech. Bull.*, 699.
Behrns, K.E., Smith, C.O., and Sarr, M.G. (1994). *Dig. Dis. Sci. 39(2)*, 315.
Bender, D.A. (1992). Nutritional Biochemistry of the Vitamins, p. 294. Cambridge University Press, Cambridge, England.
Black, A.K., Allen, L.H., Pelto, G.H., DeMata, M.P., and Chávez, A. (1994). *J. Nutr. 124*, 1179.
Campbell, J.E., and Phillips, P.H. (1952). *J. Nutr. 47*, 621.
Carmel, R. (1994). *Dig. Dis. Sci. 12*, 2516.
Casterline, J.E., Allen, L.H., and Ruel, M.T. (1997). *J. Nutr. 127*, 1966.
Catron, D.V., Richardson, D., Underkofler, L.A., Maddock, H.M., and Friedland, W.C. (1952). *J. Nutr. 47*, 461.
Clark, R., Daly, L., Robinson, K.H., Naughtey, E., Cahalane, S., Fowler, B., and Graham, I. (1991). *N. Engl. J. Med. 324*, 1149.
Coelho, M.B. (1994). *In* BASF Technical Symposium, p. 60. Clarion, Arkansas.
Corrêa, R. (1957). *Arquivos do Instituto Biologicos 24*, 199.
Cunha, R.J. (1977). Swine Feeding and Nutrition. Academic Press, New York.
Dagnelie, P.C., VanStaveren, W.A., and VandenBerg, H. (1991). *Am. J. Clin. Nutr. 53*, 695.
Davies, M.E. (1971). *Br. Vet. J. 127*, 34.
Dostalova, J. (1994). *Vyzivay 49*, 43.
Ellenbogen, L., and Cooper, B.A. (1991). *In* Handbook of Vitamins (L.J. Machlin, ed.), p. 491. Marcel Dekker, New York.
Ellenbogen, L., and Highley, D.R. (1970). *Fed. Proc. Fed. Am. Soc. Exp. Biol. 29*, 633(Abstr.).
Farquharson, J., and Adams, J.F. (1976). *Br. J. Nutr. 36*, 127.
Ferguson, E.G.W., Mitchell, G.B., and MacPherson, A. (1988). *Vet. Rec. 124*, 20.

Ferguson, R.M., and Couch, J.R. (1954). *J. Nutr. 54,* 361.
Fie, M., Zee, J.A., and Amiot, J. (1994). *Lait 74,* 461.
Filmer, J.F. (1933). *Aust. Vet. J. 9,* 163.
Fisher, G.E.J., and MacPherson, A. (1990). *Br. Vet. J. 146,* 120.
Fisher, G.E.J., and MacPherson, A. (1991). *Res. Vet. Sci. 50,* 319.
Flavin, M., and Ochoa, S. (1957). *J. Biol. Chem. 229,* 965.
Folkers, K. (1982) *In* B$_{12}$ (D. Dolphin, ed.), p. 1. Wiley, New York.
Frederick, G.L., and Brisson, G.J. (1961). *Can. J. Anim. Sci. 41,* 212.
Friesecke, H. (1980). Vitamin B$_{12}$. Hoffmann-La Roche, Basel, Switzerland.
Fyfe, J.C., Jezyk, P.F, Giger, U., and Patterson, D.F. (1989). *J. Am. Anim. Hosp. Assoc. 25,* 533.
Fyfe, J.C., Ramanujam, K.S., Ramaswamy, K., Patterson, D.F., and Seetharm, B. (1991). *J. Biol. Chem. 266,* 4489.
Gadient, M. (1986). *Proc. Nutr. Conf. Feed Mfr.,* p. 73. University of Maryland, College Park.
Graham, S.M., Arvela, O.M., and Wise, G.A. (1992). *J. Pediatr. 121,* 710.
Graham, T.W. (1991). *Vet. Clin. North Am. Food Anim. Proc. 7,* 153.
Henderickx, H.K., Teague, H.S., Redman, D.R., and Grifo, A.P. (1964). *J. Anim. Sci. 23,* 1036.
Herbert, V. (1990). Nutrition Reviews: Present Knowledge in Nutrition (R.E. Olson, H.P. Broquist, C.O. Chichester, W.J. Darby, A.C. Kolbye, and R.M. Stalvey, eds.), 5th Ed., p. 170. Nutrition Foundation, Washington D.C.
Herbert, V., and Zalusky, R. (1962). *J. Clin. Invest. 41,* 1263.
Herzlich, B.C., Lichstein, E., Schulhoff, N., Weinstock, M. Pagala, M., Ravindran, K., Namba, T., Nieto, F.J., Stabler, S.P., Allen, R.H., and Malinow, M.R. (1996). *J. Nutr. 126,* 1249S.
Hesselink, J.W., and Vellema, P. (1990). *Tijdschrift-voor-Diergeeneskunde 115,* 789.
Higginbottom, M., Sweetman, L., and Nyhan, W. (1978). *N. Engl. J. Med. 299,* 317.
Hussein, H.S., Fahey, G.C., Wolf, B.W., and Berger, L.L. (1994). *J. Dairy Sci. 77,* 3432.
John, M.J., and Mahajan, C.L. (1979). *J. Fish Biol. 14,* 127.
Jorgensen, B.B., Pedersen, N.T., and Worning, H. (1991). *Aliment. Pharmacol. Ther. 5,* 207.
Judson, G.J., Brown, T.H., Kempe, B.R., and Turnbull, R.K. (1988). *Aust. J. Exp. Agr. 28.* 299.
Keen, C.L., and Graham, T.W. (1989). *In* Clinical Biochemistry of Domestic Animals (J.J. Kaneko, ed.), 4th Ed., p. 753. Academic Press, San Diego California.
Keesling, P.T., and Morris, J.G. (1975). *J. Anim. Sci. 41,* 317(Abstr.).
Kennedy, D.G., Blanchflower, W.J., Scott, J.M., Weir, D.G., Molloy, A.M., Kennedy, S., and Young, P.G. (1992a). *J. Nutr. 122,* 1384.
Kennedy, D.G., Blanchflower, W.J., Young, P.G., and Davidson, W.B. (1992b). *Biol. Trace Elem. Res. 35,* 153.
Kennedy, D.G., Kennedy, S., Blanchflower, W.J., Scott, J.M., Weir, D.G., Molloy, A.M., and Young, P.B. (1994a). *Brit. J. Nutr. 71,* 67.
Kennedy, D.G., Young, P.B., Blanchflower, W.J., Scott, J.M., Weir, D.G., Molloy, A.M., and Kennedy, S. (1994b). *Int. J. Vit. Nutr. Res. 64,* 270.

Kieburtz, K.D., Giang, D.W., Schiffer, R.B., and Vakil, N. (1991). *Arch. Neurol.* 48, 312.

Lachance, A.P. (1998). *Nutr. Rev. 56*, 34S.

Lassiter, C.A., Ward, G.M., Huffman, C.F., Duncan, C.W., and Webster, H.D. (1953). *J. Dairy Sci. 36*, 997.

Latteur, J.P. (1962). Cobalt Deficiencies and Subdeficiencies in Ruminants. Centre d'Information du Cobalt, Brussels, Belgium.

Lee, H.J. (1963). *In* Animal Health, Production and Pasture (A.H. Worden, K.O. Sellers, and D.E. Tribe, eds.), p. 662. Longmans, New York.

Lewis, N.M., Kies, C., and Fox, H.M. (1986). *Nutr. Rep. Int. 34*, 495.

Lindenbaum, J., Rosenberg, I., Wilson, P., Stabler, S.P., and Allen, R.H. (1994). *Am. J. Clin. Nutr. 60*, 2.

Loosli, J.K. (1991). *In* Handbook of Animal Science (P.A. Putnam, ed.), p. 25. Academic Press, San Diego, California.

Lopez-Guisa, J.M., and Satter, L.D. (1992). *J. Dairy Sci., 75*, 247.

MacPherson, A. (1982). Roche Vitamin Symposium: Recent Research on the Vitamin Requirements of Ruminants, p. 1. Hoffmann-La Roche, Basel, Switzerland.

Marks, J. (1975). A Guide to the Vitamins. Their Role in Health and Disease, p. 73. Medical and Technical Publ., Lancaster, England.

Marston, J.R. (1970). *Br. J. Nutr. 24*, 615.

Mburu, J.N., Kamau, J.M.Z., and Badamana, M.S. (1993). *Int. J. Vit. Nutr. Res. 63*, 135.

Mburu, J.N., Kamau, J.M.Z., Badamana, M.S., and Mbugua, P.N. (1994). *Bull. Anim. Health Prod. Africa 42*, 141.

McDowell, L.R. (1985). *In* Nutrition of Grazing Ruminants in Warm Climates (L.R. McDowell, ed.), p. 329. Academic Press, Orlando, Florida.

McDowell, L.R. (1992). Minerals in Animal and Human Nutrition Academic Press, San Diego, California.

McDowell, L.R., Conrad, J.H., and Ellis, G.L. (1984). *In* Symposium on Herbivore Nutrition in Subtropics and Tropics-Problems and Prospects (F.M.C. Gilchrist and R.I. Mackie, eds.) p. 67. The Science Press, Pretoria, South Africa.

McDowell, L.R. (1997). Minerals for Grazing Ruminants in Tropical Regions, 3rd Ed. University of Florida Press, Gainesville, FL.

Metz, J. (1992). *Annu. Rev. Nutr. 12*, 59.

Metz, J. (1993). *Nutr. Rev. 51*, 12.

Mohammed, R. (1983). Sub-clinical Cobalt Deficiency in Sheep. Ph.D. dissertation, Univ. of Clermont, Clermont, France.

Mohammed, R., and Lamand, M. (1986). *Ann. Res. Vet. 17*, 447.

Morris, J.G. (1977). *In* Kal Kan Symposium for Treatment of Dog and Cat Diseases, p. 15. Ohio State University, Wooster.

Morris, J.G., and Gartner, R.J.W. (1967). *Agric. Sci. 68*, 1.

Muhammad, K., Briggs, D., and Jones, G. (1993). *Food Chem. 48*, 431.

Naber, E.C., and Squires, M.W. (1993). *Poult. Sci. 72*, 1046.

Norman, E.J., and Morrison, J.A. (1993). *Am J. Med. 94*, 589.

NRC. Nutrient Requirements of Domestic Animals. National Academy of Sciences-National Research Council, Washington, D.C.
(1977). Nutrient Requirements of Rabbits, 2nd Ed.

(1978). Nutrient Requirements of Nonhuman Primates.

(1981). Nutrient Requirements of Goats.

(1982a). Nutrient Requirements of Mink and Foxes.

(1985a). Nutrient Requirements of Dogs, 2nd Ed.

(1985b). Nutrient Requirements of Sheep, 5th Ed.

(1986). Nutrient Requirements of Cats, 3rd Ed.

(1989a). Nutrient Requirements of Dairy Cattle, 6th Ed.

(1989b). Nutrient Requirements of Horses, 5th Ed.

(1993). Nutrient Requirements of Fish.

(1994). Nutrient Requirements of Poultry, 9th Ed.

(1995). Nutrient Requirements of Laboratory Animals, 4th Ed.

(1996). Nutrient Requirements of Beef Cattle, 7th Ed.

(1998). Nutrient Requirements of Swine, 10th Ed.

NRC. (1982b). United States-Canadian Tables of Feed Composition, 3rd Ed. National Academy of Sciences-National Research Council, Washington, D.C.

NRC. (1987). Vitamin Tolerance of Animals. National Academy of Sciences-National Research Council, Washington, D.C.

Olcese, O., Couch, J.R., Quisenberry, J.H., and Pearson, P.B. (1950). *J. Nutr. 41*, 423.

Paerregaard, A., Hjelt, K., and Krasilnikoff, P.A. (1990). *J. Pediatr. Gastroenterol. Nutr. 11*, 351.

Pannevis, M.C., and Earle, K.E. (1994). *J. Nutr. 124*(Suppl.), 2633S.

Paterson, J.E., and MacPherson, A. (1990). *Vet. Rec. 126*, 329.

Pezacka, E.H., Jacobsen, D.W., Luce, K., and Green, R. (1992). *Biochem. Biophys. Res. Comm. 184*, 832.

Polak, D.M., Elliot, J.M., and Haluska, M. (1979). *J. Dairy Sci. 62*, 697.

Ramoz, J.J., Saez, T., Bueso, J.P., Sanz, M.C., and Fernandez, A. (1994). *Vet. Res. 25*, 405.

Raun, N.S., Stables, G.L., Pope, L.S., Harper, O.F., Waller, G.R., Renbarger, R., and Tillman, A.D. (1968). *J. Anim. Sci. 27*, 1695.

RDA. (1989). Recommended Dietary Allowances, 10th Ed. National Academy of Sciences-National Research Council, Washington, D.C.

Reinisch, F., and Gebhardt, G. (1987). *In* Symposium Vitamin and Ergotropika und Podiumsdiskussion zur Verzehrsregulation Reinhardsbrunn, E. Germany.

Ritchie, N.S., Lawson, D.C., and Parkins, J.J. (1991). *In* Tracae Elem. Man Anim. Proc. Int. Symp. (TEMA-7), p. 15. Dubrovnik, Yugoslavia.

Rothenberg, S.P., and Cotter, R. (1978). *In* Handbook Series in Nutrition and Food, Section E: Nutritional Disorders (M. Rechcigl Jr., ed.), Vol. 3, p. 69. CRC Press, Boca Raton, Florida.

Sato, K., Wang, X., and Mizoguchi, K. (1997). *J. Dairy Sci. 80*, 2701.

Savage, D.G., and Lindenbaum, J. (1995). *In* Folate in Health and Disease (L.B. Bailey, ed.), p. 237. Marcel Dekker, New York.

Savage, D.G., Lindenbaum, J., Stabler, S.P., and Allen, R.H. (1994). *Am. J. Med. 96*, 239.

Scheid, H.E., McBride, B.H., and Schweigert, B.S. (1950). *Proc. Soc. Exp. Biol. Med. 75*, 236.

Scott, J.M., Weir, D.G., and Kirke, P.N. (1995). *In* Folate in Health and Disease

(L.B. Baily, ed.), p. 329. Marcel Dekker, New York.

Scott, M.L. (1966). *Proc. Cornell Nutr. Conf.*, p. 35. Cornell University, Ithaca, New York.

Scott, M.L., Nesheim, M.C., and Young, R.J. (1982). Nutrition of the Chicken, p. 119. Scott, Ithaca, New York.

Sebrell, W.H. Jr., and Harris, R.S. (1968). The Vitamins, p. 119. Academic Press, New York.

Sewell, R.F., Cunha, T.J., Shawver, C.B., Ney, W.A., and Wallace, H.D. (1952). *Am. J. Vet. Res. 13*, 186.

Shiau, S.Y., and Lung, C.Q. (1993a). *Comp. Biochem. Phys. A. 105*, 147.

Shiau, S.Y., and Lung, C.Q. (1993b). *Aquaculture 117*, 157.

Shinton, N.K. (1972). *Br. Med. J. 1*, 556.

Simpson, K.W., Morton, D.B., and Batt, R.M. (1989). *Am. J. Vet. Res. 50*, 1233.

Squires, M.W., and Naber, E.C. (1992). *Poult. Sci. 71*, 2075.

Stabler, S.P., Lindenbaum, J., and Allen, R.H. (1996). *J. Nutr. 126*, 1266s.

Sugita, H., Kuruma, A., Hirato, C., Ohkoshi, T., Okada, R., and Deguchi, Y. (1994). *Aquaculture 119*, 425.

Sugita, H., Miyajima, C., and Deguchi, Y. (1991). *Aquaculture 92*, 267.

Surtees, R., Leonard, J., and Austin, S. (1991). *Lancet 338*, 1550.

Suttle, N.F., and Jones, D.G. (1989). *J. Nutr. 119*, 1055.

Sutton, A.L., and Elliot, J.M. (1972). *J. Nutr. 102*, 1341.

Toenniessen, J.G., and Morin, D.E. (1995). *Compendium Cont. Ed. Pract. Vet. 17*, 217.

Tokarnia, C.H., Guimaraes, J.A., Canella, C.F.C., and Döbereiner, J. (1971). *Pesqui. Agropecu. Bras. 6*, 61.

Toskes, P.P., Deren, J.J., Fruiterman, J., and Conrad, M.E. (1973). *Gastroenterology 65*, 199.

Tungtrongchitr, R., Pongpaew, P., Prayurahong, B., Changbumrung, S., Vudhivai, N., Migasena, P., and Schelp, F.P. (1993). *Int. J. Vit. Nutr. Res. 63*, 201.

Underwood, E.J. (1977). Trace Elements in Human and Animal Nutrition, Academic Press, New York.

Underwood, E.J. (1979). *In* Proc. Nutr. Conf., p. 203. University of Florida, Gainesville, Florida.

Underwood, E.J. (1981). The Mineral Nutrition of Livestock, Commonwealth Agricultural Bureaux, London, England.

Vaden, S.L., Wood, P.A., Ledley, F.D., Cornwell, P.E., Miller, R.T., and Page, R. (1992). *J. Am. Vet. Med. Assoc. 200*, 1101.

Verbeeck, J. (1975). *Feedstuffs 47(36)*, 4, 45.

Vestal, C.M., Beeson, W.M., Andrews, P.N., Hutchings, L.M., and Doyle, L.P. (1950). *Purdue Agric. Exp. Stn. Mimeo* No. 50. Purdue University, Lafayette, Indiana.

Vieira-Makings, E., Van-der Westhuyzen, J., and Metz, J. (1990). *Int. J. Vitam. Nutr. Res. 60*, 41.

Wagle, S.R., Mehta, R., and Johnson, B.C. (1958). *J. Biol. Chem. 230*, 137.

West, R. (1948). *Science 107*, 398.

Worthington-White, D.A., Behnke, M., and Gross, S. (1994). *Am J. Clin. Nutr. 6*, 930.

CHOLINE

INTRODUCTION

Choline is considered essential to the animal organism and is utilized both as a building unit and as an essential component in regulation of certain metabolic processes. Choline is tentatively classified as one of the B-complex vitamins even though it does not entirely satisfy the strict definition of a vitamin. Choline, unlike B vitamins, can be synthesized in the liver, is required in the body in greater amounts, and apparently functions as a structural constituent rather than as a coenzyme. Also, existence of choline in essential body constituents was recognized long before the first vitamin was discovered. Regardless of classification, choline is an essential nutrient for all animals and a required dietary supplement for some species (e.g., poultry, swine, and fish). Choline is likewise an essential nutrient for humans, and studies have investigated the benefits of choline treatment for certain diseases, such as cancer and Alzheimer's disease.

14

HISTORY

Choline was isolated by Streker from the bile of pigs in 1849 and by Von Balb and Hirschbrunn from an alkaloid of white mustard seed (*Sinapis alba*) in 1852 (Griffith and Nyc, 1971). Streker isolated the compound from lecithin, to which he gave the name "choline." The chemical structure of choline was established in 1867 by Bayer (Scott et al., 1982). Choline's acceptance as a biologically essential compound resulted from studies in 1929 in which acetylcholine was isolated from the spleen of a horse (Dale and Dudley, 1929).

Choline's role in nutrition was not known until the 1930s, following the discovery of insulin in 1922 by Banting and Best. It was observed that fatty degeneration of the liver associated with insulin deprivation in dogs could be corrected by feeding either raw pancreas or lecithin. In 1932 choline was discovered to be the active component of pure lecithin previously shown to prevent fatty livers ("lipotropic effect") in rats (Best et al., 1934). Betaine, considered to be only a methyl donor, was found to have a similar lipotropic effect in rats and dogs. Various studies in the late 1930s and early 1940s determined that the lipotropic activity of choline related to transfer of methyl groups and interrelationships and sparing effects of choline on dietary methionine, folacin, and vitamin B_{12}.

In 1940, Jukes showed that choline is required for normal growth and the prevention of perosis, a leg disorder in turkeys; he found that the amount required to prevent perosis was greater than that required for normal growth. Choline was found to prevent a "spraddled-leg" condition in swine in the 1950s and 1960s. More recently, choline has been found to be effective for various human conditions involving mobilization of liver lipids, and studies have investigated the role of choline (and other methyl donors) on carcinogenesis and the neurotransmitter-related syndromes (e.g., senile dementia and Alzheimer's disease).

CHEMICAL STRUCTURE AND PROPERTIES

Choline is a β-hydroxyethyltrimethylammonium hydroxide and is depicted in Fig. 14.1. The prominent feature of choline's chemical structure is its triplet of methyl groups, which enables it to serve as a methyl donor. Pure choline is a colorless, viscid, strongly alkaline liquid that is notably hygroscopic. Choline is soluble in water, formaldehyde, and alcohol and has no definite melting or boiling point. The chloride salt of this compound, choline chloride, is produced by chemical synthesis for use in the feed industry, although other forms exist. Choline chloride exists as deliquescent white crystals that are very soluble in water and alcohols. Aqueous solutions are almost pH neutral.

Choline is ubiquitously distributed in all plant and animal cells, mostly in the form of the phospholipids phosphatidylcholine (lecithin, see Fig. 14.1), lysophosphatidylcholine, choline plasmalogens, and sphingomyelin-essential components of all membranes (Zeisel, 1990). Lecithin is the predominant phospholipid (> 50%) in most mammalian membranes. In the lung, disaturated lecithin is the major active component of surfactant (Brown 1964), lack of which results in a respiratory distress syndrome in premature infants. Choline is a precursor for the biosynthesis of the neurotransmitter acetylcholine (Fig. 14.1). Glyc-

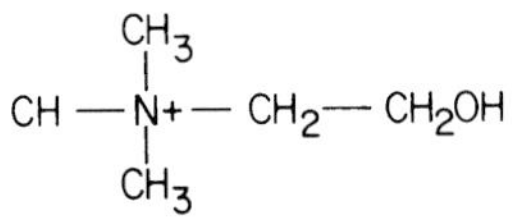

$$CH \underset{\underset{CH_3}{|}}{\overset{\overset{CH_3}{|}}{-N^+-}} CH_2 - CH_2OH$$

Choline

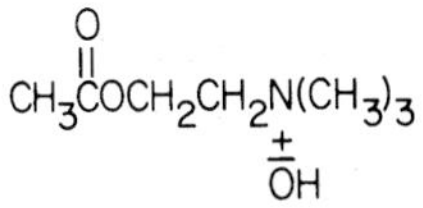

$$CH_3\overset{O}{\overset{||}{C}}OCH_2CH_2\underset{\overset{+}{OH^-}}{N(CH_3)_3}$$

Acetylcholine

$$\begin{aligned} &CH_2O\overset{O}{\overset{||}{C}}-R' \\ &| \\ &CHO\overset{O}{\overset{||}{C}}-R \\ &| \quad\quad\quad\; O \\ &CH_2O-\underset{O_-}{\overset{||}{P}}-OCH_2CH_2N(CH_3)_3 \end{aligned}$$

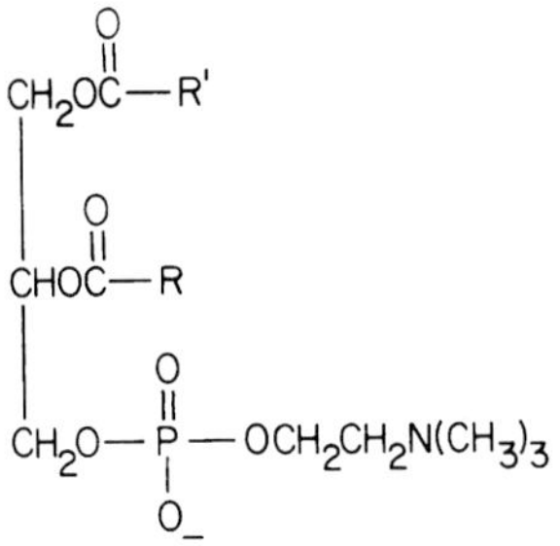

Lecithin

Fig. 14.1 Structural formulas for free choline, acetylcholine, and lecithin. R' refers to any fatty acid.

erophosphocholine and phosphocholine are storage forms for choline within the cytosol and principal forms found in milk (Rohlfs et al., 1993).

ANALYTICAL PROCEDURES

Determination of choline is complicated by its various forms in biological materials. Free choline can be extracted with water or alcohol, but more precise procedures must be used for extraction of total choline. Precautions have to be taken for the preparation of biological tissues, which contain enzymes that rapidly hydrolyze phosphate esters of choline in nervous tissues when animals die (Chan, 1991). Much of the evidence for presence of free choline in biological materials is unreliable owing to delay in the preparation of extracts, with resulting release of choline by autolysis (Griffith and Nyc, 1971). For example, dog liver contained 0 to 43 mg choline per kilogram if extracted immediately after death of the animal and 136 to 164 mg choline per kilogram if extracts were made 5 hours postmortem.

The classic and most widely used procedure for quantitative determination of choline is the colorimetric reineckate method (AOAC, 1984). This procedure involves the precipitation of choline as a reinecke salt for a colorimetric reaction. Other methods of analysis include enzymatic, fluorometric, gas chromatographic, photometric, and polarographic techniques. Analyses by high-performance liquid chromatograhy and gas chromatography-mass spectrometry (Pomfret et al., 1989; Zeisel and da Costa, 1990) have permitted the measurement of choline-containing compounds in tissues. Enzymatic radioisotopic assay and gas chromatography provide high sensitivity and specificity and have been widely used in recent years (Chan, 1991). Microbiological assay for choline generally employs *Neurospora crassa*, while biological assay methods make use of conversion of choline to acetylcholine in isolated tissues, as well as growth response of chicks. Growth response may be an unreliable measure of choline concentration as it is influenced by other constituents (e.g., methionine) in choline-limiting diets (Pesti et al., 1981).

METABOLISM

Choline is present in the diet mainly in the form of lecithin, with less than 10% present as either the free base or sphingomyelin. Choline is released from lecithin and sphingomyelin by digestive enzymes of the gastrointestinal tract, although 50% of ingested lecithin enters the thoracic duct intact (Chan, 1991).

Choline is released from lecithin by hydrolysis in the intestinal lumen. Both pancreatic secretions and intestinal mucosal cells contain enzymes capable of hydrolyzing lecithin in the diet. Phospholipase A_2 (which cleaves the β-fatty acid moiety) is found in pancreatic juice and in the intestinal brush border. Within the gut mucosal cell, phospholipase A_1 cleaves the α-fatty acid, and phospholipase B cleaves both fatty acids. Quantitatively, digestion by pancreatic lipase is the most important process (Zeisel, 1990). The net result is that most ingested lecithin is absorbed as lysophosphatidylcholine (deacylated in the β position). Within the cells of the gut wall, lysophosphatidylcholine can be deacylated to form glycerophosphocholine, or it can be acylated to reconstitute lecithin.

Choline is absorbed from the jejunum and ileum mainly by an energy- and sodium-dependent carrier mechanism. In the guinea pig, choline was taken up by ileal cells about three times faster than by jejunal cells (Hegazy and Schwenk, 1984). Preferential location of the transport system in ileal cells supports earlier findings in the rat and hamster (Sanford and Smyth, 1971). These results are expected since choline is released from lecithin in the proximal and middle small intestine.

Only one-third of ingested choline appears to be absorbed intact. The remaining two-thirds is metabolized by intestinal microorganisms to trimethylamine, which is excreted in the urine between 6 and 12 hours after consumption (De La Huerga and Popper, 1952). In contrast, when an equivalent amount of choline is consumed as lecithin, less urinary trimethylamine is excreted, with most of the metabolite appearing in urine 12 to 24 hours after consumption. Dietary choline is the principal factor governing excretion, with presence or absence of other sources of protein and of fat having relatively little effect. Absorbed choline is transported into the lymphatic circulation primarily in the form of lecithin bound to chylomicra, it is transported to the tissues predominantly as phospholipids associated with the plasma lipoproteins.

Choline is present in all tissues as an essential component of phospholipids in membranes of all types. All tissues accumulate choline, but uptake by liver, kidney, mammary gland, placenta, and brain are of especial importance. Uptake of choline by mammary cells enables this tissue to concentrate choline almost 70-fold versus maternal blood (Chao et al., 1988). Most species can synthesize choline, as lecithin, by the sequential methylation of phosphatidylethanolamine (Fig. 14.2) by phosphatidylethanolamine-N-methyltransferase. This activity is actually due to enzymes that use S-adenosylmethionine (SAM) as the methyl donor. Choline synthesis activity is low in male rats and absent from chicks until about the thirteenth week of age. The activity is greatest in liver, but is also found in many other tissues.

Choline is released in free form in the tissues by the actions of phospholipase C, which cleaves the circulating form (lecithin) to yield a diglyceride and phosphorylcholine. Free choline can be oxidized by the mitochondrial enzyme choline dehydrogenase to yield betaine aldehyde, which is then converted by the cytosolic enzyme betaine aldehyde dehydrogenase to betaine. Betaine is the actual source of methyl groups. Only a small fraction of choline is acetylated, but that amount provides the important neurotransmitter acetylcholine. This step involves the reaction of choline with acetyl CoA and is catalyzed by choline acetyltransferase localized in cholinergic nerve terminals, as well as in certain other nonnervous tissues (e.g., placenta).

In ruminants, dietary choline is rapidly and extensively degraded in

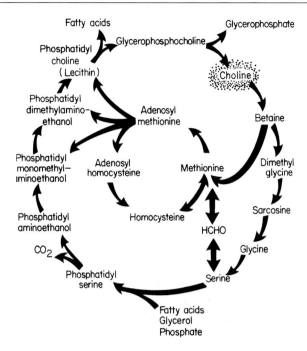

Fig. 14.2 Metabolic pathway for the synthesis of choline and related compounds. Folacin and vitamin B_{12} are required for synthesis of methyl groups and metabolism of the one-carbon unit. (Adapted from Scott et al., 1982.)

the rumen from studies with both sheep (Neill et al., 1979) and cattle (Atkins et al., 1988; Sharma and Erdman, 1988). In sheep fed forage diets, choline is rapidly degraded to trimethylamine with only 10 to 15% of the dietary choline escaping rumen degradation; however, the degree of degradation in different diets is unknown (Neill et al., 1979). Estimates of rumen degradation have ranged from 85 to 99%. In vivo studies with dairy cows, in which choline intake was increased up to 303 g/day over controls, there was an increase of only 1.3 g/day in choline flow to the duodenum (Sharma and Erdman, 1988).

Work with sheep (Neill et al., 1979) and goats (Emmanual and Kennelly, 1984) suggests that ruminants must metabolize and utilize choline in a different manner than monogastric animals. Choline absorption must be very limited in all ruminants because of (1) almost complete degradation of dietary choline in the rumen, (2) only limited supplies from any rumen protozoa that might escape rumen degradation, and (3) rumen bacteria, which are devoid of choline.

FUNCTIONS

Choline functions in four broad categories in the animal body:

1. Choline is a metabolic essential for building and maintaining cell structure. As a phospholipid it is a structural part of lecithin (phosphatidylcholine), certain plasmalogens, and the sphingomyelins. Choline is incorporated into phospholipid by being converted to phosphoryl choline, then to cytidine diphosphate choline, and finally reacting with phosphatidic acid to lecithin. The phospholipids and total fatty acids present are affected by nutritional state and the type of fatty acids present in the diet. Lecithin is a part of animal cell membranes and lipid transport moieties in cell plasma membranes. Phospholipids exist in the cell membrane bilayers, and it is thought that one of the primary roles of phospholipids is to regulate cell membrane porosity by changing the ionic characteristics of the membrane. Lecithin is also an essential component of very-low-density lipoprotein, the blood transport molecule for hepatic triacylglycerol (Lombardi et al., 1966). In the prevention of perosis, choline is required as a constituent of the phospholipids needed for normal maturation of the cartilage matrix of the bone. Various metabolic functions and synthesis of choline are depicted in Fig. 14.2.

2. Choline plays an essential role in fat metabolism in the liver. The first discovered function of dietary choline dealt with prevention of fatty liver in depancreatized dogs, and later in rats, chicks, and other species. Owing to the basic function of choline in membrane structure, the lack of choline is manifested in a variety of phospholipid-related functions, such as fatty liver and lesions of the kidney and impairment of lipoprotein metabolism. Choline prevents abnormal accumulation of fat (fatty livers) by promoting its transport as lecithin or by increasing the utilization of fatty acids in the liver itself. Choline is thus referred to as a lipotropic factor because of its function of acting on fat metabolism by hastening removal or decreasing deposition of fat in liver.

3. Choline is essential for the formation of acetylcholine, the agent released at the termination of the parasympathetic nerves (Wauben and Wainwright, 1999). It makes possible the transmission of nerve impulses from presynaptic to postsynaptic fibers of the sympathetic and parasympathetic nervous systems. For example, acetylcholine released by the stimulated vagus nerve causes a slowing of heartbeat, and oviduct contraction results from the action of acetylcholine. Acetylcholine is the most common neurotransmitter in the nervous system. Apparently, brain tissue lacks the ability to synthesize sufficient choline (Ansell and Spanner, 1971) for neural func-

tion. However, apparently circulating choline is the major source of choline for acetylcholine synthesis.

4. A fourth function of choline is as a source of labile methyl groups for formation of methionine from homocystine and of creatine from guanidoacetic acid. However, practical significance of the choline-homocystine interrelationship is of no real importance to feeding animals since natural proteins contain very little of the metabolic intermediate homocystine (Ruiz et al., 1983). Methyl groups also function in the synthesis of purine and pyrimidine, which are used in the production of DNA. Methionine is converted to S-adenosylmethionine in a reaction catalyzed by methionine adenosyl transferase. S-adenosylmethionine is the active methylating agent for many enzymatic methylations. A disturbance in folacin or methionine metabolism results in changes in choline metabolism and visa versa (Zeisel, 1990). The involvement of folacin, vitamin B_{12}, and methionine in methyl group metabolism, and of methionine in de novo choline synthesis, may allow these substances to substitute in part for choline. Severe folacin deficiency has been shown to cause secondary liver choline deficiency in rats (Kim et al., 1994).

The demand for choline as a methyl donor is probably the major factor that determines how rapidly a diet deficient in choline will induce pathology. The pathways of choline and 1-carbon metabolism intersect at the formation of methionine from homocysteine. Methionine is regenerated from homocysteine in a reaction catalyzed by betaine-homocysteine methyltransferase, in which betaine, a metabolite of choline, serves as the methyl donor (Finkelstein et al., 1982). Large increases in chick hepatic betaine-homocysteine methyltransferase can be produced under methionine-deficient conditions, especially in the presence of excess choline or betaine (Emmert et al., 1996). To be a source of methyl groups, choline must be converted to betaine, which has been shown to perform methylation functions as well as choline in some cases. However, betaine fails to prevent fatty livers and hemorrhagic kidneys. A diagram of the choline cycle, including related compounds and donations to the body's methyl pool, is shown in Fig. 14.3.

Since choline contains biologically active methyl groups, methionine can partly be spared by choline and homocysteine. Research with lactating dairy cattle suggests that a high proportion of dietary methionine is used for choline synthesis (Erdman and Sharma, 1991). Discoveries in signal transduction are beginning to reveal other important roles for choline phospholipids. Signal transduction is a new area of cell biology research and is the process by which hormones and other substances

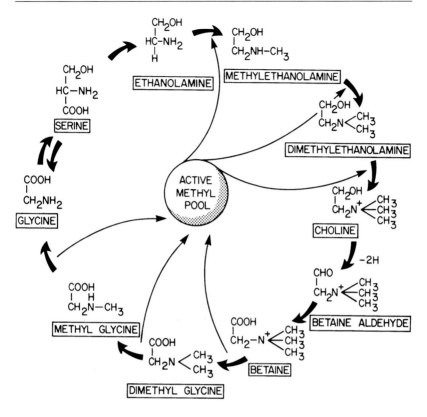

Fig. 14.3 Choline cycle showing metabolic generation and use of active methyl groups. (Adapted from Umbrett, 1960.)

transmit messages from the cell's surface to its interior, and by which a broad spectrum of cell activities—such as growth, gene expression, ion transport, and energy utilization—are regulated. Evidence shows that choline phospholipids play a central role in this process. Disruptions in phospholipid metabolism can interfere with this process and may underlie certain disease states, such as cancer and Alzheimer's disease (Canty and Zeisel, 1994).

The choline phospholipid metabolite plasmalogen has been studied in relation to myocardial infarction. High levels of plasmalogen are found in the sarcolemma, the cell membrane of heart muscle. An adverse effect of acute myocardial ischemia may be the result of plasmalogen breakdown during an ischemic attack (Canty and Zeisel, 1994).

REQUIREMENTS

Choline, unlike most vitamins, can be synthesized by most species, although in many cases not in sufficient amounts or rapidly enough to satisfy all the animal's needs. For example, when intake of precursors or accessory factors—such as methionine, vitamin B_{12}, or folacin—is insufficient, poultry, dogs, cats, monkeys, pigs, rabbits, and certain fish (e.g., bass, catfish, carp and trout) have been shown to require exogenous choline. Also, young animals show a higher need for choline than adults. Dietary factors such as methionine, betaine, *myo*-inositol, folacin, and vitamin B_{12}, or the combination of different levels and composition of fat, carbohydrate, and protein in the diet, as well as the age, sex, caloric intake, and growth rate of animals, all have influence on the lipotropic action of choline and thereby on the requirement of this nutrient (Mookerjea, 1971). Dietary betaine can spare choline, since choline functions as a methyl donor by forming betaine. In relation to protein level, a larger choline effect on litter size and piglet and litter weight was observed for gilts fed a 12% protein diet than for those fed a 16% protein diet (Maxwell et al., 1987).

Studies have shown that vitamin B_{12} and folacin reduce requirement for choline in chicks and rats (Welch and Couch, 1955). Folacin and vitamin B_{12} are required for the synthesis of methyl groups and metabolism of the one-carbon unit. Biosynthesis of labile methyl from a formate carbon requires folacin, while B_{12} plays a role in regulated transfer of the methyl group from tetrahydrofolic acid. Therefore, marked increases in choline requirement have been observed under conditions of folacin and/or vitamin B_{12} deficiency.

The two principal methyl donors functioning in animal metabolism are choline and methionine, which contain biologically labile methyl groups that can be transferred within the body. This phenomenon is called transmethylation. Methionine furnishes a methyl group that can combine with ethanolamine to form choline and, in reverse, methyl groups from choline (du Vigneaud et al., 1939). Therefore, dietary adequacy for both methionine and choline directly affect requirements of each other. Other than exogenous sources of methyl groups from choline and methionine, methyl group formation from de novo synthesis of formate carbons is reduced with folate and/or vitamin B_{12} deficiencies.

Most animals can synthesize sufficient choline for their needs provided enough methyl groups are supplied. As an example, methionine in the pig can completely replace that portion of the choline needed for

574

transmethylation. Thus, at methionine levels in excess of the physiological requirement, 4.3 mg of methionine—or 3.69 mg with hydroxyl (OH) group considered in molecular weight of choline—provides the same methylating capacity as 1 mg of choline (NRC, 1998). Kroening and Pond (1967) fed 5-kg pigs a low-protein diet (12%) supplemented with three levels of dl-methionine—0, 0.11, and 0.22%. The addition of 1,646 mg of choline per kilogram of diet improved the weight gain and feed conversion of pigs fed the control and the 0.11% but not the 0.22% methionine-supplemented diet. Young poultry, on the contrary, are unable to benefit from methionine or betaine as a dietary replacement for choline unless methylaminoethanol or dimethylaminoethanol is in the diet, as they appear unable to methylate aminoethanol when fed a purified diet (Jukes, 1947). Later studies showed that the chick can synthesize microsomal methylaminoethanol and choline from S-andenosylmethionine, but, unlike the pig, at an insufficient rate to cover its needs (Norvell and Nesheim, 1969).

Calculations from lactating dairy goats on rates of methyl group transfer revealed that only 6% of methionine methyl groups were derived from choline, while 28% of choline methyl groups were derived from methionine (Emmanual and Kennelly, 1984). This suggests that considerable dietary methionine is used for choline synthesis.

The metabolic needs for choline can be supplied in two ways: by dietary choline or by choline synthesis in the body, which makes use of labile methyl groups. For selected species, body synthesis sometimes cannot take place fast enough to meet choline needs for rapid growth, and thus clinical signs of deficiency result. Since choline functions in the prevention of fatty livers, hemorrhagic kidneys, and perosis, it does not act as a true vitamin since it is incorporated into phospholipids (via cytidine diphosphocholine). Therefore, unlike a typical B vitamin, the choline molecule becomes an integral part of the structural component of liver, kidney, or cartilage cells (Scott et al., 1982).

In general, males are more sensitive to choline deficiency than females (Wilson, 1978). Growth hormone seemed to increase the choline requirement in rats independent of its ability to promote growth and increase food intake (Hall and Bieri, 1953). Cortisone and hydrocortisone have been reported to decrease severity of renal necrosis, and hydrocortisone reduced the amount of hepatic lipid in choline-deficient rats (Olson, 1959).

Excess dietary protein increases the young chick's choline requirement. Ketola and Nesheim (1974) observed that over three times as much choline was needed for maximum growth of chicks fed a diet containing 64% protein versus 13%. Diets high in fat aggravate choline deficiency and thus increase requirement. Fatty liver is generally enhanced by fats containing a high proportion of long-chain saturated fatty acids (Hartroft, 1955). Choline deficiency develops to a greater degree in rapidly growing animals with deficiency lesions more severe in these animals.

Use of antibiotics or prevention of coprophagy in rats decreases dietary choline requirement (Barnes and Kwong, 1967). Likewise, dietary requirement of choline is reduced in germ-free rats. Intestinal flora convert choline to trimethylamine, a lipotropically inactive compound that is excreted in urine. Suppression of intestinal flora by antibiotics would result in choline being more available than as inactive trimethylamine.

Recommended dietary allowances for choline or amounts typically fed for a number of animal species are listed in Table 14.1. Requirements for choline have generally been determined through the use of purified diets, and recommendations often do not take into account bioavailability from feedstuffs, individual animal variation, or effects of other dietary factors. Typical choline requirements for monogastric animals range from 1,000 to 2,000 mg/kg of feed. In contrast to monogastric animals, no requirements for choline have been established for ruminant animals except for milk-fed calves, in which 260 mg of choline per liter of synthetic milk prevented choline deficiency signs. The NRC (1989a) suggests that milk replacers for calves should contain 0.26% choline.

Choline is an essential nutrient for humans on the basis of deficiency signs for those receiving experimental diets low in choline (Zeisel et al., 1991) and for individuals receiving total parenteral nutrition devoid of choline (Buchman et al., 1992). Choline is likely not essential when diets contain excess methionine and folacin. Human choline requirements have not been established (RDA, 1989). Based on a caloric intake of 2,000 kcal/day, one might expect the typical human diet to range in choline content from 410 to 1375 mg/kg dry matter. When compared to requirements for other animal species and, in particular, mature animals, it seems unlikely that choline deficiency would occur (DuCoa L.P., 1994).

NATURAL SOURCES

All naturally occurring fats contain some choline, and thus it is supplied by all feeds that contain fat. Choline is almost always found in the form of lecithin or sphingomyelin in most foods. Egg yolk (1.7%), glandular meats (0.6%), and brain and fish (0.2%) are the richest animal

■ Table 14.1 Choline Requirements for Various Animals and Humans

Animal	Purpose or Class	Requirement[a]	Reference
Beef cattle	Adult	Tissue synthesis	NRC (1984a)
Dairy cattle	Calf milk replacer	2,600 mg/kg liter	NRC (1989a)
	Adult	Tissue synthesis	NRC (1989a)
Chicken	Leghorn, 0–6 weeks	1,300 mg/kg	NRC (1994)
	Leghorn, 6–12 weeks	900 mg/kg	NRC (1994)
	Broilers, 0–3 weeks	1,300 mg/kg	NRC (1994)
	Broilers, 6–8 weeks	750 mg/kg	NRC (1994)
Japanese quail	Starting and growing	2,000 mg/kg	NRC (1994)
	Breeding	1,500 mg/kg	NRC (1994)
Turkey	Growing, 0–4 weeks	1,600 mg/kg	NRC (1994)
	Growing, 8–16 weeks	950 mg/kg	NRC (1994)
Sheep	Adult	Tissue synthesis	NRC (1985b)
Swine	Growing, 3–5 kg	0.6 g/kg	NRC (1998)
	Growing, 5–120 kg	0.3–0.5 g/kg	NRC (1998)
	Adult	1.00–1.25 g/kg	NRC (1998)
Horse	Adult	Tissue synthesis	NRC (1989b)
Goat	Adult	Tissue synthesis	NRC (1981b)
Cat	Adult	2,400 mg/kg	NRC (1986)
Dog	Growing	1,250 mg/kg	NRC (1985a)
Rabbit	All classes	0.12% choline chloride	NRC (1977)
Rat	All classes	1,000 mg/kg	NRC (1978a)
Fish	Catfish	400 mg/kg	NRC (1993)
	Lake trout	1,000 mg/kg	NRC (1993)
	Common carp	1,500 mg/kg	NRC (1993)
Human	All classes	Unknown	RDA (1989)

[a]Expressed as per unit of animal feed on either as-fed (approximately 90% dry matter) or dry basis (see Appendix, Tables A1a,b) (except for dairy calf).

sources, and germ of cereals (0.1%), legumes (0.2 to 0.35%), and oilseed meals are the best plant sources (DuCoa L.P., 1994). Most oil seeds, such as peanuts, cottonseed, and soybeans, are good sources of choline because of their relatively high phospholipid content. Choline content in foods is extremely variable, and much of this variation can be attributed to biological variation. However, a large portion of the reported variability may be due to differences in procedures for choline analysis.

Corn is low in choline, with wheat, barley, and oats containing approximately twice as much choline as corn. Since betaine can spare the requirements of choline, it would be useful to know the concentrations of betaine in feeds. Unfortunately, most feedstuffs contain only small amounts of betaine. However, wheat and wheat by-products apparently contain over twice as much betaine as choline. Thus, the choline needs of swine or poultry fed wheat-based diets would be much lower than those fed diets based on other grains. Sugar beets are also high in betaine.

Choline is largely absent in most fruits and vegetables. However, other foods consumed by animals and humans can be good sources. Infant formulas based on soy protein have much less choline than human or cow's milk (Zeisel et al., 1986). Choline content of typical foods and feedstuffs is shown in Table 14.2.

Little is known of the biological availability of choline in natural feedstuffs. Using a chick assay method, soybean, canola, and peanut meals were found to contain a substantial proportion of unavailable choline (Emmert and Baker, 1997). Dehulled regular soybean meal and whole soybeans were tested and appeared to range in availability from 60 to 75% (Molitoris and Baker, 1976). However, soybean lecithin products were found to be equivalent to choline chloride in bioavailability (Emmert et al., 1997). March and MacMillan (1980) presented evidence that choline bioavailability in rapeseed meal is lower than in soybean meal. Canola meal, although three times as rich in total choline as soybean meal, was found to have less bioavailable choline (Emmert and Baker, 1997). In chicks, production of trimethylamine (resulting from bacterial degradation of choline) in the intestine was greater in chicks fed rapeseed meal than in those fed soybean meal.

DEFICIENCY

The most common signs of choline deficiency include poor growth, fatty liver, perosis, hemorrhagic tissue (particularly in the kidney and certain joints), and hypertension. In general, severity of clinical signs in

■ Table 14.2   Typical Choline Concentrations in Foods and Feedstuffs (ppm, dry basis)

Alfalfa meal, dehydrated	1,370	Meat and bone meal	1,996
Bakery waste, dehydrated	1,005	Liver meal	12,281
Barley	1,177	Milk, skim, dehydrated	1,480
Blood meal, dehydrated	848	Molasses, sugarcane	1,012
Brewer's grains, dehydrated	1,757	Oats	1,116
Buttermilk (cattle), dehydrated	1,891	Peanut meal	2,120
Chicken	6,288	Potato, dehydrated	2,879
Citrus pulp, dehydrated	867	Rice	1,076
Copra (coconut) meal	1,036	Rice bran	1,357
Corn, yellow	620	Sesame	1,655
Corn gluten feed	1,518	Sorghum	737
Cottonseed meal	2,965	Soybean meal	2,916
Crab meal	2,179	Wheat	1,053
Fish meal, anchovy	4,036	Wheat bran	1,797

Sources: Selected from United States-Canadian Tables of Feed Composition (NRC, 1982) and DuCoa L.P. (1994).

animal species is influenced by other dietary factors, including methionine, vitamin B_{12}, folacin, and dietary fat (see Requirements). When feed intake—and consequently growth—are depressed by choline deficiency, severity of choline deficiency is then reduced. Clinical signs and lesions in choline-deficient animals are summarized in Table 14.3.

Effects of Deficiency

Ruminants

The ability of ruminants to synthesize the B vitamins including choline is well known. In cattle and sheep, orally ingested choline is rapidly degraded in the rumen, but rumen microbes synthesize choline. It has been found that ruminal synthesis and/or the unsupplemented diet do not always supply enough choline to meet feedlot cattle demands. Improved performance of feedlot cattle has been related to use of dietary choline, although not consistently in all experiments. Reports from Washington (Swingle and Dyer, 1970) and Maryland (Rumsey, 1975) showed increased gains by as much as 6 to 7% and improved feed efficiency by 2.5 to 8% for finishing cattle when supplemented with 500 to 750 ppm dietary choline. In other experiments with growing cattle, no response occurred after addition of dietary choline (Wise et al., 1964; Harris et al., 1966). Thus, choline, under certain conditions of high-concentrate feeding, may be limiting in the diet.

Researchers have shown interest in choline in view of its possible lipotropic effect in high-producing dairy cows. Atkins et al. (1983) and Erdman et al. (1984) studied the effects of supplementing choline on roughage adequate diets for dairy cattle and concluded that added choline had little effect on milk production, although slight increases were seen in feed intake and milk fat percentage. Limited research indicates that supplemental choline may be needed to obtain optimum milk fat, possibly through its effect on hepatic lipid metabolism. Lactating cows fed supplemental choline showed an increase in milk fat percentage and fat-corrected milk (Erdman et al., 1984). In a later experiment, Erdman and Sharma (1991) were unable to show a positive effect on milk fat percentage from choline by postruminal infusion. However, these experiments confirm earlier postruminal infusion studies in which increasing postruminal choline increased milk yield up to 3.1 kg/day.

An apparent choline deficiency syndrome was produced with a synthetic milk diet containing 15% casein (Johnson et al., 1951). Within 6 to 8 days, calves developed extreme weakness with labored breathing

■ Table 14.3 Clinical Signs and Lesions in Choline-Deficient Animals

Signs and Lesions	Rat	Mouse	Hamster	Fish	Rabbit	Monkey	Dog	Cat	Calf	Pig	Chicken	Duck	Turkey
Fatty Liver	+	+	+	+	+	+	+	+	+	+	+	+	+
Cirrhosis	+	+[a]			+[a]	+	+						
Hemorrhagic kidney	+	+[b]			+[b]				+[b]	+[b]			
Growth failure	+	+	+	+	+	+	+	+	+	+	+	+	+
Hypolipemia	+						+						
Perosis											+	+	+
Impaired reproduction	+	+	+							+			
Impaired lactation	+		+						+				
Reduced egg production													
Muscle defects	+				+			+	+	+			
Spraddled hind legs										+			
Hemorrhagic lesions	+	+											
Arterial sclerosis	+	+					+						
Myocarditis and necrosis	+	+									+		
Bradycardia	+												
Hypertension	+												
Anemia	+			+	+		+			+			
Edema, ascites	+												

Sources: Modified from Wilson (1978). Information also from NRC (1988, 1993).
Note: In many cases, lesions have not been studied or reported in various species.
[a]Produced with difficulty; see text.
[b]Renal degeneration only.

and were unable to stand. Supplementation with 260 mg of choline per liter of milk replacer prevented these deficiency signs.

Swine

Choline deficiency in the young pig results in unthriftiness, poor conformation (short-legged and pot-bellied), lack of coordination in movements, characteristic lack of proper rigidity in joints (particularly the shoulders), fatty infiltration of liver, characteristic renal glomerular occlusion, and some tubular epithelial necrosis (Cunha, 1977). These clinical signs resulted from low-methionine diets (0.8%) and were prevented with 1.6% dietary methionine.

Spraddled-leg condition is a problem occasionally seen in newborn pigs, and some evidence suggests that incidence has a strong genetic component. However, the condition is often attributed to choline deficiency and is prevented by supplementation of the vitamin. Whether folacin and B_{12} are involved in the condition is unknown, but under conditions of deficiencies of these vitamins, choline requirements are increased. Spraddled legs can be described as a congenital disorder in which the newborn pig cannot stand or walk because of the leg condition (Fig. 14.4). Nursing is also hindered, thereby affecting weaning weights.

Spraddled-leg condition started to appear when swine producers began to decrease feed allowances given sows during gestation from 2.7 to 3.2 kg to 1.4 to 2.0 kg daily (Cunha, 1977), which resulted in reduced intakes of both choline and methionine. Studies from Colombia, South America (J.H. Maner, personal communication to Cunha, 1977), revealed death losses due to spraddled-leg condition. Some of these pigs recuperated by the tenth day after birth, which could indicate that the condition can be corrected through the sow's milk. Other reports have indicated that a high proportion of baby pigs affected by spraddled legs were able to recover after a few days, especially if the hind legs were bound temporarily to allow them to move and suckle.

Protein, methionine, and sulfate concentrations of the diet influence choline requirements. A study of the effects of protein level and supplemental choline on the reproductive performance of gilts indicated that choline increases pig weight and litter weight (Maxwell et al., 1987). When dietary methionine is high, often there is no demonstrated response to supplementation of choline. This may be expected due to their mutual sparing effect. Kroening and Pond (1967) showed increased gain for 3-week-old pigs fed synthetic diets containing 1,640 ppm choline and less than 0.31% methionine; although choline tended to improve

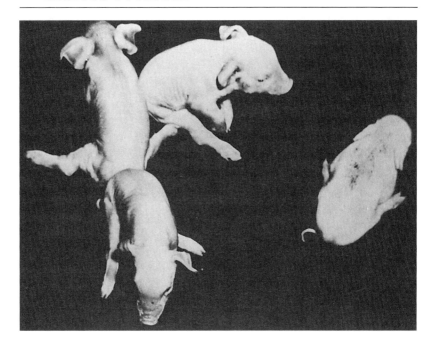

Fig. 14.4 Choline deficiency. Spraddled hind legs—the condition shown here—has been produced with a purified ration and is prevented by choline supplementation. Other factors may be involved. (Courtesy of T.J. Cunha and Washington State University.)

feed per gain in all diets containing up to 0.42% methionine. An investigation of the relationship of methionine, choline and sulfate in the diet of weanling swine indicated that choline and sulfate or methionine and sulfate improved performance (Lovett et al., 1985).

Research reports have shown that sows without choline have a significantly lower conception rate and farrowing rate and farrow significantly fewer total pigs and fewer live pigs per litter. No difference was found in the average birth weight, but sows with choline supplementation weaned significantly more pigs per litter, and sows without choline farrowed a slightly higher percentage of pigs with spraddled legs. Pigs from choline-deficient sows were unthrifty in appearance and became increasingly so with age (Ensminger et al., 1947).

The NRC-42 committee on swine nutrition in 1976 evaluated the effects of supplemental choline (770 mg/kg of diet) during gestation and lactation on litter size at birth and at weaning. Nine stations participated, with 22 trials and 551 sows. The diet was a 15.0% protein corn-soybean meal type during gestation, and 7.5% beet pulp was substituted for an equal amount of corn during the lactation period. Results indicated that sows fed supplemental choline farrowed more pigs per litter (10.54 versus 9.89) and more live pigs per litter (9.33 versus 8.64), and weaned more pigs per litter (7.72 versus 7.29).

Betaine, the methyl donor derived from choline, has been shown to be beneficial to swine (Odle, 1996). Shurson et al. (1994) concluded that inclusion of betaine for more than 30 days prior to slaughter could, in most cases, produce positive carcass effects, specifically reduced back fat and increased yield. On the contrary, however, Øverland et al. (1999) fed swine high fat diets supplemented with betaine but failed to improve growth performance, carcass quality, or nutrient digestibility.

Haydon et al. (1995) reported positive betaine effects only with low lysine:calorie feeds. Campbell et al. (1995) reported that when a methionine-deficient basal diet was supplemented with 0.125% betaine, feed efficiency was improved to the same degree as when methionine was supplemented at 0.23%.

Poultry

Growth retardation and perosis result from choline deficiency in young poultry. Perosis is the primary clinical sign of choline deficiency in chicks and turkey poults, whereas bobwhite quail develop enlarged hocks and bowed legs (NRC, 1994). Perosis is characterized first by pinpoint hemorrhages about the hock joint, followed by an apparent flattening of the tibiometatarsal joint (Scott et al., 1982). Progressively, the Achilles tendon slips from its condyles, thus rendering the bird relatively immobile. Some studies indicated that in prevention of perosis, choline is required for the phospholipids needed for normal maturation of the cartilage matrix of bone.

Adult chickens probably synthesize sufficient choline to meet requirements for egg production. Minimal dietary choline does not affect hatchability with either chickens or turkeys, but Japanese quail and their developing embryos readily express general signs of deficiency (Latshaw and Jensen, 1972; NRC, 1994). Supplementary choline may be necessary for maintenance of egg size in quail (NRC, 1994). Contrary to some reports, 500 ppm supplemental choline to Leghorn hens increased egg weight while reducing specific gravity (Tapia Romero et al., 1985). Also, the choline growth requirement for quail is apparently higher than that for chicks or poults.

Choline requirement of growing chicks decreases with age, and it is generally not possible to produce a deficiency at an age over 8 weeks. It

583

was observed that methylation of aminoethanol to methylaminoethanol seems to be the rate-limiting step in choline biosynthesis for young birds. High levels of dietary methionine or other methyl donors, therefore, cannot completely spare the chick's requirement for dietary choline, which is in contrast to the situation with growing mammals such as the pig or the rat.

Apparently, choline requirement of laying hens can be influenced by choline level in the diet of the growing pullet (Scott et al., 1982). Hens that received choline-free diets after 8 weeks of age were able to synthesize all the choline required for good egg production. Those that received choline supplements in the growing diet required supplemental choline in the laying diet for maximum egg production. The deficiency signs noted in these hens were a reduction in egg production and an increase in fat content of liver. Even with choline deficiency, however, choline content of the egg was not affected by low dietary choline.

Despite lack of evidence that laying chickens require a dietary source of choline for maximum egg production, addition of choline to practical diets markedly reduces the amount of fat in the liver (NRC, 1994). However, a number of reports with chicks and turkey poults did not find fatty livers in chicks deficient in choline (Ruiz et al., 1983). A choline response in laying chickens is likely to occur only if inadequate daily sulfur amino acid is provided.

Addition of 0.1% of supplemental methionine resulted in no response in laying hens to supplemental choline (Crawford et al., 1969). It appears that benefits from supplemental choline in layer diets occur mainly when supplemental methionine is just adequate to meet methionine requirements. Miles and Harms (1983) demonstrated that the addition of 0.11% choline plus 0.1% sulfate could essentially spare all supplemental methionine in broiler diets. However, in turkey poult diets (Harms and Miles, 1984), responses to sulfate and choline addition were not equivalent to the addition of supplemental methionine. Pesti et al. (1980), using young chicks, found that supplementation with methyl donors from either 0.23% choline or 0.23% betaine was equivalent to supplementation with 0.23% methionine in 21-day chick experiments, using basal diets containing 0.31% methionine and 0.43% cystine. Spires et al. (1982) found that supplemental choline could replace up to two-thirds of the supplemental methionine required in broiler diets from 0 to 47 days in diets containing 0.30% methionine and 0.43% cystine in the starter phase, and 0.25 and 0.42% methionine and cystine, respectively, in the finisher phase.

Horses

No studies of choline requirements or deficiencies have been undertaken in the horse.

Other Animal Species

DOGS AND CATS

In growing cats, choline deficiency results in perilobular infiltration of the liver, hypoalbuminemia, and decreased growth (NRC, 1986). In young puppies, choline deficiency results in reduced appetite and growth rate, fatty metamorphosis of the liver, and atrophic changes of the thymus. Choline-deficient dogs with fatty livers show an increased rate of hepatic phospholipid synthesis following choline supplementation (NRC, 1985a).

FISH

Dietary choline is required for optimum growth; feed utilization; and prevention of fatty livers, anemia, hemorrhages (in liver, kidney, and intestine), and other clinical signs in striped bass, salmon, trout, carp, catfish, and bream (NRC, 1993; Griffin et al., 1994). Severity and nature of choline deficiency signs, as well as the time required for them to appear, seem to be highly variable and may depend on species or diet or both (Ketola, 1976). Channel catfish fed casein-gelatin diets containing excess methionine did not develop signs of choline deficiency; however, catfish fed diets adequate but not excessive in methionine did develop deficiency signs (Wilson and Poe, 1988).

Rainbow trout fed a choline-deficient diet developed light yellow-colored livers, protruded eyes, anemia, and extended abdomens (Kitamura et al., 1967), while lake trout fed a choline-deficient diet for 12 weeks had depressed growth rate and increased liver fat content (Ketola, 1976). Common carp were found to grow normally on a choline-deficient diet but had 10% higher liver lipid content (Ogino et al., 1970). Contrary to other fish and different species, the red drum had reduced liver lipid rather than high accumulation with choline deficiency (Craig and Gatlin, 1996). Choline-deficient Japanese eels became anorexic, had poor growth, and exhibited a white-gray intestine. After 4 weeks, shrimp fed a choline-deficient diet were significantly smaller than controls (NRC, 1993).

LABORATORY ANIMALS

Guinea pigs, like young poultry, easily develop choline deficiency even with adequate dietary methionine. Clinical signs of choline deficiency in young guinea pigs include poor growth, anemia, muscular weakness, and some adrenal subcutaneous hemorrhages (NRC, 1995). In guinea pigs, choline supplementation altered carnitine homeostasis by decreasing urinary excretion of carnitine (Daily and Sachan, 1995). Hamsters showed poor appetite, reduced growth, and fatty livers on a peanut meal diet deficient in choline (Handler and Bernheim, 1949).

Both rats and mice exhibit fatty livers, but rats—unlike mice—also develop cirrhosis or fibrosis of the liver. In young rats the kidney becomes hemorrhagic, owing presumably to a deficiency of choline for the phospholipid required to build cell structure at this critical growth period. Mice, on the other hand, develop hemorrhagic kidneys only with more difficulty and diet manipulation. Administration of lecithin increased brain acetylcholine concentration and improved memory in mice with dementia (Chung et al., 1995). Severe folate deficiency caused secondary depletion of choline and phosphocholine in rat liver (Kim et al., 1994).

MONKEYS

Cebus monkeys, rhesus monkeys, and baboons fed choline-deficient diets for 1 to 2 years developed fatty changes in the liver and varying degrees of hepatic fibrosis (NRC, 1978).

RABBITS

The signs of choline deficiency in rabbits have been described as retarded growth, fatty and cirrhotic liver, and necrosis of the kidney tubules. Progressive muscular dystrophy was reported in rabbits fed a low-choline diet for more than 70 days (NRC, 1977).

Humans

In humans, as in experimental animals, dietary choline can arrest cirrhosis of the liver and reverse the fatty infiltration. However, these conclusions are not definite, and some reports show no benefit of choline in the treatment of cirrhosis (Kuksis and Mookerjea, 1984). It remains uncertain whether alcoholic cirrhosis in humans and animals is caused by one or more nutritional deficiencies, but accepted dietary regimens for treatment involve a high-calorie, high-protein, low-fat diet supplemented with choline and perhaps other lipotropic factors, such as methionine and inositol.

Choline is an essential nutrient for humans when excess methionine and folacin are not available in the diet. Healthy male subjects fed a choline-deficient diet for 3 weeks had depleted stores of choline in tissues and developed signs of incipient liver dysfunction (Zeisel et al., 1991). People receiving total parenteral nutrition have developed fatty infiltration of the liver and hepatocellular damage. One study in humans fed parenterally showed that supplemental choline (in the form of lecithin) could reverse fatty livers (Buchman et al., 1992).

The relationship of choline to atherosclerosis has been under study for a number of years. Choline-deficient diets can result in arterial damage, with a high percentage of young rats maintained on low-choline diets developing pathological changes in the major arterial trunks and in the coronary arteries. These changes are similar to those observed in early stages of atherosclerosis of the aorta and large arteries in humans. In a 3-year study of coronary thrombosis patients, there was a significant reduction in death rates and lowered blood cholesterol in atheromatous patients administered choline (DuCoa L.P., 1994). During acute myocardial ischemia, plasmalogen (a choline phospholipid found in the cell membranes of heart muscle) was broken down (Canty and Zeisel, 1994). Further observations have included increases in high-density lipoprotein and decreases in low-density lipoprotein following lecithin treatment in hypercholesterolemic humans (Childs et al., 1981).

Deficiency of choline enhances the initiating potency of several carcinogens (Mikol et al., 1983) and exerts a strong promoting effect with liver carcinogens. Choline deficiency alone can also lead directly to liver tumor formation (Mikol et al., 1983). A number of possible mechanisms have been proposed to account for the development of cancer as a result of choline deficiency, including increased cell death followed by increased proliferation and regeneration, deceased DNA methylation and repair, increased lipid peroxidation and free radical damage, and decreased methylation and detoxification of carcinogens (Canty and Zeisel, 1994).

Reports indicate that lecithin and/or choline supplements may be useful in preventing age-related memory deficits and certain neurological diseases (Kuksis and Mookerjea, 1984). Evidence suggests that dietary choline and lecithin produce clinical improvement by supplying precursors for formation of the neurotransmitter acetylcholine. Notable but sometimes limited success has been achieved with choline or lecithin therapy for tardive dyskinesia syndrome (jerky involuntary movements of face and extremities), Huntington's disease (rapid involuntary and purposeless movements), and Friedreich's ataxia disease (loss of coordination in muscles of the extremities). Studies of both Alzheimer's disease (deficiency of hippocampal cholinergic neurons) and senile dementia (forgetfulness) patients given choline or lecithin have shown mixed results (Wood and Allison, 1982). Smith et al. (1978), in a controlled experiment, noted some improvement in about 40% of the cases with advanced Alzheimer's syndrome. In general, studies have found that patients with less severe symptoms show greater response to choline supplementation. Thus, the use of choline in severe cases of Alzheimer's disease does not appear to be very helpful, but may be of value in early stages of memory-loss disorders (DuCoa L.P., 1994).

Assessment of Status

Research information is very limited on detection methods to determine choline status of animals. Often the best indicator of status or need for choline is observation of clinical signs attributable to choline deficiency (e.g., fatty livers or perosis) in particular species as well as beneficial performance responses when diets are supplemented with the vitamin.

Tissue levels of choline or its functional metabolites can be determined to evaluate choline status. There is evidence of a reduction of acetylcholine in brains, kidneys, and intestines of rats deprived of choline 6 days after weaning. Choline administered to rats either by injection or by diet caused a dose-related increase in brain acetylcholine (Kuksis and Mookerjea, 1984). Studies on mechanism of liver fat accumulation have suggested that this is related to a lack of phosphatidylcholine synthesis. With choline deficiency, the hepatic phosphatidylcholine:phosphatidylethanolamine ratio is reduced, and is thus a means of evaluating choline status.

Plasma choline levels in humans reflect dietary consumption (Hirsch et al., 1978). There is the suggestion that fall of free plasma choline below the normal range may be related to a choline-deficiency state. After consumption of 3 g of choline chloride in a meal, serum choline rose by 86% over the mean fasting level of 11.7 nmol/ml.

SUPPLEMENTATION

Choline is made synthetically, and, in the majority of cases, diet supplementation is from synthesized choline salts. Choline is synthesized from natural gas via methanol and ammonia, which are reacted to produce trimethylamine (Griffith and Nyc, 1971). This trimethylamine is subsequently reacted with ethylene oxide to produce choline. For feed supplementation purposes, a chloride salt is produced by reacting the alkaline base with hydrochloric acid. Choline is available for feed use as the 70 or 75% liquid or 25 to 60% dry powder. Choline chloride can be available on a cereal carrier; the product is obtained by spraying and thoroughly mixing aqueous choline chloride on a suitable cereal carrier and then drying to a low moisture content. The 70 to 75% liquid is very corrosive and requires special storage and handling equipment. It is not suitable for inclusion in concentrated vitamin premixes, but rather is most generally added singly to concentrate mixtures.

A variety of lecithin products that are derived from soybeans are available for use in feeds. The products range from crude fluid lecithin to 50% lecithin codried with corn syrup solids to a dry deoiled soy lecithin (Meyers, 1990). The advantage of a deoiled soybean lecithin is that it can be handled as a dry feed ingredient. The dry deoiled lecithin product also possesses those advantageous properties of soybean lecithin in general that impart important dietary formulation features, including vitamin stabilization (thus protecting vitamins from oxidation); improvement of fat and vitamin utilization; and a source of choline, inositol, and growth-stimulating compounds.

Some research has shown that supplemental betaine, a product of choline oxidation, is beneficial to swine and poultry production (Lowry et al., 1987; Odle, 1996). Supplemental betaine is available as betaine hydrochloride (98.0% betaine on an anhydrous basis).

Response to dietary supplementation of choline will be most dependent on species, age of animals, protein and sulfur amino acid intake, dietary choline, and other choline-sparing nutrients. Unlike most vitamins, choline can be synthesized by various animals, although often in insufficient amounts. It appears that choline deficiency in the young of some species (e.g., chick) may not be due to lack of ability to synthesize choline but more likely to lack of ability to synthesize it at a rate sufficient for animal needs. Age is an important consideration; for example, it is difficult to produce choline deficiency in growing chicks more than 8 weeks of age.

The young of many species (e.g., pig and rat) do not require supplementary choline if dietary methionine level is sufficiently high. On a synthetic milk diet containing 1.6% methionine, young pigs were found not to require supplemental choline (Firth et al., 1953). Neumann et al. (1949) reported that the young pig requires 0.1% dietary choline when methionine is present at 0.8 to 1.0% of the diet.

Methionine can furnish methyl groups for choline synthesis for most species. Choline, however, is effective only in sparing methionine that otherwise would be used to make up for a choline shortage. Methionine is not used for choline synthesis if there is an adequate level of dietary choline. In formulating typical poultry and swine diets, methionine is frequently one of the most limiting amino acids. Therefore, it would be impractical for marginal quantities of methionine to be wasted for synthesis of the vitamin when supplemental choline can be provided more economically.

Interrelationships of choline and methionine are discussed in the Functions and Requirements sections. In providing supplements of methionine and/or choline (or betaine), an additional nutrient, sulfur, must be considered. Significance of a four-way interrelationship among methionine, choline, betaine, and sulfate has been reviewed (Ruiz et al., 1983; Miles et al., 1986; Miles and Butcher, 1997). Sulfur is present in a number of body metabolites (e.g., mucopolysaccharides) and, if not adequately supplied in the diet, sulfur amino acids would likely be degraded. In feeding broilers, supplemental sulfate accompanied by choline or methionine achieved a greater growth response than when either was fed alone (Miles et al., 1983). Data suggest that sulfate must be present for choline to spare a maximum amount of methionine. The practical implication is that sulfate and choline need to be adequately provided in diets so that the more expensive and often marginally deficient nutrient methionine is not used to provide either of these nutrients.

Most choline supplementation studies emphasize production benefits from providing the vitamin to young animals. However, research and observations with adult swine have demonstrated improved litter size at weaning, and supplementation may keep sows in the producing herd longer (Cunha, 1977). The exact level of choline needed for sow rations is unknown. Until more research data are available, Cunha (1972) suggested the following levels in situations where spraddled hind legs are likely to occur: (1) during the first part of gestation, a daily level of 3,000 mg per sow and (2) the last month of gestation, when daily choline should be increased to 4,200 to 4,500 mg.

Supplemental choline has been shown to be beneficial to young ruminants, such as young calves prior to ruminal development. However, it is apparent that traditional supplements of choline in the form of choline chloride are extensively degraded in the rumen. For lactating dairy cows or other ruminants that may have need for supplemental choline, it should be protected from rumen degradation and available for absorption in the small intestine. A rumen-protected choline product that could potentially be used as supplemental choline for ruminants is available. In vitro studies showed that at least 87% of the choline was protected from rumen degradation (Erdman and Sharma, 1991). Studies of postruminal choline infusion and studies with rumen-protected forms of choline at 31 to 45 g/day supported a 1.9-kg increase in milk production (Erdman and Sharma, 1991; Erdman, 1992).

It is likely that a large portion of methionine is used as a methyl donor for choline synthesis in ruminants. This suggests that choline would be a more likely candidate for rumen-protected supplementation than methionine (Erdman and Sharma, 1991). Diets in which methionine or, indirectly, protein was most limiting, would most likely benefit from rumen-protected choline addition.

For humans, in view of the widespread occurrence of choline and methionine in plant and animal foodstuffs, choline supplementation is most warranted for individuals on special dietary regimens, including infants and young children fed diets deficient in protein and high in highly refined products and patients on total parenteral nutrition. Also, supplemental choline has been used with some success to diminish short-term memory loss associated with Alzheimer's disease and certain other neurological diseases. Supplemental choline has a positive benefit in reducing cancer and atherosclerosis (see Deficiency, Effects of Deficiency, Humans). Cancer patients receiving methotrexate treatment should consider receiving choline supplementation, as some data suggest that fatty infiltration of the liver associated with methotrexate treatment occurs because of a disturbance in choline metabolism (Pomfret et al., 1990).

Because 5 to 14 mg of total choline per deciliter is present in human milk and is tolerated with no adverse reactions, and because deficiency in young animals produces serious effects, it is recommended that at least 7 mg of choline per 100 kcal be included in infant formulas not based on milk (Kuksis and Mookerjea, 1984). Commercially prepared infant formulas and milk products have been supplemented with choline at these levels to ensure the presence of choline in an amount approximating that naturally occurring in milk.

The most widely used supplemental form of choline is choline chloride, which is stable in multivitamin premixes but is highly destructive to various other vitamins in the premix (Frye, 1978; Coelho, 1991). Choline is stable during processing and storage in pressure-pelleted and extruded feeds. Since the material is hygroscopic, containers of choline should be kept closed when not in use.

TOXICITY

Experimental animal toxicity data on clinical signs of choline over-dosage include salivation, trembling, jerking, cyanosis, convulsions, and respiratory paralysis. Estimates of the oral LD_{50} of choline chloride in rats varied from 3.4 to 6.7 g/kg (Chan 1991). Bell (1985) reported that when rats were exposed perinatally to 22 mg of soy lecithin preparation daily, sensorimotor development and brain cell maturation were altered. Choline levels somewhat above the requirement (868 to 2,000 ppm) were shown to reduce rate and efficiency of gain in swine (Neumann et al., 1949; Southern et al., 1986). Derilo and Balnave (1980) reported reduced gain and efficiency in young broiler chicks fed a level of choline only slightly in excess of the requirement. Studies with chickens suggest that dietary choline double the requirement is safe, with swine having a higher tolerance for choline (NRC, 1987). Work by Southern et al. (1986) showed that excess choline, up to 2,000 mg/kg above the recommended level, had no adverse effect on swine performance.

In humans, high intakes of lecithin or choline produced acute gastrointestinal distress, sweating, salivation, and anorexia (Wood and Allison, 1982). However, therapeutic doses of choline chloride and of choline dihydrogen citrate administered in amounts ranging from 3 to 12 g/day have been used in the treatment of alcoholic cirrhosis for up to 4 months with no toxic effects reported. In treatment of tardive dyskinesia (a movement disorder generally associated with the intake of antipsychotic medication), up to 16 g/day of choline has been used; in other cases, lecithin at doses greater than 100 g/day for more than 4 months has been used with no evidence of ill effects (Kuksis and Mookerjea, 1984).

■ REFERENCES

Ansell, G.B., and Spanner, S. (1971). *Biochem J. 122*, 741.

AOAC (Association of Official Agricultural Chemists), (1984). Official Method of Analysis. AOAC, Washington, D.C.

Atkins, K.B., Erdman, R.A., and Vandersall, J.H. (1983). *J. Dairy Sci. 66*(Suppl. 1), 175.

Atkins, K.B., Erdman, R.A., and Vandersall, J.H. (1988). *J. Dairy Sci. 71*, 109.

Barnes, R.H., and Kwong, E. (1967). *J. Nutr. 92*, 224.

Bell, J.M. (1985). *Devel. Psychobiol. 18*, 383.

Best, C.H., Channon, H.J., and Ridout, J.H. (1934). *J. Physiol. (Lond.) 78*, 409.

Brown, E.S. (1964). *Am J. Physiol. 207,* 402.

Buchman, A.L., Dubin, M., Jenden, D., and Moukarzel, A. (1992). *Gastroenterology 102,* 1363.

Campbell, R.G., Cadogan, D.J., Morley, W.C., Uusitalo, R., and Virtanen, E. (1995). *J. Anim. Sci.* 73(Suppl. 1), 82(Abstr.).

Canty, D.J., and Zeisel, S.H. (1994). *Nutr. Rev. 52,* 327.

Chan, M.M. (1991). *In* Handbook of Vitamins (L.J. Machlin, ed.), 2nd Ed., p. 537. Marcel Dekker, New York.

Chao, C.K., Pomfret, E.A., and Zeisel, S.H. (1988). *Biochem. J. 254,* 33.

Childs, M.T., Bowlin, J.A., Ogilvie, J.T., Hazzard, W.R., and Albers, J.J. (1981). *Atherosclerosis 38,* 217.

Chung, S., Moriyama, T., Uezu, E., Uezu, K., Hirata, R., Yohena, N., Masuda, Y., Kokubu, T., and Yamamoto, S. (1995) *J. Nutr. 125,* 1484.

Coelho, M.B. (1991). Vitamin Stability in Premixes and Feeds: A Practical Approach, p. 56. BASF Technical Symposium, Bloomington, Minnesota.

Craig, S.R., and Gatlin, D.M. III (1996). *J. Nutr. 126,* 1696.

Crawford, J.S., Griffith, M., Teekell, R.A., and Watts, A.B. (1969). *Poult. Sci. 38,* 620.

Cunha, T.J. (1972). *Feedstuffs 44,* 27.

Cunha, T.J. (1977). Swine Feeding and Nutrition, Academic Press, New York.

Daily, J.W. III, and Sachan, D.S. (1995). *J. Nutr. 125,* 1938.

Dale, H.H., and Dudley, H.W. (1929). *J. Physiol. (Lond.) 68,* 97.

De La Huerga, J., and Popper, H. (1952). *J. Clin. Invest. 31,* 598.

Derilo, Y.L., and Balnave, D. (1980). *Poult. Sci. 21,* 479.

DuCoa L.P. (1994). *In* Choline Functions and Requirements, p. 91. DuPont/ConAgra Co., Higland, Illinois.

Du Vigneaud, V., Chandler, J.P., Moyer, A.W., and Keppel, D.M. (1939). *J. Biol. Chem. 131,* 57.

Emmanual, B., and Kennelly, J.J. (1984). *J. Dairy Sci. 67,* 1912.

Emmert, J.L., and Baker, D.H. (1997). *J. Nutr. 127,* 745.

Emmert, J.L., Garrow, T.A., and Baker, D.H. (1996). *J. Nutr. 126,* 2050.

Emmert, J.L., Garrow, T.A., and Baker, D.H. (1997). *J. Anim. Sci. 74,* 2738.

Ensminger, M.E., Bowland, J.P., and Cunha, T.J. (1947). *J. Anim. Sci. 6,* 409.

Erdman, R.A. (1992). Vitamins. Abstracted Proc. Large Dairy Herd Management Symposium, p. 24. Gainesville, Florida.

Erdman, R.A., and Sharma, B.K. (1991). *J. Dairy Sci. 74,* 1641.

Erdman, R.A., Shaver, R.D., and Vandersall, J.H. (1984). *J. Dairy Sci. 67,* 410.

Finkelstein, J.D., Martin, J.J., Harris, B.J., and Kyle, W.E. (1982). *Arch, Biochem. Biophys. 218,* 169.

Firth, J., James, M., Chang, S., Mistry, P., and Johnson, B.C. (1953). *J. Anim. Sci. 12,* 915(Abstr.).

Frye, T.M. (1978). *In* Proc. Roche Vitam. Nutr. Update Meet., Arkansas Nutr. Conf., p. 54. Hoffmann-La Roche, Nutley, New Jersey.

Griffin, M.E., Wilson, K.A., White, M.R., and Brown, P.B. (1994). *J. Nutr. 124,* 1685.

Griffith, W.H., and Nyc, J.F. (1971). *In* The Vitamins (W.H. Sebrell Jr., and R.S. Harris, eds.), Vol. 3, p. 3. Academic Press, New York.

Hall, C.E., and Bieri, J.G. (1953). *Endocrinology 53,* 661.

Handler, P., and Bernheim, F. (1949). *Proc. Soc. Exp. Biol. Med. 72*, 569.

Harms, R.H., and Miles, R.D. (1984). *Poult. Sci. 63*, 1464.

Harris, R.R., Yeates, H.F., and Barrett, J.E. Jr. (1966). *J. Anim. Sci. 25*, 248 (Abstr.).

Hartroft, W.S. (1955). *Proc. Am. Soc. Exp.Biol. 14*, 655.

Haydon, K.D., Campbell, R.G., and Prince, T.J. (1995). *J. Anim. Sci. 73*,(Suppl. 1), 83(Abstr.)

Hegazy, E., and Schwenk, M. (1984). *J. Nutr. 114*, 2217.

Hirsch, M.J., Growdon, J.H., and Wurtman, R.J. (1978) *Metabolism 27, 953.*

Johnson, B.C., Mitchell, H.H., Pinkos, J.A., and Merrill, C.C. (1951). *J. Nutr. 43*, 37.

Jukes, T.H. (1947). *Annu. Rev. Biochem. 16*, 193.

Ketola, H.G. (1976). *J. Anim. Sci. 43*, 474.

Ketola, H.G., and Nesheim, M.C. (1974). *J. Nutr. 104*, 1484.

Kim, Y., Miller, J.W., Da Costa, K., Nadeau, M. Smith, D. Selhub, J., Zeisel, S.H., and Mason, J.B. (1994). *J. Nutr. 124*, 2197.

Kitamura, S., Suwa, T., Ohara, S., and Nakagawa, K. (1967). *Bull. Jpn. Soc. Sci. Fish. 33*, 1126.

Kroening, G.H., and Pond, W.G. (1967). *J. Anim. Sci. 26*, 352.

Kuksis, A., and Mookerjea, S. (1984). *In* Present Knowledge in Nutrition (R.E. Olson, H.P. Broquist, C.O. Chichester, W.J. Darby, A.C. Kolbye, and R.M. Stalvey, eds.), p. 383. Nutrition Foundation, Washington, D.C.

Latshaw, J.D., and Jensen, L.S. (1972). *J. Nutr 102*, 749.

Lombardi, B., Ugazio, G., and Raick, A. (1966). *Am. J. Physiol. 210*, 31.

Lovett, T.D., Coffey, M.T., and Miles, R.D. (1985). *J. Anim. Sci. 63*, 467.

Lowry, K.R., Izquierdo, O.A., and Baker, D.H. (1987). *Poult. Sci. 66*(Suppl. 1), 135.

March, B.E., and MacMillan, C. (1980). *Poult. Sci. 59*, 611.

Maxwell, C.V., Johnson, R.K., and Luce, W.G. (1987). *J. Anim. Sci. 64*, 1044.

Meyers, S.P. (1990). *Feed Manage. 41*(8), 12.

Mikol, Y.G., Hoover, K.L., Creasia, D., and Poirier, L.A. (1983). *Carcinogenesis. 4*, 1619.

Miles, R.D., and Butcher, G.D. (1997). *Industria Avicola 44*(2), 29.

Miles, R.D., and Harms, R.H. (1983). *In* Proc. 1983 Florida Nutrition Conference, p. 75. Gainesville, Florida.

Miles, R.D., Ruiz, N., and Harms, H. (1983) *Poult. Sci. 62*, 495.

Miles, R.D., Ruiz, N., and Harms, R.H. (1986). *Prof. Anim. Sci. 2*, 33.

Molitoris, B.A., and Baker, D.H. (1976). *J. Anim. Sci. 47*, 481.

Mookerjea, S. (1971). *Proc. Fed. Am. Soc. Exp. Biol. 30*, 143.

Neill, A.R., Grime, D.W., Snoswell, A.M., Northrop, A.J., Lindsey, D.B., and Dawson, R.M.C. (1979). *Biochem. J. 180*, 559.

Neumann, A.L., Krider, J.L., James, M.F., and Johnson, B.C. (1949). *J. Nutr. 38*, 195.

Norvell, M.J., and Nesheim, M.C. (1969). Proc. Cornell Nutr. Conf., p. 321. Ithaca, New York.

NRC. Nutrient Requirements of Domestic Animals. National Academy of Sciences-National Research Council, Washington, D.C.
(1977). Nutrient Requirements of Rabbits, 2nd Ed.

(1978). Nutrient Requirements of Nonhuman Primates.
(1981). Nutrient Requirements of Goats.
(1985a). Nutrient Requirements of Dogs, 2nd Ed.
(1985b). Nutrient Requirements of Sheep, 5th Ed.
(1986). Nutrient Requirements of Cats, 3rd Ed.
(1989a). Nutrient Requirements of Dairy Cattle, 6th Ed.
(1989b). Nutrient Requirements of Horses, 5th Ed.
(1993). Nutrient Requirements of Fish.
(1994). Nutrient Requirements of Poultry, 9th Ed.
(1995). Nutrient Requirements of Laboratory Animals, 4th Ed.
(1996). Nutrient Requirements of Beef Cattle, 7th Ed.
(1998). Nutrient Requirements of Swine, 10th Ed.
NRC. (1982b). United States-Canadian Tables of Feed Composition, 3rd Ed. National Academy of Sciences-National Research Council, Washington, D.C.
NRC. (1987). Vitamin Tolerance of Animals. National Academy of Sciences-National Research Council, Washington, D.C.
NRC. (1976). Committee on Swine Nutrition. *J. Anim. Sci. 42*, 1211.
Odle, J. (1996). *Feed Manage. 47*(1), 25.
Ogino, C., Uki, N., Watanabe, T., Iida, Z., and Ando, K. (1970). *Bull. Jpn. Soc. Sci. Fish. 36*, 1140.
Olson, R.E. (1959). *Annu. Rev. Biochem. 28*, 467.
Øverland, M., Røvik, K.A., and Skrede, A. (1999). *J. Anim. Sci. 77*, 2143.
Pesti, G.M., Benevenga, N.J., Harper, A.E., and Sunde, M.L. (1981). *Poult. Sci. 60*, 425.
Pesti, G.M., Harper, A.E., and Sunde, M.L. (1980). *Poult. Sci. 59*, 1073.
Pomfret, E.A., da Costa, K.A., Schurman, L.L., and Zeisel, S.H. (1989). *Anal. Biochem. 180*, 85.
Pomfret, E.A., da Costa, K., and Zeisel, S.H. (1990). *J. Nutr. Biochem. 1*, 533.
RDA. (1989). Recommended Dietary Allowances, 9th Ed. National Academy of Sciences-National Research Council, Washington, D.C.
Rohlfs, E.M., Garner, S.C., Mar, M., and Zeisel, S.H. (1993). *J. Nutr. 123*, 1762.
Ruiz, N., Miles, R.D., and Harms, R.H. (1983). *WPSA J. 39*, 185.
Rumsey, T.S. (1975). *Feedstuffs 47*, 30.
Sanford, P.A., and Smyth, D.H. (1971). *J. Physiol. (Lond.) 215*, 769.
Scott, M.L., Nesheim, M.C., and Young, R.J. (1982). Nutrition of the Chicken, p. 119. Scott, Ithaca, New York.
Sharma, B.K., and Erdman, R.A. (1988). *J. Dairy Sci. 71*, 2670.
Shurson, J., Salzer, T., Johnston, L., White, M., Hathaway, M., Dayton, W., and Walker, B. (1994). *In* Proc. Minnesota Nutrition Conference and Roche Technical Symposium, Bloomington, Minnesota.
Smith, C.M., Swase, M., Exton-Smith, A.N., Phillips, M.J., Overstall, P.W., Piper, M.E., and Bailey, M.R. (1978). *Lancet. 2*, 318.
Southern, L.L., Brown, D.R., Werner, D.D., and Fox, M.C. (1986). *J. Anim. Sci. 62*, 992.
Spires, H.R., Botts, R.L., and King, B.D. (1982). Syntex Research Report, Series A, No. 1.
Swingle, R.S., and Dyer, I.A. (1970). *J. Anim. Sci. 31*, 404.
Tapia Romero, E., Rojas, R.E., Arias, L.E., and Avila, G.E. (1985). *In* Re-

sumenes ALPA 85 (C.F.Chicco, ed.), p. 49 (Abstr.). Acapulco, Mexico.

Wauben, P.M., and Wainwright, P.E. (1999). *Nutr. Rev. 57*, 35.

Welch, B.E., and Couch, J.R. (1955). *Poult. Sci. 34*, 217.

Wilson, R.B. (1978). *In* Handbook Series in Nutrition and Food, Section E: Nutritional Disorders (M. Rechcigl, Jr., ed.), Vol. 2, p. 95. CRC Press, Boca Raton, Florida.

Wilson, R.P., and Poe, W.E. (1988). *Aquaculture 68*, 65.

Wise, M.B., Blumer, T.N., and Barrick, E.R. (1964). North Carolina Agri, Exp. Sta. ANS Report 139. A.H. Series 10, 22.

Wood, J.L., and Allison, R.G. (1982). *Fed. Proc. 41*, 3015.

Zeisel, S.H. (1990). *J. Nutr. Biochem. 1*, 332.

Zeisel, S.H., and da Costa, K.A. (1990). *J. Nutr. Biochem. 1*, 55.

Zeisel, S.H., Char, D., and Sheard, N.F. (1986). *J. Nutr. 116*, 50.

Zeisel, S.H., Costa, K.A., Franklin, P.D., Alexander, E.A., Lamont, J.T., Sheard, N.F., Beiser, A., and Costa, K.A. (1991). *FASEB J. 5*, 2093.

VITAMIN C

INTRODUCTION

Scurvy, a potentially fatal condition resulting from inadequate vitamin C (ascorbic acid), has been known and feared since ancient times. Its prevention and cure were associated with consumption of fresh fruits, especially citrus, but it was not until 1928 that the antiscorbutic factor was identified. Vitamin C is synthesized in almost all species, the exceptions being the primates, including humans, guinea pigs, fish, fruit-eating bats, insects, and some birds. Animals that cannot synthesize this vitamin need a dietary source for their normal maintenance.

The concept that the sole function of vitamin C is to prevent scurvy has been revised in recent years. Small quantities of vitamin C are sufficient to prevent and cure scurvy; however, larger quantities may be required to maintain good health during conditions of adverse environment, physiological stress, and certain diseases. Antioxidant vitamins (vitamin C, vitamin E, and β-carotene) have received a great deal of attention in that they play important roles in animal and human health by inactivating harmful free radicals produced through normal cellular activity and from various stressors.

HISTORY

Several historical reviews of scurvy and vitamin C are available (Marks, 1975; Vilter, 1978; Moser and Bendich, 1991). Carpenter (1986) wrote a fascinating book, *The History of Scurvy and Vitamin C,* that deals with the problems of scurvy throughout history. A historical record is presented in Table 15.1 (Vilter, 1978).

If famine is excluded, scurvy is probably the nutritional deficiency

15

1550 B.C.	Scurvy described in *Eber's Papyrus* (Thebes).
600 B.C.	Hippocrates described soldiers afflicted with scurvy.
A.D. 1200	Crusaders weakened by scurvy.
1492–1600	World exploration threatened by scurvy.
	—Magellan lost four-fifths of his crew.
	—Vasco de Gama lost 100 of his 160 men.
1536	Jacques Cartier's expedition immobilized by scurvy; learned from Indians the curative value of pine needles and bark.
1570	Captain James Lancaster prevented scurvy by giving crew members two jiggers of lemon juice daily.
1593	Sir Richard Hawkins used oranges and lemons to treat scurvy in the British Navy; Ponsseus referred to the therapeutic use of scurvy grass, watercress, and oranges.
1650	Infantile scurvy described by Glisson but was confused with rickets.
17th century	Lime juice used experimentally on ships of the East India Company.
1734	Backstrom related scurvy to a deficiency of fresh fruits and vegetables.
1740–1744	Lord Anson lost three-fifths of his crew of 1,950 men to scurvy.
1747	James Lind performed controlled shipboard experiment on the preventive effect of oranges and lemons (published 1753).
1768–1771	Captain James Cook demonstrated that prolonged sea voyages were possible without ravages of scurvy.
1789	William Stark induced scurvy in himself by a diet of bread and water for 60 days.
1795	Lemon juice made a regular ration in British Navy.
1854	Lemon juice made a regular ration in British Merchant Marines.
1863	Scurvy epidemic occurred in the opposing armies during the American Civil War.
1883	Sir Thomas Barlow differentiated infantile scurvy from rickets.
1895	Antiscorbutic ration became official in U.S. Army.
1900	Boiling and pasteurization of infant formula increased incidence of scurvy.
1906	Hopkins suggested that infantile scurvy was a deficiency disease.
1907	Hoist and Frolich produced experimental scurvy in guinea pigs by feeding a deficient diet, with pathological changes resembling those in humans.
1912	Explorer Captain Scott and his team died of scurvy during their expedition to the South Pole.
1928	Szent-Györgyi isolated hexuronic acid from orange juice, cabbage juice, and cattle adrenal glands.
1932	Waugh and King isolated hexuronic acid from lemons and identified it as vitamin C.
1933	Haworth determined structure of vitamin C.
1933	Reichstein synthesized vitamin C.
1971	Linus Pauling published book on relationship of vitamin C to the common cold, which stimulated research on therapeutic and prophylactic uses of megadoses of vitamin C on the common cold, resistance, and various diseases.

Source: Adapted and modified from Vilter (1978).

disease that has caused the most suffering in recorded history (Carpenter, 1986). Scurvy was one of the earliest diseases known, with historical evidence of its existence in Egypt, Greece, and Rome. In the Middle Ages scurvy was endemic in northern Europe during the late winter months and early spring, because at that time the foodstuffs that provided the chief source of vitamin C (green vegetables) had not been introduced. During this period scurvy was common among the seafaring Vikings and the land-dwelling northern Europeans. Between 1556 and 1857, 114 scurvy epidemics were reported in Europe, occurring during winter when fruits and vegetables were not available. For hundreds of years it was known or suspected that a dietary factor would protect against scurvy. Real progress was made toward identification of the dietary factor involved when in 1907 Holst and Frolich discovered that guinea pigs could develop scurvy, thus providing an experimental animal.

World exploration and military operations were severely hampered during the era prior to the seventeenth century by ravages of scurvy. On the long sea voyages in explorations of the late 1400s and 1500s, scurvy frequently occurred. Knowledge of the curative value of certain foods had been known for a considerable time, and American Indians had used an infusion of spruce or pine needles to prevent scurvy for at least four centuries. As early as 1536, Jacques Cartier learned from these Indians that scurvy could be cured and prevented by consuming a drink made from pine needles and bark. Previously, 107 cases of scurvy in 110 men resulted from Cartier's expedition up the St. Lawrence River. Before the relationship of scurvy to diet was found, there was a tendency to associate scurvy with venereal disease. Mercury was used as a treatment, with disastrous results.

In 1747 James Lind, a British fleet physician, carried out one of the first examples of a controlled clinical experiment, in which he showed that patients consuming lemon juice recovered from scurvy, while others failed to do so. Indeed, Lind was responsible for the relief of both scurvy and typhus in the fleet and probably helped as much as Lord Nelson to break the power of Napoleon. By the eighteenth century, it was realized that fresh fruit and vegetables and lime or lemon juice would protect sailors on long voyages. The term limey, colloquially applied to the English population, stems from lime juice given to sailors in the British Navy. Lemon juice had become a routine part of the British Navy diets by 1795. However, scurvy was an epidemic problem during the American Civil War, and it was not until 1895 that an antiscorbutic diet became official in the U.S. Army.

In the nineteenth century, 104 country epidemics of scurvy were registered. Infantile scurvy (Barlow's disease) was a severe problem in the late 1800s and early 1900s; it came about from bottle-feeding, and breast-fed babies were not affected. The problem arose because infant milk was not pasteurized but rather sterilized by boiling, thus destroying vitamin C.

In 1928, Szent-Györgyi isolated a substance (which he called hexuronic acid) from orange juice, cabbage juice, and ox adrenal glands. The isolated substance was acidic, with the formula $C_6H_{12}O_6$, and was strongly reducing. The same year, King isolated an antiscorbutic substance in crystalline form from orange juice and demonstrated that it cured scurvy; thus Szent-Györgyi tried his hexuronic acid, found it also cured scurvy, and concluded it must be vitamin C. It was not readily accepted that it represented a vitamin because amounts required were large relative to amounts required of other vitamins (up to 100 mg). But finally, in 1933, when hexuronic acid was synthesized by Richstein and shown to have the true activity of the natural product, ascorbic acid was recognized as a vitamin.

CHEMICAL STRUCTURE, PROPERTIES, AND ANTAGONISTS

Vitamin C primarily occurs in two forms (Fig. 15.1), namely, the reduced ascorbic acid and the oxidized dehydroascorbic acid. The L-isomer of ascorbic acid has activity. Although most of the vitamin exists as ascorbic acid, both forms are biologically active. In foods the reduced form of vitamin C may reversibly oxidize to the dehydro form, with dehydroascorbic acid further oxidized to the inactive and irreversible compound of diketogulonic acid. This change takes place readily; thus vitamin C is very susceptible to destruction through oxidation, a change that is accelerated by heat and light. Diketogulonic acid can be further oxidized to oxalic acid and L-threonic acid.

There are four stereoisomers of ascorbic acid; in addition to the L-isomer, only erythorbic acid (D-araborascorbic acid) has activity. Erythorbic acid has only 1/20 the activity of L-ascorbic acid and is often used in the food industry for addition to meats or canning operations as an antioxidant. This antioxidant property is used in the addition of the vitamin in canning of certain fruits (e.g., erythorbic acid) to prevent oxidation changes that cause darkening. Ascorbic acid is so readily oxidized to dehydroascorbic acid that other compounds may be protected against oxidation. Reversible oxidation-reduction of ascorbic acid with

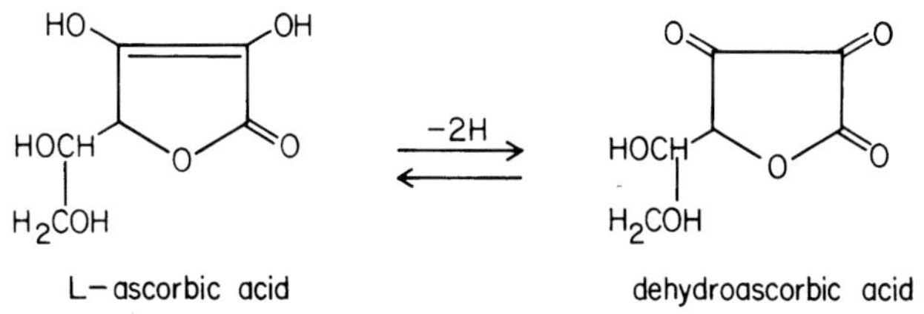

Fig. 15.1 Structures of vitamin C: L-ascorbic acid (reduced form) and dehydroascorbic acid (oxidized form).

dehydroascorbic acid is the most important chemical property of vitamin C and the basis for its known physiological activities and stabilities (Moser and Bendich, 1991). Vitamin C is the least stable, and therefore most easily destroyed, of all vitamins.

Ascorbic acid is a white to yellow-tinged crystalline powder. It crystallizes out of water solution as square or oblong crystals and is slightly soluble in acetone and lower alcohols. A 0.5% solution of ascorbic acid in water is strongly acid, with a pH of 3. The vitamin is more stable in an acid than an alkaline medium. It is not found in dry foods and is markedly destroyed by cooking, particularly when the pH is alkaline. Cooking losses also result because of its solubility. A number of chemical substances—such as air pollutants, industrial toxins, heavy metals, tobacco smoke, and several pharmacologically active compounds, among them some antidepressants and diuretics—are antagonistic to vitamin C and can lead to increased requirements of the vitamin.

Crystalline ascorbic acid is relatively stable in air without moisture, and small concentrations of metal ions will accelerate destruction of ascorbic acid. Various derivatives and analogs of vitamin C have been prepared that have little if any antiscorbutic activity. Glycoascorbic acid acts as an antimetabolite for vitamin C, which is an ascorbic acid homolog, and contains an added CHOH group that has undergone optical inversion.

ANALYTICAL PROCEDURES

Analysis of vitamin C includes biological, chemical, and physical methods. The biological method is specific for antiscorbutic activity and, as such, can be accepted as the final standard of reference when it is suspected that accuracy of chemical or physical procedures may be affected by presence of interfering substances. The biological test measures total amount of vitamin C present, that is, in both the reduced form of ascorbic acid itself and the reversibly oxidized form of dehydroascorbic acid. Applicability of the biological method may be limited only if potency of the test material is too low for it to be measured accurately. Rats cannot be used as test animals for vitamin C assay because of their ability to synthesize the vitamin, but guinea pigs have proved satisfactory. Biological methods are based on prevention or cure of scurvy in guinea pigs, in addition to dental histology, curative growth, and serum concentrations of alkaline phosphate associated with the deficiency. Procedures with guinea pigs require about 10 weeks for completion. Bioassays based on microorganisms have not been developed because no organism has been found that has an absolute requirement for L-ascorbic acid (Moser and Bendich, 1991).

Biological analytical procedures have largely been replaced by chemical and physical methods, which provide precise, faster, and less expensive assays. Chemical and physical methods require precautions to prevent oxidation (e.g., homogenize under nitrogen and avoid copper and other metallic ions). Dye methods are widely used with the reagents, 2,6-dichlorophenolindophenol for reduced ascorbic acid and 2,4-dinitrophenylhydrazine for the oxidized form and for total ascorbic acid after oxidation. L-Ascorbic acid absorbs strongly in the ultraviolet, which is the basis of spectrophotometric methods (Tono and Fujita, 1982). Both gas-liquid chromatography and high-performance liquid chromatography (HPLC) have been developed for L-ascorbic acid determination (Rose and Nahrwold, 1982; Liau et al., 1993). The HPLC technology allows a rapid separation and detection of ascorbic acid as well as of erythorbic acid.

METABOLISM

Vitamin C is absorbed in a manner similar to that of carbohydrates (monosaccharides). Intestinal absorption in vitamin C-dependent animals appears to require a Na^+-dependent active transport system. It is assumed that those species that are not prone to scurvy have an absorption mechanism by diffusion (Spencer et al., 1963). Ascorbic acid is readily absorbed when quantities ingested are small, but limited intestinal absorption by active transport occurs when excessive amounts of ascorbic acid are ingested. However, uptake by passive diffusion occurs at higher vitamin C intakes.

Bioavailability of vitamin C in foods is limited, but apparently 80 to

90% appears to be absorbed (Kallner et al., 1977). The site of absorption in the guinea pig is in the duodenal and proximal small intestine, whereas the rat showed highest absorption in the ileum (Hornig et al., 1984). In humans, ascorbic acid is absorbed predominantly in the distal portion of the small intestine and, to a lesser extent, in the mouth, stomach, and proximal intestine (Moser and Bendich, 1991).

In its metabolism, ascorbic acid is first converted to dehydroascorbate by a number of enzyme or nonenzymatic processes and is then reduced in cells (Rose et al., 1986). Vitamin C is transported in the plasma in association with the protein albumin. Absorbed vitamin C readily equilibrates with the body pool of the vitamin.

Ascorbic acid is widely distributed throughout the tissues, both in animals capable of synthesizing ascorbic acid as well as in those dependent on an adequate dietary amount of vitamin C. In experimental animals, highest concentrations of vitamin C are found in the pituitary and adrenal glands, with high levels also found in the liver, spleen, brain, and pancreas. The vitamin tends to localize around healing wounds. Tissue levels are decreased by virtually all forms of stress, which also stimulates the biosynthesis of the vitamin in those animals capable of synthesis.

Humans receiving adequate intakes of vitamin C have a body pool of approximately 1.5 to 5 g of the vitamin, with 3 to 4% of the existing body pool utilized daily. The major quantities of vitamin C are found in the liver and muscles by virtue of their large masses. The half-life of ascorbic acid is inversely related to daily intake and is 13 to 40 days in humans and 3 days in guinea pigs, which correlates with the longer time needed by a human to develop scurvy: 3 months for a human on a vitamin C-free diet compared with 3 weeks for the guinea pig.

Absorbed ascorbic acid is excreted in urine, sweat, and feces. Fecal loss is minimal, and even with large intakes in humans, only 6 to 10 mg/day is excreted by this route (Marks, 1975). Loss in sweat is also probably low. In guinea pigs, rats, and rabbits, CO_2 is the major excretory mechanism for vitamin C. Primates do not normally utilize the CO_2 catabolic pathway, with the main loss occurring in the urine. However, because of the limits on absorption, as dietary ascorbic acid increases above 180 mg/day, it is broken down by intestinal bacteria, with 30% or more recovered as carbon dioxide (Kallner et al., 1985). Urinary excretion of vitamin C depends on the body stores, intake, and renal function. Mechanism and mode of elimination are a function of glomerular filtration rate of ascorbic acid and are dependent on plasma ascorbate concentration. Substantial quantities of L-ascorbic acid are excreted in urine after concentration in blood plasma exceeds its usual threshold of approximately 1.4 mg/100 ml.

Urine contains numerous metabolites of ascorbic acid, including dehydroascorbic acid, diketogulonic acid, ascorbate-2-sulfate, oxalate, methyl ascorbate, and 2-ketoascorbitol (Sauberlich, 1990). In humans, with physiological vitamin C doses of 60 to 100 mg/day, urinary oxalate is the major metabolite, with 30 to 50 mg/day being formed. But when given in large doses, up to 10 g/day, urinary oxalate is increased by only 10 to 30 mg/day, and the vitamin is excreted largely unmetabolized in urine and feces (Moser and Bendich, 1991). Excretion of ascorbic acid in urine declines to undetectable levels with inadequate intakes of the vitamin or in the case of scurvy.

FUNCTIONS

Ascorbic acid has been found to be involved in a number of biochemical processes that involve donation of one or two electrons. Function of vitamin C is related to its reversible oxidation and reduction characteristics; however, the exact role of this vitamin in the living system is not clearly known since a coenzyme form has not been reported. Nevertheless, vitamin C plays important roles in many biochemical reactions, such as mixed-function oxidation involving incorporation of oxygen into the substrate. Biochemical and physiological functions of vitamin C have been reviewed (Chatterjee, 1978; Hornig et al., 1984; Sauberlich, 1990; Moser and Bendich, 1991; Padh, 1991; Gershoff, 1993).

Collagen Synthesis

The most clearly established functional role for vitamin C involves collagen biosynthesis. Collagens are the tough, fibrous, intercellular materials (proteins) that are principal components of skin and connective tissue, the organic substances of bones and teeth, and the ground substances between cells. Impairment of collagen synthesis in vitamin C deficiency appears to be due to lowered ability to hydroxylate lysine and proline. Syntheses of collagens involve enzymatic hydroxylations of proline to form a stable extracellular matrix and of lysine for glycosylation and formation of cross-links in the fibers (Barnes and Kodicek, 1972). Hydroxyproline residues contribute to the stiffness of the collagen triple helix, and hydroxylysine residues bind (via their hydroxyl groups) carbohydrates and form intramolecular cross-links that give collagen structural integrity.

In addition to the relationship of ascorbic acid to hydroxylase enzymes, Franceschi (1992) suggests that vitamin C is required for differentiation of mesenchyme (embryonic cells capable of developing into connective tissue)-derived connective tissues such as muscle, cartilage, and bone. It is proposed that the collagen matrix produced by ascorbic acid-treated cells provides a permissive environment for tissue-specific gene expression. A common finding in all studies is that vitamin C can alter the expression of multiple genes as cells progress through specific differentiation programs (Ikeda et al., 1997).

The requirement for ascorbic acid is specific, probably protecting the hydroxylase enzymes by oxidation of both the ferrous ions and thiol groups present. It may be that ascorbic acid is not required for the hydroxylation reaction per se but is required to keep the enzyme-bound iron in the ferrous state. Hydroxyproline is found only in collagen (14%) and arises from hydroxylation of proline. In its absence, a nonfibrous collagen precursor is formed instead of fibrous collagen and would result in scurvy.

Beneficial effects result from ascorbic acid in the synthesis of "repair" collagen. Alteration of basement membrane collagen synthesis and its integrity in mucosal epithelia during vitamin C restriction explains the mechanism by which the capillary fragility is induced in scurvy and increased incidences of periodontal disease under vitamin C deprivation (Chatterjee, 1978). Failure of wounds to heal and gum and bone changes resulting from vitamin C undernutrition are direct consequences of reduction of insoluble collagen fibers.

Antioxidant and Immunity Role

Free radicals can be extremely damaging to biological systems (Padh, 1991). Free radicals, including hydroxy, hypochorite, peroxy, alkoxy, superoxide, hydrogen peroxide, and singlet oxygen are generated by auto-oxidation, radiation, or from activities of some oxidases, dehydrogenases, and peroxidases. Also, phagocytic granuylocytes undergo respiratory burst to produce oxygen radicals to destroy the intracellular pathogens. However, these oxidative products can, in turn, damage healthy cells if they are not eliminated. Antioxidants serve to stabilize these highly reactive free radicals, thereby maintaining the structural and functional integrity of cells (Chew, 1995). Therefore, antioxidants are very important to immune defense and health of humans and animals.

Tissue defense mechanisms against free-radical damage generally include vitamin C, vitamin E, and β-carotene as the major vitamin antioxidant sources. In addition, several metalloenzymes, including glutathione peroxidase (selenium), catalase (iron), and superoxide dismutase (copper, zinc, and manganese), are also critical in protecting the internal cellular constituents from oxidative damage. The dietary and tissue balance of all these nutrients are important in protecting tissue against free-radical damage. Both in vitro and in vivo studies show that the antioxidant vitamins generally enhance different aspects of cellular and noncellular immunity. The antioxidant function of these vitamins could, at least in part, enhance immunity by maintaining the functional and structural integrity of important immune cells. A compromised immune system will affect human health and will result in reduced animal production efficiency through increased susceptibility to diseases, thereby leading to increased animal morbidity and mortality.

Vitamin C is the most important antioxidant in extracellular fluids (Stocker and Frei, 1991). Vitamin C can protect biomembranes against lipid peroxidation damage by eliminating peroxyl radicals in the aqueous phase before the latter can initiate peroxidation (Frei et al., 1989; Mukhopadhyay et al., 1995). In one study, vitamin C and E supplementation resulted in a 78% decrease in the susceptibility of lipoproteins to mononuclear cell-mediated oxidation (Rifici and Khachadurian, 1993).

Ascorbic acid is reported to have a stimulating effect on phagocytic activity of leukocytes, on function of the reticuloendothelial system, and on formation of antibodies. Vitamin C can stimulate the production of interferons, the proteins that protect cells against viral attack (Siegel, 1974). Some of the most controversial topics regarding the interactions of vitamin C with immune functions have been the reduction of common cold symptoms and favorable responses to cancer treatment. In guinea pigs, vitamin C was shown to be important in maintaining normal primary and secondary antibody responses and was important for neutrophil function (Anderson and Lukey, 1987). Ascorbic acid is very high in phagocytic cells, with these cells using free radicals and other highly reactive oxygen containing molecules to help kill pathogens that invade the body. In the process, however, cells and tissues may be damaged by these reactive species. Ascorbic acid helps to protect these cells from oxidative damage.

One of the protective effects of vitamin C may partly be mediated through its ability to reduce circulating glucocorticoids (Degkwitz, 1987). The suppressive effect of corticoids on neutrophil function in cattle is alleviated with vitamin C supplementation (Roth and Kaeberle, 1985). In addition, ascorbate can regenerate the reduced form of α-tocopherol, perhaps accounting for observed sparing effects of these vitamins (Jacob, 1995). In the process of sparing fatty acid oxidation, toco-pherol is oxidized to the tocopheryl free radical. Ascorbic acid can do-nate an electron to the tocopheryl free radical, regenerating the reduced antioxidant form of tocopherol.

Research findings in humans have suggested that "oxidative stress" may be a causal factor in the etiology of diverse and important disorders of aging, such as cancer, cardiovascular disease, and cataract formation. Cancers of the oral cavity, larynx, esophagus, stomach, colon, and rec-tum appear most related to low vitamin C intake compared to other can-cer types (Gershoff, 1993). Several lines of evidence support a role for oxidized low-density lipoprotein (LDL) in the genesis of the atheroscle-rotic lesion. Vitamin C has been shown to inhibit LDL oxidation. Also, there is evidence that vitamin C increases high-density lipoproteins (HDLs) and may lower total cholesterol. Ascorbic acid may also have beneficial effects on blood pressure, and there are epidemiological stud-ies associating subjects with cardiovascular disease with lower vitamin C intakes than normal case controls (Simon, 1992). A number of reports suggest that ascorbic acid will reduce the risk of cataracts (Gershoff, 1993; Jones and Hothersall, 1993).

The functional importance of vitamin C—other than the previously mentioned roles in collagen synthesis and in immunity, and as an an-tioxidant—includes the following:

1. Because of the ease with which ascorbic acid can be oxidized and re-versibly reduced, it is probable that it plays an important role in reactions involving electron transfer in the cell. Almost all terminal oxidases in plant and animal tissues are capable of directly or indirectly catalyzing the oxida-tion of L-ascorbic acid. Such enzymes include ascorbic acid oxidase, cy-tochrome oxidase, phenolase, and peroxidase. In addition, its oxidation is readily induced under aerobic conditions by many metal ions, hemochro-mogens, and quinones.

2. Metabolic oxidation of certain amino acids, including tyrosine, oc-curs. Tyrosyluria is observed when high levels of tyrosine are being metab-olized. Vitamin C appears to prevent the inhibition of the enzyme p-hy-droxyphenylpyruvic acid oxidase by its substrate, p-hydroxyphenylpyruvic acid, in the tyrosine metabolism sequence.

3. Ascorbic acid has a role in metal ion metabolism because of its re-ducing and chelating properties. The function of ascorbic acid is to provide electrons to keep prosthetic metal ions in their reduced forms. This includes cuprous ions in monooxygenases and ferrous ions in dioxygenases. Ascor-bic acid can result in enhanced absorption of minerals from the diet and

their mobilization and distribution throughout the body. Ascorbic acid promotes nonheme iron absorption from food (Olivares et al., 1997) and acts by reducing the ferric iron at the acid pH in the stomach and by forming complexes with iron ions that stay in solution at alkaline conditions in the duodenum. It appears to also function in the reduction and release of ferric iron from its tight linkage with plasma protein and its incorporation into ferritin. There is a postabsorption role for ascorbate for cross-membrane transport of copper ions into cells (Harris and Percival, 1991). Ascorbic acid also tends to alleviate toxic effects of transition metals in the body. Ascorbic acid, alone or in combination with chelators, lowers the concentration of lead in the tissues of the body.

4. Carnitine is synthesized from lysine and methionine and is dependent on two iron-containing hydroxylases for which ascorbic acid is a cofactor. Vitamin C deficiency can reduce the formation of carnitine, which can result in accumulation of triglycerides in blood, and in the physical fatigue and lassitude associated with scurvy (Ha et al., 1994).

5. Interrelationships of vitamin C to B vitamins are known as tissue levels, and urinary excretion of vitamin C is affected in animals with deficiencies of thiamin, riboflavin, pantothenic acid, folacin, and biotin. Vitamin C is active in changing the form of folacin to the tetrahydro derivative, a reduced form. It may also affect the ability of the body to store folacin. When vitamin C is deficient, utilization of folacin and vitamin B_{12} is impaired, resulting in anemia.

6. Vitamin C has a role in diabetes. In one study, the pancreas from scorbutic guinea pigs contained 2.4 times more insulin than that from control guinea pigs, suggesting that the decreased insulin release from the scorbutic islets was not due to decreased insulin synthesis but due to abnormal insulin secretion (Wells et al., 1995). From a different aspect of diabetes, excessive production of sorbitol from glucose is believed to play a role in the causation of some of the complications of diabetes. It was reported that supplementation with vitamin C (100 mg/day) could correct the elevated sorbitol levels seen in diabetes (Cunningham et al., 1994). Vitamin C may exert its effect by inhibiting the activity of the enzyme aldose reductase.

7. Vitamin C has been demonstrated to be a natural inhibitor of nitrosamines, which are potent carcinogens. Action of ascorbate in preventing formation of nitrosamines is reported to result from its direct reaction with nitrate.

8. Ascorbic acid is found in up to a 10-fold concentration in seminal fluid (versus serum levels). Decreasing levels have caused nonspecific sperm agglutination. It has been hypothesized that the vitamin may help to protect sperm from effects of harmful oxidation. In a review of ascorbic acid and

fertility, Luck et al. (1995) suggested how three of ascorbic acid's principal functions—its promotion of collagen synthesis, its role in hormone production, and its ability to protect cells from free radicals—may explain its reproductive actions.

9. Other physiological effects of vitamin C include detoxification of histamine, metabolism of drugs (e.g., to detoxify), expression of acetylcholine receptor, leukotriene biosynthesis, and a relationship to periodontal disease and rheumatoid arthritis (Padh, 1991).

REQUIREMENTS

A wide variety of plant and animal species can synthesize vitamin C from carbohydrate precursors, including glucose and galactose. The missing step in the pathway of ascorbic acid biosynthesis in all vitamin C-dependent species has been traced to inability to convert L-gulonolactone to 2-keto-L-gulonate, which is transformed by spontaneous isomerization into its tautomeric form, L-ascorbic acid. Vitamin C dietary-dependent species, therefore, lack the enzyme L-gulonolactone oxidase.

Metabolic need for ascorbic acid is a general one among species, but a dietary need is limited to humans, subhuman primates, guinea pigs, fruit-eating bats, some birds (including the red-vented bulbul and related *Passeriformes* species), insects, fish (such as coho salmon, rainbow trout, and carp), and perhaps certain reptiles. Inherited ascorbic acid deficiency reported in pigs (Kristensen et al., 1986) and rats (Horio et al., 1985) was related to the lack of L-gulonolactone oxidase enzyme activity. Even for species that synthesize vitamin C, the synthesizing capacity of liver microsomal preparations was shown to vary strongly from animal to animal (Chatterjee, 1978), suggesting possible dietary need for the vitamin for individuals within a species. Circumstances in which vitamin C deficiencies may occur in domestic animals are discussed in the Deficiency and Supplementation sections.

In general, domestic animals such as poultry, ruminants, swine, horses, dogs, and cats have the ability to biosynthesize ascorbic acid within their body, and hence there is no recommended requirement established by the National Research Council. However, Marks (1975) proposed the following vitamin C requirements for poultry and swine, per kilogram of diet: poultry, 50 to 60 mg; starting pigs, 300 mg; and finishing pigs, 150 mg. Itze (1984) suggested 250 mg of ascorbic acid daily for young calves. The ascorbic acid requirements of fish vary with species, size, environment, and health status of the animals. Rainbow trout require 70 to 100 mg of L-ascorbic acid per kilogram of diet for normal growth and 500 mg/kg for wound repair (Halver, 1972). For channel catfish, Li and Lovell (1985) determined a requirement of 30 mg/kg for maximum growth and 150 mg/kg for disease resistance. Likewise, increased vitamin C intakes are required for subjects exposed to cold or elevated temperatures and other acute stresses, including surgery and trauma (Sauberlich, 1990). Others for whom dietary vitamin C requirement is increased include elderly individuals, alcoholics, and users of oral contraceptives.

For humans, the RDA (1989) recommends 30 to 95 mg of vitamin C depending on body weight and physiological function (Table 15.2). The human requirement for vitamin C has been the subject of considerable debate, with diversity of opinion that seems to be irreconcilable. This controversy is reflected in the wide range of recommended daily allowances established by different countries (20 to 200 mg). These values are based on whether the allowance should prevent scurvy and permit a margin of safety, or whether more complete tissue saturation is preferable. Human scurvy can be prevented and cured with daily intake of 10 mg of vitamin C. This level of intake, however, permits little or no reserves. Approximately 18 to 25 mg/day keeps tissues half saturated.

Requirements are increased by pregnancy, lactation, thyrotoxicosis, increased metabolism, or decreased absorption. Individuals may require increased vitamin C as a result of stress or unfavorable environmental situations. Cigarette smokers with vitamin C intakes comparable to those of nonsmokers have serum vitamin C levels lower than those of nonsmokers. Smoker requirements for ascorbic acid were estimated to be increased by as much as 50%.

Research that previously established that the sole function of ascorbic acid was to prevent scurvy must be revised. There is evidence suggesting that ascorbic acid participates in extra "antiscorbutic" functions for which a higher requirement than necessary to protect against overt

■ Table 15.2   Recommended Vitamin C Daily Dietary Allowances for Humans

Group	Amount (mg)
Under 1 year	30–35
1–10 years	40–45
11–14 years	50
15–51+ years	60
Pregnancy	70
Lactation	90–95

Source: RDA (1989).

scurvy is needed. Pauling's 1971 book stimulated widespread interest in self-medication with megavitamin doses of ascorbic acid. There are reports in the literature concerning the beneficial effects of megadoses of vitamin C on the common cold, resistance, and various diseases. Pauling (1971) suggested that for optimum health, daily intake of ascorbic acid for an adult man should be 2.3 g, which could be increased to 9 to 10 g in presence of some ailments. There is great individual variation in vitamin C requirements; some people in excellent health need 250 mg/day, most people need 4 to 5 g, and for many, 10 g is best. Ten grams is more than 100 times the daily requirement suggested by the RDA (1989).

Intake of vitamin C far in excess of physiological requirements have been reported to have beneficial effects, including the following (Moser and Bendich, 1991; Pauling, 1971; Ausman and Mayer, 1999):

1. Prevention and reduction of severity of the common cold.
2. Prevention of cancer and prolonged life of cancer patients.
3. Lowering of serum cholesterol and severity of atherosclerosis.
4. Increased wound repair and normal healing processes.
5. Increased immune response for prevention and treatment of infections.
6. Control of schizophrenia.
7. Inactivation of disease viruses.
8. Prevention of megaloblastic anemia of formula-fed infants.

The efficacy of pharmacological levels of the vitamin remains controversial because many of the claims are difficult to substantiate. Many controlled studies will be required to establish which claims for megadoses of vitamin C are valid. In view of the controversy, some authorities suggest not taking large amounts of vitamin C without medical counsel. However, in recent years, health benefits arising from using vitamin C as one of the antioxidant vitamins have become more accepted.

NATURAL SOURCES

The main sources of vitamin C are fruits and vegetables, but some foods of animal origin contain more than traces of the vitamin (Table 15.3). Nearly 90% of vitamin C in the human diet is obtained from fruits and vegetables as ascorbic and dehydroascorbic acids. Vitamin C is present in relatively large amounts in fresh, canned, and frozen citrus fruits and in smaller but important amounts in other fruits, tomatoes, potatoes, and leafy vegetables (Nobile and Woodhill, 1981). Potatoes

■ Table 15.3   Vitamin C Concentrations in Various Foods (mg/100 g, as-fed basis)

Vegetables		Blackberries	20
Asparagus, canned	15	Cherries	5
Beans, runner	5	Cranberries	12
Brussels sprouts	90	Grapefruit	34–45
Cabbage, red	55	Guavas	300
Carrots	2–6	Lemons	80
Cauliflower, raw	50–90	Limes	250
Celery, raw	7	Melons (cantaloupe)	25
Corn	12	Olives	0
Oats, whole	0	Oranges	40–60
Onions, raw	10	Peaches	7–14
Parsley	170	Pineapple	25
Peas, frozen	13	Rose hips	1,000
Peppers, raw	100	Strawberries	40–90
Potatoes, new	18	Tangerines	30
Radishes	25		
Rice	0	Animal Products	
Rye, whole	0	Fish	5–30
Spinach	10–60	Kidney, lamb	9
Wheat, whole	0	Kidney, pig	11
		Liver, calf	13
Fruit		Liver, pig	15
Apples, unpeeled	10–30	Milk, cow	1–2
Bananas	6–12	Milk, human	3–6

Sources: Adapted from Nobile and Woodhill (1981) and Moser and Bendich (1991).

and cabbage are probably the most important sources of vitamin C for the majority of the Western population, at least during winter (Moser and Bendich, 1991). Vitamin C occurs in significant quantities in animal organs such as liver and kidney, but in only small quantities in meat. In untreated fruits and vegetables, content varies extremely in skin and pulp, and even between two leaves of the same vegetable or adjacent plants of the same variety. Other factors affecting vitamin C content include variety, maturity, fertility, and season (Snehalatha Reddy and Lakshmi Kumari, 1988). Postharvest storage values vary with time, temperature, damage, and enzyme content (Zee, 1991). In Nigeria, significant losses (between 21 and 83%) of ascorbic acid were observed after 4 and 8 weeks storage of garri and cassava, respectively (Ukhun and Dibie, 1991).

Fresh tea leaves, some berries, guava, and rose hips are accumulators of ascorbic acid and consequently are rich sources. For practical purposes, raw citrus fruits are good daily sources of ascorbic acid since appreciable amounts in other foods can be destroyed during processing. Ascorbic acid in foods is easily destroyed by oxidation; therefore, undue exposure to oxygen, copper, and iron, and prolonged cooking at high temperatures in the presence of oxygen, should be avoided. However, quick heating methods can protect food vitamin C by inactivating plant oxidases. Vitamin C is relatively stable to normal boiling, but losses are substantial with greater oxidation by steaming or pressure cooking. Often there is only a small vitamin C loss for foods during freezing or dehydration. However, in one report, frozen storage destroyed about 28% of the vitamin C content in black currants and 34% in strawberries (Hagg et al., 1995). No significant loss of vitamin C from microwave heating of infant formula has been reported (Sigman-Grant et al., 1992).

Bioavailability of vitamin C for humans using a depletion-repletion technique revealed that ascorbic acid from oranges, orange juice, and cooked broccoli is similar to that of synthetic ascorbic acid (Mangels et al., 1993). However, the bioavailability of ascorbic acid in raw broccoli was 20% lower than the other sources. A study to simulate home conditions for vitamin C in orange juice showed that juice retained an average of 88% of the original ascorbic acid after 1 week and 67% after 2 weeks in opened containers stored at typical home refrigerator temperatures (Shaw and Moshonas, 1991).

DEFICIENCY

Effects of Deficiency

Under practical feeding situations, only humans, nonhuman primates, guinea pigs, and fish will develop vitamin C deficiency if diets are lacking in the vitamin. Farm livestock synthesize ascorbic acid from glucose in either the liver or the kidney, and vitamin C deficiency usually does not occur in such animals. In the case of well-balanced nutrition, their tissues receive endogenous ascorbate continuously, and the level in blood and tissues can only with difficulty be affected by exogenous vitamin C. However, with nutritionally unbalanced diets, relative vitamin C deficiency may be induced in ascorbate-synthesizing animals as well (Ginter, 1970). Low blood ascorbic acid can be caused by various types of stress, including metabolic disorders, improper nutrition, insufficient vitamin A or β-carotene intake, and various infectious diseases. Under such conditions, exogenous vitamin C can have a positive effect in ascorbic acid-synthesizing species.

Ruminants

All known ruminants can synthesize ascorbic acid; however, clinical cases of scurvy in ruminants have been described. Death of cows and calves due to scurvy was characterized by changes in the oral cavity mucosa, muzzle, and skin, accompanied by weight loss and general unthriftiness (Cole et al., 1944; Duncan, 1944). In calves there was an extensive dermatosis accompanied by hair loss and thickening of skin in animals receiving insufficient milk. Blood ascorbic acid was low, and the condition was successfully treated with vitamin C injections. Scurvy and lowered blood ascorbic acid content in weaned calves were reported by Martynjuk (1952). Studies of blood vitamin C concentrations in calves receiving the same diet have revealed great individual differences, with variations related to genetic background (Palludan and Wegger, 1984).

Positive effects of ascorbic acid supplementation on milk yield and milk quality were reported by Kuemyj (1955). Studies with bulls housed differently showed a lowering of vitamin C stores as a result of cold stress (Hidiroglou et al., 1977). Ruminants can actually be considered more prone to vitamin C deficiency because of impaired synthesis than monogastric animals since they cannot rely on exogenous supplies of this vitamin, which is rapidly destroyed by ruminal microflora (Cappa, 1958; Itze, 1984).

Hypovitaminosis C is most often observed in winter and spring and tends to reduce general resistance of the animals, causing infertility, high incidence of retained placenta, low viability of progeny, and several other pathological conditions that can result in economic losses, particularly with calves (Soldatenkov and Suganova, 1966). Some data from the literature indicate that ascorbic acid-synthesizing capacity of calves during the first phases of life is insufficient to satisfy their requirements. Some researchers even suggested that calves do not synthesize vitamin C before 2 to 3 weeks after birth (Itze, 1984). However, Bouda et al. (1980) established that adult levels of vitamin C were not present in the calf until after 3 months of age. Evidence suggests that serum vitamin C content is dependent on nutrition of the dam but also on age and health of the calves. Yashin (1985) diagnosed marked scurvy clinical signs in neonatal calves whose mothers had low ascorbic acid levels in the blood and colostrum.

Jagos et al. (1977) found considerably lower plasma vitamin C content in calves with bronchopneumonia than in healthy animals. A relationship has been reported between hypovitaminosis C and skeletal muscle pain and subcutaneous hemorrhages in calves (Pribyl, 1963). Dobsinska et al. (1981) studied the relationship between ascorbemia and body weight gains of calves in a large-capacity calf-house facility and found a negative correlation between the two parameters in 2- to 22-week-old bull calves.

Studies tend to show that low plasma ascorbic acid levels are likely in animals experiencing gastrointestinal, respiratory, or other health ailments. Calves supplemented with vitamin C had lower incidence of scouring (Cummins and Brunner, 1989). In calves with respiratory disease signs, Bouda et al. (1980) found significantly lower plasma ascorbic acid levels than in healthy calves. Podgornova and Donskova (1972) found markedly reduced ascorbic acid concentrations in the organs of cattle infested with tapeworm. Scott (1981) described a skin disorder in calves that had low plasma ascorbic acid levels and could be cured by administration of vitamin C.

Calves from herds characterized by poor health status generally also had reduced ascorbic acid status during the critical period from birth to 2 weeks of age. When calves were given doses of 1.25 to 2.5 g/day, infectious disease resistance appeared to increase, and respiratory diseases were almost totally eliminated (Itze, 1984; Palludan and Wegger, 1984).

In conclusion, it is generally accepted that healthy adult ruminants under normal dietary and environmental conditions are able to meet their vitamin C requirements by body synthesis. However, young ruminants are susceptible to deficiency during the first few weeks of life, particularly when subjected to stress conditions, including cold, damp environments and disease, and/or if limited in colostrum consumption.

Swine

The signs of vitamin C deficiency in swine include weakness; fatigue; dyspnea; pain in the bones; and hemorrhages of the skin, musculature, adipose tissue, and certain organs (Zintzen, 1975). Swine nutritionists have generally formulated diets without vitamin C because the young pig can synthesize ascorbic acid within a week of birth, and both sow colostrum and milk provide a plentiful source of the vitamin to the nursing pig (Wegger and Palludan, 1984). After it is weaned, the pig becomes dependent on its own tissue synthesis of the vitamin to meet its metabolic needs. Although most farm species synthesize adequate quantities of ascorbic acid, some evidence suggests that the rate of synthesis in swine may be inadequate during adverse environmental conditions, after a disease insult, and during other periods of stress. Mahan et al. (1994) reported a growth response the initial 2 weeks postweaning but not thereafter.

Swine researchers have indicated that under certain situations, pigs may need supplemental vitamin C for maximum weight gain and feed use (Mahan et al., 1966; Yen and Pond, 1981); however, nearly an equal number of reports are negative (Brown et al., 1970; Yen and Pond,

1984, 1987; NRC, 1998). Reasons for this inconsistency may be that unpredictable environmental and psychological stresses imposed on swine may increase requirements for ascorbic acid.

The level of available dietary energy is a major factor in determining the amount of ascorbic acid available to the pig (Brown et al., 1975; Brown, 1984). Serum ascorbic acid concentrations as well as urinary output are directly related to the level of energy in the diet. It was also found that a minor stress such as individual penning will evoke a positive growth response from supplementary ascorbic acid, especially in animals fed a "low-energy" diet. Dietary energy is able to cause a shift in ascorbic acid synthesis because of restrictions on amount of free glucose available for this synthesis.

If a need for dietary vitamin C exists in swine, the newly weaned pig would seem to be the class of swine most likely to be deficient. Sow's milk contains a high concentration of vitamin C at parturition, but the level drops dramatically with time toward weaning. For the baby pig, the general consensus is that ascorbic acid blood level increases with colostrum intake, drops at weaning, and slowly increases after 7 weeks to the mature level (Wegger and Palludan, 1984).

A specific clinical leg-weakness syndrome in growing pigs manifests itself mainly as crooked and/or deviated forelegs. These signs are indicated by contracted flexor tendons and weak joint ligaments that become apparent in pigs weighing 30 to 45 kg and seem to indicate impaired development in growing connective tissues (Nielsen and Vinther, 1984). Vitamin C administered to boars during the growing period from 39 to 105 kg body weight resulted in straightness of front legs compared to controls (Cleveland et al., 1987).

Ivos et al. (1971) reported an inverse relationship between ambient temperature and conception rate in sows. Additionally, these authors reported that average conception rate in sows increased when boars were supplemented with either 1 or 2 g daily of ascorbic acid compared to controls. Lin et al. (1985) observed increased sperm concentration per ejaculate in heat-stressed working boars that received 300 mg of ascorbic acid per day compared to unsupplemented boars. Boars that received the supplemental ascorbic acid also had fewer abnormal sperm cells per ejaculate.

Handling practices at weaning (especially early weaning)—which are generally considered to be stressful and include transport and mixing with unfamiliar pigs—have been shown to deplete body ascorbate. In view of decreased plasma vitamin C concentration and dramatic changes in nutritional, social, and other environmental factors associated with weaning, it was suggested that beneficial response from supplemental vitamin C with weanling pigs may be related to suppression of postweaning subclinical disease (Yen and Pond, 1981). In a study with growing pigs between the ages of 4 and 7 weeks, Park and Harrison (1990) reported an improvement in nursing pig performance (6% improvement in daily gain, 5% improvement in gain/feed) resulting from vitamin C supplementation in tap drinking water.

Spontaneous scurvy as a result of a genetic defect was observed in a swine production herd among 2- to 3-week-old piglets (Jensen and Basse, 1984). Closer observation revealed that all pigs were from the same boar. Analysis of their blood and tissues revealed only a very small concentration of vitamin C. The 3:1 ratio between normal and affected pigs was characteristic of simple autosomal recessive inheritance in matings between nonaffected carriers. Liver microsomes were shown to be incapable of synthesizing ascorbic acid in vitro even with L-gulonolactone as substrate (Jensen and Basse, 1984).

The influence of maternal vitamin C deficiency on fetal development was studied in swine with a hereditary lack of ability to synthesize ascorbic acid (Wegger and Palludan, 1994). Severe pathological changes were seen in the uterus and fetuses. Characteristic findings were hemorrhages and hematomas in both fetal and maternal placenta, and general edema and subcutaneous hemorrhages in the fetuses. Ossification of the fetal skeleton was severely deranged.

Poultry

Like swine, poultry are able to synthesize vitamin C, and thus it is assumed they do not require dietary sources of the vitamin. However, in newly hatched poultry, there is a slow rate of ascorbate synthesis, and this, combined with encountered stress, increases probability of vitamin C deficiency. The chick is subject to considerable stress conditions, such as rapid growth, exposure to hot or cold temperatures, starvation, vaccination, and disease conditions such as coccidiosis. Pardue and Williams (1990) reported that plasma ascorbic acid levels in poults were depressed significantly by cold stress, beak trimming, and injection at 1 and 14 days of age. Supplemental vitamin C (150 ppm) enhanced performance of broiler chicks exposed to multiple concurrent environmental stressors (McKee and Harrison, 1995).

For both stressed mature and newly hatched poultry, several reports have documented a beneficial effect of supplementing the feed with ascorbic acid on growth rate, egg production, eggshell strength and thickness, fertility and spermatozoa production, counteracting unfavorable climate and housing conditions, and intoxication or disease (Mc-Donald et al., 1981; Pardue, 1987). On the contrary, many researchers have found no beneficial effect of vitamin C supplementation under any conditions.

For heat-stressed chickens, supplemental vitamin C provided definite improvements in egg production, eggshell strength, and interior egg quality (El-Boushy and Van Albada, 1970; Cheng et al., 1988). Peebles and Brake (1985) also reported that supplemental ascorbic acid holds promise for increased production during high environmental temperatures or for nutritionally marginal diets. When ascorbic acid was used at levels of 100 ppm or less for commercial layers, there was improvement in livability, egg production, and eggshell quality. Perek and Kendler (1963) carried out experiments in the Jordan Valley, where hens were subjected to hot temperatures, and reported increases in egg production of 23 and 11.2% in two experiments in which the birds were given supplemental ascorbic acid. They also reported increased egg weights, decreased culls and mortality, and no shell quality differences. Other researchers were not able to confirm the positive effects of ascorbic acid supplementation.

Male reproduction is favored by vitamin C supplementation. Monsi and Onitchi (1991) supplemented the feed of heat-stressed broiler breeders with 0, 125, 250, or 500 ppm of ascorbic acid. Semen volume, total sperm per ejaculate, and motile sperm per ejaculate were significantly increased due to the addition of ascorbic acid. Semen volume and sperm concentration of turkey toms were found to be increased by 28% by the supplementation of 150 ppm of ascorbic acid to the breeder ration (Dobrescu, 1987). When Noll (1993) supplemented the feed of male breeder turkeys with 200 ppm of ascorbic acid for 8 weeks, ascorbic acid supplementation increased semen volume 16% and sperm concentration 18%.

Vitamin C is necessary for bone development and eggshell quality. Supplementing ascorbic acid to molted laying hens was beneficial to egg production and eggshell quality (Zapata and Gernat, 1995). Orban et al. (1993) reported that large doses of ascorbic acid (2,000 ppm) in the diet influenced calcium metabolism, affecting bone and eggshell mineralization in chickens. Vitamin C is a necessary cofactor for the bioconversion of vitamin D_3 to its active form, $1,25(OH)_2D_3$. Weiser et al. (1990) reported that 100 ppm of ascorbic acid in the diet of chicks increased plasma concentrations of $1,25(OH)_2D_3$, which led to elevated activities of duodenal calcium-binding protein and greater weights and breaking strength of bones. It is possible that the many cases of "field rickets" in poults may be due to stress-induced deficiency of vitamin C.

Njoku (1986) concluded that during periods of heat stress in the tropics, dietary supplementation of broiler diets with 200 ppm of ascorbic acid was necessary and economically advantageous as body weight and feed; gain responses were improved. Other researchers have not been able to confirm the positive effects of vitamin C supplementation. In a study supplementing 2,600 ppm of ascorbic acid, egg production, eggshell thickness, egg weight, and mortality were not affected, but interior quality was improved (Nockels, 1984).

Pardue et al. (1985) were unable to find significant vitamin C effects of heat stress in broiler performance, except that heat-associated mortality was markedly reduced in supplemented females. When acute heat stress was imposed on broilers, vitamin C reduced adrenal corticosteroid concentration in the plasma of birds associated with the stress. Apparently, high levels of ascorbic acid in the adrenal gland regulates glucocorticoid synthesis, thus limiting some of the deleterious responses associated with stress and delaying the depletion of steroid hormone precursors.

Disease conditions have been found to affect vitamin C metabolism in poultry. When chicks were infected with fowl typhoid, their plasma vitamin C concentrations were reduced (Hill and Garren, 1958). The vitamin C concentrations in plasma and tissue were also reduced in chicks infected with intestinal coccidiosis (Kechik and Sykes, 1979). Dietary ascorbate was shown to prevent this and contributed to intestinal repair.

In addition to performance, evidence also suggests an association between vitamin C and the animal's ability to tolerate or resist bacterial infection. In early work, chickens infected with fowl typhoid had reduced blood ascorbic acid, and the administration of vitamin C at 1,000 ppm in feed resulted in reduced early mortality from typhoid infection (Satterfield et al., 1940). Chickens fed a diet containing supplemental ascorbic acid showed increased resistance to a combined Newcastle disease virus–*Mycoplasma gallissepticum* infection and to a secondary *E. coli* infection, as well as to a primary *Escherichia coli* challenge infection (Takahashi et al., 1991).

Leghorn-type chickens aged 6 weeks, supplemented with 330 ppm of vitamin C and exposed to air-sac challenge with *E. coli*, had a 19% incidence of *E. coli* infection versus 76% in controls (Gross et al., 1988). The authors hypothesized that the response to vitamin C may be attributed to the vitamin increasing the synthesis of superoxide anion that kills phagocytized bacteria. Dietary level of ascorbic acid appears to be important since too little vitamin C results in too little superoxide anion production, and excessive vitamin C may result in reduction of super-oxide anion in the phagocytic cells.

Since ascorbic acid can be synthesized at the tissue level by domestic fowl, it has been held by many nutritionists that exogenous supplementation of vitamin C to poultry would be senseless. Over the past several decades, the relationship between stress and vitamin C in poultry was recognized; however, research data have been inconsistent and conflicting, making it difficult to establish requirements for this nutrient under all conditions. Some data suggest that supplementation with vitamin C should be considered as a management alternative to prevent vitamin C deficiency when poultry are stressed (Quarles and Adrian, 1989; Quarles et al., 1989).

Horses

Horses, like other farm species, synthesize vitamin C, but stress situations such as bacterial and viral infection (e.g., influenza, rhinopneumonia) have been reported to lower vitamin C serum levels (Jaeschke, 1984). This is further associated with blood parameters, indicating delayed and/or disturbed collagen metabolism in young horses. Studies have shown that horses of all ages that suddenly show poor performance often have a reduced ascorbic acid serum level (Jaeschke, 1984). Performance of these horses improved after intravenous administration of ascorbic acid. Despite early suggestions that supplementary ascorbic acid (vitamin C) improved the sperm quality of stallions and the breeding performance of mares (Davis and Cole, 1943), other workers have been unable to repeat those results.

Other Animal Species

Dogs and Cats

The dog is able to synthesize vitamin C. Naismith (1958) showed that this synthetic ability is present in puppies during the first weeks of postnatal life. Chatterjee et al. (1975) demonstrated that dogs synthesized ascorbic acid in the liver at an hourly rate of 5 µg/mg of protein. However, this rate is low compared with the hourly rate in other mammals, such as cows (68 µg/mg of protein), rats (39 µg/mg of protein), and rabbits (23 µg/mg of protein).

There is controversy about the therapeutic use of ascorbic acid in canine diseases. Vitamin C has been used in treatment of canine viral infections. Some clinicians stated that 1,000 to 2,500 mg of ascorbic acid given intravenously once daily for at least 3 days was beneficial in the treatment of canine distemper (Belfield, 1967; Leveque, 1969).

Vitamin C deficiency also has been reported to be associated with canine hypertrophic osteodystrophy (Grondalen, 1976). Meier et al. (1957) found that dogs with hyperbaric oxygen drenching had low plasma ascorbic acid concentration, and large doses of vitamin C (100 to 200 mg) given orally or intramuscularly enhanced healing. Vitamin C supplementation of 50 to 100 mg/day may be beneficial in combating arthritis in older dogs (Lewis and Morris, 1983).

Some trials failed to demonstrate a need for dietary ascorbic acid in cats (Carvalho da Silva, 1950). Successful growth and reproduction are routinely obtained with commercial and purified (NRC, 1986) diets containing no supplemental ascorbic acid.

As in the dog, vitamin C synthesis in the cat is lower than in other species, including the cow, sheep, rat, and rabbit (Rucker et al., 1980). Pietronigro et al. (1983) reported that central nervous system function following spinal cord injury in the cat is associated with large losses of ascorbic acid from the region of the injury. Treatment of injury with two drugs (naloxone or methyl-prednisolone) preserved neurologic function and prevented ascorbate loss.

FISH

Deficiency of vitamin C in most aquaculture species results in poor formation of connective tissue. Intensively fed, caged channel catfish grew slowly and exhibited scoliosis and lordosis (Fig. 15.2), broken-back syndrome, and elevated mortality from bacterial infection while receiving an ascorbic acid-deficient diet (Lovell, 1973). Other signs of ascorbic acid deficiency in channel catfish are internal and external hemorrhage, fin erosion, dark skin color, and reduced formation of bone collagen. Similar structural deformities such as scoliosis and lordosis due to vitamin C deficiency have been observed in Indian major carp, common carp, roach, blue tilapia, Nile tilapia, and yellowtail (NRC, 1993). Vitamin C-deficient salmon and trout exhibited structural deformities (scoliosis, lordosis, and abnormal support cartilage of the eye, gill, and fins) and internal hemorrhaging, usually preceded by nonspecific signs such as anorexia and lethargy (NRC, 1993).

Japanese eels fed a vitamin C-deficient diet had reduced growth after 10 weeks and hemorrhage in the head and fins after 14 weeks (Arai et al., 1972). Vitamin C-deficient shrimp exhibited black death syndrome, a condition characterized by melanized lesions in connective tis-

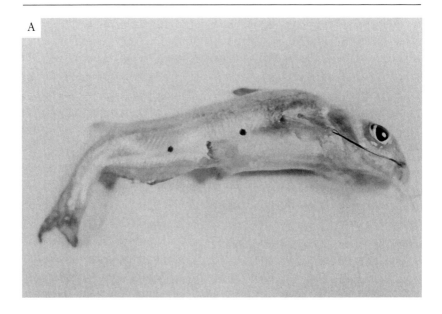

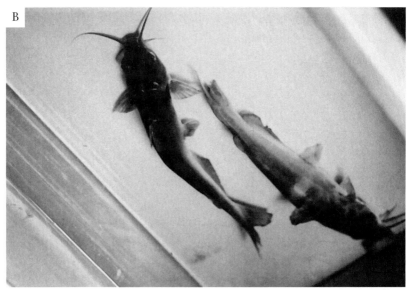

Fig. 15.2 Vitamin C deficiency in catfish. (A) Fingerling channel catfish fed a diet devoid of vitamin C for 8 weeks. Note scoliosis and lordosis. (B) Channel catfish from commercial cage culture where the regular diet was devoid of vitamin C. Fish at left shows lateral curvature of the spine (scoliosis); fish at right shows vertical curvature (lordosis) and a vertical depigmented band at the point of spinal injury, which is characteristic. (Courtesy of R.T. Lovell and Auburn University, Alabama.)

sue under the exoskeleton as well as on the gills, abdomen, and gut (Magarelli et al., 1979).

The immune system and reproduction are dependent on vitamin C. Vitamin C appears to protect phagocytic cells and surrounding tissues from oxidative damage. An increased immune response due to high concentrations of vitamin C supplementation has been demonstrated in channel catfish (Li and Lovell, 1985) and rainbow trout (Navarre and Halver, 1989). Reduced reproductive performance has been reported in tilapia and rainbow trout (NRC, 1993).

FOXES AND MINK

Helgebostad (1984) indicated that the fox and mink are able to synthesize sufficient vitamin C.

LABORATORY ANIMALS

Because of body synthesis, the rat, mouse, and hamster do not require dietary vitamin C, and classic studies on scurvy have been conducted with the guinea pig (NRC, 1995). Early signs of vitamin C deficiency in guinea pigs are reduced feed intake and weight loss, followed by anemia and widespread hemorrhages. Additional signs include enlarged costochondral junction, disturbed epiphyseal growth centers of long bones, bone demineralization, altered dentine, and gingivitis (NRC, 1995; Kip et al., 1996). Vitamin C deficiency in guinea pigs also results in hypertriglyceridemia, hypercholesterolemia, and decreased vitamin E concentrations in liver and lungs.

A number of studies using guinea pigs as a laboratory animal requiring vitamin C are examining new functional roles of the vitamin. As examples, ascorbic acid has been shown to prevent lipid peroxidation and prevent damage of proteins in guinea pig extrahepatic tissue microsomes (Mukhopadhyay et al., 1995), and ascorbic acid was found to be essential for the release of insulin from scorbutic guinea pig pancreatic islets (Wells et al., 1995).

NONHUMAN PRIMATES

Unless dietary vitamin C content is adequate, scurvy is apt to occur in all species of nonhuman primates. In fact, along with vitamin D_3 deficiency in New World monkeys, scurvy is the most frequently diagnosed specific nutrient deficiency in captive primates (NRC, 1978). Lesions of vitamin C deficiency states include gingival hemorrhage, loose teeth, subperiosteal hemorrhage, normocytic normochromic anemia, and epiphyseal fractures (Banerjee and Bal, 1959).

623

RABBITS

The rabbit does not require dietary vitamin C (NRC, 1977). Harris et al. (1956) demonstrated that young rabbits kept for periods as long as 25 weeks on vitamin C-free diets gained weight normally and continued to excrete considerable amounts of ascorbic acid in their urine.

Humans

In humans, gross vitamin C deficiency results in scurvy, a disease characterized by multiple hemorrhages (Fig. 15.3). In adults, manifest scurvy is often preceded by lassitude, fatigue, anorexia, muscle pain, and greater susceptibility to infection and stress. Scurvy is characterized by anemia and alteration of protein metabolism; weakening of collagenous structures in bone, cartilage, teeth, and connective tissue; swollen, bleeding gums, with loss of teeth; fatigue and lethargy; rheumatic pain in the legs; degeneration of muscles; massive "sheet" hematomas in the thighs; and skin lesions. Bleeding gums gingivitis and loosening of the teeth are usually the earliest objective signs (Marks, 1975; Vilter, 1978; Moser and Bendich, 1991). Structural defects characteristic of scurvy include the following:

1. Bones and cartilage—the cartilage cells cease to form matrix.
2. Teeth—odontoblasts, predentine, dentine, and enamel are not formed; interrelated with bone and collagen formation.
3. Muscles—atrophy and necrosis occur, with calcium deposits.
4. Connective tissues—collagen fibers are not formed by fibroblasts.
5. Capillaries and vascular system—capillary walls are fragile.
6. Blood—hemorrhage causes anemia because red blood cells are rapidly destroyed.
7. Liver and other organs—liver atrophies and is infiltrated with fat; bile secretion is impaired; kidney atrophies; and spleen enlarges.
8. Reproductive organs—degeneration of ovaries or germinal epithelium of testes occurs but may be nonspecific.
9. Other endocrines—thyroid shows hyperemia, hypersecretion, and irregularity of structure; adrenals are abnormal.

Scurvy may be fatal, particularly in infants and otherwise debilitated adults. Well-defined scurvy is not common in more developed countries, and occurs chiefly in infants fed diets deficient in ascorbic acid. Scurvy is an epidemic disease in underdeveloped areas of the world, where poverty, wars, and great migrations produce situations of malnutrition.

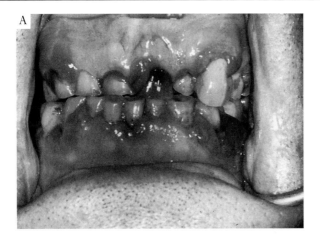

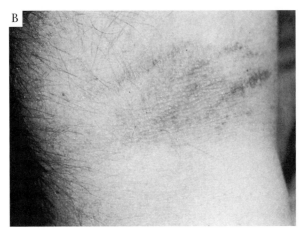

Fig. 15.3 Scurvy in a vitamin C-deficient human. (A) Severe scurvy, with swelling, bleeding, and receding gums. (B) Capillary fragility, with small hemorrhagic areas (ecchymoses). (Courtesy of Howerde E. Sauberlich, University of Alabama.)

Dietary levels were found to be deficient for 41 to 48% of children in a region of Russia (Krasnopevtsev et al., 1993) and for 30 to 41% of adults in Warsaw, Poland (Pardo et al., 1991). In urban and rural regions of Turkey, 43% of school-age children had deficient plasma vitamin C concentrations.

Infantile scurvy (Barlow's disease), which is usually due to lack of vitamin C in artificial foods, generally occurs between the ages of 6 and

18 months. In the United States in the late 1800s and early 1900s, many children died from infantile scurvy due to the practice of boiling or sterilizing milk, which completely destroyed the vitamin C. As a rule, infantile scurvy is first noticed when the infant cries on being handled, is irritable, and loses appetite and weight. Tenderness of extremities and pain on movement are almost invariably present (Marks, 1975). Manifestations of scurvy appear insidiously, usually after 5 to 6 months of severe deprivation of vitamin C.

Scurvy is a rare disease in developed countries and appears sporadically in elderly individuals who live alone, in smokers, in alcoholics, in infants with prolonged artificial feeding without a complementary diet, and in a miscellaneous group of patients with unusual diets, some of whom have psychiatric problems (Moser and Bendich, 1991; Gomez-Carrasco et al., 1994). Other risk groups include diabetics, rheumatoid arthritis patients, oral contraceptive users, and individuals exposed to petrochemicals in the workplace (Moser and Bendich, 1991).

Vitamin C and the other antioxidant vitamins (vitamin E and β-carotene) convert highly active radicals to less active species and thereby reduce certain disease incidence. A large body of evidence has been accumulated, including the results of recently published epidemiological studies that consistently report an association of dietary intake of vitamins C and E and of β-carotene and a risk reduction for coronary heart disease and cancer (Weber, 1994). Vitamin C alone has been related to dramatic reduction of coronary heart disease risk factors (Kranowski, 1991; Jacques, 1992; Singh et al., 1995; Duell, 1996; Toohey et al., 1996; Jacob, 1998) and cancer (Block, 1991; Gershoff, 1993; Kune et al., 1993). In addition to reduction of cancer and heart disease, vitamin C is reported beneficial in eliminating cataracts, reducing complications of diabetes, maintaining normal sperm, lowering hypertension, and reducing infectious disease by maintaining a normal immune response (see Functions).

Assessment of Status

Completely satisfactory and reliable procedures to assess vitamin C nutritional status have not been developed because of limited knowledge concerning the vitamin's metabolic functions. However, information concerning adequacy has been determined by an analysis of vitamin C concentrations in serum, leukocytes, whole blood, or urine. Leukocyte vitamin C concentrations provide information concerning body stores of ascorbic acid (Turnbull et al., 1981). Precautions need to be taken to protect the vitamin in solution, and to select an assay that measures the vitamin itself and not other substances present.

Methods of biochemical detection of deficiency include the following:

1. Tissue content—28 mg/100 g of liver is the saturation level for humans and guinea pigs; lower concentrations will reveal reduced intake.

2. Leukocytes—ascorbate concentration in leukocytes with adequate diets is about 25 mg/100 ml, with less than 20 mg/100 ml in deficiencies.

3. Serum—the normal range of ascorbate (0.5 to 2.2 mg/100 ml) is often too variable to permit reliable estimation of deficiencies.

4. Urinary excretion—the load test and saturation test generally indicate immediate past intake and not overall nutritional status; nevertheless, amount of a given dose that is excreted is indicative of the tissue stores. Amount of ascorbate excreted during 3 hours following a 100-mg dose will be 50% for a normal, saturated person; 15% for a depleted person; and 5% for a scorbutic patient.

5. Other tests include (a) intradermal test, which involves rate of decoloration of 2,6-dichlorophenolindophenol injected intradermally; (b) decolorization of dye on the tongue; and (c) serum alkaline phosphatase, excretion of tyrosine metabolism products, and urinary creatine, which are not specific.

SUPPLEMENTATION

Supplementation with vitamin C is not normally recommended for common livestock species (ruminants, poultry, swine, and horses) under normal management and feeding regimens. As previously mentioned, stress conditions affect vitamin C synthesis, and supplementation considerations must take this into account. Kolb (1984) summarized various types of stress that apparently increase demands while reducing animals' capability to synthesize vitamin C, as follows:

1. Dietary conditions—deficiencies of energy, protein, vitamin E, selenium, iron, etc.

2. Production or performance stress—high production or performance (e.g., rapid growth rates, high milk production, racehorse running).

3. Transportation, animal handling, and new environmental location stress—animals being driven or transported to market, animals placed in new surroundings (e.g., weaned pigs from different litters placed together),

627

and stressful management practices (e.g., castration, vaccination).

4. Temperature—high ambient temperature or cold trauma.

5. Diseases and parasites—fever and infection reduce blood ascorbic acid, while parasites, particularly of the liver, disturb ascorbic acid synthesis and increase requirements for the vitamin.

The stress associated with confinement calf housing decreased immune response to a specific antigen and decreased plasma ascorbate concentrations (Cummins and Brunner, 1991). The health of young calves supplemented with vitamin C improved, as reflected by decreased navel infections, peritonitis, pneumonia, enteritis, respiratory disease, scouring, and mortality (Blair and Cummins, 1984; Itze, 1984; Cummins and Brunner, 1989).

During the first weeks of life, the calf's requirement for ascorbic acid must be covered by colostrum and milk concentrations and from the inborn storages of the vitamin. One calf study in which reared calves were denied colostrum found that all but one of the experimental animals died of umbilical infections and peritonitis (Palludan and Wegger, 1984). That survivor had a high content of ascorbic acid in its blood at birth. Further investigations showed positive results from supplementation of calves with ascorbic acid. Calves fed 1.75 g/day of vitamin C that were colostrum-deprived had lower clinical scores for diarrhea, and at 14 days of age, plasma IgG concentrations were higher than those of controls not fed ascorbate (Cummins and Brunner, 1989).

It is important to note that reserves of ascorbic acid are high at birth but decline rapidly afterward unless exogenous supply is furnished until synthesis can handle the load (Itzeova, 1984; Palludan and Wegger, 1984). Plasma ascorbic acid level in calves fed fresh colostrum twice a day and frozen colostrum of the first milking once a day was high, with indications that the decrease in ascorbic acid content usually seen after birth can be avoided by this practice (Itzeova, 1984). Itze (1984) recommended supplementation with vitamin C for calves reared on milk diets. The initial days of calf rearing are critical, for the calf must adapt itself to a new environment, feeding practice, and housing at an age when its resistance is minimal. Of various programs tested, the author recommends daily oral supplementation with 2.5 g of ascorbic acid in combination with parenteral application of 500 mg of ascorbic acid in two doses immediately after moving animals into their new rearing facilities. Lehocky (1981), in his work with dairy calf supplementation, found that only 50% of a calf's requirement for vitamin C is covered when feeding various milk replacers.

Various studies have demonstrated beneficial effects of low doses of 50 to 100 mg of ascorbic acid per kilogram to diets of broilers or laying hens exposed to heat stress (Kolb, 1984). Njoku (1984) reported that 200 mg of ascorbic acid per kilogram fed to broilers helped alleviate heat stress. Eggshell thickness increased for hens (El-Boushy et al., 1968), while livability, weight gain, and immune response improved in broilers (Pardue and Thaxton, 1982) when heat-stressed birds received supplemental vitamin C. Peebles and Brake (1985) fed vitamin C to broiler breeders throughout a complete production cycle. They found fertility improved at dietary levels of 50 mg/kg, with improvement in hatch of fertile eggs due to a decrease in early embryonic mortality. There was no further benefit at 100 mg/kg. In turkeys, toms given 150 mg/kg increased semen volume by 31% per ejaculate. It is thought that vitamin C stimulates testicular activity by its involvement in the synthesis of steroid hormones (Dobrescu, 1987).

Since vitamin C can be synthesized at the tissue level by swine, it has been held by many nutritionists that supplemental vitamin C to swine would be senseless. Data suggest that supplementation with ascorbic acid should be considered as a management alternative to prevent vitamin C deficiencies when swine are stressed.

The literature reports concerning efficacy of supplementation of swine diets with ascorbic acid is conflicting. Young pigs seem to be more likely than adults to respond to supplementation, much the same as was reported for ruminants. Perhaps the inconsistency of results is due to uncontrolled stress or genetic differences (Brown, 1984).

Early weaning (0 to 3 weeks) of piglets has been shown to decrease ascorbic acid levels in liver, and tests seem to indicate that maximal synthesizing capacity is not developed until about 8 weeks, thus indicating a possible advantage in supplementing milk replacer products with vitamin C (Wegger and Palludan, 1984). Sandholm et al. (1979) reported that umbilical hemorrhages (Fig. 15.4) occurring in piglets immediately after birth can be prevented by supplementing the sows' feed with 1 g of ascorbic acid per day during the last week of gestation.

The intensive selection that has taken place for several decades in the swine industry may have altered the enzymatic constitution of animals so that ability to synthesize vitamin C has changed. Furthermore, modern intensive production systems and continuous demand for higher productivity may have increased the requirement of ascorbic acid for swine. Feeding practice in pig production has also changed; the tendency is to use more processed feedstuffs that, practically speaking, contain no ascorbic acid.

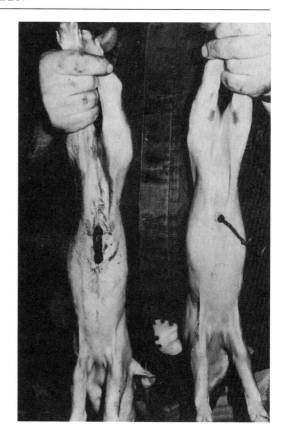

Fig. 15.4 Navel bleeding syndrome. Umbilical cords of a bleeding piglet (*left*) and a normal piglet (*right*), age 10 hours. Navel bleeding has been prevented by preparturient administration of ascorbic acid. (Courtesy of Markus Sandholm, College of Veterinary Medicine, Helsinki, Finland.)

Therapeutic, as distinguished from nutritional, use of ascorbic acid has been useful in treating infectious diseases of the horse and dog (Kolb, 1984). The importance of ascorbic acid for defense against infections and for phagocytosis has been stressed. Beneficial effects of supplemental vitamin C have been reported for puppies with disorders in bone development accompanied by painful swelling of joints when the vitamin is deficient (Kolb, 1984).

L-Ascorbic acid is the most important of the several compounds that have vitamin C activity. Ascorbic acid is commercially available as 100% crystalline, 50% fat-coated, and 97.5% ethylcellulose-coated products and their dilutions. The more soluble sodium salt of ascorbic acid (sodium ascorbate) is also commercially available. Various derivatives of ascorbic acid, which are more stable than the parent compound, have been shown to provide antiscorbutic activity. These include L-ascorbate-2-sulfate, L-ascorbyl-2-monophosphate, magnesium-L-ascorbyl-2-phosphate, and L-ascorbyl-2-polyphosphate. When providing supplemental ascorbic acid, it is advisable to use a stabilized form, and coating ascorbic acid crystals with ethylcellulose is a suitable stabilization method. In storage experiments, ascorbic acid protected in this manner was found to be four times more stable than untreated ascorbic acid crystals (Kolb, 1984).

Adams (1982) reported that coated (ethylcellulose) ascorbic acid showed a higher retention after processing than the crystalline form (84 versus 48%). Retention of ascorbic acid in mash feed was fairly good, but with elevated storage time and temperature, stability was poor in crumbled feeds. Although retention of vitamin C activity in feed containing the ethylcellulose-coated product was low, it was 19 to 32% better than that of the crystalline form. Cows dosed orally with vitamin C coated with ethylcellulose had higher plasma ascorbic acid concentrations than did cows that received vitamin C in the form of fine powder (Hidiroglou, 1999).

Reports have evaluated polyphosphorylated L-ascorbic acid in fish (Chen and Chang, 1994; Matusiewicz et al., 1995), and found it to be more stable against oxidation and extrusion. Approximately 50% of the supplemental ascorbic acid is destroyed during the manufacture of extruded catfish feeds (Lovell and Lim, 1978), and excess ascorbic acid is added to commercial formulations to ensure that an adequate concentration of the vitamin is retained during processing. The form of the vitamin selected depends on how the fish feed is to be manufactured and how long it is to be stored before being fed to the fish. It may be more economical to overfortify channel catfish feeds with the ethycellulose-coated product than to use the phosphate derivatives of ascorbic acid; price-to-benefit relationships must be considered. Crystalline L-ascorbic acid and L-ascorbyl-2-polyphosphate were of similar bioavailability in broiler chicks (Pardue et al., 1993). Magnesium-L-ascorbyl-2-phosphate is a stable form of vitamin C that was shown to be available in swine diets (Mahan et al., 1994).

Supplementation of vitamins E (see Chapter 4, Supplementation) and C have been shown to improve oxidation stability of beef, improving lipid and color stability. Jugular infusion of sodium ascorbate 10 minutes prior to slaughter extended color display of fresh beef by 2 to 4 days (Schaefer et al., 1995). Contrary to feeding supplemental vitamin E, providing supplemental vitamin C to stabilize lipid and beef color will likely not be practical until a ruminally stable vitamin C product is developed.

The food industry uses ascorbic acid as a natural antioxidant. For certain human foods, enrichment or fortification with vitamin C is practiced, and vitamin C is also used in the food industry for its antioxidant activity. The antioxidant—that is, the reducing property of ascorbic acid—is exploited for preservation of flavor, color, and appearance of certain foods (Nobile and Woodhill, 1981). It is used in commercial preparation of beer, fruit juices, and canned and frozen vegetables and fruits; in meat curing; and in the flour industry to enhance baking qualities and appearance of bread. In meat processing, ascorbic acid makes it possible to reduce both the amount of added nitrite and the residual nitrite content in the product. In the stomach, nitrites are transformed into potentially carcinogenic nitrosamines. The addition of ascorbic acid to fresh flour improves its baking qualities, thus saving the 4 to 8 weeks of maturation flour would normally have to undergo after milling. As a result of food fortification and antioxidant uses in the food industry, food that is characteristically low in vitamin C will have higher levels than expected, provided processing methods have not destroyed the added vitamin.

Scurvy remains an important consideration, especially for underdeveloped countries, where crop failure and malnutrition remain real concerns due to droughts, floods, pestilence, wars, and general poverty. In more developed countries, cases of scurvy still occur occasionally (despite improved standards of living) due to inadequate diets and food faddism. Infants receiving artificial diets, alcoholics, and elderly individuals—especially elderly men living alone with low incomes—are at risk of developing overt signs of vitamin C deficiency. Vitamin C deficiency is likely to develop in individuals who do not consume optimum quantities of fruits (particularly citrus) and vegetables.

For humans in developed countries, large quantities of supplemental vitamin C are taken as part of multivitamin pills and separately, sometimes in megavitamin doses. There are significant new views on the health benefits of megavitamin doses, particularly the antioxidant vitamins (C, E, and β-carotene). Megadoses (e.g., more than 0.5 g/day) of vitamin C have been reported beneficial for preventing or modifying heart disease, cancer, cataracts, diabetes, and other disease conditions (see Deficiency, Humans). The beneficial effects of megadoses of vitamin C seem obvious; however, more studies are needed to further clarify these effects. For some subjects, excess supplemental vitamin C may be unwise (e.g., individuals with hemochromatosis). Of lesser consideration is the method of administering large doses of vitamin C (e.g., 0.5 g or greater) in tablets that are swallowed or chewable. Chewing large doses of the vitamin regularly can raise the acidity level in the mouth. This may dissolve the enamel and lead to tooth damage.

TOXICITY

The reported benefits of gram doses of vitamin C have led to widespread ingestion of vitamin C supplements by many individuals, thus raising issues of the safety of such practices. In general, high intakes of vitamin C are considered to be of low toxicity. Safety and tolerance of ascorbic acid in humans at levels as high as 10 g/day have been demonstrated (Koemer and Weber, 1972). Reported toxic effects include possible acidosis, gastrointestinal complaints, glycosuria or sensitivity reactions, mutagenic activity, and adverse effects concerning the metabolism of some minerals. Barness (1977) reports that toxic effects of megadoses of vitamin C are insignificant, rare, or troublesome but of little consequence. Effects demonstrated by in vitro experiments have often later been found to be nonexistent once definitive in vivo studies were conducted. Danger for vitamin C toxicity is minimized and unlikely in humans because of limited intestinal absorption capacity and efficient renal elimination. Nevertheless, prolonged megadose intakes of vitamin C should be avoided as adverse effects may result, particularly for patients with inborn errors of metabolism (e.g., cytinuria, oxalosis, and hyperuricemia).

The two greatest concerns with excess vitamin C for humans relate to (1) elevated oxalate production, which increases the risk of urinary calculi formation, and (2) ascorbic acid-enhancing iron absorption, which may lead to iron accumulation (e.g., hemochromatosis). In actuality, with excessive intake, the absorbed ascorbic acid is largely excreted into the urine. Only a small amount is metabolized to oxalate regardless of the level of dietary vitamin C. Methodological pitfalls account for many discrepancies in findings of varying oxalate levels after vitamin C intake. Inappropriate handling and storage of the samples favor an in vitro conversion of ascorbic acid to oxalic acid. Wandzilak et al. (1994) fed diets of 1, 5, and 10 g/day of ascorbic acid to healthy subjects and concluded that increasingly large doses of vitamin C did not increase urinary oxalates excretion, and thus do not increase the risk of kidney stone formation in healthy individuals. Contrary to the majority of scientists, Herbert (1996) believes that most free radical damage is produced by catalytic iron and that free radical release from high body iron slowly and insidiously promotes heart disease, cancer, and premature aging in individuals with hemochromatosis. Such an effect is not to be expected, however, as optimal iron absorption is effected with rather low doses of vitamin C (25 to 50 mg of ascorbic acid per meal). It can be concluded that vitamin C cannot be considered a risk factor for oxalate stones or excess iron absorption in healthy persons. Nevertheless, prudence dictates the avoidance of megadoses of vitamin C for individuals with a history of forming renal stones or patients with hemochromatosis or other forms of excess iron accumulation.

Few studies on potential vitamin C toxicity in domestic animal species have been carried out (NRC, 1987). Chronic toxicity studies generally indicate that ascorbic acid is well tolerated in animals. Oral ascorbic acid may be administered to most laboratory animals at doses of several grams per kilogram of body weight without appearance of any obvious general effect on health. Rabbits showed only transient subconjunctival hemorrhages without other manifestations after 4 months of daily parenteral injections of 200 mg/kg body weight. Guinea pigs tolerated daily doses of 8.9 g/kg body weight, equivalent to 1,800 times the normal requirement of 4 to 5 mg/kg body weight per day. Male guinea pigs fed 8.7% ascorbic acid for 6 weeks had decreased bone density and decreased urinary hydroxyproline compared to controls (Bray and Briggs, 1984). Helgebostad (1984) reported that high doses of 100 to 200 mg/kg body weight daily were harmful to mink with pronounced anemia in pregnant females and reduced the number and size of kits. A dietary ascorbic acid concentration of 1 g/kg of feed appears to pose no hazard to chickens, pigs, dogs, cats, or, probably, horses. Dietary supplementation of vitamin C even at levels as high as 3% had no appreciable effects on body weight gain, feed intake, or feed efficiency of growing chicks (Nakaya et al., 1986).

■ REFERENCES

Adams, C.R. (1982). *In* Vitamins–The Life Essentials. Nutrition Institute, National Feed Ingredient Association. NI-82, 1-9, Des Moines, Iowa.

Anderson, R., and Lukey, P.T. (1987). *Ann. N. Y. Acad. Sci. 49,* 229.

Arai, S., Nose, T., and Hashimoto, Y. (1972). *Bull. Freshwater Res. Lab. Tokyo 22,* 69.

Ausman, L.M., and Mayer, J. (1999). *Nutr. Rev. 57,* 222.

Banerjee, S., and Bal, H. (1959). *Indian J. Med. Res. 47,* 646.

Barnes, M.J., and Kodicek, K. (1972). *Vitam. Horm. 30,* 1.

Barness, L.A. (1977). *In* Re-evaluation of Vitamin C (A. Hanck and G. Ritzel, eds.), p. 23. Huber, Bern.

Belfield, W.O. (1967). *Vet. Med. Small Anim. Clin.* 62, 345.

Blair, L., and Cummins, K.A. (1984). *J. Dairy Sci.* 67(Suppl. 1), 138(Abstr.).

Block, G. (1991). *Am. J. Clin. Nutr.* 54, 1310S.

Bouda, J., Jagos, P., Dvorak, R., and Ondrova, J. (1980). *Acta Vet. Brno.* 49, 53.

Bray, D.L., and Briggs, G.M. (1984). *J. Nutr.* 114, 920.

Brown, R.G. (1984). *In* Proc. Ascorbic Acid in Domestic Animals (I. Wegger, F.J. Tagwerker, and J. Moustgaard, eds.), p. 60. Danish Agriculture Society, Copenhagen.

Brown, R.G., Sharma, V.D., and Young, L.G. (1970). *Can. J. Anim. Sci.* 50, 605.

Brown, R.G., Buchanan-Smith, J.G., and Sharma, V.D. (1975). *Can. J. Anim. Sci.* 55, 353.

Cappa, C. (1958). *Rev. Zooiatr.* 31, 299.

Carpenter, K.J. (1986). The History of Scurvy and Vitamin C. Cambridge University Press, Cambridge.

Carvalho da Silva, A. (1950). *Acta Physiol. Lat. Am.* 1, 26.

Chatterjee, G.C. (1978). *In* Handbook Series in Nutrition and Food, Section E: Nutritional Disorders (M. Rechcigl Jr., ed.), Vol. 2, p. 149. CRC Press, Boca Raton, Florida.

Chatterjee, I.B., Majumder, A.K., and Nandi, B.K. (1975). *Ann. N.Y. Acad. Sci.* 258, 24.

Chen, H., and Chang, C. (1994). *J. Nutr.* 124, 2033.

Cheng, T.C., Coon, C.N., and Hamre, M.L. (1988). *Poult. Sci.* 67(Suppl. 1), 67(Abstr.).

Chew, B.P. (1995). *J. Nutr.* 125, 1804S.

Cleveland, E.R., Bondari, K., and Newton, G.L. (1987). *Livestock Prod. Sci.* 17, 277.

Cole, C.L., Rasmussen, R.A., and Thorp, F. (1944). *Vet. Med.* 39, 204.

Cummins, K.A., and Brunner, C.J. (1989). *J. Dairy Sci.* 72, 129.

Cummins, K.A., and Brunner, C.J. (1991). *J. Dairy Sci.* 74, 1582.

Cunningham, J.J., Mearkle, P.L., and Brown, R.G. (1994). *J. Am. Coll. Nutr.* 13, 344.

Davis, G.K., and Cole, C.L. (1943). *J. Anim. Sci.* 2, 53.

Degkwitz, E. (1987). *Ann. N.Y. Acad. Sci.* 498, 470.

Dobrescu, O. (1987). *Feedstuffs* 54(9), 18.

Dobsinska, E., Sova, Z., Kopak, V., and Trhon, M. (1981). *Vet. Med. Praha.* 26, 203.

Duell, P.B. (1996). *J. Nutr.* 126, 1067S.

Duncan, C.W. (1944). *J. Dairy Sci.* 27, 636.

El-Boushy, A.R., and Van Albada, M. (1970). *Neth. J. Agric. Sci.* 18, 62.

El-Boushy, A.R., Simons, P.C.M., and Wiert, G. (1968). *Poult. Sci.* 47, 456(Abstr.).

Franceschi, R.T. (1992). *Nutr. Rev.* 50, 65.

Frei, B., England, L., and Ames, B.N. (1989). *Proc. Natl. Acad. Sci.* 86, 6377.

Fumihiko, H., Shibata, T., Makino, S., Machina, S., Hayashi, Y., Hattori, T., and Yoshida, A. (1993). *J. Nutr.* 123, 2075.

Gershoff, S.N. (1993). *Nutr. Rev.* 51, 313.

Ginter, E. (1970). *Acta Med. Acad. Sci. Hung.* 27, 23.

Gomez-Carrasco, J.A., Lopez-Herce, C.J., and Bernabe de Frutos, C. (1994). *J.*

Pediatr. Gastroenterol. Nutr. 19. 118.

Grondalen, J. (1976). *J. Small Anim. Prac. 17,* 721.

Gross, W.G., Jones, D., and Cherry, J. (1988). *Avian Dis. 32,* 407.

Ha, T.Y., Otsuka, M., and Arakawa, N. (1994). *J. Nutr. 124,* 732.

Hagg, M., Ylikoski, S., and Kumpulainen, J. (1995). *J. Food Compos. Anal. 8,* 12.

Halver, J.E. (1972). *Bull. Jpn. Soc. Sci. Fish 38,* 79.

Harris, E.D., and Percival, S.S. (1991). *Am. J. Clin. Nutr. 54,* 1193S.

Harris, L., Constable, B.J., Howard, A.N., and Leader, A. (1956). *Br. J. Nutr. 10,* 373.

Helgebostad, A. (1984). *In* Proc. Ascorbic Acid in Domestic Animals (I. Wegger, F.J. Tagwerker, and J. Moustgaard, eds.) p. 169. Danish Agriculture Society, Copenhagen.

Herbert, V. (1996). *J. Nutr. 126,* 1197S.

Hidiroglou, M. (1999). *J. Dairy Sci. 82,* 1831.

Hidiroglou, M., Ivan, M., and Lessard, J.R. (1977). *Can. J. Anim. Sci. 57,* 519.

Hill, C.H., and Garren, H.W. (1958). *Poult. Sci. 37,* 236.

Horio, F., Ozaki, K., Yoshida, A., Makino, S., and Hayashi, Y. (1985). *J. Nutr. 115,* 1630.

Hornig, D., Glatthaar, B., and Moser, U. (1984). *In* Proc. Ascorbic Acid in Domestic Animals (I. Wegger, F.J. Tagwerker, and J. Moustgaard, eds.) p. 3. Danish Agriculture Society, Copenhagen.

Ikeda, S., Tahasu, M., Matsuda, T., Kakinuma, A., and Horio, F. (1997). *J. Nutr. 127,* 2173.

Itze, L. (1984). *In* Proc. Ascorbic Acid in Domestic Animals (I. Wegger, F.J. Tagwerker, and J. Moustgaard, eds.) p. 120. Danish Agriculture Society, Copenhagen.

Itzeova, V. (1984). *In* Proc. Ascorbic Acid in Domestic Animals (I. Wegger, F.J. Tagwerker, and J. Moustgaard, eds.) p. 139. Danish Agriculture Society, Copenhagen.

Ivos, J., Doplihar, C., and Muhaxhiri, G. (1971). *Veteriwarski. Arhiv. Zagreb. Knjiga. 41*(7-8), 202.

Jacob, R.A. (1998). *Nutr. Rev. 56,* 334.

Jaeschke, G. (1984). *In* Proc. Ascorbic Acid in Domestic Animals (I. Wegger, F.J. Tagwerker, and J. Moustgaard, eds.) p. 153. Danish Agriculture Society, Copenhagen.

Jacob, R.A. (1995). *Nutr. Res. 15,* 755.

Jacques, P.F. (1992). *J. An. Coll. Nutr. 11,* 139.

Jagos, P., Bouda, J., and Dvorak, R. (1977). *Vet. Med. Praha. 22,* 133.

Jensen, P.T., and Basse, A. (1984). *In* Proc. Ascorbic Acid in Domestic Animals (I. Wegger, F.J. Tagwerker, and J. Moustgaard, eds.) p. 87. Danish Agriculture Society, Copenhagen.

Jones, R.H.V., and Hothersall, J.S. (1993). *Biochem. Med. Metab. Biol. 50,* 197.

Kallner, A., Hartman, D., and Hornig, D. (1977). *Int. Vitam. Nutr. Res. 47,* 383.

Kallner, A., Hornig, D., and Pelikha, R. (1985). *Am. J. Clin. Nutr. 41,* 609.

Kechik, I.T., and Sykes, A.H. (1979). *Br. J. Nutr. 42,* 97.

Kip, D.E., Grey, C.E., McElvain, M.E., Kimmel, D.B., Robinson, R.G., and Lukert, B.P. (1996). *J. Nutr. 126,* 2044.

Koemer, W.F., and Weber, F. (1972). *Int. J. Vitam. Nutr. Res. 42*, 528.

Kolb, E. (1984). *In* Proc. Ascorbic Acid in Domestic Animals (I. Wegger, F.J. Tagwerker, and J. Moustgaard, eds.) p. 162. Danish Agriculture Society, Copenhagen.

Kranowski, J.J. (1991). *J. Fla. Med. Assoc. 78*, 435.

Krasnopevtsev, V.M., Istomin, A.V., Grishina, T.I., and Chizhov, S.S. (1993). *Gigiena. I. Sanitariya 6*, 34.

Kristensen, B., Thomsen, P.D., Palludan, B., and Wegger, I. (1986). *Acta Vet. Scand. 27*, 486.

Kuemyj, A. (1955). *Vopr. Pitan. 14*, 3.

Kune, G.A., Kune, S., Field, B., Watson, L.F., Cleland, H., Merenstein, D., and Vitetta, L. (1993). *Nutr. Cancer 20*, 61.

Lehocky, J. (1981). *Veterinarstvi 31*, 388.

Leveque, J.I. (1969). *Vet. Med. Small Anim. Clin. 64*, 997.

Lewis, L.D., and Morris, M.R. (1983). Small Animal Clinical Nutrition. Mark Morris Associates, Topeka, Kansas.

Li, Y., and Lovell, R.T. (1985). *J. Nutr. 115*, 123.

Liau, L.S., Lee, B.L., New, A.L., and Ong, C.N. (1993). *J. Chromatogr. 612*, 63.

Lin, H.K., Chen, S.Y., Huang, C.Y., Kuo, M.H., and Wung, L.C. (1985). *Ann. Res. Rep. Anim. Ind. Res. Inst. TSC*, 59.

Lovell, R.T. (1973). *J. Nutr. 103*, 134.

Lovell, R.T., and Lim, C. (1978). *Trans. Am. Fish Soc. 107*, 321.

Luck, M.R., Jeyaseelan, I., and Scholes, R.A. (1995). *Biol. Reprod. 52*, 262.

Magarelli, P.C., Hunter, B., Lightner, D.V., and Colvin, L.B. (1979). *Comp. Biochem. Physiol. 63*, 103.

Mahan, D.C., Lepine, A.J., and Dabrowski, K. (1994). *J. Anim. Sci. 72*, 2354.

Mahan, D.C., Pickett, R.A., Perry, T.W., Curtin, T.M., Featherson, W.R., and Beeson, W.M. (1966). *J. Anim. Sci. 25*, 1019.

Mangels, A.R., Block, G., Frey, C.M., Patterson, B.H., Taylor, P.R., Norkus, E.P., and Levander, O.A. (1993). *J.Nutr. 123*, 1054.

Marks, J. (1975). A Guide to the Vitamins. Their Role in Health and Disease, p. 73. Medical and Technical Publ., Lancaster, England.

Martynjuk, B.F. (1952). *Med. Veter. 29*, 21.

Matusiewicz, M., Dabrowski, K., Volker, L., and Matusiewicz, K. (1995). *J. Nutr. 125*, 3055.

McDonald, P., Edwards, R.A.,and Greenhalgh, J.F.D. (1981). Animal Nutrition, 3rd Ed., p. 83. Longman, New York.

McKee, J.S., and Harrison, P.C. (1995). *Poult. Sci. 74*, 1772.

Meier, H., Clark, S.T., and Schnelle, G.B. (1957). *Am. Vet. Med. Assoc. 130*, 483.

Monsi, A., and Onitchi, D.O. (1991). *Anim. Feed Sci. Tech. 34*, 141.

Moser, U., and Bendich, A. (1991). *In* Handbook of Vitamins, 2nd Ed. (L.J. Machlin, ed.) p. 195. Dekker, New York.

Mukhopadhyay, C.K., Ghosh, M.K., and Chatterjee, I.B. (1995). *Mol. Cell Biochem. 142*, 71.

Naismith, D.H. (1958). *Proc. Nutr. Soc. 17*, xlii.

Nakaya, T., Suzuki, S., and Watanabe, K. (1986). *Jpn. Poult. Sci. 23*, 276.

Navarre, O., and Halver, J.E. (1989). *Aquaculture 79*, 207.

Nielsen, N.C., and Vinther, K. (1984). *In* Proc. Ascorbic Acid in Domestic Animals (I. Wegger, F.J. Tagwerker, and J. Moustgaard, eds.) p. 39. Danish Agriculture Society, Copenhagen.

Njoku, P.C. (1984). *Feedstuffs 56*(52), 23.

Njoku, P.C. (1986). *Anim. Feed Sci. Tech. 16*, 17.

Nobile, S., and Woodhill, J.M. (1981). Vitamin C. MTP Press (International Medical Publ.), Boston.

Nockels, C.F. (1984). *In* Proc. Ascorbic Acid in Domestic Animals (I. Wegger, F.J. Tagwerker, and J. Moustgaard, eds.) p. 175. Danish Agriculture Society, Copenhagen.

Noll, S. (1993). Personal communication to Tillman, P.B. *Feed Manage. 44*(10), 31.

NRC. Nutrient Requirements of Domestic Animals. National Academy of Sciences-National Research Council, Washington, D.C.

(1977). Nutrient Requirements of Rabbits, 2nd Ed.

(1978). Nutrient Requirements of Nonhuman Primates.

(1985). Nutrient Requirements of Dogs, 2nd Ed.

(1986). Nutrient Requirements of Cats.

(1993). Nutrient Requirements of Fish.

(1995). Nutrient Requirements of Laboratory Animals.

(1998). Nutrient Requirements of Swine, 10th Ed.

NRC. (1987). Vitamin Tolerance of Animals. National Academy of Sciences-National Research Council, Washington, D.C.

Olivares, M., Pizarro, F., Pineda, O., Name, J.J., Hertrampf, E., and Walter, T. (1997). *J. Nutr. 127*, 1407.

Orban, J.I., Roland, D.A., Cummins, K., and Lovell, R.T. (1993). *Poult. Sci. 72*, 691.

Padh, H. (1991). *Nutr. Rev. 49*, 65.

Palludan, B., and Wegger, I. (1984). *In* Proc. Ascorbic Acid in Domestic Animals (I. Wegger, F.J. Tagwerker, and J. Moustgaard, eds.) p. 131. Danish Agriculture Society, Copenhagen.

Pardo, B., Sygnowska, E., Rywik, S., Kulesza, W., and Waskiewicz, A. (1991). *Appetite 16*, 1.

Pardue, S.L. (1987). Proc. The Role of Vitamins on Animal Performance and Immune Response, p. 18. Hoffmann-La Roche, Nutley, New Jersey.

Pardue, S.L., and Thaxton, J.P. (1982). *Poult. Sci. 61*, 1522(Abstr.).

Pardue, S.L., and Williams, S.H. (1990). *In* Proc. 2nd Symp. Ascorbic Acid in Domestic Animals. Kartause Ittingen, Switzerland, Oct. 9.

Pardue, S.L., Thaxton, J.P., and Brake, J. (1985). *Poult. Sci. 64*, 1334.

Pardue, S.L., Brake, J., Seib, P.A., and Wang, X.Y. (1993). *Poult. Sci. 72*, 1330.

Park, T.F., and Harrison, P.C. (1990). Growth performance of nursery pigs provided tap and carbonated drinking water sources supplemented with monopotassium ascorbate. Personal communication. Dept. of Anim. Sci., Univ. of Illinois, Urbana, Illinois.

Pauling, L. (1971). Vitamin C and the Common Cold. Freeman, San Francisco.

Peebles, E.D., and Brake, J. (1985). *Poultry Sci. 64*, 2041.

Perek, M., and Kendler, J. (1963). *Br. Poult. Sci. 4*, 191.

Pietronigro, D.D., Hovsepian, M., Demopoulos, H.B., and Flamm, E.S. (1983).

J. Neurochem. 41, 1072.

Podgornova, G.P., and Donskova, T.J. (1972). *Voprosy Mofologii Ekologii i Parazitologii Zhivotnykh 1*, 137.

Pribyl, E. (1963). Diseases of Young Cattle, 230 p. SZN, Praha.

Quarles, C.L., and Adrian, W.J. (1989). *In* The Role of Vitamin C in Poultry Stress Managment, p. 37. RCD 7839. Hoffmann-La Roche, Inc., Nutley, New Jersey.

Quarles, C.L., Adrian, W.J., and Krautmann, B.A. (1989). Tenth Ann. Mtg. South. Poult. Sci. Soc. p. 34(Abstr.).

RDA. (1989). Recommended Dietary Allowances 9th Ed. National Academy of Sciences-National Research Council, Washington, D.C.

Rifici, V.A., and Khachadurian, A.K. (1993). *J. Am. Coll. Nutr. 12*, 631.

Rose, R.C., and Nahrwold, D.L. (1982). *Anal. Biochem. 123*, 389.

Rose, R.C., McCormick, D.B., Li, T.K., Lumeng, L., Haddad, J.G., and Spector, R. (1986). *Fed. Proc. Fed. Am. Soc. Exp. Biol. 45*, 30.

Roth, J.A., and Kaeberle, M.L. (1985). *Am. J. Vet. Res. 46*, 2434.

Rucker, R.B., Dubick, M.A., and Mouritsen, J. (1980). *Am. J. CLin. Nutr. 33*, 961.

Sandholm, M., Honkanen-Buzalski, R., and Rasi, V. (1979). *Vet. Rec. 104*, 337.

Satterfield, G.H., Mosley, M.A., Gauger, H.C., Holmes, A.D., and Tripp, F. (1940). *Poult. Sci. 19*, 337.

Sauberlich, H.E. (1990). *In* Nutrition Reviews, Present Knowledge in Nutrition: (R.E. Olson, ed.), p. 132. Nutrition Foundation, Washington, D.C.

Schaefer, D.M., Liu, Q., Faustman, C., and Yin, M. (1995). *J. Nutr. 125*, 1792S.

Scott, D.W. (1981). *Bov. Practice 2*, 22.

Shaw, P.E., and Moshonas, M.G. (1991). *J. Food Sci. 56*, 867.

Siegel, B.V. (1974). *Infect. Immunol. 10*, 409.

Sigman-Grant, M., Bush, G., and Anantheswaran, R. (1992). *Pediatrics 90*, 412.

Simon, J.A. (1992). *J. Am. Coll. Nutr. 11*, 107.

Singh, R.B., Niaz, M.A., Agarwal, P., Begom, R., and Rastogi, S.S. (1995). *J. Am. Diet. Assoc. 95*, 775.

Snehalatha Reddy, N., and Lakshmi Kumari, R. (1988). *Nutr. Rep. Int. 37*, 77.

Soldatenkov, P.F., and Suganova, N.M. (1966). *Selskochoz. Biol. 1*, 446.

Spencer, R.P., Purdy, S., Hoeldtke, R., Bow, T.M., and Markulis, M.A. (1963). *Gastroenterology 44* 768.

Stocker, R., and Frei, B. (1991). *In* Oxidative Stress (H. Sies, ed.), p. 213. Academic Press, United Kingdom.

Takahashi, K., Akiba, Y., and Horiguchi, M. (1991). *Br. Poult. Sci. 32*, 545.

Toohey, L., Harris, M.A., Allen, K.G.D., and Melby, C.L. (1996). *J. Nutr. 126*, 121.

Tono, T., and Fujita, S. (1982). *Agric. Biol. Chem. 46*, 2953.

Turnbull, J.D., Sudduth, J.H., Saberlich, H.E., and Omaye, S.T. (1981). *Int. J. Vitam. Nutr. Res. 51*, 47.

Ukhun, M.E., and Dibie, E.N. (1991). *Food-Chem Essex 41*, 277.

Vilter, R.W. (1978). *In* Handbook Series in Nutrition and Food. Section E: Nutritional Disorders (M. Rechcigl Jr., ed.), Vol. 3, p. 91. CRC Press, Boca Raton, Florida.

Wandzilak, T.R., D'Andre, S.D., Davis, P.A., and Williams, H.E. (1994). *J. Urol.*

151, 834.

Weber, P. (1994). *In* Proc. Roche Technical Seminar, Antioxidant Vitamins, p. 134. Hoffmann-La Roche Inc., Nutley, New Jersey.

Wegger, I., and Palludan, B. (1984). *In* Proc. Ascorbic Acid in Domestic Animals (I. Wegger, F.J. Tagwerker, and J. Moustgaard, eds.), p. 68. Danish Agriculture Society, Copenhagen.

Wegger, I., and Palludan, B. (1994). *J. Nutr. 124,* 241.

Weiser, H., Schlachter, M., Probst, H.P., and Kormann, A.W. (1990). *In* Proc. 2nd Symp. Ascorbic Acid in Domestic Animals. Kartause Ittingen, Switzerland, Oct. 9.

Wells, W.W., Dou, C.Z., Dybas, L.N., Jung, C.H., Kalbach, H.L., and Xu, D.P. (1995). *Proc. Natl. Acad. Sci. 92,* 11869.

Wetherilt, H., Ackurt, F., Brubacker, G., Okan, B., Aktas, S., and Turdu, S. (1992). *Int. J. Vitam. Nutr. Res. 62,* 21.

Yashin, A.V. (1985). *Veterinariya (Moscow) 1,* 57.

Yen, J.T., and Pond, W.G. (1981). *J. Anim. Sci. 53,* 1291.

Yen, J.T., and Pond, W.G. (1984). *J. Anim. Sci. 58,* 132.

Yen, J.T., and Pond, W.G. (1987). *J. Anim. Sci. 64,* 1672.

Zapata, L.F., and Gernat, A.G. (1995). *Poult. Sci. 74,* 1049.

Zee, J.A., Carmichael, L., Codere, D., Poirier, D., and Fournier, M. (1991). *J. Food Compos. Anal. 4,* 77.

Zintzen, H. (1975). A Guide to the Nutritional Management of Breeding Sows and Pigs No. 1465. Hoffmann-La Roche & Co. Ltd., Basel, Switzerland.

CARNITINE

INTRODUCTION

Under most conditions for the majority of species, carnitine would not be considered a vitamin as it is adequately synthesized in body tissues. However, the need for supplemental carnitine has been demonstrated in mammals in circumstances in which the biosynthesis is limited by nutritional deprivation of the precursor amino acids lysine and methionine. Dietary carnitine is essential for some insect species, including beetles of the family *Tenebrionidai* (mealworms), the beetle *Oryzaephilus surinamensis*, and the fly *Drosophila melanogaster*. For these species it is appropriate to refer to carnitine as a vitamin.

16

HISTORY

Carnitine was isolated from meat extracts and identified in 1905. In 1948, Fraenkel's research on dietary requirements of the mealworm *(Tenebrio molitor)* led to recognition of a new B vitamin, which in 1932 was identified as carnitine (Friedman and Fraenkel, 1972). Since it was a small water-soluble compound required in the diet of *T. molitor*, it was given the name vitamin B_T (sometimes referred to as vitamin B_7). It was not until the 1960s that carnitine was recognized as a biologically active substance (Borum, 1991).

CHEMICAL STRUCTURE AND PROPERTIES

Carnitine is a quaternary amine, β-hydroxy-γ-trimethylaminobutyrate (Fig. 16.1). It is a very hygroscopic compound, easily soluble in water, and has a molecular weight of 161.2. Carnitine is found in biological

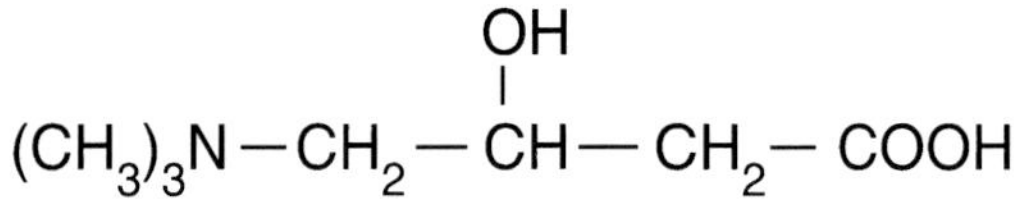

Fig. 16.1 Chemical
structure of carnitine.

$$(CH_3)_3N-CH_2-\overset{\overset{\displaystyle OH}{|}}{CH}-CH_2-COOH$$

samples both as the free carnitine and as the ester of a wide variety of acyl compounds. Of the two types of carnitine, L- and D-carnitine, only L-carnitine is biologically active.

ANALYTICAL PROCEDURES

Methods of analysis first utilized the bioassay technique using *T. molitor*. Other methods developed for carnitine determination include chemical, enzymatic, gas chromatographic, and radioisotopic procedures (Chan, 1984). The most commonly used methodology to determine the carnitine concentration in biological samples is the radioenzymatic assay (Rossle et al., 1985). Methods such as radioisotopic assays are sensitive; the radioactive acylcarnitine formed is separated from residual acetyl CoA by cation exchange filtration, and radioactivity is counted (Deufel, 1990).

Development and use of high-performance liquid chromatography (HPLC) is common (Minkler and Hoppel, 1993) for carnitine analysis, as is the use of radioisotopic exchange/HPLC methods (Schmidt-Sommerfeld et al., 1992). Recently, enzyme spectrophotometer assays (Indyk and Woollard, 1995) and a modified enzyme-spectrophotometry method (Tuan and Chou, 1995) have been used to determine carnitine in milk and infant formulas.

METABOLISM

Under normal conditions in omnivores, about 70 to 80% of dietary carnitine is absorbed (Rebouche and Chenard, 1991). Carnitine appears to be absorbed across the proximal small intestine by an active process dependent on Na$^+$ as well as by a passive diffusion, which may be important for the absorption of large doses of the factor. The uptake of carnitine from the intestinal lumen into the mucosa is rapid, and about one-half of the carnitine taken up is acetylated in that tissue. Carnitine is not carried in blood in any tightly bound forms, in contrast to many water-soluble vitamins. Tissues such as cardiac and skeletal muscle require carnitine for normal fuel metabolism but cannot synthesize carnitine and are totally dependent on the transport of carnitine from other tissues. Cantrell and Borum (1982) reported that carnitine uptake by the heart is facilitated by a cardiac carnitine-binding protein.

Carnitine is synthesized in liver and kidney and stored in skeletal muscle; free carnitine is excreted mainly in the urine (Tanphaichitr and Leelahagul, 1993). The product is trimethylamine oxide (Mitchell, 1978). Carnitine is highly conserved by the human kidney, which reabsorbs more than 90% of filtered carnitine, thus playing an important role in the regulation of carnitine concentration in blood.

Carnitine synthesis depends on two precursors, L-lysine and methionine, as well as ascorbic acid, nicotinamide, vitamin B_6, and iron (Borum, 1991). Deficiency in any cofactor will cause L-carnitine deficiency. In rats, total acid-soluble carnitine and free carnitine in plasma and tissues were reduced in a vitamin B_6 deficiency but increased when vitamin B_6 was provided in a repletion diet (Cho and LeKlem, 1990; Ha et al., 1994). It has been suggested that early features of scurvy (fatigue and weakness) may be attributed to carnitine deficiency. Vitamin C is a cofactor for two α-ketoglutarate-requiring dioxygenase reactions (epsilon-N-trimethyllysine hydroxylase and γ-butyrobetaine hydroxylase) in the pathway of carnitine biosynthesis. Carnitine concentrations are variably low in some tissues of vitamin C-deficient guinea pigs (Rebouche, 1991). The results of studies of enzyme preparations and perfused liver in vitro, and of scorbutic guinea pigs in vivo, provide compelling evidence for participation of ascorbic acid in carnitine biosynthesis (Rebouche, 1991). Results reported by Ha et al. (1991) suggest that ascorbic acid is specifically required for the hydroxylation of γ-butyrobetaine and, furthermore, that ascorbic acid can regulate carnitine synthesis in primary cultured liver cells from guinea pigs.

Choline has also been shown to affect carnitine homeostasis in humans and guinea pigs (Daily and Sachan, 1995). Choline supplementation resulted in decreased urinary excretion of carnitine in young adult women, and choline resulted in a conservation of carnitine in guinea pigs. In choline-deficient rats, a single injection of choline raised the concentration of liver carnitine within 1.5 hours (Carter and Frenkel, 1978). This suggests that choline was capable of facilitating carnitine release from some storage pool, as de novo synthesis would require more time.

In the rat, about 1/15 to 1/20 of the body pool turns over each day, consistent with the slow rate of turnover in muscle, where most of the body carnitine is stored (Bremer, 1983). For the dog, 95 to 98% of the carnitine body pool is in skeletal muscle and heart (Rebouche and Engel, 1983). Flores et al. (1996) reported that the small intestine in rats is a considerable and previously unrecognized proportion of the carnitine pool of suckling animals.

FUNCTIONS

Carnitine is an important cofactor for normal cellular metabolism. Optimal utilization of fuel substrates for adenosine triphosphate (ATP) generation by skeletal muscle during exercise is dependent on adequate carnitine stores. Carnitine is required for transport of long-chain fatty acids into the matrix compartment of mitochondria from cytoplasm for subsequent oxidation by the fatty acid oxidase complex for energy production. The oxidation of long-chain fatty acids in animal tissues is dependent on carnitine because it allows long-chain acyl-CoA esters to cross the mitochondrial membrane, which is otherwise impermeable to CoA compounds. Carnitine facilitates the β-oxidation of long-chain fatty acids in the mitochondria by transporting the substrate into the mitochondria. Carnitine acyltransferase is the enzyme responsible for this shuttle mechanism. It exists in two forms, carnitine acyltransferase I and carnitine acyltransferase II. After the long-chain fatty acid is activated to acyl-CoA, it is converted to acylcarnitine by the enzyme carnitine acyltransferase I and crosses to the matrix side of the inner mitochondrial membrane. Carnitine acyltransferase II then releases carnitine and the acyl-CoA into the mitochondrial matrix. Acyl-CoA is then catabolized via β-oxidation (Mitchell, 1978; Borum, 1991). Thus, utilization of long-chain fatty acids as a fuel source depends on adequate concentrations of carnitine.

The role of carnitine in the transport of long-chain fatty acids across the inner mitochondrial membrane is known. However, liver medium-chain fatty acid (MCFA) metabolism has been considered carnitine independent because of their passive diffusion through the inner mitochondrial membrane and intramitochondrial activation (Bremer, 1990). However, evidence suggests that MCFA metabolism may be affected by supplemental carnitine (Rebouche et al., 1990; Van Kempen and Odle, 1993, 1995).

Another role of carnitine may be to protect cells against toxic accumulation of acyl-CoA compounds of either endogenous or exogenous origin by trapping acyl groups such as carnitine esters, which may then be transported to the liver for catabolism or to the kidney for excretion in the urine. It has been reported that nicotinamide and L-carnitine protect human cells from oxygen free radical-induced damage and that this makes these compounds possible antiaging substances (Monti et al., 1992). Carnitine also has functions in other physiological processes critical to survival, such as lipolysis, thermogenesis, ketogenesis, and possibly regulation of certain aspects of nitrogen metabolism (Borum, 1985). Carnitine administration has significant benefits in patients with disorders of ammonia metabolism, including urea cycle defects, chronic valproic acid therapy, liver failure, organic acidemias, and Reye's syndrome (Rebouche, 1992). Carnitine plays a role in ammonia detoxification (Sakemi et al., 1992; Freeman et al., 1994; Melegh et al., 1994). Propionyl-L-carnitine protects the ischemic heart from reperfusion injury, perhaps by scavenging free radicals or preventing their formation by chelating iron necessary for generation of hydroxyl radicals. Its function as an antiarrhythmic agent for the heart has been reported (Pande and Murthy, 1989; Reznic et al., 1992). An additional function of carnitine is as a memory- and alertness-enhancing agent in Alzheimer's disease (Kendler, 1986; Corrigan et al., 1995).

REQUIREMENTS

Carnitine is an essential growth factor for some insects, such as the mealworm. However, most insects and higher animals, as well as mammals, can synthesize carnitine. For common species there are no established nutritional requirements for carnitine. Studies have indicated that the biosynthesis of carnitine may be limited or inadequate in certain classes of humans and animals. Because the young of several species, including humans, have been found to have low tissue carnitine when fed low-carnitine diets, it is likely that the total carnitine biosynthetic capacity may be immature in newborns, thus they are dependent on their diets for preformed carnitine.

In omnivores, carnitine synthesis normally provides only about one-eighth to one-half of total carnitine available to the organism, whereas in strict vegetarians, endogenous carnitine synthesis provides more than 90% of total available carnitine. Normal adult humans both synthesize and ingest carnitine in amounts totaling 100 mg/day. Healthy children and adults can synthesize up to 20 mg of endogenous carnitine daily (Anonymous, 1985). In mammals, γ-butyrobetaine (YBB), the immediate precursor of carnitine, can be synthesized from the essential amino acids lysine and methionine in most tissues. The four-carbon chain comes from lysine; the methyl groups come from methionine. The ultimate conversion of YBB to carnitine occurs in the liver (Olson and Rebouche, 1987).

NATURAL SOURCES

In general, foods of plant origin are low in carnitine, whereas animal-derived foods are rich in carnitine (Table 16.1) (Mitchell, 1978). Red meats and dairy products are particularly rich sources. The carnitine concentration increases in the order of fish, poultry, pork, and beef. In general, the redder the meat, the higher the concentration of carnitine. Typical concentrations of carnitine could be 600 µg/kg in beef, 45 to 90 µg/kg in chicken, and 75 µg/kg in lamb (Mitchell, 1978). On the contrary, grains such as barley, corn, and wheat have undetectable or negligible concentrations.

Carnitine is located principally in skeletal muscle, which has about 40 times the concentration of carnitine in blood. Average muscle content of total carnitine ranges from 10.75 to 19.06 nmol/mg of noncollagen protein. Most plant foods that are low in carnitine are also likely to be low in lysine and methionine, the precursors of carnitine. Therefore, a pure vegetarian diet may lack both preformed carnitine and its precursors. Strict vegetarian diets contain less than 10% as much carnitine as typical omnivorous diets of the developed nations. Nevertheless, vegetarian diets furnishing adequate lysine, methionine, and micronutrients for carnitine biosynthesis should theoretically maintain normal carnitine nutrition in the healthy individual.

Milk is essential for the nursing mammal to supply carnitine. Although carnitine is synthesized in growing young and adult animals, previous studies in humans provide evidence that exogenous carnitine is necessary to maintain normal fat metabolism during infancy. Healthy full-term infants fed formulas devoid of carnitine show reduction in the products of ketogenesis and accumulation of fatty acid precursors in plasma compared with infants provided carnitine in either cow's milk formula or breast milk (Novak et al., 1983). Studies by Davis (1989) indicated that up to 50% of tissue carnitine in suckling rats is derived from the mother's milk. Studies with neonatal rabbits (Penn and Schmidt-Sommerfeld, 1988) and rats (Flores et al., 1996) demonstrated that body tissues of carnitine are greatly diminished in newborns deprived of milk during early life. Coffey et al. (1991) showed that diminished dietary intake is associated with decreased levels of carnitine in the liver, but not heart or muscle, in neonatal piglets receiving low levels of dietary carnitine compared with piglets receiving carnitine supplementation. These observations indicate the importance of milk. The demand for carnitine during the suckling period may exceed the capacity for its synthesis.

■ Table 16.1   Typical Carnitine Concentrations in Various Foods and Feedstuffs (μg/100 g)

Plant Derived[a]	
Alfalfa concentrate	2.00
Avocado	1.25
Cauliflower	0.13
Peanut	0.76
Torula yeast	1.60–3.29
Animal Derived	
Beef, muscle	59.8–67.4
Beef heart	19.3
Beef kidney	1.8
Beef liver	2.6
Chicken, muscle	4.6–9.1
Cow's milk	0.53–3.91
Lamb, muscle	78.0

Source: Mitchell (1978).
[a]Carnitine was not detected in analyses of cabbage, orange juice, spinach, corn, or egg.

DEFICIENCY

In carnitine deficiency, fatty acid oxidation is reduced, and fatty acids are diverted into triglyceride synthesis, particularly in the liver. Mitochondrial failure develops in carnitine deficiency when there is insufficient tissue carnitine available to buffer toxic acyl-coenzyme (acyl-CoA) metabolites. Toxic amounts of acyl-CoA impair the citrate cycle, gluconeogenesis, the urea cycle, and fatty acid oxidation. Carnitine replacement treatment is safe and induces excretion of toxic acyl groups in the urine (Stumpf et al., 1985).

If carnitine deficiency involves the liver, the supply of ketones and the utilization of long-chain fatty acids during starvation are cut off; all tissues become glucose dependent. When liver carnitine is depleted, starvation tends to cause nonketotic, insulinopenic hypoglycemia. Because liver hepatocytes depend on fatty acids for their energy requirements during fasting, carnitine depletion may also cause clinical liver dysfunction, shown by hyperammonemia, encephalopathy, and hyperbilirubinemia (Feller and Rudman, 1988). Skeletal muscles are generally involved, with weakness, lipid myopathy, and myoglobinuria often aggravated or precipitated by fasting or exercise. The heart, like skeletal muscle, is dependent on fatty acids for energy during fasting, and heart failure and arrhythmias are frequent manifestations of systemic carnitine deficiency.

647

The heart derives approximately 60% of its ATP supply from β-oxidation of fatty acids. Carnitine concentrations in the heart are normally very high in many species (Rebouche and Paulson, 1986).

Effects of Deficiency
Ruminants

Research conducted with both steers and heifers fed high-roughage diets supplemented with soybean meal resulted in increased weight gains when supplemented with carnitine, while other studies have showed no effect (Hill et al., 1995). Diets high in forage or roughage content generally shift the ruminal volatile fatty acid profile in the direction of more acetate production and less propionate production, and carnitine is reported to be important in the regulation of liver and blood acetate levels.

Feeding veal male Holstein calves from 140 days with or without supplement of 1, 3, or 5 g/day of L-carnitine resulted in mean daily weight gains of 1.12, 1.14, 1.19, and 1.23 kg, while carcass yield was 64.1, 64.7, 65.5, and 66.4%, respectively. The auxinic effect of carnitine is attributed to its hyperglycemic activity and favorable effect on lipid metabolism (Bonomi et al., 1991). Intravenous L-carnitine significantly lowered plasma ammonia N levels in ewes given oral urea (Chapa et al., 1998). Addition of L-carnitine to ruminant feeds could alleviate hyperammonemia experienced by ruminants that consume a high level of nonprotein N.

The most popular topic of carnitine research in ruminants has been that dealing with ketonemia, an economically important problem commonly known as pregnancy toxemia in sheep, and ketosis, acetonemia, and ketoacidosis in cattle. Ketosis occurs when body reserves are mobilized for productive functions; the condition is exacerbated by restriction of energy or protein intake. It is hypothesized that ketosis is the result of the derepression of carnitine acyltransferase, which allows large, uncontrolled amounts of fatty acids to enter the liver mitochondria, where they are metabolized to acetoacetate and subsequently form β-hydroxybutyrate, both of which accumulate.

In lactating dairy cows, carnitine supplementation increased concentrations of carnitine in plasma and liver and improved lipid digestibility (La Count et al., 1995). However, in three dairy cattle experiments, supplemental carnitine (6 to 12 g/day) did not benefit milk yield or milk composition but was effective at increasing the concentrations of carnitine in liver, plasma, and milk of dairy cows during early lactation (La Count et al., 1995, 1996a,b).

Swine

The capacity of swine to synthesize carnitine has not been directly examined. However, plasma and tissue concentrations of carnitine are reduced in neonatal pigs reared on formulas devoid of carnitine (Baltzell et al., 1987). Supplementation with carnitine in 4-kg mini-pigs during total parenteral nutrition was shown to increase their energy gain from exogenous fat and to increase their nitrogen retention fourfold (Bohles et al., 1984). Supplemental carnitine resulted in increased growth rate at moderately high lysine intakes, but tended to depress growth rate when lysine levels were near, below, or in considerable excess of published requirements (Newton and Burtle, 1992). Additionally, it was found that pigs that were lightweight at weaning (generally 5 kg or less) were more likely to have a positive growth response to supplemental carnitine over the 4-week nursery period than heavier pigs. Hoffman et al. (1993) found no benefit from supplemental L-carnitine to young pigs. Likewise, addition of L-carnitine to the lactation diet had little effect on the performance of the first parity sow. However, decreased feed intake during the first week of lactation and a tendency toward fewer days to estrus were observed (Musser et al., 1997).

Dietary L-carnitine has been found to improve the gain:feed ratio and reduces carcass lipid accretion in early weaned pigs fed 1,000 ppm of L-carnitine (Owen et al., 1996). In newborn pigs, medium-chain fatty acid (MCFA) oxidation accounted for 40% of the MCFA infused, and carnitine, independent of the level, increased the fatty acid oxidation by as much as 20% if the energy provided as MCFA exceeded 50% of the metabolic needs of the pig (Van Kempen et al., 1993).

From results of trials with finishing pigs, there was a curvilinear response in growth rate for the first 14 days, and in back-fat thickness at slaughter weight, due to carnitine intake. Growth rate and back fat were both increased at higher carnitine intakes (greater than 0.4 mg/kg of body weight per day). There was also a differential response due to sex, with female pigs responding to a much greater degree than male castrates (Newton and Haydon, 1989).

Poultry

The increases in plasma and hepatic acylcarnitines in broilers fed 0.5% L-carnitine indicated that supplementary carnitine lessens the load of free acyl groups in the liver by eventual oxidation or excretion (Smith et al., 1994). In another study, Barker and Sell (1994) found that carnitine intake (0, 50, and 100 mg/kg) did not affect body weight, feed conversion efficiency, or proximate composition at 21 days in turkeys and at 45 days in broilers. L-Carnitine significantly increased cholesterol in egg yolk when added with or without nicotinic acid at 500 mg/kg. With 50 and 100 mg/kg in the feed of layer hens, hatchability increased by 4 and 2.9%, respectively (Leibetseder, 1995).

Horses

Working with horses in combined training, the animals were tested in exercise trials and were given 5 g/day of L-carnitine with oats. It was found that carnitine did not improve performance, but there was a lower increase of lactate in the carnitine group during exercise and a lower increase of enzyme activity of lactate dehydrogenase. It was concluded that carnitine, besides its function in mitochondria energy-linked processes, also improves membrane stability (Iben et al., 1992). In brood mares supplemented with 10 g/day of L-carnitine, it was found that the decline in milk carnitine after foaling was reversed in supplemented animals but not in unsupplemented ones. The drop in foal plasma carnitine was also reversed in foals from supplemented mares, and there were no apparent side effects of carnitine supplementation (Benamou and Harris, 1993).

Other Animal Species

DOGS

In dogs with dilated cardiomyopathy (DCM), myocardial concentrations of L-carnitine are sometimes very low. Carnitine deficiency associated with DCM was documented in Doberman pinschers (Keene et al., 1989) and a family of boxers (Keene et al., 1986). A few years later, Keene (1992) reported DCM in a wide range of dog breeds and found that myocardial free L-carnitine deficiency occurred in 50 to 90% of dogs with DCM. In these dogs, the myocardial concentrations of carnitine were very low, and substantial clinical improvement after intravenous or oral therapy with L-carnitine was observed. The possible explanation is that these dogs have a membrane transport defect that prevents adequate quantities of carnitine from moving into the heart from the plasma (Keene, 1991; Keene et al., 1991). McEntee et al. (1995) reported DCM in a female Labrador, whose diet was exclusively from vegetables and cereals because of a presumed allergy to animal proteins. The dog had a poor appetite, coughing, abdominal distention, exercise intolerance, and a peculiar body odor. After 4 days of carnitine supplementation, the dog showed spectacular improvement in appetite, increased tolerance to exercise, and reduction of the body odor. The peculiar body odor was also described in children with carnitine deficiency (Waber et al., 1982).

Grandjean et al. (1993) demonstrated the need of supplemental carnitine for working husky dogs. After exercise, carnitine-supplemented dogs showed better utilization of lipids, lower free fatty acid blood levels, more stable blood glucose levels, and less accumulation of lactate residues.

Systemic and myopathic forms of L-carnitine deficiency are well known etiologies of DCM in human medicine. Evidence suggests that congestive heart failure caused by rapid ventricular pacing in dogs is also associated with myocardial carnitine deficiency (Keene, 1994).

FISH

Accelerated growth and reduced body fat have been reported for hatchery-reared sea bass (Santulli and D'Amelio, 1986; Santulli et al., 1988) and African catfish fed carnitine (Torreele et al., 1993). Atlantic salmon fed L-carnitine exhibited altered intermediary metabolism and reduced tissue lipid, but no change in growth rate (Ji et al., 1996). These results implicated induction of pyruvate carboxylase (or a reduction in turnover) and enhanced protein synthesis in the mechanism for carnitine-induced changes in gluconeogenesis and nitrogen metabolism.

Supplementation of carnitine (500 mg/kg of diet) in catfish fingerlings produced a nonsignificant increase in growth rate; 1,000 mg/kg produced a significant increase in growth rate and feed efficiency, and the response to 2,000 mg/kg was approximately equal to that observed with 500 mg/kg. Fish fed 2,000 mg/kg, however, had significantly less lipid in their fillets than fish fed the control diet (Newton and Burtle, 1992).

LABORATORY ANIMALS

Rats have not been reported to be deficient in carnitine. However, rats fed diets deficient in lysine or methionine were shown to develop mild depressions in tissue carnitine concentrations and to suffer growth depression and fatty liver, both of which are at least partially alleviated by feeding carnitine. In guinea pigs, vitamin C deficiency was linked to impairment in carnitine synthesis, increased urinary carnitine excretion, and prolonged survival time with carnitine supplementation (Alkonyi et al., 1990).

Humans

It was formerly assumed that because humans have the ability to synthesize carnitine, this compound is not an essential nutrient. However, since 1973 it has been described as "conditionally essential" because it was discovered that certain segments of the human population—mainly preterm infants, normal infants, adults on total parenteral nutrition, and adults and children with a variety of genetic, infectious, and injury-related illnesses—have a need for carnitine.

Borum (1981) presented evidence that newborns have a critical need for carnitine since they have not attained the full biosynthetic capacity for carnitine, and their plasma and tissue concentrations are low. Newborn infants depend heavily on lipids as a concentrated source of fuel to achieve rapid growth during the first months of life (Shenai and Borum, 1984; Nakano et al., 1989). It has been estimated that the amount of carnitine in skeletal muscle of very premature infants, indexed to whole-body weight, is about 10 times less than that of adults (Schmidt-Sommerfeld and Penn, 1990). In premature infants, Helms et al. (1990) observed increased nitrogen balance and weight gain in intravenously fed infants supplemented with carnitine.

Bonner et al. (1995) concluded that very low birth weight infants requiring prolonged parenteral nutrition have carnitine deficiency with impaired ketogenesis. Parenteral administration of carnitine appears to alleviate this metabolic disturbance. In low birth weight infants, lowered plasma-free carnitine produced a higher blood ammonia (Nakamura et al., 1990).

Human carnitine deficiency can be hereditary or acquired. Hereditary carnitine deficiency can be grouped into three clinical entities: myopathic carnitine deficiency, systemic carnitine deficiency, and organic acidurias. Acquired carnitine deficiency is due to inadequate intake, increased requirement, and increased loss of carnitine (Tanphaichitr and Leelahagul, 1993).

Myopathic and systemic abnormalities are classified as autosomal recessive disorders (DiMauro, 1979). A defective transport system for carnitine uptake has been proposed as the cause of the myopathic disorder (Engel, 1980; Bremer, 1983). It is not known what biochemical defect causes the systemic disorder. In both cases, the muscle is infiltrated with fat, and there is general weakness. The organic acidemias are inborn errors of metabolism in which fatty and organic acids accumulate, causing growth retardation, muscle hypotonia, protein intolerance, hyperammonemia, and ketoacidosis. Metabolic improvement has been observed with oral L-carnitine (Roe and Bohan, 1982; Seccombe et al., 1982).

Assessment of Status

Most carnitine status assessment relates to plasma or serum concentrations compared with normal values for a particular species. Assessment of the carnitine status in humans is difficult because plasma carnitine concentrations and urinary carnitine excretion are not good indicators of tissue carnitine status (Borum, 1991). An individual with low carnitine concentrations in plasma may have normal concentrations in muscle or liver. It is also difficult to know how low a carnitine concentration must be before it is pathological.

SUPPLEMENTATION

Although carnitine has been studied in humans and under laboratory conditions for many years, its effectiveness in promoting the performance and well-being of domestic animals has only recently received attention. A role for carnitine in swine and fish diets has been established, and continued research may find that it has a place in the production of poultry, horses, and ruminants. Some studies have found production responses for supplemental carnitine in poultry, cattle, and horse diets, while other reports have found no benefits.

Supplementation of weanling pigs with carnitine appears to have commercial potential. The major response may be improved growth rate with lower-energy diets and improved feed efficiency with added-fat diets. Optimum dietary carnitine levels would appear to be between 800 and 1,200 mg/kg of feed for the first 1 or 2 weeks postweaning, with the level dropped to 50 to 500 mg/kg after that (Newton and Burtle, 1992). Supplemental levels of carnitine for fish to accelerate growth and reduce body fat have ranged from 500 to 2,000 mg/kg of feed.

Carnitine has been observed to be beneficial in the treatment of dilated cardiomyopathy in certain families of dogs (Keene et al., 1986, 1988), but ineffective in others (Costa and Labuc, 1994). A carnitine level of 50 mg/kg of body weight has been used as preventive therapy. Working dogs have been shown to have a need for supplemental carnitine (Grandjean et al., 1993).

In the dog, maintenance requirements of endogenous L-carnitine appear sufficient, while in certain physiological states (exercise, exposure to cold, reproduction) or deficiencies (myopathies, muscle damage), in which mobilization of fatty acids is desirable, L-carnitine supplementation has been suggested at a level of 50 mg/kg of body weight (Pelletier, 1992). On the basis of physiology tests (e.g., cardiac frequency, free fatty acids, and lactic acid) after exercising Alaskan husky dogs, Grandjean et al. (1993) concluded that supplemental carnitine was beneficial.

Normal adult humans both synthesize and ingest carnitine in amounts totaling 100 mg/day. Under a variety of circumstances, however, carnitine deficiency may become manifest. Individuals particularly vulnerable are newborn infants, premature infants, persons with inborn metabolic defects, individuals receiving peritoneal dialysis or hemodialysis, alcoholics with liver disease, malnourished infants, and persons receiving total parenteral nutrition (Anonymous, 1985; Rebouche, 1986). Hemodialysis patients can also be depleted of carnitine due to the loss of carnitine in the dialysate, which greatly exceeds the amount normally lost in the urine. This can be prevented if carnitine is added to the dialysate. Oral carnitine has also been found effective in correcting the hypertriglyceridemia that is frequent in uremic patients undergoing hemodialysis. The most economical and practical method of supplementing L-carnitine is ingestion of 660 to 990 mg/day or 2 to 3 g just prior to hemodialysis (Golper and Ahmad, 1992). Hypocarnitinemia and tissue carnitine depletion are common in patients with advanced cirrhosis, who not only tend to have marginal intakes of carnitine and its precursors, but also have loss of liver function, including the capacity to synthesize carnitine.

Some segments of the human population, such as vegetarians and Third World rural Asians, who consume diets high in grains and low in animal products, were found to have slightly lower serum or plasma carnitine concentrations than their omnivorous counterparts, but no clinical abnormalities (Rebouche, 1986; Lombard et al., 1989). The need for supplemental carnitine for this population group has yet to be established; however, if intake of lysine and methionine are inadequate, supplemental carnitine may be beneficial.

Acetyl-L-carnitine has been shown to be effective in slowing the progression of mental deterioration in Alzheimer's disease by improving the ability of patients to handle tasks requiring attention and concentration (Spagnoli et al., 1991). In a double-blind, randomized, controlled clinical trial, progression of Alzheimer's disease was significantly reduced in patients who received acetyl-carnitine (2 g/day) for 1 year (Bowman, 1992).

Dietary carnitine deficiency may be a cause of smooth muscle dysmotility of the gastrointestinal tract. After dietary supplementation of carnitine, gastrointestinal symptoms resolved, oesophageal manometry returned to normal, and serum carnitine increased to 37.2 mmol/L (Weaver et al., 1992).

The consequences of suboptimal carnitine status would appear to be great for the infant who, at birth, changes from a pattern of energy metabolism based on glucose as the major fuel to one based on utilization of fats. Infants have compromised endogenous carnitine synthesis; their carnitine status is dependent on that of the mother, on the placental transfer of carnitine in utero, and on the availability of exogenous sources after birth. However, milk or infant formula prepared from cow's milk contains appreciable amounts of carnitine, which is adequate to meet daily requirements. Soybeans, on the other hand, lack carnitine, hence infants fed an infant formula prepared from soy protein receive no carnitine unless it is added by the manufacturers. Many infant formulas contain low concentrations of carnitine, and supplemental carnitine is recommended to be added to these formulas (Sugiyama et al., 1984). Likewise, preterm infants have often been maintained on total parenteral nutrition containing no carnitine.

TOXICITY

Studies to determine maximum tolerance for carnitine in animals are lacking. Carnitine supplementation at dosages that far exceed the usual dietary intake of carnitine have been administered in humans (Goa and Brogden, 1987). Oral dosages such as 100 mg/kg body weight per day for infants and children with failure to thrive and 1 to 3 g of carnitine per day for adults with muscle weakness have been frequently used. Some patients have experienced diarrhea, but not if they started with smaller dosages and then increased gradually (Borum, 1991). Administration of the D-isomer may interfere with the normal functions of the L-isomer.

■ REFERENCES

Alkonyi, I., Cseko, J., and Sandor, A. (1990). *J. Clin. Chem. Clin. Biochem. 28*, 319.
Anonymous (1985). *Nutr. Rev. 43*, 23.
Baltzell, J.K., Bazer, F.W., Miguel, S.G., and Borum, P.R. (1987). *J. Nutr. 117*, 754.
Barker, D.L., and Sell, J.L. (1994). *Poult. Sci. 73*, 281.
Benamou, A.E., and Harris, R.C. (1993). *Equine Vet. J. 25*, 49.
Bohles, H., Segerer, H., and Fekl, W. (1984). *JPEN 8*, 9.

Bonner, C.M., DeBrie, K.L., Hug, G., Landrigan, E., and Taylor, B.J. (1995). *J. Pediatr. 126*, 287.

Bonomi, A., Quantarelli, A., Sabbioni, A., Mazzali, I., Cabassi, E., Corradi, A., and Cantoni, A.M. (1991). *Riv. Soc. Ital. Sci. Alim. 20*, 401.

Borum, P.R. (1981). *Nutr. Rev. 39*, 385.

Borum, P.R. (1985). *Can. J. Physiol. Pharmacol. 63*, 571.

Borum, P.R. (1991). *In* Handbook of Vitamins (L.J. Machlin, ed.), p. 557. Marcel Dekker, New York.

Bowman, B.A.B. (1992). *Nutr. Rev. 50*, 142.

Bremer, J. (1983). *Physiol. Rev. 63*, 1420.

Bremer, J. (1990). *J. Clin. Chem. Clin. Biochem. 28*, 297.

Cantrell, C.R., and Borum, P.R. (1982). *J. Biol. Chem. 257*, 10599.

Carter, A.L., and Frenkel, R. (1978). *J. Nutr. 108*, 1748.

Chan, M.M. (1984). *In* Handbook of Vitamins (L.J. Machlin, ed.), p. 549. Marcel Dekker, New York.

Chapa, A.M., Fernandez, J.M, White, T.W., Bunting, L.D., Gentry, L.R., Ward, T.L., and Blum, S.A. (1998). *J. Anim. Sci. 76*, 2930.

Cho, Y.O., and LeKlem, J.F. (1990). *J. Nutr. 120*, 258.

Coffey, M.T., Shireman, R.B., Herman, D.L., and Jones, E.E. (1991). *J. Nutr. 121*, 1047.

Corrigan, F.M., Rhijn, A.G., Best, P.V., Besson, J.A., Cooper, M.B., and Van Rhijn, A.G. (1995) *J. Nutr. Med. 5*, 35.

Costa, N.D., and Labuc, R.H. (1994). *J. Nutr. 124*, 2687S.

Daily, J.W., and Sachan, D.S. (1995). *J. Nutr. 125*, 1938.

Davis, A. (1989). *J. Nutr. 119*, 262.

Deufel, T. (1990). *J. Clin. Chem. Clin. Biochem. 28*, 307.

DiMauro, G. (1979). *In* Handbook of Clinical Neurology (P.J. Vinken and G.W. Bruyn, eds.), p. 271. Academic, New York.

Engel, A.G. (1980). *In* Carnitine Biosynthesis, Metabolism and Functions (R.A. Frenkel and J.D. McGarry, eds.), p. 271. Academic Press, New York.

Feller, A.G., and Rudman, D. (1988). *J. Nutr. 118*, 541.

Flores, C.A., Hu, C., Edmond, J., and Koldovsky, O. (1996). *J. Nutr. 126*, 1673.

Freeman, J.M., Vining, E.P., Cost, S., and Singhi, P. (1994). *Pediatrics 93*, 893.

Friedman, S., and Fraenkel, G.S. (1972). *In* The Vitamins (W.H. Sebrell Jr. and R.S. Harris, eds.), Vol. 5, 2nd Ed., p. 329. Academic Press, New York.

Goa, K.L., and Brogden, R.N. (1987). *Drugs, 34*, 1.

Golper, T.A., and Ahmad, S. (1992). *Semin. Dialysis, 5*, 94.

Grandjean, D., Valette, J.P., Jougln, M., Gabillard, C., Barque, H., Bene, M., and Guillaud, J.P. (1993). *Recueil de Medecine Veterinaire, 169*, 543.

Ha, T.Y., Otsuka, M., and Arakawa, N. (1991). *J. Nutr. Sci. Vitaminol. 37*, 371.

Ha, T.Y., Otsuka, M., and Arakawa, N. (1994). *J. Nutr. 124*, 732.

Helms, R.A., Mauer, E.C., Hay, W.W., Christensen, M.L., and Storm, M.C. (1990). *JPEN 14*, 448.

Hill, G.M., Newton, G.L., and Mathis, M.J. (1995). The University of Georgia, College of Agriculture, Department of Animal and Dairy Science 1995 Annual Report, p. 52.

Hoffman, L.A., Ivers, D.J., Ellersieck, M.R., and Veum, T.L. (1993). *J. Anim. Sci. 71*, 132.

Iben, C., Bergmeister, G., Sadila, E., and Leibetseder, J. (1992). *In* European Conference on the Nutrition of the Horse. Physiology and Pathology of the Digestive Tract, p. 150. Hanover, Germany.

Indyk, H.E., and Woollard, D.C. (1995). *J. Assoc. Off. Anal. Chem. Int. 78*, 69.

Ji, H., Bradley, T.M., and Tremblay, G.C. (1996). *J. Nutr. 126*, 1937.

Keene, B.W. (1991). *Vet. Clin. North Am. Small Anim. Pract. 21(5)*, 1005.

Keene, B.W. (1992). *In* Current Veterinary Therapy XI: Small Animal Practice (R.W. Kirk and J.D. Bonagura, eds.). W.B. Saunders, Philadelphia.

Keene, B.W. (1994). Abstract of 4th Annual ESVIM, p. 20. Congress, Brussels, Belgium.

Keene, B.W., Atkins, C.E., Kittleson, M.D., Rush, J.E., and Shug, A.L. (1988). *ACVIM* (Abstr.), p. 26. American College of Veterinary Internal Medicine, Washington, D.C.

Keene, B.W., Kittleson, M.D., Rush, J.E., Plan, P.D., Atkins, C.E., DeLellis, L.D., Meurs, K.M., and Shug, A.L. (1989). *J. Vet. Intern. Med. 3*, 126.

Keene, B.W., Panciera, D.P., Atkins, C.E., Regitz, V., Schmidt, M.J., and Shug, A.L. (1991). *J. Am. Vet. Med. Assoc. 198(4)*, 647.

Keene, B.W., Panciera, D.L., Regitz, V., Noonan, J.J., Subramanian, R., and Shug, A.L. (1986). *ACVIM* (Abstr.), p. 22. American College of Veterinary Internal Medicine, Washington, D.C.

Kendler, E. (1986). *Prev. Med. 15*, 373.

La Count, D.W., Drackley, J.K., and Weigel, D.J. (1995). *J. Dairy Sci. 78*, 1824.

La Count, D.W., Emmert, L.S., and Drackley, J.K. (1996a). *J. Dairy Sci. 79*, 591.

La Count, D.W., Ruppert, L.D., and Drackley, J.K. (1996b). *J. Dairy Sci. 79*, 260.

Leibetseder, J. (1995). *Arch. Anim. Nutr. 48*, 97.

Lombard, K.A., Olson, A.L., Nelson, S.E., and Rebouche, C.J. (1989). *Am. J. Clin. Nutr. 50*, 301.

McEntee, K., Clercx, C., Snaps, F., and Henroteaux, M. (1995). *Canine Pract. 20(2)*, 12.

Melegh, B., Pap, M., Morava, E., Molnar, D., Dani, M., and Kurucz, J. (1994). *J. Pediatr. 125*, 317.

Minkler, P.E., and Hoppel, C.L. (1993). *J. Chromatogr. 613*, 203.

Mitchell, M. (1978). *Am. J. Clin. Nutr. 31*, 293.

Monti, D., Troiano, L., Tropea, F., Grassilli, E., Cossarizza, A., Barozzi, D., Pelloni, M., Tamassia, M.G., Bellomo, G., and Franceschi, C. (1992). *Am. J. Clin. Nutr. 55* (6, Suppl.), 1208.

Musser, R.E., Goodbund, R.D., Tokack, M.D., Neissen, J.L., Owens, K.Q., and Blum, S.A. (1997). *J. Anim. Sci. 75*(Suppl. 1), 194.

Nakamura, T., Nakamura, S., Kondo, J., Ikeda, T., Ogata, T., Endo, F., and Matsuda, I. (1990). *J. Pediatr. Gastroenterol. Nutr. 10*, 66.

Nakano, C., Takashima, S., and Takeshita, K. (1989). *Early Hum. Dev. 19*, 21.

Newton, G.L., and Burtle, G.J. (1992). *In* Current Concepts in Carnitine Research (A.L. Carter, ed.), p. 59. CRC Press, Boca Raton, Florida.

Newton, G.L., and Haydon, K.D. (1989). *J. Anim. Sci. 67*(Suppl. 1), 267.

Novak, M., Monkus, E., Buch, M., Lesmes, H., and Silverio, J. (1983). *Acta Chir. Scand. 517*(Suppl), 149.

Olson, A.L., and Rebouche, C.J. (1987). *J. Nutr. 117*, 1024.

Owen, K.Q., Nelssen, J.L., Goodband, R.D., Weeden, T.L., and Blum, S.A. (1996) *J. Anim. Sci. 74,* 1612.

Pande, S.V., and Murthy, M.S. (1989). *Biochem. Cell Biol. 67,* 671.

Pelletier, B. (1992). *Action Veterinaire 1210,* 19.

Penn, D., and Schmidt-Sommerfeld, E. (1988). *J. Nutr. 118,* 1535.

Rebouche, C.J. (1986). *Ann. Rev. Nutr. 61,* 41.

Rebouche, C.J. (1991). *Am. J. Clin. Nutr. 54*(6 Suppl.), 1147S.

Rebouche, C.J. (1992). *FASEB J. 6,* 3379.

Rebouche, C.J., and Chenard, C.A. (1991). *J. Nutr. 121,* 539.

Rebouche, C.J., and Engel, A.G. (1983). *Arch. Biochem. Biophys. 220,* 60.

Rebouche, C.J., and Paulson, D.J. (1986). *Ann. Rev. Nutr. 6,* 41.

Rebouche, C.J., Panagides, D.D., and Nelson, S.E. (1990). *Am. J. Clin. Nutr. 52,* 820.

Reznic, A.Z., Kagan, V.E., Ramsey, R., Tsuchiya, M., Khwaja, S., Serbinova, E.A., and Packer, L. (1992). *Arch. Biochem. Biophys. 296,* 394.

Roe, C.R., and Bohan, T.P. (1982). *Lancet 1,* 1411.

Rossle, C., Kohse, K.P., Franz, H.E., and Furst, P. (1985). *Clinica Chimica Acta, 149,* 263.

Sakemi, K., Hayasaka, K., Tahara, M., Sanada, Y., and Takada, G. (1992). *Tohoku J. Exp. Med. 167,* 89.

Santulli, A., and D'Amelio, V. (1986). *Aquaculture 59,* 177.

Santulli, A., Modica, A., Curatolo, A., and D'Amelio, V. (1988). *Aquaculture 68,* 345.

Schmidt-Sommerfeld, E., and Penn, D. (1990). *Biol. Neonate 58*(Suppl. 1), 81.

Schmidt-Sommerfeld, E., Penn, D., Rinaldo, P., Kossack, B.D., Li, B.U.K., Huang, Z.H., and Gage, D.A. (1992). *Pediatr. Res. 31,* 545.

Seccombe, D.W., Snyder, F., and Parsons, H.G. (1982). *Lancet 2,* 1401.

Shenai, J.P., and Borum, P.R. (1984). *Pediatr. Res. 18,* 679.

Smith, M.O., Cha, Y.S., and Sachan, D.S. (1994). *Comp. Biochem. Physiol. 109,* 177.

Spagnoli, A., Lucca, U., Menasce, G., and Bandera. L. (1991). *Neurology 41,* 1726.

Stumpf, D.A., Parker, W.D., and Angelini, C. (1985). *Neurology 35,* 1041.

Sugiyama, N., Suzuki, K., and Wada, Y. (1984). *Jpn. Pediatr. Soc. 88,* 1968.

Tanphaichitr, V., and Leelahagul, P. (1993). *Nutrition 9,* 246.

Torreele, E., Van Der Sluisgen, A., and Verreth, J. (1993). *Br. J. Nutr. 69,* 289.

Tuan, S., and Chou, C.C. (1995). *J. Chi. Nutr. Soc. 20,* 73.

Van Kempen, T., and Odle, J. (1993). *J. Nutr. 123,* 1531.

Van Kempen, T., and Odle, J. (1995). *J. Nutr. 125,* 238.

Waber, I.J., Valle, D., Neill, C., Dimauro, S., and Shug, A. (1982). *J. Pediatr. 191*(5), 700.

Weaver, L.T., Rosenthal, S.R., Gladstone, W., and Winter, H.S. (1992). *Acta Pediatr. 81,* 79.

VITAMIN-LIKE SUBSTANCES

17

INTRODUCTION

In addition to the 15 vitamins discussed in previous chapters, other substances have been classed with the vitamins although their true vitamin character has not been established. For various reasons, the term vitamin has been applied to many substances that do not meet criteria for vitamin status. Vitamins are regarded as essential organic micronutrients that must be supplied in the diet. What is a vitamin for some species may only be an essential metabolite for others, as dietary sources are not needed because of tissue synthesis (e.g., vitamin C). *myo*-Inositol fits this category, but apparently for only a few species, including fish, gerbils, and perhaps other species.

Many compounds described as vitamins in the scientific literature of the 1930s and 1940s have since proven to be identical to other essential nutrients or to be mixtures of various compounds. Many of the substances referred to as vitamins, growth factors, or accessory factors in early research literature are no longer considered to be vitamins (Cody, 1991). Some compounds, such as *myo*-inositol, lipoic acid, coenzyme Q, and polyphenols, exhibit biological activity without being dietary essentials (or vitamins) for most species. The term vitamin denotes dietary need. Pyrroloquinoline quinone is a potential new vitamin, with additional evidence needed for its establishment as a vitamin. Another group of substances is called vitamins by potential promoters for profit; these substances, including pangamate, laetrile, gerovital, and cabagin, are not dietary essentials and are more properly called pseudovitamins (Cody, 1991). The present chapter will emphasize *myo*-inositol since this substance is a vitamin to some species, with only brief mention allotted to other vitamin-like substances.

MYO-INOSITOL (INOSITOL)

Introduction

myo-Inositol, also referred to as inositol, is a water-soluble growth factor for which no coenzyme function is known. It was first isolated from muscle in 1850 and was identified as a growth factor for yeast and molds, though not for bacteria. *myo*-Inositol deficiency in mice, characterized by inadequate growth, alopecia, and death, was reported. However, these results were challenged as the diets were ill defined and were apparently deficient in some of the B-complex vitamins (Kukis and Mookerjea, 1978). Most evidence suggests that *myo*-inositol is not a true vitamin for most species. Nevertheless, signs of *myo*-inositol deficiency have been demonstrated in fish and gerbils (Kroes, 1978). Difficulty in demonstrating deficiency is related to endogenous synthesis, highly variable turnover rates, and interactions of *myo*-inositol with certain vitamins or other nutrients.

Chemical Structure and Properties

Inositol exists in nine forms. It is a cyclohexane compound, with only *myo*-inositol (Fig. 17.1) demonstrating any biological activity. *myo*-Inositol is an alcohol, similar to a hexose sugar. It is a white, crystalline, water-soluble compound with a sweet taste, and is stable in acids, alkalines, and heat up to about 250°C. Because of hydroxyl groups, it forms various ester, ethers, and acetals. The hexaphosphoric acid ester (combined with six phosphate molecules) of *myo*-inositol is phytic acid, a compound that complexes with phosphorus and other minerals, making them less available for absorption (Fig. 17.1). Methods of analysis include the traditional microbiological method, which is being replaced by more rapid methods of gas-liquid, paper, and thin-layer chromatography.

Metabolism and Functions

Ingested *myo*-inositol is absorbed by rats and humans at a rate of over 99%, with *myo*-inositol from phytate absorbed at less than 50% in the presence of high dietary calcium (Cody, 1991). *myo*-Inositol is absorbed by active transport from dietary sources, or it may be synthesized de novo from glucose. Based on animal studies, *myo*-inositol may also be converted to glucose. *myo*-Inositol appears to have three metabolic fates: oxidation to CO_2, use in gluconeogenesis, and synthesis of phospholipids.

The function of *myo*-inositol is not completely understood, al-

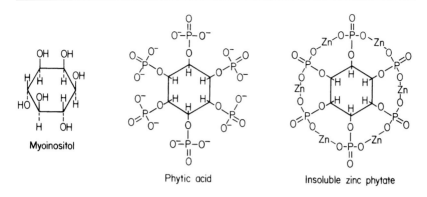

Fig. 17.1 Chemical structures of *myo*-inositol, phytic acid, and phytic acid combined with zinc.

though its biochemical functions probably relate to its role as a phospholipid component of membranes and lipoproteins. Assuming that *myo*-inositol is bound as liposirol, it makes up over 25% of total lipid and almost 50% of phospholipid in microsomes of the liver cell. *myo*-inositol is a structural component of phosphoinositides, with many of the possible functions associated with its role as a membrane component. In addition to the general role of maintaining selective permeability of plasma membranes, phosphatidylinositol and its highly charged phosphorylated forms are hypothesized to regulate cell-surface phenomena, such as binding of hormones and transfer of nervous impulses (Michell, 1975). Inositol 1,4,5-triphosphate has been shown to release intracellular Ca^{2+} from the endoplasmic reticulum, providing a link between receptor activation and cellular Ca^{2+} mobilization (Putney et al., 1986). Examples of cellular processes controlled by the phosphoinositides include amylase secretion, insulin release, smooth muscle contraction, liver glycogenolysis, platelet aggregation, histamine secretion, and DNA synthesis in fibroblasts and lymphoblasts. Under certain conditions, *myo*-inositol is lipotropic, with the lipotropic activity usually synergistic with that of choline. *myo*-Inositol reduces liver lipids for diets low in protein and fat, while choline is lipotropic also for diets containing lipids.

Sources, Requirements, and Deficiency

All plants and animals contain measurable amounts of *myo*-inositol (Clements and Darnell, 1980; Cody, 1991). The most concentrated dietary sources of *myo*-inositol are foods that consist of seeds, such as beans, grains, and nuts; cantaloupe and citrus fruits are also good plant sources. Most *myo*-inositol from plant sources occurs bound to phosphate as phytate. The best animal sources are the organ meats, which contain *myo*-inositol in free form or as a component of phospholipids (primarily phosphatidyl inositol). High concentrations are found in heart, kidney, liver, spleen, and thyroid.

There are no known dietary requirements for *myo*-inositol in humans or most species of animals studied. This is most likely due to the availability of *myo*-inositol from dietary sources, from endogenous synthesis, and from bacterial synthesis. Early work suggested that *myo*-inositol was an essential nutrient for several animal species. Effects of *myo*-inositol deficiency included alopecia in rats and mice; fatty liver and "spectacle eye" in rats; and retarded growth in guinea pigs, hamsters, and chickens. Subsequent work using more complete and defined diets with these species failed to show any *myo*-inositol requirement. Early reports of deficiency were in fact deficiencies of biotin, choline, vitamin E, or other nutrients.

For ruminants, synthesis of *myo*-inositol by microorganisms in the digestive tract, in addition to dietary sources, is presumably sufficient to meet the animals' needs. Since *myo*-inositol deficiency has been associated with failure of lipid transport in a number of species, it was suggested that *myo*-inositol supplementation might be beneficial in alleviating fatty liver syndrome (hepatic lipidoses) in dairy cattle. However, *myo*-inositol supplementation (17 g daily) to dairy cows was ineffective in altering liver *myo*-inositol concentrations or in improving liver lipoprotein output (Gerloff et al., 1986).

From a review of the *myo*-inositol literature, Kroes (1978) reported that there is little or inconclusive evidence that *myo*-inositol is required for cats, poultry, ruminants, dogs, guinea pigs, hamsters, mice, pigs, or rats. For rats and other species, however, reports show relative requirements for *myo*-inositol when diets are deficient in single other nutrients, such as choline, or in multiple vitamin and mineral deficiencies (Yagi et al., 1965). The deficiency signs were lipid accumulation for simultaneous choline deficiency and depressed growth if vitamin and mineral imbalance existed.

Under typical feeding conditions, most evidence indicates that pigs and poultry have no requirement for dietary *myo*-inositol. Lindley and Cunha (1946) demonstrated that addition of 100 mg of *myo*-inositol per 100 g of a diet deficient in biotin and supplemented with sulfathalidine could partially relieve signs of biotin deficiency. Presumably, the added *myo*-inositol stimulated intestinal synthesis of biotin. In some studies, *myo*-inositol has promoted growth in chicks, decreased liver fat, and increased egg production. These results have been refuted by other investigators (Kroes, 1978).

Animal species that have shown a dietary need for *myo*-inositol are fish and gerbils. In fish, deficiency of *myo*-inositol results in anorexia, dark skin coloration, fin degeneration, edema, anemia, reduced growth, and inefficient feed conversion, as well as a decreased rate of gastric emptying and activity of cholinesterase and certain transaminases (Halver, 1982). Decreased cholinesterase and certain aminotransferase activities were observed in trout, red sea bream, Japanese eel, Japanese parrot fish, and yellowtail with *myo*-inositol deficiency (NRC, 1993). Rainbow trout fed a diet deficient in *myo*-inositol had large accumulations of neutral lipids in the liver and increased levels of cholesterol and triglycerides, but decreased amounts of total phospholipid, phosphotidylcholine, phosphotidylethanolamine, and phosphotidylinositol (Holub et al., 1982).

myo-Inositol is synthesized in common carp intestine (Aoe and Masuda, 1967), but not in amounts sufficient to sustain normal growth of young fish without dietary source of this vitamin, because younger carp require a higher level of *myo*-inositol than older fish. Burtle and Lovell (1989) demonstrated de novo synthesis of *myo*-inositol in the liver of channel catfish, as well as intestinal synthesis. A tentative recommended allowance for young salmon and trout is 350 to 500 mg/kg of feed (McLaren et al., 1947).

Female gerbils with *myo*-inositol deficiency were characterized with intestinal lipodystrophy, with a resulting hypocholesterolemia, debilitation, and eventual death (Hegsted et al., 1973). Male gerbils were apparently protected by testicular synthesis of *myo*-inositol. Requirement of *myo*-inositol for female gerbils varied from 20 mg/kg of diet when the diet contained predominantly unsaturated fats (20% safflower oil) to 120 mg/kg of diet with saturated fats (20% coconut oil) (Kroes et al., 1973).

A number of factors affect *myo*-inositol status, and it is apparent that under certain conditions, a need for *myo*-inositol can be shown for various species. The reasons for the need under those conditions is not exactly known; however, administration of antibiotics, dietary stress, and physiological stress may influence the need for *myo*-inositol (Cunha, 1971; Cody, 1991). Antibiotics kill *myo*-inositol-producing intestinal flora, thus reducing the exogenous supply of *myo*-inositol to the body. Increasing levels of dietary saturated fatty acids may stress *myo*-inositol-requiring lipid transport systems. For humans, impaired *myo*-

inositol metabolism occurs in diabetics, uremic individuals, and premature infants (Cody, 1991).

Detrimental Effects of *myo*-Inositol as Phytates

myo-Inositol is of greatest significance to livestock and human nutrition because of its hexaphosphate ester phytic acid (Fig. 17.1). Phytic acid, which is formed from six phosphate molecules combined with *myo*-inositol, hinders intestinal absorption of phosphorus, calcium, and other minerals, including zinc, copper, cobalt, iron, manganese, and magnesium. In grains and plant protein supplements, about two-thirds of the phosphorus is in the less available phytate form. Utilization of phytate phosphorus is influenced by phytase present in plant materials or synthesized by rumen microflora, and by intake of vitamin D, calcium, and zinc, as well as by such factors as alimentary tract pH and dietary ratio of calcium to phosphorus. Calcium exaggerates the inhibition of zinc absorption by phytate, while vitamin D needs are higher to counteract high phytate intakes.

Phytin is especially high in bran of cereal grains and oilseed meals. About 20 to 50% of phytin phosphorus is available to the pig. A good guide is to assume that no more than about 50% of the phosphorus in plant feeds is available to the pig (Cunha, 1977). There is disagreement concerning the ability of poultry to utilize phytin phosphorus (NRC, 1994). Most data, however, indicate that the utilization of phytin phosphorus by young or adult poultry is negligible if dietary calcium concentrations are sufficient to meet the birds' requirements. Some reports suggest, however, that the older bird has ability to use most of the phytin phosphorus. Many cereal grains contain the enzyme phytase, which is capable of splitting phosphorus from *myo*-inositol and leaving the phosphorus, calcium, and other minerals attached to it available for absorption. Rye in particular, and also wheat, contain enough phytase to lead to considerable destruction of phytic acid. Thus, although 50% or more of the phosphorus in the original whole grain may be in the form of phytic acid, the amount in the final product may be very much less. At the other extreme, oats contain little phytase. Phytin phosphorus may be almost totally unavailable to the pig unless the phytase of grains or other sources is present in the diet. Ruminants utilize phytin phosphorus quite satisfactorily because of consumption of dietary phytases and phytase production by rumen microorganisms (Morse et al., 1992).

Low availability of phytate phosphorus poses two problems: (1) the need to add inorganic phosphorus supplements to diets, and (2) the excretion of large amounts of phosphorus in manure. Land application of manure has been the primary method of disposal of livestock and poultry waste due to its fertilizing value. There is a potential environmental impact from excessive phosphorus buildup in soil, with surface runoff and erosion of soil phosphorus into rivers, lakes, and streams. Excess phosphorus causes algae and other aquatic plants to have unchecked growth, which reduces and/or changes the oxygen and carbon dioxide levels in water and causes other aquatic life to suffer. Because of this, many state and local governments have enacted or are enacting legislation to reduce phosphorus pollution. Providing phytases to monogastric diets makes plant sources of phosphorus more available, with less inorganic phosphorus required and less of the mineral in feces to be detrimental to the environment.

Great strides have been made to develop microbial phytases to break down phytate in natural feed sources. The addition of microbial phytase produced from a genetically modified *Aspergillus niger* strain to high phytate corn-soybean meal diets fed to poultry (Denbow et al., 1995; Yi et al., 1996) and swine (Simons et al., 1990; Cromwell et al., 1993; Lei et al., 1993) have been beneficial. Some studies have shown the bioavailability of phytate phosphorus to be improved by 20 to 30%. Lei et al. (1993) reported that supplemental microbial phytase improved phytate phosphorus utilization by pigs and reduced fecal phosphorus excretion. Cereal phytase from wheat bran fed to pigs from weaning through finishing was shown to be almost as effective as microbial phytase in improving phytate phosphorus utilization for body weight gain, but not for bone mineralization (Han et al., 1997).

Many human nutritionists feel that the two minerals most likely to be deficient in typical diets are calcium and iron, both of which are affected by plant phytates. In human nutrition, the amount of calcium absorbed is dependent on bread type. Calcium is much less freely absorbed from diets consisting largely of brown bread than from those consisting largely of white, because whole wheat flour contains much higher levels of phytate. Inhibitory effects of soybean-derived food products and cereal grains on iron absorption as a result of phytates have caused concern among nutritionists and food scientists (Morris, 1983). For pigs, phytase was shown to improve iron bioavailability from soybean meal for hemoglobin synthesis (Stahl et al., 1999).

The high use of soy protein or soybean meal in human and monogastric diets has led to zinc deficiency. During extraction of soy protein, phytic acid forms a complex with zinc to form zinc phytate (Fig. 17.1), which is insoluble in the intestinal tract. The zinc requirement of growing pigs receiving semipurified diets containing isolated soybean protein or natural corn-soybean meal diets containing the recommended calcium level is about 50 ppm. However, in the absence of plant phytates, pigs receiving a casein-glucose diet require only 15 ppm zinc (NRC, 1988). Higher levels of calcium are known to further exaggerate the inhibition of zinc absorption by phytate, resulting in the formation of zinc-calcium-phytate complexes (Forbes et al., 1983).

PYRROLOQUINOLINE QUINONE (PQQ)

In 1979 studies of specialized bacteria, the methylotrophs, resulted in the discovery of a new enzyme cofactor, pyrroloquinoline quinone (PQQ) (Salisbury et al., 1979). Structural analysis showed that PQQ had a molecular weight of 424 and an empirical formula of $C_{17}H_{12}N_2O_9 \cdot 2H_2O$.

Pyrroloquinoline quinone has been identified in several other important enzymes (now collectively called quinoproteins) in yeasts, plants, and animals. However, three laboratories were unable to confirm PQQ as a cofactor in three mammalian enzymes previously shown to contain it (Harris, 1992). Nevertheless, PQQ is reported as part of the enzyme lysyl oxidase (Williamson et al., 1986).

Pyrroloquinoline quinone functions as the redox center in the quinoprotein enzymes (Bishop et al., 1998) The redox behavior of PQQ involves its ability to facilitate both one- and two-electron transfers. There is substrate oxidation by a two-electron transfer to PQQ, followed by single-electron transfer to acceptors such as copper-containing proteins and cytochromes. The two forms of the cofactor—the semiquinone PQQH and the catechole $PQQH_2$ (Fig. 17.2)—have been found in the bacterial quinoproteins.

Pyrroloquinoline quinone and copper are cofactors for lysyl oxidase, an enzyme required for cross-linking of collagen and elastin (Killgore et al., 1989). Mice deficient in PQQ showed friable skin, mild alopecia, and hunched posture. About one-fifth of the PQQ-deprived mice died within 8 weeks of feeding, with aortic aneurysms or abdominal hemorrhages. Pregnant mice fed chemically defined diets apparently devoid of PQQ exhibited reproductive failure.

Little information is available on dietary sources of PQQ. Some reports indicate PQQ to be present in egg yolk, adrenal tissue, and many citrus fruits in the range of 500 to 20,000 ppb. It is ubiquitous in dietary components, including water, and may be produced in mammalian cells at less than optimal levels, making it difficult to determine if it is an es-

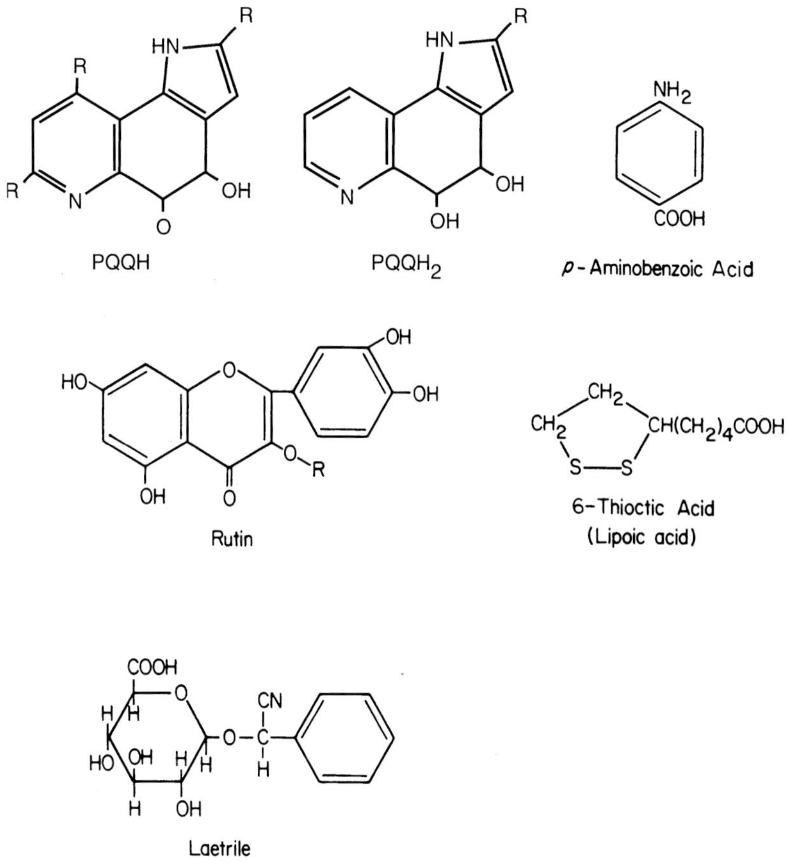

Fig. 17.2 Chemical structures off the semiquinone PQQH, the catechole PQQH$_2$, p-aminobenzoic acid, rutin, lipoic acid, and laetrile.

sential nutrient. Further studies with PQQ may result in its establishment as a vitamin.

p-AMINOBENZOIC ACID (PABA)

p-Aminobenzoic acid (PABA) (Fig. 17.2) was originally identified as a growth factor for many species of bacteria and as a required nutrient for lactation in rats and growth for the chick. The only role of PABA in higher animals would appear to be as part of the folacin molecule (see Chapter 12). When sufficient dietary folacin is available, there is little evidence that

PABA plays a direct role in the nutrition of higher animals or humans, and therefore it cannot be classified as a vitamin. If folacin is lacking, PABA may have its main effect by providing a building block for intestinal synthesis of the vitamin. One of the better recognized properties of PABA is its ability to counteract the bacteriostatic effects of sulfonamides. The chemical structure of PABA is very similar to that of some sulfonamides, which explains why it can counteract inhibition of microbial growth by these drugs. Therefore, ingestion of PABA can worsen infection. Of interest, PABA is the protective component in sunscreen.

FLAVONOIDS (POLYPHENOLS)

In 1936, Rusznyak and Szent-Györgyi reported the presence of a substance in citrus fruits, different from vitamin C, that is essential to prevent fragility of capillaries. The substance was designated as vitamin P. Several reports have shown that quercetin, catechol, rutin (Fig. 17.2), hesperidin, chalcone, and other nonspecific polyphenols, or flavonoids, can provide some protection against capillary fragility under certain conditions. This effect, which would appear to spare vitamin C, may be due to the ability of flavonoids to chelate divalent metal cations (e.g., Cu^{++}, Fe^{++}), thus performing antioxidant functions. Some of these compounds may have value as a supplement to limited vitamin C intake, particularly under conditions of stress (Maynard et al., 1979).

Flavonoids are colored phenolic substances found in all higher plants; more than 3,000 different flavonoids have been isolated (Cody, 1991). They are the major sources of red, blue, and yellow pigments (except for carotenoids) in the plant kingdom. Flavonoids are ubiquitous throughout the plant kingdom, with higher flavonoid concentrations found in colored exterior tissues, such as peels and skins, than in interior tissues (Herrmann, 1976). They are widely distributed in fruits and vegetables, and in beverages such as tea and wine (Cao et al., 1998). The greatest source of flavonoids in the diet is fruit juice, with orange juice supplying approximately 22 mg of hesperidin per capita per day and grapefruit juice supplying approximately 5.6 mg of naringin per capita per day (Cody, 1991). Hertog et al. (1993b) reported in a food-consumption survey in the Netherlands that the most important flavonoid was quercetin (mean intake 16 mg/day). Important sources of flavonoids were tea (48% of total intake), onions (29%), and apples (7%). On a milligram-per-day basis, the intake of the antioxidant flavonoids exceeded that of the antioxidants β-carotene and vitamin E. Thus flavonoids represent an important source of antioxidants in the human diet.

In addition to reducing capillary fragility, numerous other biological effects of flavonoids have been claimed (Vlietinck et al., 1988; Bravo, 1998; Yang et al., 1998). They are believed to lower blood cholesterol and to prevent cancer, hypertension, viral infection, and allergic reactions. Other potentially important reports of the flavonoid activities include the in vitro inhibition of aldose reductase, which converts glucose and galactose to their polyols (Varma and Kinoshita, 1976). These metabolic products have been implicated in the neuropathy of diabetes and in cataract formation.

Although a number of polyphenols exhibit biological activities, including reduction of capillary fragility and protection of biologically important compounds through antioxidant activity, none of the polyphenols has been demonstrated to be essential or to be capable of causing deficiency signs when removed from the diet. However, epidemiological data from the Netherlands (Hertog et al., 1993a) indicated a reduced risk of coronary heart disease in men associated with increased ingestion of flavonoids. Relative risk of mortality from coronary heart disease and incidence of a first myocardial infarction were about 50% lower for the higher flavonoid intake groups. Red wine is a significant source of flavonoids in the diet of some cultures, and its antioxidant properties may contribute to a possible explanation of reduced risk of coronary heart disease in wine drinkers—the so-called French paradox (Frankel et al., 1993).

LIPOIC ACID (THIOCTIC ACID)

Lipoic acid (thioctic acid) (Fig. 17.2) plays an important role in the growth of certain microorganisms. It also is essential in oxidative decarboxylations of α-keto acids, such as pyruvic acid, in carbohydrate metabolism. There is, however, no clear evidence for an established need in animal nutrition that enables it to be classed as a vitamin, despite several experiments with rats and chicks (Maynard et al., 1979).

COENZYME Q (UBIQUINONES)

Coenzyme Q is a collective name for a number of ubiquinones, such as Q_4 and Q_{10}, that play an established role in the respiratory chain in mitochondrial systems. It is an electron carrier between flavoproteins and cytochromes. In addition, the coenzyme appears to have beneficial effects in certain disease states, including muscular dystrophy, periodontal disease, hypertension, and congestive heart failure (Basu and Dicker-

669

son, 1996). The importance of coenzyme Q as a ubiquitous catalyst for respiration ensures its status as an essential metabolite. There is evidence that specific ubiquinones have a sparing effect on vitamin E, resulting in remission of some clinical signs of the vitamin deficiency. Dietary ubiquinone seems on the whole to be unimportant unless it provides the aromatic nucleus for endogenous synthesis. There is no proof that justifies classification of coenzyme Q as a separate vitamin.

VITAMIN B₁₃ (OROTIC ACID)

Vitamin B₁₃ (orotic acid) was isolated from distiller's solubles, with the purified compound orotic acid, which is an intermediate in pyrimidine metabolism. It has been found to stimulate the growth of rats, chicks, and pigs under certain conditions, but evidence remains uncertain whether it plays an essential role in an otherwise adequate diet (Cody, 1991). It has no known coenzyme function.

VITAMIN B₁₅ (PANGAMIC ACID)

Vitamin B₁₅ (pangamic acid) is found in rice bran, yeast, blood meal, and other feeds. It is not a chemically defined substance, and there is no evidence that pangamic acid preparations have vitamin activity or offer therapeutic benefit.

VITAMIN B₁₇ (LAETRILE)

Vitamin B₁₇, or laetrile (amygdalin), is a β-cyanogenic glucoside occurring naturally in the kernels or seeds of most fruits (e.g., apricot). Although many unsupported claims have been made for the therapeutic benefit of laetrile treatment, most publicized claims are for its use in treating cancer. In these claims, the two major lines of argument advanced are that (1) the cyanide in laetrile acts specifically to destroy cancer cells and (2) cancer is a nutritional deficiency disease requiring laetrile treatment for dietary control (Cody, 1991). In a clinical study involving 178 terminally ill cancer patients conducted at four U.S. cancer centers, no differences were observed in terms of cure, disease progression, improvement of symptoms, or extension of life span in patients with or without laetrile therapy (Moertel et al., 1982). Most nutritionists do not consider laetrile a vitamin.

VITAMIN H₃ (GEROVITAL)

Vitamin H_3 (gerovital) is a buffered solution of procaine hydrochloride better known as novocaine, which is used as a pain killer by dentists. It is promoted as a nutritional substance that alleviates symptoms of diseases associated with aging. These claims have not been supported by scientific studies, and it is therefore not recognized as a vitamin.

VITAMIN U (CABAGIN)

Vitamin U (cabagin) is claimed to be an antiulcer factor and occurs naturally in cabbage and other green vegetables. The actual active substance is a methylsulfonium salt of methionine. The claims as an antiulcer factor have not been supported by some studies.

GLUCOSE TOLERANCE FACTOR

Glucose tolerance factor contains the element chromium, which has been reported to be involved in maintaining normal serum cholesterol and in regulating glucose metabolism (Williams and McDowell, 1985). The glucose tolerance factor qualifies as a vitamin since it contains chromium, organic components of nicotinic acid, glycine, glutamic acid, and cysteine and has much greater biological activity than inorganic sources of chromium alone. This would be comparable to vitamin B_{12} being more metabolically effective than the element cobalt.

OTHER VITAMIN-LIKE FACTORS

In 1972, Cheldelin and Baich listed unidentified growth factors (UGFs) and the organisms utilizing them. A total of 255 references were noted. In particular, many references involved unidentified factors present in fish products, alfalfa meal, liver, and whey. Thus, we have such terms as whey factor, fish solubles factor, grass juice factor, and many others.

With the discovery of folacin in the early 1940s, many believed that all of the unidentified factors had been discovered and that no more factors were needed for optimum nutrition. One reason for this supposition was the fact that completely synthetic diets of known nutrient composition, containing all recognized vitamins and mineral nutrients and adequate in the essential amino acids, would support growth and development in young weanling rats (Scott et al., 1982). However, in 1948 the discovery of vitamin B_{12} as the unknown activity—termed the animal protein factor—responsible for special growth-promoting effects was an excellent example of the fallacy of assuming that no more factors exist simply because animals can survive on synthetic diets.

With the discovery of vitamin B_{12} in 1948, the period of active identification and isolation of the major vitamins appeared to be ending. However, even since 1948 many field reports have suggested that practical diets containing sources of UGF are superior to purified or commercial diets. Typically, the unidentified factors found in certain feed ingredients have not been isolated and identified. These factors could be providing vitamins, trace minerals, or a better amino acid balance, or counteracting antagonists in the regular diet. In poultry, many of the growth responses obtained from UGF involved relationships between known nutrients, such as natural chelates in corn distiller's dried solubles that improved zinc utilization in a purified diet containing soybean (Scott et al., 1982).

Fish solubles, dried whey, brewer's dried yeast, corn distiller's dried solubles, and other fermentation residues are the major special ingredients often added to poultry diets as potential sources of unrecognized nutritional factors. In swine studies, Cunha (1977) reported that high-quality alfalfa meal and pasture, animal protein concentrates, liver, soil, dried distiller's solubles, fish solubles, grass juice concentrate, dried whey, and other feeds have been shown to contain a factor or factors useful either for the growing pig or for the sow during gestation and lactation.

The use of short, lush, green leafy pastures will minimize vitamin deficiencies in swine (Cunha, 1977). Likewise, most nutritionists recognize the possible benefits of using some UGF supplementation to ensure optimal performance of diets for broilers and breeding hens (Scott et al., 1982). This practice, in addition to pasture use, may have a twofold advantage in providing possible unidentified growth factor responses and, at the same time, supplying additional amounts of some of the known vitamins, as UGF supplements usually are good sources of many vitamins. The additional vitamins in the diet may prevent serious losses when there is a loss of potency or omission of an important vitamin from the vitamin premix (Scott et al., 1982).

■ REFERENCES

Aoe, H., and Masuda, I. (1967). *Bull. Jpn. Soc. Sci. Fish, 33,* 674.

Basu, T.K., and Dickerson, J.W.T. (1996). *In* Vitamins in Human Health and Disease, p. 249. CAB International, Wallingford, United Kingdom.

Bishop, A., Gallop, P.M., and Karnovsky, M.L. (1998). *Nutr. Rev. 56,* 287.

Bravo, L. (1998). *Nutr. Rev. 56,* 317.

Burtle, G.J., and Lovell, R.T. (1989). *Can. J. Fish. Aquat. Sci. 46,* 218.

Cao, G., Russell, R.M., Lischner, N., and Prior, R.L. (1998). *J. Nutr. 128,* 2383.

Cheldelin, V.H., and Baich, A. (1972) *In* The Vitamins (W.H. Sebrell Jr. and R.S. Harris, eds.), Vol. 5, 2nd Ed., p. 398. Academic Press, New York.

Clements, R.S., and Darnell, B. (1980). *Am. J. Clin. Nutr. 33,* 1954.

Cody, M.M. (1991). *In* Handbook of Vitamins (L.J. Machlin, ed.), p. 565. Marcel Dekker, New York.

Cromwell, G.L., Stahly, T.S., Coffey, R.D., Monegue, H.J., and Randolph, J.H. (1993). *J. Anim. Sci. 71,* 1831.

Cunha, T.J. (1971). *In* The Vitamins (W.H. Sebrell Jr. and R.S. Harris, eds.), Vol. 3, 2nd Ed., p. 394. Academic Press, New York.

Cunha, T.J. (1977). Swine Feeding and Nutrition. Academic Press, New York.

Denbow, D.M., Ravindran, V., Kornegay, E.T., Yi, Z., and Hulet, R.M. (1995). *Poult. Sci. 74,* 1831.

Forbes, R.M., Erdman, J.W., Parker, H.M., Kondo, H., and Ketelsen, S.M. (1983). *J. Nutr. 113,* 205.

Frankel, E.N., Kanner, J., German, J.B., Parks, E., and Kinsella, J.E. (1993). *Lancet 341,* 454.

Gerloff, B.J., Herdt, T.H., Wells, W.W., Liesman, J.S., and Emery, R.S. (1986). *J. Anim. Sci. 62,* 1682.

Halver, J.E. (1982). *Comp. Biochem. Physiol. 73,* 43.

Han, Y.M., Yang, F., Zhou, A.G., Miller, E.R., Ku, P.K., Hogberg, M.G., and Lei, X.G. (1997). *J. Anim. Sci. 75,* 1017.

Harris, E.D. (1992). *Nutr. Rev. 50,* 263.

Hegsted, D.M., Hayes, K.C., Gallagher, A., and Hanford, H. (1973). *J. Nutr. 103,* 302.

Herrmann, K. (1976). *J. Food Techol. 11,* 433.

Hertog, M.G.L., Feskens, E.J.M., Hollman, P.C.H., Katan, M.B., and Kromhout, D. (1993a). *Lancet. 342,* 1007.

Hertog, M.G.L., Hollman, P.C.H., Katan, M.B., and Kromhout, D. (1993b). *Nutr. Cancer 20,* 21.

Holub, B.J., Bregeron, B., and Woodward, T. (1982). *J. Nutr. 113*(6), xxi(Abstr.).

Killgore, J., Smidt, C., Duich, L., Romero-Chapman, N., Tinker, D., Reiser, K., Melko, M., Hyde, D., and Rucker, R. (1989). *Science 245,* 850.

Kroes, J. (1978). *In* Handbook Series in Nutrition and Food, Section E: Nutritional Disorders (M. Rechcigl Jr., ed.), Vol. 2, p. 143. CRC Press, Boca Raton, Florida.

Kroes, J.F., Hegsted, D.M., and Hayes, K.C. (1973). *J. Nutr. 103,* 1448.

Kukis, A., and Mookerjea, S. (1978). *Nutr. Rev. 36,* 233.

Lei, X.G., Ku, P.K., Miller, E.R., and Yokoyama, M.T. (1993). *J. Anim. Sci. 71*, 3359.

Lindley, D.C., and Cunha, T.J. (1946). *J. Nutr. 32*, 47.

Maynard, L.A., Loosli, J.K., Hintz, H.F., and Warner, R.G. (1979). Animal Nutrition, 7th Ed, p. 283. McGraw-Hill, New York.

McLaren, B.A., Keller, E., Donnell, D.J., and Elvehjem, C.A. (1947). *Arch. Biochem. Biophys. 15*, 169.

Michell, R.H. (1975). *Biochem. Biophys. Acta 415*, 81.

Moertel, C.G., Fleming, T.R., Rubin, J., Kvols, L.K., Sarna, G., Koch, R., Currie, V.E., Young, C.W., Jones, S.E., and Davignon, J.P. (1982). *N. Engl. J. Med. 306*, 201.

Morris, E.R. (1983). *Fed. Proc. Fed. Am. Soc. Exp. Biol. 42*, 1716.

Morse, D., Head, H.H., and Wilcox, C.J. (1992). *J. Dairy Sci. 75*, 1979.

NRC. (1988). Nutrient Requirements of Domestic Animals: Nutrition Requirements of Swine, 9th Ed. National Academy of Sciences-National Research Council, Washington, D.C.

NRC. (1993). Nutrient Requirements of Domestic Animals: Nutrition Requirements of Fish. National Academy of Sciences-National Research Council, Washington, D.C.

NRC. (1994). Nutrient Requirements of Domestic Animals: Nutrition Requirements of Poultry, 9th Ed. National Academy of Sciences-National Research Council, Washington, D.C.

Putney, J.W., Aub, D.L., Taylor, C.W., and Merritt, J.E. (1986). *Fed. Proc. Fed. Am. Soc. Exp. Biol. 45*, 263.

Rusznyak, S., and Szent-Györgyi, A. (1936). *Nature (London) 138*, 27(Abstr.).

Salisbury, S.A., Forrest, H.S., Cruse, W.B.T., and Kennard, O. (1979). *Nature 280*, 843.

Scott, M.L., Nesheim, M.C., and Young, R.J. (1982). Nutrition of the Chicken, p. 119. Scott, Ithaca, New York.

Simons, P.C.M., Versteegh, H.A.J., Jongbloed, A.W., Kemme, P.A., Slump, P., Bos, K.D., Wolters, M.G.E., Beudeker, R.F., and Verschoor, G.J. (1990). *Br. J. Nutr. 64*, 525.

Stahl, C.H., Han, Y.M., Roneker, K.R., House, W.A., and Lei, X.G. (1999). *J. Anim. Sci. 77*, 2135.

Varma, S.D., and Kinoshita, J.H. (1976). *Biochem. Pharm. 25*, 2505.

Vlietinck, A.J., Berghe, D.A.V., and Haemers, A. (1988). *In* Plant Flavonoids in Biology and Medicine II (V. Cody, E. Middeton Jr., J.B. Harborne, and A. Beretz, eds.), p. 283. Alan R. Liss, New York.

Williams, S.N., and McDowell, L.R. (1985). *In* Nutrition of Grazing Ruminants in Warm Climates (L.R. McDowell, ed.), p. 317. Academic Press, New York.

Williamson, P.R., Moog, R.S., Dooley, D.M., and Kagan, H.M. (1986). *J. Biol. Chem. 261*, 16302.

Yagi, K., Kotaki, A., and Yamamoto, Y. (1965). *J. Vitaminol. 11*, 14.

Yang, F., de Villiers, J.S., McClain, C.J., and Varilek, G.W. (1998). *J. Nutr. 128*, 2334.

Yi, Z., Kornegay, E.T., Ravindran, V., and Denbow, D.M. (1996). *Poult. Sci. 75*, 240.

ESSENTIAL FATTY ACIDS

INTRODUCTION

Although essential fatty acids (EFA) are not vitamins by definition, a deficiency disease or condition with dietary insufficiency does result, and in some ways, a similarity to vitamin deficiencies can be seen. The finding that components of fat, other than the fat-soluble vitamins, are dietary essentials is of nutritional and medical importance. Excellent reviews in the literature of EFA have been prepared by Holman (1978a,b) and Hansen (1994).

Knowledge that carbohydrates can be readily converted into fat and that essential lipid constituents such as phospholipids and cholesterol can be made in the body led to the view that dietary lipids were not required. In 1926, Evans and Burr changed this viewpoint by reporting that the total deprivation of fat in the diet of rats induced a syndrome of deficiency that could be corrected by certain components of fat. The EFAs originally included linoleic, linolenic, and arachidonic acids. However, arachidonic was later found to be synthesized from linoleic acid. Most species have a dietary requirement for linoleic acid, while others (e.g., fish) require linolenic acid. Studies are reevaluating the beneficial effects of linolenic acid in species that previously were considered to need only linoleic acid as a dietary essential.

HISTORY

Historical aspects of EFAs have been reviewed (Aaes-Jørgensen, 1982; Mead, 1982). The earliest report that components of fat other than fat-soluble vitamins are dietary essentials for rats was made by Evans and Burr (1926). Burr and Burr (1929, 1930) first demonstrated

18

an essential dietary requirement by the rat for a specific unsaturated fatty acid configuration that could not be synthesized by the animal. The name "essential fatty acids" was coined to describe these unsaturated fatty acids of linoleic and linolenic. Hume et al. (1940) reported that arachidonic acid was also an EFA.

Most of the history of EFA is associated with Dr. R.T. Holman, of the Hormel Institute, University of Minnesota, who has contributed more to the knowledge of essential fatty acids than any other individual. He is responsible for the delineation of metabolic conversions of polyunsaturated fatty acids, interactions among families of fatty acids, and determining quantitative requirements for linoleic and linolenic acids in animals and humans.

CHEMICAL STRUCTURE AND PROPERTIES

Chemical structures of linoleic, linolenic, and arachidonic acids as well as other fatty acids associated with EFA, are shown in Fig. 18.1. There are three common families of unsaturated 18-carbon fatty acids and one family of unsaturated 16-carbon fatty acids. The exact structure of an unsaturated fatty acid is given by three numbers: (1) the number of carbon atoms in the chain, (2) the number of double bonds, and (3) the omega (ω) number, which indicates the number of carbon atoms from the terminal methyl group to the carbon atom of the first double bond. The omega system, which was originated by Holman, designated those unsaturated fatty acids belonging to each series. Another system (not used in this book) substitutes n for ω (e.g., n-6 versus ω-6). The ω-9 and ω-7 series can be derived from endogenously synthesized oleic acid (18:1ω-9) and palmitoleic acid (16:1ω-7), respectively. The ω-6 series is derived from linoleic acid (18:2ω-6) and the ω-3 series from linolenic acid (18:3ω-3). These latter two fatty acids are considered essential as they are products of plants and cannot be synthesized by animals. Thus, it appears that linoleic acid (18:2ω-6) is essential for most species because of the inability of animals to synthesize a double bond between carbons 6 and 7 counting from the terminal methyl group.

The polyunsaturated fatty acids are liquids at room temperature. Double bonds of natural fatty acids would normally be found in nature as the *cis*-form. Ruminant animals ingest unsaturated fatty acids with their plant foods. Subsequently, bacteria in the rumen use these unsaturated fatty acids as acceptors for excess hydrogen produced during bacterial anaerobic fermentation, thus resulting in saturation of the fatty acids. However, in some cases, the end product is not a saturated bond

Palmitoleic (9,hexadecenoic)(16:1ω7)

CH₃-CH₂-CH₂-CH₂-CH₂-CH₂-CH=CH-CH₂-CH₂-CH₂-CH₂-CH₂-CH₂-CH₂-COOH

Oleic acid (9,octadecenoic)(18:1ω9)

CH₃-CH₂-CH₂-CH₂-CH₂-CH₂-CH₂-CH₂-CH=
CH-CH₂-CH₂-CH₂-CH₂-CH₂-CH₂-CH₂-COOH

5,8,11 - Eicosatrienoic (20:3ω9)

CH₃-CH₂-CH₂-CH₂-CH₂-CH₂-CH₂-CH₂-CH=CH-CH₂-CH=
CH-CH₂-CH=CH-CH₂-CH₂-CH₂-COOH

Linoleic acid (9,12 octadecadienoic acid) (18:2ω6)

CH₃-CH₂-CH₂-CH₂-CH₂-CH=CH-CH₂-CH=
CH-CH₂-CH₂-CH₂-CH₂-CH₂-CH₂-CH₂-COOH

γ-Linolenic acid (6,9,12 octadecatrienoic acid) (18:3ω6)

CH₃-CH₂-CH₂-CH₂-CH₂-CH=CH-CH₂-CH=
CH-CH₂-CH=CH-CH₂-CH₂-CH₂-CH₂-COOH

8,11,14-Eicosatrienoic acid (20:3ω6)

CH₃-CH₂-CH₂-CH₂-CH₂-CH=CH-CH₂-CH=
CH-CH₂-CH=CH-CH₂-CH₂-CH₂-CH₂-CH₂-CH₂-COOH

Arachidonic acid (5,8,11,14 eicosatetraenoic acid)(20:4ω6)

CH₃-CH₂-CH₂-CH₂-CH₂-CH=CH-CH₂-CH=
CH-CH₂-CH=CH-CH₂-CH=CH-CH₂-CH₂-CH₂-COOH

Linolenic acid (9,12,15 octadecatrienoic acid) (18:3ω3)

CH₃-CH₂-CH=CH-CH₂-CH=CH-CH₂-CH=
CH-CH₂-CH₂-CH₂-CH₂-CH₂-CH₂-CH₂-COOH

4,7,10,13,16,19-Docosahexaenoic (22:6ω3)

CH₃-CH₂-CH=CH-CH₂-CH=CH-CH₂-CH=CH-CH₂-CH=
CH-CH₂-CH=CH-CH₂-CH=CH-CH₂-CH₂-COOH

Fig. 18.1 Structures of essential fatty acids and other unsaturated fatty acids.

but an unsaturated one with a different configuration—*trans* instead of *cis*—or in a different position, or both. As a consequence, the body and milk fat of ruminants contain *trans*-fatty acids, about 2 to 9% in the case of butterfat.

A similar process, which uses hydrogen gas and a nickel catalyst, is employed industrially to turn liquid edible oils into solid fats. During the hydrogenation process, some of the naturally occurring *cis*-double bonds are isomerized to the *trans*-conformation, resulting in a decreased bond angle and an acyl chain resembling a saturated fatty acid (Lichtenstein, 1993). Hydrogenation also results in the saturation of a portion of the existing double bonds in the fatty acyl chain, thereby decreasing the polyunsaturated fatty acid (PUFA) and increasing the saturated and monounsaturated fatty acid content of the fat. The *trans*-fatty acid content of commercial edible fats may vary from 0% for diet margarines high in linoleic acid to more than 50% of fatty acids for certain shortenings and frying fats (Katan and Mensink, 1992).

One school of thought regarding *trans*- versus *cis*-fatty acids is that dietary substitution of vegetable fats for animal fats reduces the risk of cardiovascular heart disease (CHD). However, all forms of vegetable fat are not alike, and research indicates that consumption of hydrogenated rather than unhydrogenated vegetable oils may negatively influence plasma lipids and risk of CHD. Low-density lipoprotein (LDL) cholesterol was raised by both *trans*-fatty acids and saturated fatty acids compared to a diet high in oleic acid (Katan and Mensink, 1992). Also, *trans*-fatty acids depressed high-density lipoprotein (HDL) cholesterol, the so-called good cholesterol," whereas saturates did not have this effect.

New forms of linoleic acid, conjugated linoleate acid (CLA) have received considerable attention as chemopreventive agents since they have been shown to inhibit rat mammary tumorigenesis, mouse forestomach neoplasia, and mouse skin carcinogenesis (Belury, 1995; Parodi, 1999). These compounds are linoleic acid derivatives with *cis*-9, *trans*-11-; *trans*-9, *cis*-11-; *trans*-9, *trans*-11-; *trans*-10, *trans*-12-; and *trans*-10, *cis*-12-octadecadienoic acids accounting for the major isomers. The CLAs are found predominantly in foods from ruminants, first identified as an anticarcinogen following isolation from grilled ground beef extracts (Ha et al., 1987).

Linoleic acid is a colorless oil that melts at −12°C. It is soluble in ether, absolute alcohol, and other fat solvents and oils. It has an iodine value of 181 and a molecular weight of 280.44. Arachidonic acid is an oil that melts at −49.5°C, has an iodine value of 333.5, and has a molecular weight of 304.46 (Scott et al., 1982).

ANALYTICAL PROCEDURES

Essential and nonessential fatty acids are now readily determined by gas-liquid chromatographic procedures (Holman et al., 1989) that are much more precise than alkaline isomerization analyses. Methyl esters of the fatty acids are formed before injection into the column; they are then distributed between a moving gas phase (nitrogen, helium, or argon) and a stationary liquid phase (Hofstetter et al., 1965). Bioassays are available in which growth rates of newly weaned rats are dependent on the linoleic acid concentrations of feeds being tested.

METABOLISM AND FUNCTIONS

Fats and fatty acid metabolism in relation to digestion, absorption, and excretion are discussed elsewhere (Dupont, 1990). Fatty acid-binding proteins (FABPs) have been identified as a family of cytosolic proteins found in heart, liver, and epithelial cells lining the small intestine (Anonymous, 1985). FABPs are believed to be integrally involved in the cellular uptake as well as intracellular transport and/or compartmentalization of fatty acids. It has been postulated that the intestinal FABPs may actually participate in cellular fatty acid transport across the intestinal mucosa, as well as in selected intracellular events.

In humans, placental transfer of fat to the fetus occurs late in pregnancy. The late second trimester or early third trimester fetus has only 1.7% of its body weight as fat, compared with 15% in the full-term infant (Sosenko, 1995).

After fat absorption in monogastric animals, fatty acid composition of body fat is directly related to fatty acid composition of the diet. In ruminants, however, polyunsaturated fatty acids are hydrogenated to a large extent by ruminal microorganisms, resulting in more saturated body fat of the animal. In all species, certain fatty acids form structural components and serve indispensable biochemical functions.

The relationship among the three common families of unsaturated 18-carbon fatty acids is shown in Fig. 18.2. Members of a particular family may be metabolically converted to more proximally unsaturated (toward the carboxyl group) or chain-elongated fatty acids, but no conversion from one ω family to another occurs in mammals. For example, linoleic acid ($18:2\omega$-6) is converted to arachidonic acid ($20:4\omega$-6) in animals, and linolenic acid ($18:3\omega$-3) may be converted to eicosapentaenoic ($20:5\omega$-3) and docosahaexenoic acid ($22:6\omega$-3). Members of the ω-6 and ω-3 families are considered essential fatty acids for mammals, because they cannot be synthesized de novo.

Linoleic acid and linolenic acid are the precursors of the entire ω-6 and ω-3 families of polyunsaturated fatty acids, respectively. All members of the ω-6 and ω-3 families are active as essential fatty acids, and many have been shown to be more active than their original precursor. Studies employing graded dose levels of arachidonic acid fed to rats have revealed that the deposition of arachidonic acid in liver is greater when arachidonic acid itself is fed in the diet than when linoleic acid is fed. This indicates that the conversion of $18:2\omega$-6 acid to arachidonic acid for deposit in tissue lipids is a less efficient process than the deposition

679

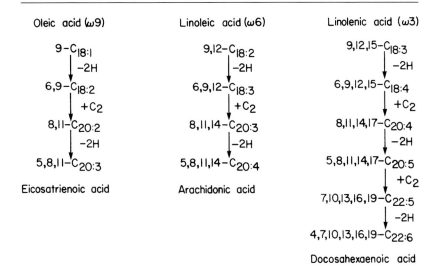

Fig. 18.2 Metabolic transformations of oleic, linoleic, and linolenic fatty acids.

of dietary 20:4ω-6 acid directly into tissue lipids, and that the potency of 20:4ω-6 is greater than that of 18:2ω-6 (Holman, 1978a).

The effect of dietary deficiency of linoleic acid on the fatty acid composition of testicular tissue lipids for swine fed different levels of linoleic acid is illustrated in Fig. 18.3 (Sewell and McDowell, 1966). The same phenomenon has been observed in a large variety of both tissues and species, the differences being mainly in magnitude (Holman, 1978a, 1986). Changes of greatest magnitude have occurred in heart and liver lipids. At zero intake of linoleic acid, the major differences in fatty acid composition are in the polyunsaturated acids themselves. In linoleic acid deficiency, 18:2ω-6, 20:4ω-6, and 22:5ω-6 are much lower than found in normal animals. Palmitoleic acid, 16:1ω-7, and oleic acid, 18:1ω-9, are higher than normal, but the most striking increase is in 20:3ω-9, which is formed endogenously from oleic acid. This acid, which is a normal component of tissue lipids in trace amounts, increases very dramatically in linoleic acid deficiency. It is found in the phospholipids in the 2 position, the same position in which arachidonic acid, 22:5ω-6, and other polyunsaturated acids are normally found.

Similar studies have been made with graded dose levels of linolenic acid as the sole fatty acid supplement to a fat-free diet (Mohrhauer and Holman, 1963). Supplementation of the fat-free diet with 18:3ω-3 causes dramatic increases in 20:5ω-3, 22:5ω-3, and 22:6ω-3 in compar-

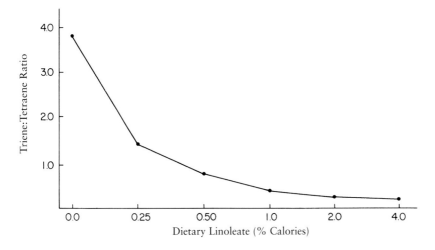

Fig. 18.3 Relationship of triene:tetraene ratio of testes tissue from young swine fed varying levels of dietary linoleic acid. (Modified from Sewell and McDowell, 1966.)

ison with the amounts found in the lipids of fat-deficient animals. Ayre and Hulbert (1996) noted that polyunsaturated fatty acids in muscle phospholipids from rats fed high ω-6 or ω-3 fatty acid diets reflected the composition of their respective diets.

Studies on dose of a single fatty acid versus response of several fatty acids in tissues have shown that each family of fatty acids suppresses metabolism of other families of fatty acids (Holman, 1964; Hwang et al., 1988).

In the absence of the main ω-6 (linoleic) and ω-3 (linolenic) families in the diet, animals are capable of synthesizing some polyunsaturated acids from endogenous precursors. Both oleic (18:1ω-9) and palmitoleic (16:1ω-7) acids themselves, and their respective families, are enhanced in the tissue lipids. None of these polyunsaturated acids is fully efficacious in meeting the requirement for polyunsaturation, for although they are present in enhanced quantity in linoleic acid deficiency, the animals often die.

The enzymatic systems that perform chain elongation, desaturation, and insertion of fatty acids into various lipid molecules apparently handle all groups of fatty acids, for there is competition between substrates at every step in each of these processes. The ω-3 family effectively suppresses metabolism of the ω-6 family. Likewise, the ω-6 family is able to suppress metabolism of the ω-3 family, but less effectively. The ω-6 family, however, suppresses the formation of polyunsaturated acids from oleic acid, as is manifested in linoleic acid deficiency. Ability of the precursor acids to compete for these enzyme systems is in the order linolenic > linoleic > oleic.

Depending on animal species, different EFAs are not equal in relationship to requirements or in ability to prevent all signs of EFA deficiency. For most species, linolenic acid does not fully relieve dermal signs of linoleic acid deficiency, even at high levels (Holman, 1978a). However, arachidonic acid (20:4ω-6) is twice as active as its precursor, linoleic acid, in reducing dermal signs attributed to the deficiency.

The eicosanoids (*eikosi* = 20 in Greek), which are important in the regulation of widely diverse physiological processes, are derived from ω-6 (e.g., 20:4) and ω-3 (e.g., 20:5) fatty acids. They have different biological activity depending on the precursor molecule. Prostaglandins, thromboxanes, prostacyclins, leukotrienes, and hydroxy fatty acids are among the eicosanoids that can be formed by enzymatic conversion of di-homo-γ-linolenic, arachidonic, and eicosapentaenoic acids. Table 18.1 shows that eicosanoids have effects related to blood pressure, capillary permeability, inflammatory reactions, and blood platelet functions.

One of the most important specific metabolic functions of EFAs is as precursors for a diverse group of "local hormones" called prostaglandins. These biologically potent compounds seem to play a regulatory role in many cellular processes. Prostaglandins have been shown to be involved in blood clotting, renal free water excretion, renal blood flow, reproduction, bronchoconstriction, gastrointestinal motility and water loss, endocrine function, and neurotransmitter release (Scott et al., 1982). Prostaglandins are intimately involved in regulation of immune function and thus resistance to infection (Boissonneault and Johnston, 1983).

Prostaglandins are formed by elongation and desaturation of linoleic acid to dihomo-γ-linoleic acid (20:3ω-6) (DHGL) and to arachidonic acid (20:4ω-6), and from long-chain fatty acids of the linolenic family (20:5ω-3), eicosapentaenoic acid. These fatty acids are found in membrane phospholipids. Practically all cells are capable either of producing or of being influenced by prostaglandins. A large number of known biologically active prostaglandins have been identified. Prostaglandins formed from DHGL without further desaturation to arachidonate comprise the 1 series of prostaglandins. Prostaglandins formed from arachidonate comprise the 2 series. The 3 series of prostaglandins is formed from eicosapentaenoic acid (20:5ω-3).

■ Table 18.1   Biological Effects of Eicosanoids Derived from Two Essential Fatty Acid Families

Cell Type	Arachidonic Acid ($20:4$, ω-6)	Eicosapentaenoic Acid ($20:5$, ω-3)
Several cells	PGE_2 Immunosuppression Vasodilating Permeability Hyperalgesia	PGE_3 Immunosuppression Inactive?
Platelets	TXA_2 Aggregating Vasoconstricting	TXA_3 Antiaggregating Inactive?
Endothelial	PGI_2 Antiaggregating Vasodilating	PGI_3 Antiaggregating Vasodilating
Leukocytes	LTB_4 (inflammatory agent) Chemotaxis Aggregating Receptor bind Permeability	LTB_5 (immunosuppressive agent) Chemotaxis Aggregating Receptor bind Permeability

Source: Modified from Drevon (1992).

The discovery of prostaglandin-like molecules in human urine and plasma (Morrow et al., 1994) pointed to a nonenzymatic peroxidation of arachidonate, resulting in many different oxygenated products with prostaglandin-like structures. They are called isoprostanes because many of them resemble the prostaglandins, with some differences in stereochemistry, for example, 8-epi-prostaglandin $F_{2\text{-}a}$ versus prostaglandin $F_{2\text{-}a}$ (Hansen, 1994).

Generally, prostaglandins and leukotrienes constitute a group of extracellular mediator molecules that are part of an organism's defense system (Calder, 1998). Prostaglandins and leukotrienes are formed during the inflammatory process, and if the inflammation is caused by invading bacteria, the formation of prostaglandins and leukotrienes will stimulate macrophages and other leukocytes to begin the process of destroying the bacteria.

Lipid sources could alter the development of autoimmune disease and the life span of short-lived animals. Many investigators have observed that polyunsaturated lipids that hinder cardiovascular disease (when compared to saturated fats) can be proinflammatory (Fernandes and Venkatraman, 1993).

Macrophages are involved in immune and inflammatory functions and possess the enzymes necessary for prostaglandin and leukotriene biosynthesis. Consuming high levels of ω-3 fatty acids may provide considerable health benefits in relation to inflammatory diseases, such as atopic dermatitis and rheumatoid arthritis (Drevon, 1992). The mechanism behind the potentially beneficial effect of ω-3 fatty acids on some inflammatory diseases may be related to altered eicosanoid formation. Reduction of eicosanoid biosynthesis by inflammatory cells is of clinical interest because of the immunosuppressive potential of elevated levels of prostaglandin E (PGE) (Kinsella et al., 1990) and possibly leukotriene B_4 (LTB$_4$) (Goodwin, 1985). For instance, production of leukotriene derived from 20:5ω-3 (e.g., LTB$_5$) is an immunosuppressive result for one of the more potent inflammatory agents (LTB$_4$), which is derived from 20:4ω-6 (Drevon, 1992).

Many age-associated diseases, including malignancy and autoimmune disease with a viral etiology, appear to be exacerbated by high-fat diets with a large proportion of vegetable oils high in ω-6 fatty acids. These oils could increase autoimmune disease by increasing free radical formation and decreasing levels of antioxidant enzyme mRNA, thus further decreasing immune function, in particular by inhibiting the development of anti-inflammatory cytokines such as interleukin (IL-2) and transforming growth factor (TGFb). In contrast, ω-3 lipids could protect against autoimmunity by enhancing TGFb mRNA levels and preventing an increase in oncogene expression (Fernandes, 1995).

Polyunsaturated fatty acids have a structural function as an integral part of phospholipids, the building unit of biomembranes. This is inferred from the specific composition of the fatty acids in these phospholipids (the β position normally being esterified with the highly unsaturated members of the EFA families) and from the fact that in EFA deficiency, these fatty acids are replaced by eicosatrienoic acid (20:3ω-9), biosynthesized from oleic acid (18:1ω-9), with the known concomitant deleterious effects on biomembrane function and integrity. The phospholipids of cell membranes will influence membrane viscosity and permeability and thereby possibly the enzyme activity of membrane proteins. Different types of eicosanoids are formed from different essential fatty acids. The general rule is that eicosanoids derived from eicosapentaenoic acid are less potent than the corresponding compounds derived from arachidonic acid (Drevon, 1992).

It has been suggested that EFA deficiency and replacement of the linoleic acid family in membrane structures may cause a disruption in spatial arrangements in mitochondria that results in less efficient oxidative phosphorylation and a derangement of basal metabolism. Such a process may be the partial uncoupling of oxidative phosphorylation in mitochondria. In poultry, presence of linoleic acid may not be absolutely necessary in the body since a deficiency will not always result in death. Fatty acids that replace the linoleic acid family in tissue lipids seem to cause a reduction in the metabolic efficiency and functioning of the animal, but life often can still be maintained (Scott et al., 1982).

A disturbed water balance is a characteristic defect of EFA deficiency and can include increased water loss through the skin, increased urinary arginine-vasopressin loss, increased water intake, and reduced urine output (Holman, 1968; Hansen and Jensen, 1986; Hansen, 1994). Increased water loss through skin results from a defect in the permeability barriers of skin, which is an indication that EFAs are involved in membrane structure. Histological studies have shown many changes in skin structure as a result of the deficiency.

Additional functions of EFAs include provision of adequate fluidity to sustain cellular function and for lipid transport (Holman, 1978a). Phospholipids and cholesteryl esters containing an abnormally high proportion of saturated fatty acids would tend to be more rigid or less fluid than would similar compounds with high proportions of polyunsaturated acids. Ethanol can penetrate the lipid bilayer of the cell membrane and can cause changes in the structure and organization of the fatty acid core, thus changing the membrane fluidity (Hoek and Rubin, 1990). Ethanol may affect the uptake of very long chain fatty acids from the diet and/or their incorporation into lipids (Swanson et al., 1995).

One of the functions of polyunsaturated acids is to provide lipids that are fluid at body temperature. Alloxan diabetes, hyperthyroidism, dietary cholesterol, saturated-fat diet, or mineral oil all involve the transport of a nonessential lipid in large quantities. These conditions have been found to accelerate EFA deficiency significantly. Studies suggest that one function of polyunsaturated acids is to provide necessary structural components for circulating lipoproteins (Holman, 1978a).

In a review, Vergroesen (1977) summarized the beneficial effects of adequate linoleic acid: (1) decreased blood cholesterol and triglyceride levels, (2) decreased thrombotic tendency of platelets, (3) preventive and curative effects in sodium-induced hypertension, (4) improvement of the physiological function of the heart, and (5) normalization of the biochemical abnormalities in obesity and maturity-onset diabetes. Mechanisms of these responses are not clearly established; however, many of the biological effects are derived from the eicosanoids synthesized from arachidonic acid ($20:4\omega$-6), including prostaglandins, thromboxanes, prostacyclins, and leukotrienes.

Linoleic and linolenic acids stimulate the growth of mammary epithelium in normal rats. Dietary linoleate seems to be necessary to the development of mammary ducts and alveoli in immature mice and to their maintenance in adult animals (Knazek and Liu, 1979). Using rats, Ollivier-Bousquet et al. (1993) suggested that only ω-6 fatty acids (versus ω-3) are required for the optimal functioning of lactating mammary epithelial cells.

CLA (see Chemical Structure and Properties) has been identified as an anticarcinogen. The CLA has several unique structural and functional properties, resulting in chemical and physiological effects that are different from those of all-*cis*- nonconjugated polyunsaturated fatty acids. In turn, these unique qualities appear to modulate cellular processes involved in carcinogenesis (Belury, 1995).

Synthesis of CLA requires the presence of free linoleic acid (the substrate), a free radical-generating species, and proteins rich in sulfur residues (Dormandy and Wickens, 1987). These conditions occur in vivo (through oxidative pathways and enzymatic isomerization) and in vitro (treatment of foods with heat) (Chin et al., 1992). The major dietary sources of CLA are foods derived from ruminants, such as beef and cheese. More than 85% of the CLA in animal tissues is the *cis*-9, *trans*-11 isomer form. They have been found in triglycerides, lipoproteins, and cell membrane phospholipids in several tissues of rodents, rabbits, and humans. Intestinal bacterial flora of rats is capable of converting free linoleic acid to *cis*-9, *trans*-11, and *trans*-9, *cis*-11 CLA isomers (Chin et al., 1994).

Increased attention has been given to the question of possible health benefits of ω-3 (linolenic family) of polyunsaturated fatty acids (Lands, 1986; Drevon, 1992; Hansen, 1994). Whatever the mechanisms involved, epidemiological studies of Greenland Eskimos (who subsist entirely on a marine diet high in ω-3 fatty acids) clearly indicated that their diet exerts potentially antithrombotic effects on platelet function, with a low death rate from coronary heart disease (Willis, 1984). In Japan, a lower death rate from coronary heart disease was also related to higher fish consumption. The Japanese studies showed a dose-response effect of fish intake, incorporation of ω-3 fatty acids in plasma lipids, and reduced cardiovascular disease. Cerebrovascular deaths were also reduced (Leaf, 1992). Similar results were obtained in human or animal studies in which fish oils rich in 20:5ω-3 were administered. The most striking result of human studies is marked prolongation of bleeding time. This clearly indicates that marine diets may reduce platelet plug formation in damaged blood vessels and may inhibit vessel-wall-induced clotting of plasma, as observed in rats (Willis, 1984).

Using isolated working heart models from rats, Pepe and McLennan (1996) reported that dietary fish oil prevented the initiation and reduced the severity of arrhythmias in the isolated hearts in response to a variety of stimuli. These results establish that irrespective of any effects on blood pressure or platelet function in vivo, dietary fish oil directly affects myocardial properties, which may contribute to observed clinical reductions in cardiac mortality associated with fish consumption.

From studies on postinfarct transcutaneous angioplasty, there are some conflicting data on the effect of very long chain ω-3 fatty acids on the frequency of re-stenosis, while a prospective study on mortality after coronary artery infarction reported a significant decrease (29%) in all-cause mortality after 2 years for patients using at least two fatty fish meals weekly (Burr et al., 1989). Sudden cardiac death accounts for about 50% of total coronary disease mortality in westernized industrial countries. The lack of early symptoms for this disorder makes prevention the preferred strategy. In a rat model of cardiac ischemia, dietary ω-6 (sunflower seed oil) and ω-3 (fish oil) polyunsaturated fatty acids were shown to protect against arrhythmia compared with saturated fat; greatest protection was observed with fish oil (Topping, 1993). Studies have shown that one aspirin every other day reduced CHD events by 47% in 5 years in 23,000 men. Aspirin interferes with platelet aggregation by inhibiting the enzyme cyclooxygenase in platelets. ω-3 Fatty acid supplements have been shown to inhibit the same enzyme and to inhibit platelet aggregation (Leaf, 1992).

The brain, as well as most of the nervous system, is a well-protected organ, especially with regard to polyunsaturated fatty acids. The nervous system has the greatest concentration of lipids after adipose tissue. Interestingly, these lipids are practically all structural and are not related to energy production; they participate directly in the functioning of cerebral membranes. Brain lipids are formed of polyunsaturated fatty acids derived from dietary essential linoleic and linolenic acids. On average, one fatty acid out of three in the brain is polyunsaturated, and these fatty acids participate in the structure of phospholipids.

The ω-6 fatty acids are required for normal fetal growth, but ω-3 fatty acids are beneficial for surfactant synthesis (Viscardi, 1995). Surfactant is a phospholipid-rich substance that lines the air-alveolar interface in the lung and prevents alveolar collapse, a major cause of mortality and morbidity in premature infants.

The long-chain ω-3 fatty acids are found in high proportions in reproductive and nervous tissues. The elongated docosahexaenoic acid (22:6ω-3) is the most abundant fatty acid in the ethanolamine phospholipids of cerebral gray matter and the retina (Carlson et al., 1986; Connor et al., 1992). The need for ω-3 fatty acids in developing visual acuity was presented as evidence for a functional requirement for ω-3 fatty acids in primates (Neuringer et al., 1984). Differences in physical activity and ability to learn have been related to low content of 22:6ω-3 in brains of rats produced by feeding a diet low in linolenic acid (Lamptey and Walker, 1976).

A diet deficient in linolenic acid alters nerve-ending fluidity and enzymatic activities, reduces the amplitude of electrophysiological parameters such as the electroretinogram, alters the resistance of the nervous system to poisons, and reduces the performance of learning tasks (Bourre et al., 1989, 1993; Enslen et al., 1991; Zerouga et al., 1991). It has been shown that changes in lipid membrane composition can modulate the binding of neurotransmitters or hormones to membrane receptors at the periphery (Murphy, 1990). Modifications of the neurotransmission pathways might induce the behavioral disturbances that are seen in animals (Delion et al., 1994).

Diets rich in PUFAs have been associated with promotion of tumor growth in rodents under certain conditions. However, studies in rats and mice (Cave, 1991) have shown that not all PUFAs should be incriminated. Increasing the fat contribution from ω-6 PUFAs (in vegetable oils) from 0 to 4% dietary energy routinely enhances tumorigenesis in rodents, while diets with equivalent levels of long-chain highly unsaturated ω-3 fatty acids found in fish oil often diminish formation of certain tumors.

Epidemiologic studies suggest that individuals who consume diets rich in fat are at higher risk for colon cancer, whereas consumption of fish products rich in ω-3 fatty acids, such as eicosapentaenoic acid (EPA) and docosahexaenoic acid (DHA), is associated with low incidence of colorectal cancer (Willett et al., 1990). Fish oil seems to protect against cancers that are most likely linked to diet—those of the colon, pancreas, breast, and ovary.

Leaf (1992) reviewed the effect of ω-3 fatty acids in reducing cardiovascular disease; additional physiologic and pharmacologic effects of fish oils were referenced as follows: (1) decreases blood pressure in normal and moderately hypertensive subjects, (2) decreases blood viscosity, (3) decreases microvascular albumin leakage in insulin-dependent diabetics, (4) decreases plasma triglycerides, (5) decreases vascular response to norepinephrine, (6) decreases ventricular fibrillation from ischemia, (7) decreases cardiac toxicity of cardiac glycosides, (8) decreases platelet adhesion, (9) decreases leucocyte-endothelium interactions, (10) increases vascular compliance, and (11) increases platelet survival.

REQUIREMENTS

The dietary essentiality of both linoleic acid (18:2ω-6) and linolenic acid (18:3ω-3) is dependent on species and, to a certain extent, on the definition of an essential nutrient. Table 18.2 provides EFA requirements for various animals and humans.

The predominant EFA for most mammals and birds is linoleic acid; the requirement for linolenic acid is much less and is unknown for many species. Determination of linoleic acid requirements have been based on observations of gross dermal lesions as well as variations in tissue polyunsaturated fatty acids. Shifts in fatty acid composition of metabolically active tissues (liver, heart, brain, etc.) that occur during onset of deficiency are very similar in all species. Similarities between EFA deficiencies induced in various species are striking when the biochemical parameters of the deficiency are considered. Quantitative requirements for several species are also strikingly similar when measured with biochemical parameters.

Triene:tetraene is the ratio of abnormally elevated endogenous metabolite of oleic acid, 20:3ω-9, to the metabolic product, 20:4ω-6, derived from linoleic acid (see Deficiency), and it has been used to estimate the minimal linoleic acid requirement (Holman, 1960). The ratio drops from a high value in deficiency to a low and rather constant value in the region between 1 and 2% of calories. The implication from these biochemical parameters is that dietary requirement for linoleic acid lies between 1 and 2% of calories.

Holman (1960) suggested a ratio of 0.4 as the point at which the minimal linoleic acid requirement of the rat, as well as other species, has been met. Fig. 18.3 illustrates the plotting of the triene-tetraene ratio versus six dietary linoleic acid levels in 3-week-old swine testes (Sewell and McDowell, 1966). The ratio decreased markedly as dietary level of linoleic acid increased from zero to 1% of dietary calories, with only a slight decrease occurring beyond this level of linoleic acid intake. Requirement for linoleic acid for pigs of this age is therefore less than 2% of dietary calories. The triene-tetraene ratio at the 1% level of linoleic acid was 0.38, which is comparable to the figure of 0.4 suggested by Holman (1960).

Contrary to most species, evidence has shown that the cat family

■ **Table 18.2** Essential Fatty Acid Requirements for Various Animals and Humans

Animal	Purpose or Class	Requirement[a]	Reference
Dairy cattle	Calf milk replacer	10% fat	NRC (1989a)
Chicken	Leghorn, 0–18 weeks	1% linoleic	NRC (1994)
	Leghorn, breeding	1% linoleic	NRC (1994)
	Leghorn, laying-breeding[b]	1–1.4% linoleic	Scott et al. (1982)
	Broilers	1% linoleic	NRC (1994)
Turkey	0–8 weeks	1% linoleic	NRC (1994)
	8–20 weeks	0.8% linoleic	NRC (1994)
Japanese quail	Growing-breeding	1% linoleic	NRC (1994)
Sheep	Growing	< 0.32 linoleic as energy	Bruckner et al. (1984)
Swine	Growing	1–2% linoleic as energy	Sewell and McDowell (1966)
Horse	All classes	0.5% linoleic	NRC (1989b)
Cat[c]	Growing[c]	0.5% 18:2 ω-6 and 0.02% 20:4 ω-6	NRC (1986)
Dog	All classes	1% linoleic	NRC (1985a)
Mink	Adult	0.5% linoleic	NRC (1982a)
	Pregnancy-lactation	1.5% linoleic	NRC (1982a)
Rat	Males	1.3% linoleic as energy	NRC (1995)
	Females	0.5% linoleic as energy	NRC (1995)
Guinea pig	Growing	0.88–1.04% linoleic as energy	NRC (1995)
Mouse	All classes	0.68% linoleic as energy	NRC (1995)
Nonhuman primates	All classes	1–2% linoleic as energy	NRC (1978)
Fish	Chum salmon	1% linoleic and 1% linolenic	NRC (1993)
	Rainbow trout	1% linoleic and 0.8% linolenic	NRC (1993)
	Yellowtail	2% 20:5ω-3 and 22:ω-6	NRC (1993)
Human	All classes	1–2% as energy	RDA (1989)

[a]Often requirements are unknown; for some species, treatments or essential fatty acid levels that have been successful are noted. Requirements are expressed either as percentage of diet or as percentage of calories (energy). Values can be on either as-fed (approximately 90% dry matter) or dry basis (see Appendix, Tables A1a.b).

[b]For laying and breeding hens, 1.4% linoleic acid is required; after maximum egg size is reached, 1% is adequate.

[c]The cat has very limited abilities to desaturate linoleic and linolenic acid to longer-chain fatty acids.

(e.g., cats and lions) is unable to desaturate linoleic and linolenic acids (NRC, 1986). As a result, these species may require a source of pre-formed longer-chain fatty acids, which means that these animals may exhibit a specific requirement for polyunsaturated lipids of animal origin. Nevertheless, linoleic acid prevents several signs of EFA deficiency, including scaly skin, increased transepidermal water loss, and enlarged fatty livers. Thus, linoleic acid has a specific role as an EFA independent of arachidonic acid synthesis.

Most fish, unlike terrestrial animals, have a definite requirement for linolenic acid (ω-3), while linoleic acid (ω-6) is often of less value. The majority of fish and shellfish species studied required 18:3ω-3, some required a combination of 18:3ω-3 and 18:2ω-6, and only a few showed a preference for 18:2ω-6 (NRC, 1993). For some fish species (e.g., rainbow trout), the metabolite of linolenic acid, 22:6ω-3, was more effective in stimulatory growth and other production parameters than linolenic acid. At least four species of fish required ω-3 fatty acids, and 22:6ω-3 best satisfied the requirement. One suggestion to explain the difference in EFA requirements for fish was that ω-3 structure permitted a greater degree of unsaturation, which was necessary in membrane phospholipids to maintain flexibility and permeability characteristics at low temperatures (NRC, 1993).

A number of factors influence development of EFA deficiency and thus requirements for EFA:

1. Age and carryover effects—Animals that had been fed normal diets for a longer time should have larger reserves of polyunsaturated fatty acids and could withstand deficiency for a longer time than weanlings. Inducing dermal signs of EFA deficiency is difficult in adult animals. Linoleic acid requirement of young chicks can be affected markedly by carryover of linoleic acid from the egg to newly hatched chicks. If chicks hatch from eggs low in linoleic acid and are fed purified diets very low in linoleic acid, the dietary requirement may be in excess of 1.4%, compared to the typical requirement of 1.0% (Scott et al., 1982).

2. Dietary fat and hormone imbalance—Animals that practice co-prophagy have an additional source of lipids not available to animals that do not. However, diets rich in saturated fatty acids or monounsaturated fatty acids are also known to moderately enhance the development of EFA deficiency. Peifer and Holman (1955) studied the effect of adding 1% cholesterol to the diet of EFA-deficient rats. An EFA deficiency syndrome, judged by growth and dermal signs, occurred within periods of 2 weeks to

1 month. Comparable EFA deficiency signs were observed only after 3 months in rats on fat-free diets without cholesterol. Substances or conditions that induce hypercholesterolemia likewise accelerate EFA deficiency.

3. Growth rate—Any animal that is called upon to grow more rapidly, and therefore to build more tissue, would have a higher requirement for EFA and would consequently exhibit deficiency signs earlier.

4. Humidity and water balance—Low atmospheric humidity hastens onset of dermal signs of EFA deficiency, probably through enhanced loss of water by evaporation, causing additional irritation of skin. Aaes-Jørgensen and Dam (1954) reported an experiment in which female rats were raised on diets with various amounts of fat for 16 weeks. They found that the water intake was higher and urine production lower in rats on diets with hydrogenated peanut oil or hydrogenated whale oil and in the absence of dietary fat than in rats on diets with lard, peanut oil, or coconut oil.

5. Sex of animal—Male animals are known to be more sensitive than females to EFA deficiency. The requirement for the female rat was found to be between 10 and 20 mg/day, while the male rat's requirement exceeded 50 mg/day (Greenberg et al., 1950; NRC, 1995). Pudelkewicz et al. (1968) estimated the linoleic acid requirement of growing female and male rats to be 0.5 and 1.3% of dietary metabolizable energy, respectively.

6. Pen arrangement—Leat (1962) concluded, from feeding pigs, that whether the animals are penned individually or in groups is important in the development of EFA-deficiency signs. He found that the skin condition was noticeably better in pigs penned in pairs than in those penned individually. He believed that keeping animals in close proximity with each other may prevent dermatitis from becoming apparent merely through physical contact.

7. Temperature and environment—For fish, EFA requirements may change with temperature and culture conditions. When rainbow trout from the same source were tested simultaneously in seawater and fresh water, the EFA deficiency was manifested more quickly in seawater (NRC, 1993). Likewise, the fatty acid composition of fish lipids, especially membrane lipids such as phospholipids, are significantly affected by acclimation temperature.

For species that require a predominance of linolenic versus linoleic acid, information is lacking on linolenic acid requirements. For pregnant rats and pups up to weaning, the minimum linoleic and linolenic acid intake should be 2.4 and 0.4% of total dietary energy, respectively (Bourre et al., 1990). For the adult rat, linolenic acid requirement is reduced to 0.26% of dietary energy (Bourre et al., 1993).

For humans, many recommendations are that a minimum intake of essential fatty acids should be 3% of total energy intake, whereas many national nutrition committees have recommended that not more than 10% of total energy should be derived from PUFA, monoenes, and saturated fatty acids (Drevon, 1992).

On the basis of human milk composition, Neuringer et al. (1988) recommend 0.7 to 1.3% of energy as linoleic acid, with the optimal ω-6:ω-3 ratio 4 to 10:1. If the diet contains an ω-6:ω-3 fatty ratio greater than 50:1, ω-3 fatty acid deficiency is expected. However, a high ω-3 level (ω-6:ω-3 1.4:1) depressed the cell-mediated immune response, PGE_2 production, and plasma vitamin E in aged dogs (Wander et al., 1997).

NATURAL SOURCES

The EFAs are widely distributed among food fats. For example, vegetable oils of corn, soybean, cottonseed, peanut, and certain others are excellent linoleic acid sources. Safflower oil contains 75% linoleic acid, whereas corn oil, soybean oil, and cottonseed oil all contain approximately 50% linoleic acid. Linseed, canola, and soybean oils contain approximately 57, 8, and 7% linolenic acid, respectively (Drevon, 1992). Linolenic acid is particularly high in forage lipids. From the lipids of pasture grasses, 61% is reported as linolenic acid (Garton, 1960).

Linoleic and arachidonic acid contents of feed ingredients are shown in Table 18.3. Linoleic acid and its dehydrogenation product 18:3ω-6 are found in highest abundance in plants, but more unsaturated and longer-chain members of this family are found principally in animals. Notable exceptions to these generalities are the occurrence of arachidonic acid and other higher members of the group in primitive plants such as ferns and algae (Schlenk and Gellerman, 1965). Concentrations of the long-chain linolenic acid (ω-3) family for marine products are listed in Table 18.4.

Arachidonic acid (20:4ω-6) is the most abundant PUFA in animal membranes; thus, when animal products are consumed as food, the arachidonic acid content varies with the amount of membrane. Crawford et al. (1989) determined the arachidonic acid composition in various species in the food chain as follows (percent of total fatty acids): wild pig (8.5), antelope (7.4), dolphin muscle (16.8), herring muscle (0.6), squid (5.8), mollusk (2.3), algae (12.4), and phytoplankton (0.7).

CLA (see Chemical Structure and Properties; Metabolism and

693

■ Table 18.3 Typical Linoleic Acid and Arachidonic Acid in Various Foods and Feedstuffs (as-fed basis)

Food or Feedstuff	Linoleic Acid (%)	Arachidonic Acid (%)
Alfalfa meal, dehydrated	0.40	—
Barley	0.83	—
Brewer's grains, dehydrated	2.94	—
Coconut oil	1.10	—
Corn gluten meal	3.83	—
Corn oil	55.40	—
Corn, yellow	1.82	—
Cottonseed meal, solvent extracted	0.80	—
Crab meal	0.33	—
Fish meal, anchovy	0.20	—
Fish meal, menhaden	0.15	—
Fish oil, menhaden	2.70	—
Fish solubles, condensed	0.20	—
Lard	18.30	0.3–1.0
Linseed oil	13.90	—
Meat meal	0.34	—
Milk, cow's, dehydrated	0.01	—
Oats	1.49	—
Peanut meal	1.25	—
Poultry by-products meal	1.72	—
Poultry fat (offal)	22.30	0.5–1.0
Rice bran oil	36.50	—
Safflower oil	72.70	—
Sorghum	1.08	—
Soybean meal, solvent extracted	0.35	—
Soybean seed	7.97	—
Tallow	4.30	0–0.2
Wheat	0.58	—
Wheat bran	2.25	—

Source: Data adapted from NRC (1982b).

Function) is a naturally occurring substance in food. Dietary sources of CLA include milk fat, meat products, and vegetable oils. In foods, CLA is highest (mg/g of fat) in ruminant meats and is found in smaller amounts in poultry and eggs (Chin et al., 1992). Dairy products such as natural cheeses, processed cheeses, and milks and yogurts that have undergone a variety of heat-processing treatments all contain considerable amounts of CLA (Lin et al., 1995). Total CLA is generally increased in foods that are heat processed (dairy pasteurization, pan frying of meats, etc.) (Shantha et al., 1992). Overall, vegetable fats are poorer sources of CLA. Concentrations of CLA in bovine milk can be increased by dietary regimen and management (Jiang et al., 1996; Chouinard et al., 1999).

■ Table 18.4   Eicosapentaenoic (20:5ω-3) and Docosahexaenoic (22:6ω-3)
Acids in Fish or Marine Products

	Total Fat (g/100 g)	20:5	22:6
Carp	5.6	0.2	0.1
Catfish, channel	4.3	0.1	0.2
Cod, Atlantic	0.7	0.1	0.2
Herring	9.0	0.7	0.9
Mackerel	13.9	0.9	1.6
Salmon (wild)	5.4	0.3	0.9
Trout (wild)	7.7	0.1	0.5
Crab, blue	1.0	0.2	0.1
Shrimp	1.5	0.3	0.2
Oyster, east	2.0	0.3	0.2
Cod liver oil	100.0	9.0	9.5
Salmon oil	100.0	8.8	11.1
Menhaden oil	100.0	12.7	7.9

Sources: Data adapted from Drevon (1992) and Sanders (1994).

DEFICIENCY

Effects of Deficiency

Induction of EFA deficiency in animals requires rigid exclusion of fat from the diet, and even with supposed low-fat diets for humans, deficiency state in adults is difficult to attain (Holman, 1978b). Clinical signs of EFA deficiency induced by a fat-free diet require almost one-eighth of a rat's normal lifetime to develop, and rarely have humans been subjected to a low-fat diet under observation for a proportionate span of time. Natural diets, even poor ones, usually contain adequate amounts of EFA; therefore, the deficiency is far rarer than deficiencies of protein, vitamins, or minerals. Nevertheless, EFA deficiency does occur when animals or humans receive insufficient dietary fat.

Linoleic acid deficiency signs and other criteria range from early classic signs such as reduced growth rate, parakeratosis, increased water permeability of skin, increased susceptibility to bacteria, and male and female sterility to more recently recognized signs such as decreased prostaglandin biosynthesis, reduced myocardial contractility, abnormal thrombocyte aggregation, and swelling of rat liver mitochondria (Vergroesen, 1977). For all land species studied, the major feature of the deficiency is impairment of the exterior covering of the animal. Mammals exhibit dermatitis, chickens exhibit faulty feathering, and moths are unable to form normal scales on their wings. All the manifestations indicate faulty membrane formation, a feature of deficiency that is common to all tissues and species (Holman, 1978a).

For land animals, EFA deficiency is a term primarily referring to linoleic acid deficiency. However, findings suggest that the linolenic family (ω-3) of fatty acids, particularly 20:5ω-6 and 22:6ω-3, are likewise important. Fish oils, rich in ω-3 fatty acids have been linked to reduction of thrombosis and heart disease in humans as well as proper brain development in children and rats (Drevon, 1992; Jumpsen et al., 1997).

Ruminants

The EFA deficiency of ruminants has been less extensively researched than that of nonruminants, with the deficiency in adult ruminants not readily demonstrated (Palmquist et al., 1977). The microbial population appears to provide enough EFA to meet the requirements; however, studies with lambs suggest that the required level of EFA may be elevated in the presence of host microflora (Bruckner et al., 1984). Gullickson et al. (1942) reported that calves fed a low-fat diet did not develop EFA deficiency signs, but growth was suppressed. Cunningham and Loosli (1954b) reported that calves receiving a fat-free synthetic milk developed leg weakness and muscular twitches within 1 to 5 weeks and died unless a source of fat was supplied. Lambert et al. (1954) also studied the effect of a "lipid-free," semisynthetic milk fed to dairy calves. They reported the following clinical signs: growth retardation after 3 weeks on trial; scaly dandruff; long dry hair; dull hair coat; excessive loss of hair on the back, shoulders, and tail; and diarrhea.

Weanling lambs fed a fat-free diet for 7 months showed no evidence of skin lesions or other clinical signs typical of fat deficiency (Cunningham and Loosli, 1954a). In a second experiment, 2-day-old lambs and kids were given fat-free synthetic milk. The lambs and kids receiving the fat-free diets became weak and died within 1 to 7 weeks, while controls were raised successfully on the same milk with 2% added lard.

Delivery of fatty acids at various levels for metabolism can influence events important in dairy cow reproduction. A soybean oil emulsion (50% linoleic acid) was infused intravenously to Holstein heifers (Lucy et al., 1990). This resulted in increased plasma concentrations of prostaglandin F 2-α(PGF$_{2\alpha}$) metabolite and increased ovarian follicles, and the size of the largest follicle was greater. In a second study, feeding rumen-protected fat to lactating dairy cows increased the numbers of 3- to 5-mm follicles and follicles greater than 15 mm in diameter, and increased the size of the preovulatory follicle of a synchronized estrus cycle during the early postpartum period (Lucy et al., 1991). Garcia-Bojalil (1993) fed rumen-protected fat (0.5 kg/day), which improved conception rates of lactating Holstein cows from 52 to 86%.

Inclusion of fish oil in the diet appears to result in an alteration in regression dynamics of the corpus luteum as evidenced by a greater proportion of cows having elevated concentration of plasma progesterone after injection of $PGF_{2\alpha}$ (Burke et al., 1996). Perhaps the increase in conception rate (39.5 versus 30.6%) could be attributable to increased survival of the embryo at the time of pregnancy recognition (e.g., when $PGF_{2\alpha}$ secretion is suppressed). It would appear that fatty acids are important to both stimulated follicles (elevated $PGF_{2\alpha}$) to bring about pregnancy but later decrease PGF_2, which would result in greater progesterone production and maintenance of pregnancy.

Swine

Witz and Beeson (1951) used a diet that contained only 0.06% lipid and produced the following signs: slower growth rate; underdeveloped digestive systems; small gallbladders; enlarged thyroid glands; delayed sexual maturity; scaly dandruff-like dermatitis on the tail, back, and shoulders; loss of hair, with the remaining hair being dull and dry; a brown, gummy exudate on the belly and sides; necrotic areas on the skin around the neck and shoulders; and an unthrifty appearance. Leat (1962) fed pigs from 4.5 to 91 kg live weight a diet consisting of 0.07% of the calories as linoleic acid. This diet resulted in pronounced scaliness of the skin, first noted after about 13 weeks on the diet. Scaliness seemed to be confined to the dorsal surface and was most severe about the shoulders. The hair was dry and appeared to stand out from the skin at all angles. When linoleic acid made up 0.5% of the dietary calories, there was little or no flakiness of skin.

Sewell and McDowell (1966) fed 3-week-old male pigs purified diets containing six levels of linoleic acid. For the 10-week experiment, no differences were noted in weight gains, but dermal lesions (Fig. 18.4) were observed after 6 to 7 weeks of the experiment. Scaly, dandruff-like desquamation of the skin over the dorsal surface was the first noticeable sign, and later, a brownish gummy exudate appeared around the ears and axillary spaces, and under the flanks. Skin eruptions were also present about the ears, axillary spaces, and flanks in the severest cases. Lesions were observed only among pigs receiving 0.5% linoleic acid or less; pigs receiving the 1% level and above were free of skin lesions.

Studies have been conducted in swine on the effect of PUFA in mod-

697

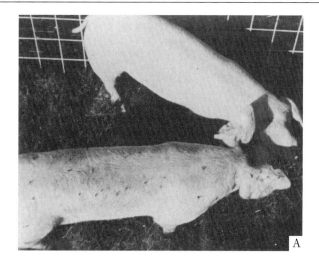

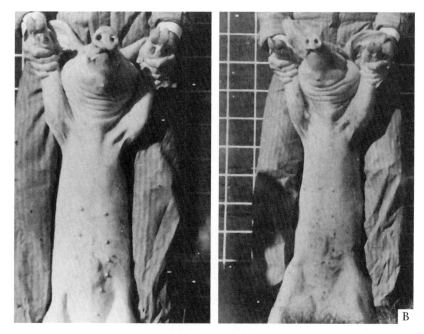

Fig. 18.4 (A) Dermal lesions of a linoleic acid-deficient pig (foreground) that was fed a diet with no linoleic acid (the black spots are flies that were attracted to the brown, gummy exudate). The other pig received 1.0% of calories as linoleic acid. (B) The same pigs as in A; the one on the right has EFA deficiency, with dermal lesions particularly severe at the axillary spaces. (Courtesy of L.R. McDowell, R.F. Sewell, and the University of Georgia.)

ulating infectious disease processes. Turek et al. (1994) found that dietary (ω-3 and ω-6) PUFAs affected alveolar macrophage tumor necrosis factor (TNF) production and leucine aminopeptidase (LAP) levels, and the production of T-cell growth factors by alveolar lymphocytes. In another study, these researchers found that dietary PUFA can affect disease pathogenesis (e.g., *Mycoplasma hyopneumonia*, the most common respiratory pathogen in swine) and that the ω3:ω6 PUFA ratio may modulate the host response (Turek et al., 1996).

Poultry

Growing chicks fed a fat-free ration did not survive the fourth week (Reiser, 1950). The most readily observed clinical sign of linoleic acid deficiency in young chicks is slow growth rate. Machlin and Gordon (1961) found that adding safflower oil or linoleic acid, but not linolenic acid, to purified diets free of unsaturated fatty acids resulted in an immediate (within 7 days) growth response in chickens. Some microbial synthesis of ω-6 fatty acids occurs in the gut of quail. On a diet deficient in linoleic acid, germ-free animals had a lower growth rate and more severe clinical signs than normal ones.

Linoleic acid deficiency in chicks has also been reported to result in an enlarged fatty liver, degeneration of testes, and subcutaneous edema, and, in some cases, general edema in the body occurs. Deficiency of linoleic acid in the male can impair spermatogenesis and affect fertility (NRC, 1994). Linoleic acid-deficient chicks are more susceptible to respiratory infections (Scott et al., 1982). High mortality resulted from an atypical respiratory infection for chicks fed linoleic acid-deficient diets from hatching to 10 to 12 weeks of age.

Fritsche et al. (1991) reported that feeding laying hens a diet rich in ω-3 PUFA (7% fish oil) significantly enhanced their primary antibody response and altered lymphocyte proliferation. Feeding broiler chickens diets rich in ω-3 PUFA reduced antibody-dependent cell cytotoxicity and altered eicosanoid release by chicken immune cells (Fritsche and Cassity, 1992).

Linoleic acid deficiency in laying hens results in depressed egg production, small egg size, a slight reduction in fertility, and a marked increase in early mortality of the embryo during incubation. Eggs from hens severely deficient in linoleic acid will not hatch. For severely deficient hens it is necessary to feed pullets diets that are very low in linoleic acid from hatching on. Linoleic acid is stored in the body for long periods by animals reared on a diet containing adequate linoleic acid.

Other Animal Species

DOGS AND CATS

Dogs deficient in EFA have low growth rates, a characteristic dermatitis, swelling and redness of the paws, and increased susceptibility to infection (NRC, 1985a). Beagle puppies fed a low-fat diet exhibited skin lesions within 2 to 3 months.

Clinical signs attributed to EFA deficiency in cats include listlessness; dry, unattractive hair coats; and severe dandruff (NRC, 1986). Growth is poor, and susceptibility to infections is increased. Histological examination of the liver reveals fatty infiltration and parenchymal disorganization. Both males and females lack libido, testes are underdeveloped, and estrus cycles are absent.

FISH

In common with other vertebrates, fish cannot synthesize either 18:2ω-6 or 18:3ω-3 de novo. One or both of these fatty acids must be supplied preformed in the diet, depending on the EFA requirements. Fish vary considerably in their ability to convert 18-carbon unsaturated fatty acids to longer-chain more highly unsaturated fatty acids of the same series. In general, freshwater fish require either dietary linoleic acid (18:2ω-6) or linolenic acid (18:3ω-3) or both, whereas marine fish require dietary EPA (20:5ω-3) and/or DHA (22:6ω-3).

The principal gross signs of EFA deficiency reported for various fishes are dermal signs (fin rot), a shock syndrome, myocarditis, reduced growth rate, reduced feed efficiency, and increased mortality (Castell et al., 1972; NRC, 1993). Essential fatty acid deficiency has also been shown to reduce the reproductive performance of common carp, rainbow trout, and Red Sea bream (NRC, 1993).

Deficiency signs specific to trout are poor growth, elevated tissue levels of ω-9 fatty acids (particularly 20:3ω-9), necrosis of the caudal fin, fatty pale liver, dermal depigmentation, increased muscle water content, syncope accentuated by stress, increased mitochondrial swelling, increased respiration rate of liver homogenates, heart myopathy, and lowered hemoglobin level. Poor growth, low feed efficiency, high mortality, and swollen pale livers were reported in chum salmon fed an EFA-deficient diet (NRC, 1993).

In certain warm-water fish—common carp, for example—it was demonstrated that dietary levels of 22:6ω-3 significantly affected egg hatchability (NRC, 1993). Shrimp would not produce eggs unless the diet contained 20:5ω-3 and 22:6ω-3. Watanabe et al. (1983) reported that ω-3 PUFAs, such as EPA and DHA, are required for normal growth and development of ayu and Red Sea bream larvae. High mortalities and abnormalities, such as underdeveloped swim bladder and scoliosis, have been observed in Red Sea bream larvae.

FOXES

Foxes on low-EFA diets showed clinical signs of hyperkeratosis and dandruff (NRC, 1982a).

LABORATORY ANIMALS

Signs of EFA deficiency in the rat are reduction in growth (which plateaus after about 12 to 18 weeks); scaly skin; rough, thin hair coat; necrosis of the tail; electrocardiographic abnormalities; fatty liver; impaired reproduction; and death. Many other less noticeable but equally severe changes have been reported, including kidney lesions and a decrease in urine volume, lipid-containing macrophages in the lung, increased metabolic rate, decreased capillary resistance, and aberrant ventricular conduction (NRC, 1995).

During fetal growth and postnatal development, large amounts of ω-3 and ω-6 are deposited in nervous system tissues, particularly in the central nervous system in rats. In rats, inadequate $22:6\omega$-3 supply to these tissues during fetal development and postnatal life is associated with abnormal retinal function, visual acuity, and behavior (Enslen et al., 1991).

Newborns from rats fed linoleic acid-deficient diets exhibit the most severe signs of deficiency and usually die within 3 days to 3 weeks after birth, depending on the duration of the EFA feeding to the dam. In young rats fed a fat-free diet, two of the earliest signs of EFA deficiency are increased transepidermal water loss and increased urinary arginine-vasopressin excretion (Hansen and Jensen, 1986).

Mice with EFA deficiency have hair loss, dermatitis with scaling and crusting of skin, and occasional diarrhea. Deficiency in older mice caused infertility without visible skin changes (NRC, 1995). In the deficient guinea pig, there is weight loss, with clinical signs including dermatitis; skin ulcers; fur loss; underdevelopment of spleen, testes, and gallbladder; and enlargement of kidneys, liver, adrenals, and heart.

NONHUMAN PRIMATES

In monkeys, EFA deficiency resulted in dryness and scaliness of the skin, with loss of hair, although many months of the deficient diet were required for appearance of clinical signs (NRC, 1978).

Signs in rabbits of EFA deficiency are reduced growth, hair loss, degenerative changes in seminiferous tubules, and impaired sperm development (Ahluwalia et al., 1967).

Humans

Essential fatty acid deficiency in humans has primarily been studied in infants. Eczema has been reported in a number of studies of infants maintained on a low-fat diet (Holman, 1978a). Hansen et al. (1958) presented data showing that young healthy infants, within a relatively short time, may develop symptoms when given diets extremely low in fat. After several weeks on trial, alterations in the skin were observed in the majority of infants. The first sign detected was dryness, then thickening, and later desquamation, with oozing in the intertriginous folds (Fig. 18.5). Addition of linoleic acid, as 2% of the caloric intake, restored the skin to normal, while the addition of saturated fatty acid had no effect.

Patients who are maintained by fat-free total parenteral nutrition (TPN) are candidates for EFA deficiency. Premature infants receiving TPN are particularly susceptible to rapid development of EFA deficiency signs (Cooke et al., 1984).

The need for ω-3 fatty acids in human diets has been established (see Metabolism and Functions). Potential benefits of ω-3 fatty acids have been found to reduce thrombosis of platelet aggregation and heart disease, as well as hypertension. There are numerous reports of potentially beneficial effects of fish oil (ω-3 fatty acids) on triglycerides, blood rheology, blood pressure, and inflammation. Studies have also revealed an anticancer effect (e.g., colon cancer) of supplemental ω-3 found in fish oils (Cave, 1991).

Essential fatty acid deficiency has been mostly related to linoleic acid deficiency, but in most situations linolenic acid deficiency coexists (Uauy and de Andraca, 1995). One study found that ω-3 fatty acids—especially docosahexaenoic acid ($22:6\omega$-3), present in human milk—are necessary for retinal and brain development in primates and humans (Uauy and Hoffman, 1991). Rod photoreceptor function and the maturation of visual acuity of human low birth weight infants are dependent on the supply of these essential nutrients (Birch et al., 1992).

Assessment of Status

In addition to various deficiency clinical signs and responses to EFA supplementation, the most accurate indicators of EFA status are bio-

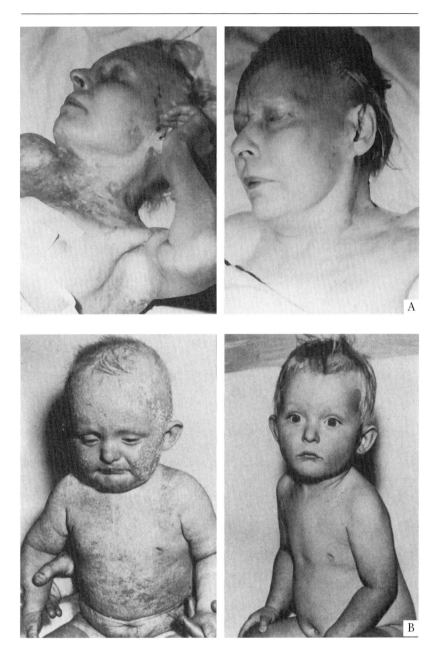

Fig. 18.5 Skin lesions associated with EFA deficiency in (A) an adult and (B) an infant before and after EFA administration. The adult received fat-free total parenteral nutrition. (Courtesy of R.T. Holman, The Hormel Institute, University of Minnesota, and M.C. Riella, J.W. Broviac, M. Wells, and B.H. Scribner (1975), *Ann. Intern. Med.* 83:786–789.)

chemical changes associated with EFA deficiency. Anatomical signs of EFA deficiency vary from species to species, but biochemical aberrations associated with deficiency in rats are found to be the same in all other species studied (Holman, 1978a). The biochemical signs of linoleic acid deficiency have been known for many years. The chief alterations in various tissues are decreased levels of linoleic (18:2ω-6), arachidonic (20:4ω-6), and docosapentaenoic (22:5ω-6) acids, and increased levels of eicosatrienoic (20:3ω-9) and docosatrienoic (22:3ω-9) acids. With the EFA-deficient diet the tissues attempt to produce unsaturated acids from the oleic acid (18:1ω-9), which results in the accumulation of the trienoic acid, eicosatrienoic acid (20:3ω-9). The triene:tetraene ratio is the ratio of the abnormally elevated endogenous metabolite of oleic acid, 20:3ω-9, to the metabolic product, 20:4ω-6, from the dietary essential linoleic acid (see Requirements). Therefore, it is the ratio of the "abnormal" to "normal" major polyunsaturated acids in tissue lipids. The curve describing the triene-tetraene ratio versus dietary linoleate had a sharp break at or near 1% of calories, suggesting that 1% of calories of linoleic acid may be a critical amount, the dietary requirement (Holman, 1960). Values of the ratio below 0.4 have been considered normal for animals. Fig. 18.6 is an example of a study in which six levels of linoleic acid were fed to young male pigs (Sewell and McDowell, 1966). As dietary linoleic acid was increased, arachidonic acid (20:4ω-6) was elevated and 20:3ω-9 was suppressed. Castell et al. (1972) suggested that the ratio of 20:3ω-9:20:5ω-3 in polar lipids from the liver of rainbow trout might be a useful index of linolenic acid status.

SUPPLEMENTATION

Linoleic acid deficiency is not likely to develop when diets contain appreciable amounts of corn. Yellow corn is the major source of linoleic acid in most feed formulas for swine and poultry. Diets composed of corn and soybean meal with no further supplementation are likely to be adequate in linoleic acid for chick growth but marginal for maximum egg size. Since linoleic acid has a marked effect on egg size, it is necessary to ensure that a sufficient amount of linoleic acid is included in the diet of laying hens to enable them to lay eggs of maximum size as early as possible during the egg production year (Scott et al., 1982). A typical dietary linoleic acid recommendation for poultry is 1% of total calories. However, for laying and breeding hens the requirement would be 1.4% of calories until egg size is reached (Scott et al., 1982).

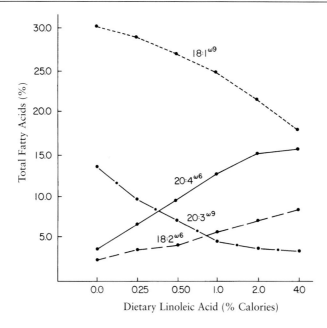

Fig. 18.6 Influence of varying levels of dietary linoleic acid on linoleic (18:2 ω-6), arachidonic (20:4 ω-6), eicosatrienoic (20:3 ω-9), and oleic (18:1 ω-9) acid content of testes tissue from young swine. (Modified from Sewell and McDowell, 1966.)

Animals fed diets containing sorghum, barley, or wheat instead of corn as the major grain may receive suboptimal quantities of linoleic acid. Even more important, when roots and tubers (such as potatoes and cassava) or processed carbohydrates (such as cane sugar) make up a major part of the energy source, and when solvent-extracted protein supplements are used exclusively, there is potential danger of skin lesions related to linoleic acid deficiency (McDowell, 1977). For young ruminants, the main supplementation concern is that milk replacers contain adequate concentrations of EFA.

Supplementing cattle with fish oils or protected fat may have a beneficial reproduction response. Typically, unsaturated fatty acids are biohydrogenated by ruminal microorganisms, therefore preventing their delivery as-is to the lower gut for absorption. However, eicosapentaenoic (20:5ω-3) and docosahexaenoic (22:6ω-3) fatty acids found in fish oil appear to escape biohydrogenation (Ashes et al., 1992; Palmquist and Kinsey, 1994). Therefore, feeding fish meal may result in uptake of these fatty acids for metabolism by reproductive tissues of the lactating cow (Smith and Marnett, 1991; Garcia-Bojalil, 1993) and result in higher reproductive rates.

Under typical conditions, EFA deficiency would not be expected in humans. The average fat content of U.S. diets is 40% of calories. Likewise, there has been a marked shift in preference from animal fat to vegetable oils, which contain high quantities of linoleic acid. Even if all dietary fat were from one source, it is unlikely that EFA content of the diet would be inadequate. Because polyunsaturated acids of the ω-6 family are nearly ubiquitous in plants and animals, and in most natural food sources they constitute more than the minimum nutrient requirement, even random selection of foods is not likely to induce EFA deficiency (Holman, 1978a).

Research suggests that human health could be improved with *cis*-versus *trans*-fatty acids and conjugated linoleic acid. *Trans*-fatty acids (hydrogenated fats) raise the undesirable LDL cholesterol and depress the favorable HDL cholesterol (Katan and Mensink, 1992). Conjugated linoleic acid from ruminant animal products have been shown to have an anticarcinogen effect (Belury, 1995).

The main concern for supplementation of EFA for humans would be for infants not receiving mother's milk, but rather a milk product low in EFA. Particular attention is needed for premature infants to ensure that parenteral nutrition includes formulas containing adequate EFA. Visual function of full-term infants fed human milk is enhanced for up to 3 years, supporting the concept of long-term benefits of human milk feeding on mental development (Birch et al., 1993). Docosahexaenoic acid ($22:6\omega$-3) is particularly required for brain development. Low birth weight infants randomized to human milk or formula tube feeding demonstrated the benefits of human milk for IQ at age 8 years (Lucas et al., 1992). Plasma $22:6\omega$-3 concentrations of full-term infants fed formula are lower than that of breast-fed infants. This suggests that present formulas provide insufficient linolenic acid, or chain elongation-desaturation enzymes are not sufficiently active during early life to support tissue accretion of $22:6\omega$-3. Also, studies of infants who were born at term and died from sudden infant death syndrome revealed that brain composition is affected by human milk feeding. The data indicated that higher $22:6\omega$-3 content was found in the brain cortex of breast-fed infants relative to infants receiving formulas based on cow's milk (Farquharson et al., 1992).

Long-chain polyunsaturated fatty acids are being included in infant formulas. It is clear that the balance between $20:4\omega$-6 and $22:6\omega$-3 in the diet is a powerful determinant of the level of these fatty acids in the developing brain. Addition of 20:4ω-6 or 22:6ω-3 alone may be inappropriate; balanced addition of both ω-6 and ω-3 long-chain PUFAs (20:4ω-6 and 22:6ω-3) seems to be required (Jumpsen et al., 1997).

Chylomicronemia (increased fat particles in blood) in patients with severe familiar hypertriglyceridemia has been shown to respond to long-term treatment with ω-3 fatty acids (Pschierer et al., 1995). Long-term supplementation of a diet with ω-3 fatty acids results in a persistent decrease of serum triglyceride concentrations, a pronounced reduction in the number of chylomicrons present in the fasting state, and an improvement in plasma viscosity.

For human diets, increasing attention is being paid to the dietary role of long-chain ω-3 PUFAs (e.g., 20:5ω-3 and 22:6ω-3). Research suggests that marine oil fatty acids (linolenic or ω-3 family) play a role in ameliorating thrombosis, heart disease, hypertension, inflammation (e.g., arthritis), and some types of cancer, and in improving the immune response. As a result, increased dietary intake of ω-3 fatty acids has been recommended as a means of reducing risk for coronary heart disease (Kromhout et al., 1985; Nair et al., 1999; Tinker et al., 1999). Table eggs enriched with ω-3 fatty acids provide an alternative to fish as a source of these proposed healthful fatty acids (Marshall et al., 1994). Inclusion of various fish oils, seeds, and seed oils in layer rations readily results in the incorporation of up to 220 mg of ω-3 fatty acids per egg yolk (Hargis and Van Elswyk, 1993). This level of ω-3 fatty acids is equivalent to that which would be consumed in a 100-g (3.5-oz.) serving of lean fish; therefore, consumption of one egg enriched with ω-3 fatty acids could replace a serving of fish (Marshall et al., 1994).

In swine, feeding diets containing canola or fish oils has resulted in increased tissue levels of the ω-3 family of fatty acids (Leskanich et al., 1997; Soler-Velásquez et al., 1998). Menhaden fish oil at 7% in a sow's late-gestation and lactation diet greatly elevated the content of ω-3 fatty acids in the nursing pig immune cells (Fritsche et al., 1993). Likewise, the desire to manipulate the fatty acid composition of ruminant tissues is motivated by human health concerns about saturated fatty acids in animal food products and by the emerging roles of unsaturated fatty acids as regulators of cell function. In cattle (Fotouhi and Jenkins, 1992) and sheep (Jenkins, 1995), the reaction of unsaturated fatty acids with primary amines produced fatty acyl amides that resisted biohydrogenation and caused less disruption of ruminal fermentation. In dairy cattle, conversion of soybean oil to butylsoyamide protected unsaturated fatty acids from ruminal biohydrogenation, causing linoleic acid to increase in the plasma and milk of dairy cows (Jenkins et al., 1996).

TOXICITY

There are nutritional disadvantages from excessive intakes of EFAs. Before the role of antioxidants and the dietary requirement for vitamin E were understood, a large amount of literature accumulated concerning the alleged toxicity of polyunsaturated fats (Holman, 1978a). These readily oxidized acids increase the requirement (see Chapter 4) for vitamin E, which functions as an antioxidant in the body. Several experiments have shown that levels of the vitamin that were normally sufficient to prevent vitamin E deficiency signs such as muscular dystrophy and encephalomalacia proved inadequate as the intakes of EFAs were increased. It is difficult to experimentally separate the effects of high levels of PUFAs from a relative deficiency of tocopherol, but it is obvious that, at least under some circumstances, high levels of PUFAs may have undesirable effects.

Not only are excess PUFAs detrimental to vitamin E, but individual fatty acids are detrimental to other fatty acids. Excess fatty acids of one family will suppress the metabolism of other families of fatty acids (Hwang et al., 1988). Suggested favorable ω-6:ω-3 fatty acid ratios for humans are 4 to 10:1, respectfully. Increased ω-3 to result in a 1.4 ω-6:1.0ω-3 ratio has been shown to depress the cell-mediated immune response and $PGE_{2\alpha}$ production in dogs (Whelan, 1996; Wander et al., 1997).

■ REFERENCES

Aaes-Jørgensen, E. (1982) *Prog. Lipid Res. 20*, 123.
Aaes-Jørgensen, E., and Dam, H. (1954) *Brit. J. Nutr. 8*, 290.
Ahluwalia, B., Pincus, G., and Holman, T. (1967) *J. Nutr. 92*, 205.
Anonymous (1985). *Nutr. Rev. 43*(11), 350.
Ashes, J.R., Siebert, B.D., Gulati, S.K., Cuthbertson, A.Z., and Scott, T.W. (1992) *Lipids 27*, 629.
Ayre, K.J., and Hulbert, A.J. (1996) *J. Nutr. 126*, 653.
Belury, M.A. (1995) *Nutr. Rev. 53*, 83.
Birch, E.E., Birch, D.G., Hoffman, D.R., and Uauy, R.D. (1992) *Ophthal. Vis. Sci. 33*, 3242.
Birch, E.E., Birch, D.G., Hoffman, D.R., Hale, L., Everett, M., and Uauy, R.D. (1993) *J. Pediatr. Ophthalmol. Strabismus 30*, 33.
Boissonneault, G.A., and Johnston, P.V. (1983) *J. Nutr. 113*, 1187.

Bourre, J.M., Francois, M., Youyou, A., Dumont, O., Piciotti, M., Pascal, G., and Durand, G. (1989) *J. Nutr. 119*, 1880.

Bourre, J.M., Piciotti, M., Dumont, O., Pascal, G., and Durand, G. (1990) *Lipids 25*, 465.

Bourre, J.M., Dumont, O., Pascal, G., and Durand, G. (1993) *J. Nutr. 123*, 1313.

Bruckner, G., Gurnewalk, K.K., Tucker, R.E., and Mitchell Jr., G.E. (1984) *J. Anim. Sci. 58*, 971.

Burke, J.M., Staples, C.R., Risco, C.A., and Thatcher, W.W. (1996) *In* 7th Annual Florida Ruminant Nutrition Symposium, p. 21. University of Florida, Gainesville.

Burr, G.O., and Burr, M.M. (1929) *J. Biol. Chem. 82*, 345.

Burr, G.O., and Burr, M.M. (1930) *J. Biol. Chem. 86*, 587.

Burr, M.L., Fehily, A.M., and Gilbert, J.F. (1989) *Lancet 2*, 757.

Calder, P.C. (1998). *Nutr. Rev. 56*, S 70.

Carlson, S.E., Carver, J.D., and House, S.G. (1986) *J. Nutr. 116*, 718.

Castell, J.D., Sinnhuber, R.O., Wales, J.H., and Lee, D.J. (1972) *J. Nutr. 102*, 77.

Cave, W.T. Jr. (1991) *FASEB J. 5*, 2160.

Chin, S.F., Liu, W., Storkson, J.M., Ha, Y.L., and Pariza, M.W. (1992) *J. Food Comp. Anal. 5*, 185.

Chin, S.F., Storkson, J.M., Liu, W., Albright, K.J., and Pariza, M.W. (1994) *J. Nutr. 124*, 694.

Chouinard, P.Y., Corneau, L., Barbano, D.M., Metzer, L.E., and Bauman, D.E. (1999). *J. Nutr. 129*, 1579.

Connor, W.E., Neuringer, M., and Reisbick, S. (1992) *Nutr. Rev. 50*, 21.

Cooke, R.J., Zee, P., and Yeh, Y.Y. (1984) *J. Pediatr. Gastroenterol. Nutr. 3*, 446.

Crawford, M.A., Doyle, W., Drury, P., Ghebremeskel, K., Harbige, L., Leyton, J., and Williams, G. (1989) *In* Dietary ω3 and ω6 Fatty Acids. Biological Effects and Nutritional Essentiality (C. Galli and A.P. Simopoulos, eds.), p. 5. Plenum Press, New York.

Cunningham, H.M., and Loosli, J.K. (1954a) *J. Anim. Sci. 13*, 265.

Cunningham, H.M., and Loosli, J.K. (1954b) *J. Dairy Sci. 37*, 453.

Delion, S., Chalon, S., Hérault, J., Guilloteau, D., Besnard, J.C., and Durand, G. (1994) *J. Nutr. 124*, 2466.

Dormandy, T.L., and Wickens, D.G. (1987) *Chem. Phys. Lipids 45*, 353.

Drevon, C.A. (1992) *Nutr. Rev. 50*, 38.

Dupont, J. (1990). *In* Present Knowledge in Nutrition (M.L. Brown, ed.), 6th ed., p. 56. International Life Science Institute, Washington, D.C.

Enslen, M., Milon, H., and Malnoe, A. (1991) *Lipids, 26*, 203.

Evans, H.M., and Burr, G.O. (1926) *Proc. Soc. Exp. Biol. Med. 24*, 740.

Farquharson, J., Cockburn, F., and Ainslie, P.W. (1992) *Lancet 340*, 810.

Fernandes, G. (1995) *Nutr. Rev. 53*, 572.

Fernandes, G., and Venkatraman, J.T. (1993) *Nutr. Res. 13*, 519.

Fotouhi, N., and Jenkins, T.C. (1992) *J. Anim. Sci. 70*, 3607.

Fritsche, K.L., and Cassity, N.A. (1992) *Poult. Sci. 71*, 1646.

Fritsche, K.L., Cassity, N.A., and Huang, S.C. (1991) *Poult. Sci. 70*, 611.

Fritsche, K.L., Alexander, D.W., Cassity, N.A., and Huang, S. (1993). *Lipids 28*, 677.

Garcia-Bojalil, C.M. (1993) Reproductive, Productive and Immunological Responses of Holstein Dairy Cows Fed Diets Varying in Concentration and Ruminal Degradability of Protein and Supplemented with Ruminally Inert Fat. Ph.D. Dissertation, University of Florida, Gainesville.

Garton, G.A. (1960) *Nature 187*, 511.

Goodwin, J.S. (1985) Prostaglandins and Immunity. Martinus Nijhoff, Boston, Massachusets.

Greenberg, S.M., Colbert, C.E., Savage, E.E., and Deuel, J. (1950) *J. Nutr. 41*, 473.

Gullickson, T.W., Fountaine, F.C., and Fitch, J.B. (1942) *J. Dairy Sci. 25*, 117.

Ha, Y.L., Grimm, N.K., and Pariza, M.W. (1987) *Carcinogenesis 8*, 1881.

Hansen, A.E., Haggard, M.E., Boelsche, A.N., Adam, D.J., and Wiese, H.F. (1958) *J. Nutr. 66*, 565.

Hansen, H.S. (1994) *Nutr. Rev. 52*, 162.

Hansen, H.S., and Jensen, B. (1986) *J. Nutr. 116*, 198.

Hargis, P.S., and Van Elswyk, M.E. (1993) *Poult. Sci. 70*, 874.

Hoek, J., and Rubin, E. (1990) *Alcohol 25*, 143.

Hofstetter, H., Sen, N., and Holman, R.T. (1965) *J. Am. Oil Chem. Soc. 42*, 537.

Holman, R.T. (1960) *J. Nutr. 70*, 405.

Holman, R.T. (1964) *Fed. Proc. Am. Soc. Exp. Biol. 23*, 1062.

Holman, R.T. (1968) *Prog. Chem. Fats Other Lipids 9*, 279.

Holman, R.T. (1978a) *In* Handbook Series in Nutrition and Food, Section E: Nutrition Disorders, Volume 3 (M. Rechcigl Jr., ed.), p. 491. CRC Press, West Palm Beach, Florida.

Holman, R.T. (1978b) *In* Handbook Series in Nutrition and Food, Section E: Nutrition Disorders, Volume 3 (M. Rechcigl Jr., ed.), p. 335. CRC Press, West Palm Beach, Florida.

Holman, R.T. (1986). *J. Am. Coll. Nutr. 56*, 303.

Holman, R.T., Johnson, S.B., and Kokmen, E. (1989). *Proc. Natl. Acad. Sci. U S A 86*, 4720.

Hume, E.M., Nunn, L.A., Smedley-MacLean, I., and Smith, H.H. (1940). *Biochem. J. 34*, 879.

Hwang, D.H., Boudreau, M., and Chanmugam, P. (1988). *J. Nutr. 118*, 427.

Jenkins, T.C. (1995). *J. Anim. Sci. 73*, 818.

Jenkins, T.C., Bateman, H.G., and Block, S.M. (1996). *J. Dairy Sci. 75*, 585.

Jiang, J., Bjoerck, L., Fonden, R., and Emanuelson, M. (1996). *J. Dairy Sci. 79*, 438.

Jumpsen, J., Lien, E.L., Goh, Y.K., and Clandinin, M.T. (1997). *J. Nutr. 127*, 724.

Katan, M.B., and Mensink, R.P. (1992). *Nutr. Rev. 50*, 46.

Kinsella, J.E., Lokesh, B., Broughton, K.S., and Whelan, J. (1990). *Nutrition 5*, 24.

Knazek, R.A., and Liu, S.C. (1979). *Proc. Soc. Exp. Biol. Med. 162*, 346.

Kromhout, D., Bosschieter, E.B., and Coulander, C. deL. (1985). *N. Engl. J. Med. 312*, 1205.

Lambert, M.R., Jacobson, N.L., Allen, R.S., and Zaletel, J.H. (1954). *J. Nutr. 52*, 259.

Lamptey, M.S., and Walker, B.L. (1976). *J. Nutr. 106*, 86.

Lands, W.E.M. (1986). *Nutr. Rev. 44*, 189.

Leaf, A. (1992). *Nutr. Rev. 50*, 150.

Leat, W.M. (1962). *Brit. J. Nutr. 16*, 559.

Leskanich, C.O., Matthews, K.R., Warkup, C.C., Noble, R.C., and Huzzledine, M. (1997). *J. Anim. Sci. 75*, 673.

Lichtenstein, A. (1993). *Nutr. Rev. 51*, 340.

Lin, H., Boylston, T.D., Chang, M.J., Luedecke, L.O., and Shultz, T. (1995). *J. Dairy Sci. 78*, 2358.

Lucas, A., Morley, R., Cole, T.J., Lister, G., and Leeson-Payne, C. (1992). *Lancet 339*, 261.

Lucy, M.C., Gross, T.S., and Thatcher, W.W. (1990). In Livestock Reproduction in Latin America, p. 119. Atomic Energy Agency, Vienna.

Lucy, M.C., Staples, C.R., Michel, F.M., and Thatcher, W.W. (1991). *J. Dairy Sci. 74*, 483.

Machlin, L.J., and Gordon, R.S. (1961). *J. Nutr. 75*, 157.

Marshall, A.C., Kubena, K.S., Hinton, K.R., Hargis, P.S., and Van Elswyk, M.E. (1994). *Poult. Sci. 73*, 1334.

McDowell, L.R. (1977). Geographical Distribution of Nutritional Diseases in Animals. Department of Animal Science, University of Florida, Gainesville.

Mead, J.F. (1982). *Prog. Lipid Res. 20*, 1.

Mohrhauer, H., and Holman, R.T. (1963). *J. Lipid Res. 4*, 151.

Morrow, J.D., Minton, T.A., Badr, K.F., and Roberts, L.J. (1994). *Biochim. Biophys. Acta 1210*, 244.

Murphy, M.G. (1990). *J. Nutr. Biochem. 1*, 68.

Nair, S.S.D., Leitch, J., Falconer, J., and Garg, M.L. (1999). *J. Nutr. 129*, 1518.

Neuringer, M., Connor, W.E., Van Petten, C., and Barstad, L. (1984). *J. Clin. Invest. 73*, 272.

Neuringer, M., Anderson, G.J., and Connor, W.E. (1988). *Annu. Rev. Nutr. 8*, 517.

NRC. Nutrient Requirements of Domestic Animals. National Academy of Sciences-National Research Council, Washington, D.C.

(1978). Nutrient Requirements of Nonhuman Primates.

(1982a). Nutrient Requirements of Mink and Foxes.

(1985a). Nutrient Requirements of Dogs, 2nd Ed.

(1986). Nutrient Requirements of Cats, 3rd Ed.

(1989a). Nutrient Requirements of Dairy Cattle, 6th Ed.

(1989b). Nutrient Requirements of Horses, 5th Ed.

(1993). Nutrient Requirements of Fish.

(1994). Nutrient Requirements of Poultry, 9th Ed.

(1995). Nutrient Requirements of Laboratory Animals, 2nd Ed.

NRC. (1982b). United States-Canadian Tables of Feed Composition, 3rd Ed. National Academy of Sciences-National Research Council, Washington, D.C.

Ollivier-Bousquet, M. Guesnet, P., Seddiki, T., and Durand, G. (1993). *J. Nutr. 123*, 2090.

Palmquist, D.L., and Kinsey, D.J. (1994). *J. Dairy Sci.*(Suppl. 1) 77, 350(Abstr.).

Palmquist, D.L., Mattos, W., and Stone, R.L. (1977). *Lipids 12*, 235.

711

Parodi, P.W. (1999). *J. Dairy Sci. 82*, 1339.

Peifer, J.J., and Holman, R.T. (1955). *Arch. Biochem. Biophys. 57*, 520.

Pepe, S., and McLennan, P.L. (1996). *J. Nutr. 126*, 34.

Pschierer, V., Richter, W.O., and Schwandt, P. (1995). *J. Nutr. 125*, 1490.

Pudelkewicz, C., Seuffert, J., and Holman, R.T. (1968). *J. Nutr. 94*, 138.

Reiser, R. (1950). *J. Nutr. 42*, 319.

Sanders, K.M. (1994). *Feed Management 45*(4), 53.

Schlenk, H., and Gellerman, J.L. (1965). *J. Am. Oil Chem. Soc. 42*, 504.

Scott, N.L., Nesheim, M.C., and Young, R.J. (1982). Nutrition of the Chicken, p. 119. Scott, Ithaca, New York.

Sewell, R.F., and McDowell, L.R. (1966). *J. Nutr. 89*, 64.

Shantha, N.C., Decker, E.A., and Ustunol, Z. (1992). *J. Am. Oil Chem. Soc. 69*, 425.

Smith, W.L., and Marnett, L.J. (1991). *Biochim. Biophys. Acta, 1083*, 1.

Soler-Velásquez, M.P., Brendemuhl, J.H., McDowell, L.R., Sheppard, K.A., Johnson, D.D., and Williams, S.N. (1998). *J. Anim. Sci. 76*, 110.

Sosenko, I.R.S. (1995). *J. Nutr. 125*, 1652S.

Swanson, R.L., Baumgardner, C.A., and Geer, B.W. (1995). *J. Nutr. 125*, 553.

Tinker, L.F., Parks, E.J., Behr, S.R., Schneeman, B.O., and Davis, P.A. (1999). *J. Nutr. 129*, 1126.

Topping, D. (1993). *Nutr. Rev. 51*, 271.

Turek, J.J., Schoenlein, I.A., Clark, L.K., and Van Alstin, W.C. (1994). *J. Leukoc. Biol. 56*, 599.

Turek, J., Schoenlein, A., Watkins, A., Van Alstine, G., Clark, L., and Knox, K. (1996). *J. Nutr. 126*, 1541.

Uauy, R., and de Andraca, I. (1995). *J. Nutr. 125*, 2278S.

Uauy, R., and Hoffman, D.R. (1991). *Semin. Perinatol. 15*, 449.

Vergroesen, A.J. (1977). *Nutr. Rev. 35*, 1.

Viscardi, R.M. (1995). *J. Nutr. 125*, 1645S.

Wander, R.C., Hall, J.A., Gradin, J.L., Du, S.H., and Jewell, D.E. (1997). *J. Nutr. 127*, 1198.

Watanabe, T., Kitajima, C., and Fujita, S. (1983). *Aquaculture 34*, 115.

Whelan, J. (1996). *J. Nutr. 126*, 1086.

Willett, W.C., Stampfer, M.J., Colditz, G.A., Rosner, B.A., and Speizer, F.E. (1990). *N. Engl. J. Med. 323*, 1664.

Willis, A.L. (1984). *In* Nutrition Reviews, Present Knowledge in Nutrition (R.E. Olson, ed.), p. 90. The Nutrition Foundation, Inc., Washington, D.C.

Witz, W.M., and Beeson, W.M. (1951). *J. Anim. Sci. 10*, 112.

Zerouga, M., Beauge, F., Niel, E., Durand, G., and Bourre, J.M. (1991). *Biochim. Biophys. Acta 1086*, 295.

VITAMIN SUPPLEMENTATION

INTRODUCTION

In the early part of this century, pasture, other forages, distiller's solubles or grains, brewer's grains, fermentation products, and meat, milk, and fish by-products were depended on as sources of the vitamins for animal feeding. As animal feeding became more sophisticated, as faster-growing and higher-producing animals were developed, and as the trend toward more intensified operations occurred, it became necessary to add an increasing number of vitamins to properly fortify animal diets.

Vitamins represent only a minute fraction of animal feeds, typically amounting to only 0.05% by weight and 1 to 2% of feed cost for swine and poultry operations depending on the diet used and the level of supplementation required (McNaughton, 1990). Yet a balanced vitamin fortification program for meeting requirements of nonruminant animals under a wide range of feeds and different production systems will more than offset the cost of adding vitamins.

Because of proper diet selection and vitamin supplementation, human deficiency diseases attributed to vitamin A (xerophthalmia and night blindness), vitamin D (rickets), vitamin C (scurvy), thiamin (beriberi), niacin (pellagra), and vitamin B_{12} (pernicious anemia) have been eliminated in varying degrees in developing countries but still pose a problem for susceptible groups. Vitamin A deficiency particularly is still a problem in many world areas. In human nutrition, vitamin supplementation should be provided to susceptible population groups, with the precaution of avoiding quantities in extreme excess, in particular vitamin A.

Supplementation guidelines specific for each vitamin have been presented in the respective chapters (Chapters 2 through 18). The present

19

chapter will discuss general supplementation considerations for both animals and humans.

FACTORS RESULTING IN INADEQUATE DIETARY INTAKES OF VITAMINS

Vitamin dietary intake and utilization is influenced by many factors,
including particular feed ingredients, bioavailability, harvesting, processing, storage, feed intake, antagonists, least-cost feed formulations,
and other factors (NRC, 1973; McDowell, 2000).

Agronomic Effects and Harvesting Conditions

Vitamin levels will vary in feed ingredients because of crop location,
fertilization, plant genetics, plant disease, and weather. Intensive crop-
ping practices and use of new crop varieties may result in reduced levels
of certain vitamins in many feedstuffs. In forage crops, factors that favor production of lush, green plants also favor production of many vitamins, particularly β-carotene, vitamin E, and vitamin K. The vitamin
C content of tomatoes depends primarily on intensity of sunlight striking the fruits of the tomato during the immediate preharvest period
(Scott, 1973).

Harvesting conditions often play a major role in the vitamin content
of many feedstuffs. Vitamin content of corn is drastically reduced when
harvest months are not conducive to full ripening. If corn has been subjected to alternate periods of freezing and thawing while it contains a
high amount of moisture, fermentation occurs in corn kernels, and there
is a loss of vitamin content, particularly of vitamin E and cryptoxanthin.
In one study, vitamin E activity in blighted corn was 59% lower than in
sound corn, and activity of the vitamin in lightweight corn averaged
21% lower than in sound corn (Hoffmann-La Roche, 1991). Young et
al. (1975) reported that the rate of oxidation of natural tocopherol was
higher in high-moisture corn than in low-moisture corn due to increased
peroxidation of the lipid. Certain legumes, particularly alfalfa and soybeans, contain the enzyme lipoxidase that, unless quickly inactivated,
readily destroys much of the carotenes.

Processing and Storage Effects

Many vitamins are delicate substances that can suffer loss of activity due to unfavorable circumstances encountered during processing or
storage of premixes and feeds. Stress factors for vitamins include humidity, pressure (pelleting), friction (abrasion), heat, light, oxidation-re-

duction, rancidity, trace minerals, pH, and interactions with other vitamins, carriers, enzymes, and feed additives (NRC, 1973).

Humidity is the primary factor that can decrease the stability of vitamins in premixes and feedstuffs. Water softens the matrix, for example, of vitamin A, thus the vitamin becomes more permeable to oxygen. Trace elements, acids, and bases are activated only by water. Humidity augments the negative effects exerted by choline chloride, trace elements, and other chemical reactions that are not found in dry feed. Thus, the water level is responsible for a higher reactivity of vitamins with other feed components. Elevated moisture content or incorrect storage of premixes and feedstuffs is the root of almost all stability problems. Christian (1983) determined the stability of vitamin A in a premix. After 3 months of storage, the vitamin A retention was 88% under low temperature and low humidity, 86% under high temperature and low humidity, and 2% under high temperature and high humidity. They concluded that humidity was significantly more stressful than temperature.

Vitamins that undergo friction or are mixed and stored with minerals are subject to loss of potency. Friction is an important factor because it erodes the coating that protects several vitamins and reduces vitamin crystals to a smaller particle size. Friction is very high in pelleting. Some abrasion is inevitable in the mixing process, but fortunately, most minerals contain little moisture, with the exception of salt, which is, of course, somewhat hygroscopic if exposed to environmental moisture. Therefore, packaging, careful transport, and storage become important, and few companies would willingly use very high levels of salt in a supplement containing fat-soluble vitamins.

Hazards to vitamins from minerals are abrasion and direct destruction by certain trace elements, particularly copper, zinc, and iron; manganese and selenium are the least reactive. Free metal ion is the most reactive (metal filings), followed by sulfate, carbonate, oxide, and the least reactive form is chelated. Chelated mineral forms become incapable of initiating formation of free radicals. In fat-soluble vitamins, esters are significantly more stable than alcohols. The hydroxy group of alcohols is extremely sensitive to oxidation. The five double bonds in retinyl acetate still make the compound sensitive to oxidation. Vitamin A is significantly more stable in vitamin premixes than in vitamin-trace mineral premixes because trace minerals catalyze oxidation of the five double bonds (Coelho, 1996). Dove and Ewan (1986) determined the stability of α-tocopherol in feeds without and with trace minerals. At the end of 3 months of storage at 25 to 30°C, α-tocopherol retention was 50 and 30%, respectively. The addition of 245 ppm copper as copper sulfate produced 0% retention after 15 days. In addition to trace minerals, choline chloride is highly destructive to vitamins (see Chapter 14) and should not be included in a vitamin premix.

Some vitamins are destroyed by light. Riboflavin is stable to most factors involved in processing; however, it is readily destroyed by either visible or ultraviolet light. Vitamin B_6, vitamin C, and folacin can also be destroyed by light. It is necessary, therefore, to protect premixes of feeds containing these vitamins from light and radiation (Stamberg and Peterson, 1946).

Sun-field curing of cut hay is essential to provide vitamin D activity but results in loss of other vitamin potency. Mangelson et al. (1949) showed that mechanical dehydration at 177°C within 1 hour after cutting produced an alfalfa meal that contained 2.5 times more carotene as did sun-cured alfalfa. There was no loss of riboflavin, pantothenic acid, niacin, or folacin during dehydration. Field-cured alfalfa was lower in riboflavin, and when alfalfa was exposed to rain, there was a large loss of pantothenic acid and niacin (Scott, 1973).

Dehydration of alfalfa at 135°C resulted in an average of 18% loss of α-tocopherol. When dehydrated alfalfa meal was stored for 12 weeks at 32°C, the α-tocopherol loss averaged 65% (Livingston et al., 1968). Corn is often dried rapidly under high temperatures, resulting in losses of vitamin E activity and other heat-sensitive vitamins. When corn was artificially dried for 40 minutes at 88°C, losses of α-tocopherol averaged 19%, and when corn was dried for 54 minutes at 107°C, losses averaged 41% (Adams, 1973).

While pelleting generally improves the value of energy and protein carriers in a feed, this is not true for some vitamins. During pelleting of feeds, four elements destructive for a number of vitamins are applied in combined action: friction, heat, pressure, and humidity. Increasing the pelleting temperature or conditioning time generally enhances redox reactions and destroys vitamins. As with friction, not all vitamins or forms of vitamins respond to these factors equally. Significant amounts of the vitamin E in the alcohol form and ascorbic acid, but very little of the vitamin E in the acetate form or choline, are destroyed as pelleting temperatures and conditioning times increase. Gadient (1986) reported that vitamins A, D_3, K_3, C, and thiamin are most likely to show stability problems in pelleted feeds. Pelleting of feed may have a beneficial effect on availability of vitamins such as niacin and biotin, which are often present in bound forms (Scott, 1973). Feed manufacturers have increased pelleting temperatures for all animal feeds in order to control

Salmonella organisms and increase digestibility, and are using steam pelleting, prepelleting conditioners, and feed expanders, which lead to increased vitamin degradation (Coelho, 1994).

In extrusion, the dominant stress factors are pressure, heat, moisture, and redox reactions. Extrusion is the most aggressive process against vitamins due to the high temperature (107 to 135°C), pressure (400 to 1,000 psi), and moisture (30%) involved in the process (Coelho, 1996).

Processing with the goal of producing better-quality fish meals and fish solubles under conditions in which putrefaction is prevented has resulted in lower levels of vitamin K and vitamin B_{12} in these feedstuffs than were present when the products were allowed to undergo a considerable degree of putrefaction. Early studies on vitamin K and vitamin B_{12} proved that fish meal and rice bran exposed to the action of microorganisms showed increased content of these vitamins. On the other hand, processing of many raw fishes with heat is required to inactivate a potent thiaminase that destroys thiamin. Also, attempts to preserve fish with nitrates led to the production of carcinogenic nitrosamines.

Each stage of human food preparation and storage results in vitamin loss. Fruits and vegetables that are harvested long before use undergo heavy vitamin losses by enzymatic decomposition. Vitamin C is particularly liable to this type of destruction. In apples stored under domestic conditions, the vitamin C content may fall to about one-third of the original value after only 2 or 3 months. Blanching vegetables before canning or freezing also results in vitamin loss. Estimates suggest that losses due to blanching fluctuate between 13 and 60% for vitamin C, 2 and 30% for thiamin, and 5 and 40% for riboflavin (Marks, 1975). Vitamin losses during heat sterilization are generally small because oxygen is excluded during this process. Thiamin is the vitamin most susceptible because of its labile nature in heat, and considerable thiamin losses have been observed in meat. Irradiation results in damage to vitamins, of which the most sensitive vitamins are thiamin, riboflavin, vitamin A, and vitamin E; niacin is relatively stable. Storage in cans, freezing, and dehydration are all relatively good methods of preservation concerning vitamin retention.

Reduced Feed Intake

When feed intake is reduced, vitamin allowances should be adjusted to ensure adequate vitamin intake for optimum performance. Restricting feed intake practices and/or improved feed conversion will decrease

717

dietary intake of all nutrients, including vitamins. Restricted feeding of broiler breeders, turkey breeder hens, and gestating sows and gilts may result in marginal vitamin intake if diets are not adequately fortified (Hoffmann-La Roche, 1989; McDowell, 2000). Reduced feed intake may also result from stress and disease.

Use of high-energy feeds such as fats to provide diets with greater nutrient density for higher animal performance requires a higher vitamin concentration in feeds. Nonruminant species provided diets ad libitum consume quantities sufficient to meet energy requirements. Thus, vitamin fortification must be increased for high-energy diets because animals will consume less total feed. Feed consumption was compared in broilers receiving metabolizable energy ranging from 2,800 to 3,550 kcal/kg of feed (Friesecke, 1975). Feed and vitamin consumption were each 19.1% lower in broilers consuming the diet with greater energy density compared to those consuming the lowest-energy diet.

Ambient temperature also has an important influence on diet consumption, as animals consume greater quantities during cold temperatures and reduced amounts as a result of heat stress. Vitamins, as well as other nutrients, must therefore be adjusted to reflect changing dietary consumption.

Vitamin Variability and Insufficient Analysis

Tables of feed and food composition demonstrate the lack of complete vitamin information, with vitamin levels varying widely within a given feedstuff. Kurnick et al. (1972) found that, of the feeds surveyed, information on the niacin and riboflavin content of feedstuffs was more complete than for any other vitamins, whereas values for vitamin B_{12} and vitamin K were most deficient. Thus, 2 to 30% of the ingredients lacked niacin, riboflavin, or pantothenic acid values, while 89 to 97% did not have values for carotene, vitamin B_{12}, or vitamin K. Information about the other vitamins was not listed for 36 to 64% of the ingredients. In more than 25 years since this report, the situation has not greatly improved; vitamin analyses of feeds are still woefully inadequate.

Variability of vitamin content within ingredients is generally large and difficult to quantify and anticipate. It is well recognized that vitamin levels shown in tables of vitamin composition of feedstuffs represent average values and that actual vitamin content of each feedstuff varies over a fairly wide range. Vitamin content of feed ingredients differs drastically from sample to sample; therefore, at least two standard deviations (average, 10%) need to be deducted from the initial content. Several months elapse between harvest, processing, and finally consumption of feed ingredients. Since most natural vitamins are not chemically protected in feed ingredients, there is considerable loss between harvesting and consumption (average, 25% loss) (BASF, 1991).

Methods of processing and storage, as previously mentioned, account for variability as well as different analysis techniques. Often, it is questionable whether the accuracy of vitamin levels from feedstuffs, calculated using tabular values, can be ensured (Kurnick et al., 1972). Proof of this is the statement by the 1982 NRC publication on U.S.-Canadian Tables of Feed Composition that ". . . organic constituents (e.g., crude protein, cell wall constituents, ether extract, and amino acids) can vary as much as $\pm y15\%$, the inorganic constituents as much as $\pm y30\%$, and the energy values as much as $\pm y10\%$." Therefore, average values in feed composition tables may vary considerably from the nutrient value in a specific group of feeds.

Vitamin Bioavailability

Even accurate feedstuff analyses of vitamin concentrations do not provide bioavailability data needed for certain vitamins. Bound forms of vitamins in natural ingredients often are unavailable to animals. Bioavailability of choline, niacin, and vitamin B_6 is adequate in some feeds but limited or variable in others. For example, bioavailability of choline is 100% in corn but varies from 60 to 75% in soybean meal; that of niacin is 100% in soybean meal but zero in wheat and sorghum and varies from 0 to 30% in corn; that of vitamin B_6 is 65% in soybean meal and varies from 45 to 56% in corn (Hoffmann-La Roche, 1991). The niacin in cereal grains and their by-products is in a bound form, which is virtually unavailable for the pig and chick (Cunha, 1982). For alfalfa meal, corn, cottonseed meal, and soybean meal, bioavailability of biotin is estimated at 100% (Cunha, 1984a). However, biotin availability is variable for other feedstuffs, for example, 20 to 50% in barley, 62% in corn gluten meal, 30% in fish meal, 20 to 60% in sorghum, 32% in oats, and 0 to 62% in wheat. Likewise, ascorbic acid in cooked cabbage is present in the bound form, ascorbinogen, a form that is absorbed very poorly by humans (Marks, 1975).

Some data obtained for the pig showed that responses to vitamins may differ depending on whether vitamins are being added to a purified or natural diet (Cunha, 1977). Requirements of the pig for niacin, riboflavin, and pantothenic acid were considerably higher on a natural diet than requirements established earlier from experiments using purified diets (McMillen et al., 1949). This shows that results obtained with purified diets must also be verified with natural diets and that bioavailability of vitamins may be greater in purified diets.

Computerized Least-Cost Feed Formulations

Vitamins are not usually entered as specifications in computerized feed formulations. Therefore, vitamin-rich feedstuffs—such as alfalfa, distiller's solubles or grains; brewer's grains; fermentation products; and meat, milk, and fish by-products—are often excluded or reduced when least-cost feed formulations are computed. The resulting least-cost diet consisting of a grain and soybean meal is usually lower in vitamins than a more complex one containing more costly vitamin-rich feeds (Roche, 1979).

FACTORS AFFECTING VITAMIN REQUIREMENTS AND UTILIZATION

Physiological Makeup and Production Function

Vitamin needs of animals and humans depend greatly on their physiological makeup, age, health, and nutritional status and function (e.g., producing meat, milk, eggs, hair or wool, or developing a fetus) (Roche, 1979). For example, dairy cows producing greater volumes of milk have higher vitamin requirements than dry cows or cows producing low quantities. Breeder hens have higher vitamin requirements for optimum hatchability, since vitamin requirements for egg production are generally less than for egg hatchability. Higher levels of vitamins A, D_3, and E are needed in diets for breeder hens than in feeds for rapidly growing broilers. Selection for faster growth rate may allow animals to reach much higher weights at much younger ages, with less feed consumed. Dudley-Cash (1994) concluded that since genetic potential has improved at the rate of 0.8% feed conversion yearly, and most of the NRC vitamin requirement data are 20 to 40 years old, vitamin requirements determined several decades ago may not apply to today's poultry. Selection for faster weight gains in swine and increased number of litters per year also demands elevated vitamin requirements (Cunha, 1980a, 1984b).

Different breeds and strains of animals have been shown to vary in their vitamin requirements. Vitamin needs of new strains developed for improved production are higher. Leg problems seen in fast-growing strains of broilers can be corrected in part by higher levels of biotin, folacin, niacin, and choline (Roche, 1979).

Confinement Rearing Without Access to Pasture

Moving swine and poultry operations into complete confinement without access to pasture has had a profound effect on vitamin nutrition (as well as mineral nutrition). Pasture could be depended on to provide significant quantities of most vitamins, since young, lush, green grasses or legumes are excellent vitamin sources. More available forms of vitamins A and E are present in pastures and green forages, which contain ample quantities of β-carotene and α-tocopherol versus lower bioavailable forms in grains. Confinement rearing to include poultry in cages and swine on slatted floors allows limited animal access to feces (coprophagy), which is rich in many vitamins. Confinement rearing requires producers to pay more attention to higher vitamin requirements needed when this management system is used (Cunha, 1984b).

Stress, Disease, or Adverse Environmental Conditions

Intensified production increases stress and subclinical disease level conditions because of higher densities of animals in confined areas. Stress and disease conditions in animals may increase the basic requirement for certain vitamins. A number of studies have indicated that nutrient levels that are adequate for growth, feed efficiency, gestation, and lactation may not be adequate for normal immunity and for maximizing the animal's resistance to disease (Cunha, 1985; Nockels, 1988). Diseases or parasites affecting the gastrointestinal tract will reduce intestinal absorption of vitamins, both from dietary sources and those synthesized by microorganisms. If they cause diarrhea or vomiting, this will also decrease intestinal absorption and increase needs. Vitamin A deficiency is often seen in heavily parasitized animals that supposedly were receiving an adequate amount of the vitamin. Mycotoxins are known to cause digestive disturbances such as vomiting and diarrhea, as well as internal bleeding, and to interfere with absorption of dietary vitamins A, D, E, and K. In broiler chickens, moldy corn (mycotoxins) has been associated with deficiencies of vitamins D (rickets) and E (encephalomalacia) in spite of the fact that these vitamins were supplemented at levels regarded as satisfactory.

In recent years, a malady dubbed "spiking syndrome" in broilers caused a sharp rise in mortality at about 14 days of age. Some nutritionists feel that this problem may be associated with *Fusarium* mycotoxins, although the exact cause is not clearly defined. Increased levels of thiamin ameliorate the rise in mortality, and it has been suggested that when either corn quality is poor or mycotoxin levels and/or mold counts are high, thiamin should be increased by 1.11 to 1.65 mg/kg in the starter feed (Coelho, 1995).

Mortality from fowl typhoid (*Salmonella gallinarum*) was reduced in chicks fed vitamin levels greater than normal (Hill, 1961). Vitamin E supplementation at a high level decreased chick mortality due to *Escherichia coli* challenge from 40 to 5% (Tengerdy and Nockels, 1975). Scott et al. (1982) concluded that coccidiosis produces a triple stress on vitamin K requirements as follows: (1) Coccidiosis reduces feed intake, thereby reducing vitamin K intake; (2) coccidiosis injures the intestinal tract and reduces absorption of the vitamin; and (3) treatment with sulfaquinoxaline or other coccidiostats causes an increased requirement for vitamin K.

Vitamin Antagonists

Vitamin antagonists (antimetabolites) interfere with the activity of various vitamins, and Oldfield (1987) summarized the action of antagonists. The antagonist could cleave the metabolite molecule and render it inactive, as occurs with thiaminase and thiamin; it could complex with the metabolite, with similar results, as happens between avidin and biotin; or, by reason of structural similarity, it could occupy reaction sites and thereby deny them to the metabolite, as with dicumarol and vitamin K. The presence of vitamin antagonists in animal and human diets should be considered in adjusting vitamin allowances, as most vitamins have antagonists that reduce their utilization (see Chapters 2 through 18). Some common antagonists are as follows:

1. Thiaminase, found in raw fish and some feedstuffs, is a thiamin antagonist. Pyrithiamin is another thiamin antagonist.
2. Dicumarol, found in certain plants, interferes with blood clotting by blocking the action of vitamin K.
3. Avidin, found in raw egg white, and streptavidin, from *Streptomyces* molds, are biotin antimetabolites.
4. Rancid fats inactivate biotin and destroy vitamins A, D, and E and possibly others.
5. Oral contraceptives and drug therapy to control tuberculosis are antagonistic to vitamin B_6.

Use of Antimicrobial Drugs

Some antimicrobial drugs will increase vitamin needs of animals by altering intestinal microflora and inhibiting synthesis of certain vitamins. Certain sulfonamides may increase requirements of biotin, folacin, vitamin K, and possibly others when intestinal synthesis is reduced. This may be of little significance except when drugs that are antagonistic toward a particular vitamin are added in excess, that is, sulfaquinoxaline versus vitamin K, amprolium versus thiamin, and sulfonamide potentiators versus folacin (Perry, 1978).

Levels of Other Nutrients in the Diet

Level of fat in the diet may affect absorption of the fat-soluble vitamins A, D, E, and K, as well as the requirement for vitamin E and possibly other vitamins. Fat-soluble vitamins may fail to be absorbed if digestion of fat is impaired. The high cost of fat as an energy source has resulted in minimal fat levels in least-cost feed formulations, which may result in reduced absorption of fat-soluble vitamins (Hoffmann-La Roche, 1991).

Many interrelationships of vitamins with other nutrients exist and therefore affect requirements. For example, prominent interrelationships exist for vitamin E with selenium, vitamin D with calcium and phosphorus, choline with methionine, and niacin with tryptophan.

Body Vitamin Reserves

Body storage of vitamins from previous intake will affect daily requirements of these nutrients. This is truer for the fat-soluble vitamins A, D, and E and for vitamin B_{12} than for the other water-soluble vitamins and vitamin K. Vitamin A may be stored by an animal in its liver and fatty tissue in sufficient quantities to meet requirements for up to 6 months or even longer.

OPTIMUM VITAMIN ALLOWANCES

The National Research Council (NRC) requirements for a vitamin are usually close to minimum levels required to prevent deficiency signs and for conditions of health and adequate performance, provided sufficient amounts of all other nutrients are supplied. Vitamin requirements for various animal species (NRC) and humans (RDA, 1989) are presented in each chapter and in the appendix, Table A1. Most nutritionists usually consider NRC requirements for vitamins to be close to minimum requirements sufficient to prevent clinical deficiency signs, and they may be adjusted upward according to experience within industry in situations in which a higher level of vitamins is needed.

Allowances of a vitamin are those total levels from all sources fed to compensate for factors influencing vitamin needs of animals. These influencing factors include (1) those that may lead to inadequate levels of the vitamin in the diet (see Factors Resulting in Inadequate Dietary Intakes of Vitamins) and (2) those that may affect the animal's ability to utilize the vitamin under commercial production conditions (see Factors Affecting Vitamin Requirements and Utilization). The higher the allowance, the greater the extent to which it may compensate for the influencing factors. Thus, under commercial production conditions, vitamin allowances higher than NRC requirements may be needed to allow optimum performance (Roche, 1979).

The optimum supplementation level is the vitamin concentration that achieves the best growth rate, feed utilization, and health (including immune competency) and provides adequate body reserves (Coelho, 1996).

The concept of optimum vitamin nutrition under commercial production conditions is illustrated in Fig. 19.1 (Roche, 1979). The marginal zone represents vitamin levels that are lower than requirements that may predispose animals to deficiency. The requirements zone represents minimum vitamin quantities that are needed to prevent deficiency signs, but may lead to suboptimum performance even though animals appear normal. The allowances in the optimum zone permit animals to achieve their full genetic potential for optimum performance. In the excess zone, vitamin levels range from levels still safe, but uneconomical, to concentrations that may produce toxic effects. Usually only vitamins A and D, under practical feeding conditions, pose the possibility of toxicity problems for livestock. Optimum allowances of any vitamin are depicted as a range in Fig. 19.1 because factors influencing vitamin needs are highly variable, and optimum allowances to allow maximum response may vary from animal to animal of the same species, type, and age within the same population and from day to day (Roche, 1979).

It should be emphasized that subacute deficiencies can exist although the actual deficiency signs do not appear. Such borderline deficiencies are both the most costly and the most difficult to cope with and often go unnoticed and unrectified, yet they may result in poor and expensive gains, impaired reproduction, or depressed production. Also, under farm conditions, one will usually not find a single vitamin deficiency. Instead, deficiencies are usually a combination of factors, and often deficiency signs will not be clear cut. If the NRC minimum requirement for a vitamin is the level that barely prevents clinical deficiency signs, then this level moves in relationship to the level required for optimum production responses. This means that if a greater quantity of a vi-

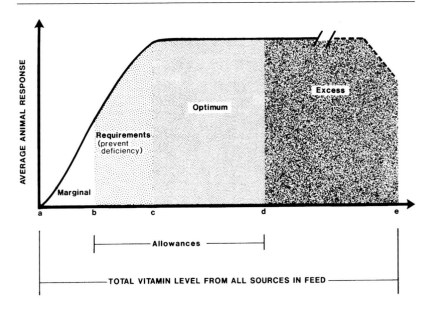

Fig. 19.1 Optimum vitamin nutrition for animals under commercial production conditions. Allowances are for total vitamin levels from all sources fed to compensate for factors affecting animals' vitamin needs. (Adapted from Roche, 1979. Printed with permission of Hoffmann-La Roche Inc., Nutley, New Jersey.)

tamin is required for an optimum response (because of the influencing factors), a greater quantity would also be required to prevent deficiency signs (Fig. 19.2). Similarly, if a lesser quantity is required for an optimum response, less would also be required to prevent deficiencies (Perry, 1978). Optimum animal performance required under modern commercial conditions cannot be obtained by fortifying diets to just meet minimum vitamin requirements. Establishment of adequate margins of safety must provide for those factors that may increase certain dietary vitamin requirements and for variability in active vitamin potencies and availability within individual feed ingredients.

The NRC requirements often do not take into account that certain vitamins have special functions in relation to disease conditions with higher than the recommended levels needed for response (Cunha, 1985). In pigs artificially infected with *Treponema hyodysenteriae*, the agent causing diarrhea, high supplementation with vitamin E (200 mg/day) in combination with selenium (0.2 mg/day) markedly reduced the number of pigs that became clinically ill (Tiege et al., 1978). Clinical signs and pathological changes were less severe compared with pigs with vitamin

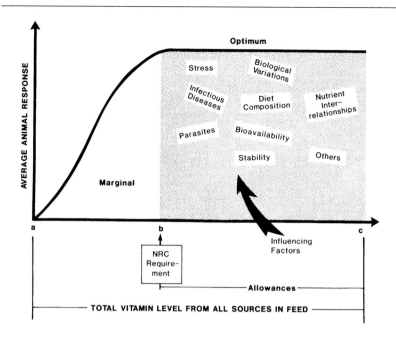

Fig. 19.2 Optimum vitamin nutrition for animals under commercial production conditions and influencing factors. (Adapted from Perry, 1978. Printed with permission of Hoffmann-La Roche Inc., Nutley, New Jersey.)

E deficiency. Thus, high doses of vitamin E increase resistance against disease. In practice, feeds contaminated with mycotoxins increase requirements for fat-soluble and other vitamins (e.g., biotin, folacin, and possibly others); therefore, supplementation should be increased above NRC minimum requirements. Apart from these fat-soluble vitamins, addition of folacin also improved performance in pigs fed moldy grain (Purser, 1981), and of biotin in pigs fed feeds containing certain molds (Cunha, 1984a). Besides other nutrients, vitamins play a major role in the immune response, the body's defense system against infectious disease. Vitamin supplementation above requirements was shown to be required for optimum immune responses (Ellis and Vorhies, 1976; Cunha, 1985; Weiss, 1998).

In relation to poultry, Kennedy et al. (1992) suggested that the NRC vitamin requirements have essentially been the same for the last 40 years. The industry vitamin average allowances have increased significantly (30 to 500%) to keep pace with greater genetic potential, faster growth rates, better feed efficiency, poorer quality ingredients, larger poultry houses, and generally higher disease levels, all of which caused increased stress in one study (McNaughton, 1990). A reasonable amount of logic would suggest that vitamin requirements determined several decades ago may not apply to today's poultry feeds (Dudley-Cash, 1994).

Dritz et al. (1995) fed sows higher vitamin concentrations than NRC requirements, with the result that 0.1 more pigs were born alive, 0.2 more pigs were weaned per litter, and weaned pigs were 1.1 kg heavier than controls. Stahly (1994) fed growing pigs under two management schemes to create a moderate or high level of antigen exposure. Within each antigen group, pigs were fed one of five dietary concentrations of B vitamins (niacin, riboflavin, pantothenic acid, B_{12}, or folacin). The addition of B vitamin concentrations of 370 to 470% above the current NRC (1998) recommendation resulted in 21% greater body weight gains and 10% improvement in feed utilization for pigs in either antigen group.

Interest has increased regarding the elimination of vitamin supplementation from poultry and swine diets for varying lengths of time. Skinner et al. (1991), for example, found that broiler performance was not impaired when vitamin supplementation was deleted from the diet for the last 21 days of the feed period. In contrast with these results, however, Gwyther et al. (1992) reported that NRC vitamin recommendations were much too low to maintain broiler performance. This latter study indicated that broiler vitamin requirements exceed those recommended by the NRC, and that the elimination of vitamin supplementation from broiler diets would severely impair performance. Teeter and Deyhim (1996) eliminated vitamins and/or minerals from broiler diets for the last 21 days of life, during which time the birds were exposed to heat stress. There was significant reduction in live bird and carcass performance. Performance tended to be poorest when the diet contained added trace minerals and no added vitamins, suggesting oxidation of the vitamins already present.

VITAMIN SUPPLEMENTATION MOST NEEDED BY LIVESTOCK

Vitamin requirements, as previously noted, are highly variable within the various species and classes of animals. Supplementation allowances need to be set at levels that reflect different management systems and are high enough to take care of fluctuations in environmental temperatures, energy content of feed, or other factors that might influence feed consumption or the vitamin requirements in other ways (McGinnis, 1986; McDowell, 1998).

A new concept of vitamin supplementation for both livestock and humans relates to providing antioxidant vitamins (carotenoids, vitamin E, and vitamin C) in excess of supposed dietary requirements (see Chapters 2, 4, and 15). These nutrients play important roles in animal health by inactivating harmful free radicals produced through normal cellular activity and from various stressors. Both in vitro and in vivo studies showed that these antioxidant vitamins generally enhance different aspects of cellular and noncellular immunity. A compromised immune system will result in reduced animal production efficiency through increased susceptibility to diseases, thereby leading to increased animal morbidity and mortality.

The following section will briefly discuss vitamins that are normally provided in ruminant, poultry, swine, and horse diets (McDowell, 2000).

Ruminants

Grazing ruminants generally need supplemental vitamin A only if pastures are low in carotene and possibly vitamin E (influenced by selenium status). Vitamin D is provided by ultraviolet light activity on the skin, while all other vitamins are provided by ruminal or intestinal, microbial, or tissue synthesis.

Ruminants housed under more strict confinement conditions generally require vitamins A and E and may require vitamin D if they are deprived of sunlight. Additional supplemental vitamin E would be needed to stabilize the meat color of finishing animals. Under specific conditions relating to stress and high productivity, ruminants may benefit from supplemental B vitamins, particularly thiamin and niacin. Future research may find a need for biotin and carnitine supplementation.

Adding a complete B-vitamin mixture to cattle entering the feedlot during the first month can reduce stress and increase gains. In one study, supplemental B vitamins given to feedlot calves tended to reduce morbidity of animals (Zinn et al., 1987). Apparently, under stress conditions of feedlots, the microbial population in the rumen is not synthesizing certain B vitamins at adequate levels.

Steer feedlot calves were feed-restricted and infected with bovine herpes virus-1 (BHV-1), with one treatment group receiving injections of B vitamins (Dubeski et al., 1996a). The IgG titers tended to be higher for the calves receiving B-vitamin injections, indicating that the humoral immune response was enhanced by B-vitamin treatment. B-vitamin status in stressed calves at the time of vaccination or disease challenge may affect the success of the immune response. The mild respiratory (BHV-1) infection in steer calves markedly decreased plasma concentrations of vitamin B_6, vitamin B_{12}, pantothenic acid, and ascorbate but not folacin (Dubeski et al., 1996b). Depletion of B-vitamin and ascorbate status during shipping and marketing may contribute to the enhanced susceptibility of cattle to infectious disease during the first few weeks after arrival at feedlots.

Poultry

Poultry managed under intensive production systems are particularly susceptible to vitamin deficiencies (Scott et al., 1982). Reasons for this susceptibility are as follows: (1) Poultry derive little or no benefit from microbial synthesis of vitamins in the gastrointestinal tract, (2) poultry have high requirements for vitamins, and (3) the high-density concentration of modern poultry operations places many stresses on the birds that may increase their vitamin requirements. Typical grain-oilseed meal (e.g., corn-soybean meal) poultry diets are generally supplemented with vitamins A, D, D_3, E, and K; riboflavin; niacin; pantothenic acid; B_{12}; and choline (Scott et al., 1982). Thiamin, vitamin B_6, biotin, and folacin are usually present in adequate quantities in the major ingredients, such as corn-soybean meal-based diets. Carnitine may be found to be of value in future studies.

Riboflavin and vitamins A, D, and B_{12} are usually low in poultry diets. However, adding other vitamins to poultry diets is good insurance. Vitamins D and B_{12} are almost completely absent from diets based on corn and soybean meal. Vitamin K is generally added to poultry diets more than to those for other species, because birds have less intestinal synthesis due to a shorter intestinal tract and faster rate of food passage. Birds in cages require more dietary K and B vitamins than those on floor housing because of more limited opportunity for coprophagy.

Swine

Vitamin supplementation of swine diets is obviously necessary (Figs. 19.3 and 19.4) because vitamin needs have become more critical as complete confinement feeding has increased. Swine in confinement, without access to vitamin-rich pasture, and housed on slatted floors, which limits vitamins available from feces consumption, have greater need for supplemental vitamins. The vitamins most likely to be marginal or deficient in corn-soybean diets are vitamins A, D, E, B_{12}, riboflavin, niacin, pantothenic acid, and occasionally vitamin K and choline.

729

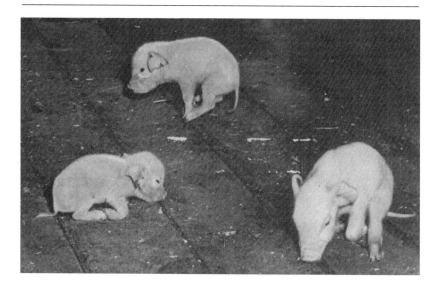

Fig. 19.3 Small, weak pigs at birth due to a lack of B vitamins. (Courtesy of T. J. Cunha and University of Florida.)

Almost all swine diets in the United Stated are now fortified with vitamins A, D, E, and B$_{12}$; riboflavin; niacin; pantothenic acid; and choline. An increasing number of feed manufacturers are adding vitamin K, and many are adding biotin and B$_6$ to diets. Diets are fortified with these vitamins even though not all experiments indicate a need for each of them. Most feed manufacturers add them as a precaution to take care of stress factors, subclinical disease level, and other conditions on the average farm that may increase vitamin needs (Cunha, 1977). It appears that carnitine supplementation of weanling pigs has potential (Newton and Burtle, 1992).

Horses

There is a lack of experimental information on the level of vitamins required in well-balanced horse diets, as well as on which vitamins need to be added (Cunha, 1980b). The vitamins most likely to be deficient in all classes of horses are vitamins A and E, with vitamin D also deficient in horses in confinement. Inadequate vitamin D may be provided to racehorses that are exercised only briefly in the early morning, when sunlight provides less antirachitic protection. Requirements for vitamins A, D, and E can be met with a high-quality (e.g., green) sun-cured hay. Deficiencies of vitamin K and the B vitamins appear to be less likely in

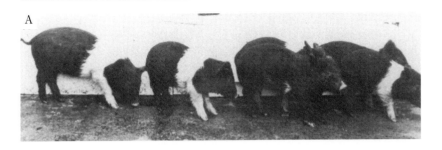

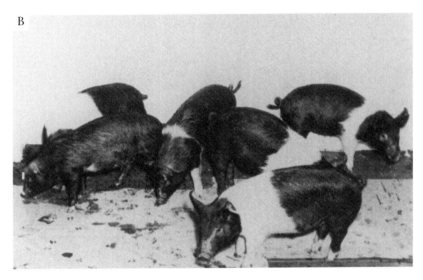

Fig. 19.4 The effect of B-vitamin supplementation on deficient pigs obtained from farms in Michigan. (A) These pigs were about 80 days old and weighed an average of 9.1 kg. (B) The same pigs after 35 days of supplementation. (Courtesy of R.W. Luecke, Michigan State University.)

the mature horse than in other monogastric species, as many vitamins occur in the cecum of the horse. It is not known, however, how much of the vitamins synthesized in the cecum is absorbed in the large intestine. Since it is difficult to depend on the intestinal synthesis, many horse owners use B-vitamin supplementation of diets for young horses and for those being developed for racing or performance purposes (Cunha, 1991).

Vitamin supplementation has become more critical for horses as the trend toward total confinement has increased. Currently, few horses receive a high level of vitamin intake from a lush, green pasture or from a high-quality leafy, green hay. Cunha (1980b) suggested that a vitamin premix for horses contain vitamins A, D, E, K, B_6, and B_{12}; thiamin; riboflavin; niacin; pantothenic acid; folacin; and choline. Biotin supplementation is also recommended since Comben et al. (1984) showed a benefit of the vitamin for hoof integrity. More recently, it has been suggested that carnitine supplementation is beneficial for horses. Vitamin E was found to have an effect on the susceptibility of horses to exercise-induced muscle damage (BASF, 1997a). Dietary levels of vitamin E greater than 80 IU/kg, and potentially 300 IU/kg, are required to maintain the blood and muscle vitamin E concentrations in horses undergoing exercise conditioning.

VITAMIN SUPPLEMENTATION FOR HUMANS

People in developed countries consume an average of 3,000 calories and almost 40 g of protein daily, while those in developing countries consume two-thirds as many calories and only one-fifth as much protein. Thus, calorie and protein deficiency are the most important problems in nutrition. In developing countries, vitamin deficiencies usually coexist with protein-calorie deficiency. In developed countries, on the other hand, inappropriate eating patterns can lead to poor nutrition and result in vitamin deficiencies (Marks, 1975).

A number of factors influence the vitamin deficiency state in humans. Diseases caused by primary or dietary deficiency result solely from inadequate quantities of the vitamin in the diet. Lack of vitamin intake can result from a number of factors (Marks, 1975), including crop failure, losses during food preparation and storage, poverty, ignorance, loss of appetite, apathy, food taboos or fads, dental problems, and chronic disease. Even social changes can affect dietary intake. For example, old people, particularly those living alone, tend to abandon ordinary meal preparation and live on small amounts of so-called easy foods (coffee, soup, and bread) that can lead to scurvy and other deficiency diseases.

However, some vitamin deficiencies occur even under conditions in which the diet would normally be considered adequate by most standards. Such deficiencies, usually referred to as secondary or conditioned deficiencies, arise from metabolic stress or organic disease. The increased metabolic demands during pregnancy and lactation are prime examples of metabolic stress states requiring extra vitamin therapy. Use of oral contraceptives and of various drugs, such as tranquilizers and antibiotics, can result in conditioned deficiencies. Particular attention to vitamin supplementation is needed for individuals with inborn errors of metabolism, for whom requirements are much higher for certain vitamins, and for hospital patients receiving total parenteral nutrition.

Certain disorders or diseases and some medications may interfere with vitamin intake, digestion, absorption, metabolism, or excretion and thus change requirements. The stress placed on carbohydrate metabolism in the alcoholic is another example of a condition requiring more than normal daily vitamin consumption. A number of B-vitamin deficiencies, including those of thiamin, niacin, B_6, B_{12}, and folacin, have resulted from alcoholism. For example, a major cause of folacin deficiency in the United States is chronic alcoholism. Diets of alcoholics are likely to contain inadequate quantities of a number of nutrients.

Another important cause of conditioned deficiency results from disease. In these cases a defect in the host results in decreased absorption of the vitamin from the diet. Pernicious anemia is a conditioned vitamin B_{12} deficiency because a lack of gastric intrinsic factor severely limits absorption of the vitamin from the gastrointestinal tract. Another example of this type is vitamin K deficiency that results from poor absorption and is caused by inadequate supplies of bile. Vitamin therapy in such cases is usually administered parenterally (e.g., intravenous injection).

Typical well-balanced diets that include ample quantities of vegetables, fruits, and animal products should provide vitamins in adequate quantities. For most individuals consuming such diets, there should be no need for supplemental vitamins. Nevertheless, many circumstances—including individual variations, lack of proper diet, older age, and physiological and emotional stress—may warrant vitamin supplementation. Many individuals also consume multiple vitamins (and sometimes minerals) daily, which gives them a sense of well-being and in essence is a type of nutritional insurance against possible deficiencies. In addition to vitamin deficiencies, it is also important to consider possible effects of excessive quantities of vitamins (hypervitaminosis) in human diets, particularly regarding vitamin A and, to a lesser degree, vitamin D.

The antioxidant nutrients—vitamin E, vitamin C, and β-carotene— have become the focus for their protective role in disease prevention, particularly cardiovascular disease (atherosclerosis) and cancer. These nutrients play important roles in health by inactivating harmful free radicals produced through normal cellular activity and from various stressors. Both in vitro and in vivo studies have shown that these antioxidant vitamins generally enhance different aspects of cellular and noncellular immunity. Many individuals, particularly those in more developed countries, take pharmacological levels of the antioxidant vitamins as well as the antioxidant mineral selenium. This trend is likely to continue because health benefits will continue to be amplified as more and more studies validate the health benefits of these nutrients.

The vitamins least likely to be needed for supplementation in human diets are choline, pantothenic acid, and biotin. Those that warrant supplementation are the following:

1. Vitamin A—Deficiency of vitamin A is widespread in the world and is most common in young children who receive inadequate green and yellow vegetables and foods derived from animals.

2. Vitamin D—In developed countries there is vitamin D fortification of human diets; however, most of the world depends on sunlight. Children not receiving sufficient sunlight are at great risk of deficiency, and older populations need to consider supplementation. Decreased ability of the kidney to convert 25-OHD to $1,25\text{-}(OH)_2D$ is a problem in the elderly (Tsai et al., 1984). Thus, even with more sunlight and more dietary intake, it is possible that elderly individuals would not maintain equivalent activity of $1,25\text{-}(OH)_2D$. Diseases and parasites that impair the ability of the liver and kidney to convert vitamin D to $1,25\text{-}(OH)_2D$ may also be problems, especially in developing countries.

3. Vitamin E—This vitamin is most likely deficient in individuals consuming low-fat diets or diets high in unsaturated fats and would be more critical in regions deficient in selenium, as vitamin E supplementation is beneficial for diverse disease conditions.

4. Vitamin K—Newborns are commonly given a single dose of vitamin K to prevent abnormal bleeding. Many persons take aspirin for pain, to minimize coronary problems, and for other reasons. There are indications that this may increase vitamin K needs.

5. Thiamin—Individuals subsisting mostly on refined grains (e.g., polished rice) are most likely in need of thiamin supplementation. In developed countries, people have for a number of years received food fortified with thiamin (e.g., bread enrichment). In Far Eastern countries, rice enriched with thiamin has dramatically reduced the incidence of beriberi.

6. Riboflavin—Often, individuals in developing countries do not have the economic resources needed to consume major dietary sources of riboflavin, such as meat, milk, and dairy products.

7. Niacin—Supplementation is important when diets are primarily based on corn and sorghum and for individuals with metabolic defects (e.g., conversion of tryptophan to niacin) or when grain has not been heated or

treated sufficiently to make niacin available. Pharmacological effects have included reduction of serum cholesterol and treatment of schizophrenia.

8. Vitamin B_6—Supplementation is most important for young, pregnant, or lactating women. Requirements are increased by oral contraceptives, certain drug therapy, radiation sickness, urinary calculi, and in errors of metabolism. Vitamin B_6 has been used to alleviate nausea during pregnancy and in megadose therapy for a wide variety of conditions, including premenstrual syndrome and behavioral disorders.

9. Folacin—A high percentage of the human population is estimated to be at a moderate to high risk for folacin deficiency (see Chapter 12) during growth, pregnancy, and old age. Supplementation is particularly needed for individuals not consuming optimum quantities of fruits and vegetables. To prevent certain birth defects, starting in 1998 certain foods (e.g., cereals and bread) in the United States were required by law to contain supplemental folacin.

10. Vitamin B_{12}—Organ meats and other animal products are the best sources of vitamin B_{12}. Vegetarians as well as individuals with the malabsorption defect of pernicious anemia need B_{12} supplementation.

11. Vitamin C—Supplementation is likely needed for individuals not consuming optimum quantities of fruits and vegetables. Megavitamin doses of vitamin C for most individuals are not harmful.

12. Essential fatty acids—Under typical conditions, linoleic acid ($18:2\omega6$) deficiency would not be expected for humans. The need for supplementing the linolenic acid family (e.g., $22:6\omega3$) has been suggested for prevention of cardiovascular disorders, hypertension, inflammation, and some types of cancer, as well as normal brain development and improvement of immune response.

PROVIDING VITAMIN SUPPLEMENTS

The physical and chemical forms of various vitamin products used to fortify feeds are usually different from the forms found in feedstuffs. Modification of these naturally occurring vitamin forms is required to improve their stability, compatibility, dispersion, and handling characteristics for feed fortification.

Various chemical and physical vitamin forms available for supplementation are presented in Table 19.1 (Adams, 1978; Hoffmann-La Roche, 1991). To obtain sufficient stability, compatibility with other feed components, and the properties required for application, vitamin producers try to devise vitamin forms according to the following methods (Schneider and Hoppe, 1986):

735

■ Table 19.1   Product Forms of Vitamins and Application Uses

Vitamin	Product Form		Application Uses
	Chemical	Physical	
A	Alcohol (retinol)	Crystalline or liquid	Liquid and dry oral pharmaceuticals
	Acetate and/or palmitate	Beadlets	Dry feeds; dry oral pharmaceuticals
		Spray- or drum-dried powders	Dry feeds; dry oral pharmaceuticals; water-dispersible vitamin products
		Liquid concentrates	Liquid feed supplements; oral and parenteral pharmaceuticals
		Oil dilutions	Nonpelleted feeds
		Oil absorbates	Nonpelleted feeds
	Propionate	Liquid concentrates	Oral and parenteral pharmaceuticals; liquid feed supplements
D (D_2 and D_3)	Ergocalciferol (D_2), or cholecalciferol (D_3)	Beadlets (with vitamin A)	Dry feeds; dry oral pharmaceuticals
		Spray- or drum-dried powders	Dry feeds; dry oral pharmaceuticals
		Liquid concentrates (with vitamin A)	Liquid feed supplements; oral and parenteral pharmaceuticals
		Oil dilutions	Nonpelleted feeds
		Oil absorbates	Nonpelleted feeds
E	d- or dl-α-tocopheryl acetate	Absorbate powder or oil	Feeds, foods, and pharmaceuticals
		Spray-dried powders	Water-dispersible vitamin products
	Mixed tocopherols	Oils	Foods and pharmaceuticals
	d-α-tocopheryl succinate	Powder	Pharmaceuticals
K	Menadione (K_3), MSB (menadione sodium bisulfite), MSBC (menadione sodium bisulfite complex), or MPB (menadione dimethyl pyrimidinol bisulfite)	Dry dilutions	Dry feeds or pharmaceuticals
		Water-dispersible powders	Water-dispersible vitamin products
	Phytomenadione (K_1)	Liquid	Parenteral pharmaceuticals

■ Table 19.1 *Continued*

	Product Form		
Vitamin	Chemical	Physical	Application Uses
Thiamin (B$_1$)	Thiamin mononitrate	Crystalline; dry dilutions	Feeds, foods, and pharmaceuticals
	Thiamin hydrochloride	Dry dilutions	Feeds
		Crystalline	Parenteral and oral pharmaceuticals; feeds
Riboflavin (B$_2$)	Riboflavin:	High-potency powder;	Feeds, foods, and dry oral pharmaceuticals
	chemically synthesized	Spray-dried powders	
	crystalline product;		
	fermentation product		
	Riboflavin-5′-phosphate	Water-soluble powder	Parenteral and liquid oral
	pharmaceuticals		
Niacin (B$_3$)	Niacin (niacinamide;	Crystalline	Feeds and pharmaceuticals
	nicotinic acid)	Dry dilutions	Feeds
Vitamin B$_6$	Pyridoxine	Dry dilution	Feeds
	hydrochloride	Crystalline	Oral and parenteral pharmaceuticals
Pantothenic acid	Calcium *d*- or *dl*-pantothenate	Powders	Feeds, foods, and pharmaceuticals
	Calcium *dl*-pantothenate-	Powder	Feeds
	calcium chloride complex		
	d-Panthenol	Liquid	Parenteral and liquid oral pharmaceuticals; cosmetics
Biotin	*d*-Biotin	Crystalline	Feeds, foods, and pharmaceuticals
		Dry dilutions	Feeds
Folacin	Folacin	Crystalline	Feeds, foods, and pharmaceuticals
		Dry dilutions	Feeds

■ Table 19.1 *Continued*

Vitamin	Product Form		Application Uses
	Chemical	Physical	
B$_{12}$	Vitamin B$_{12}$ (cyanocobalamin):		
	(a) Crystalline product from fermentation	Dry dilutions	Feeds
	(b) Chemically synthe-sized crystalline product	Water-soluble dilutions oral and parenteral pharmaceuticals	Water-dispersible vitamin products;
C	Ascorbic acid	Dry dilutions	Feeds
		Coated products	Feeds and foods
		Crystalline	Parenteral pharmaceuticals; feeds
	Sodium ascorbate	Powder	Antioxidant-preservative for foods
Choline	Choline chloride	70% liquid	Feeds
		25–60% dry powders	Feeds
		Crystalline	Pharmaceuticals
	Choline bitartrate	Water-soluble powders	Water-dispersible vitamin products; pharmaceuticals

Sources: Modified from Adams (1978) and Hoffmann-La Roche (1991).

- Synthesis of stable derivatives
- Addition of stabilizing agents
- Coating
- Absorption of liquid vitamins on suitable carriers
- Transformation of fat-soluble or poorly soluble vitamins into water-soluble or dispersible forms
- Transformation of water-soluble vitamins or derivatives into poorly water-soluble or fat-soluble forms
- Standardization of content
- Providing high bioavailability

In view of the nutritional importance of vitamins A, D, and E, many commercial vitamin producers have succeeded in enhancing stability of these vitamins in two ways: (1) by mechanical means, enveloping minute droplets of the vitamin or vitamins in a stable fat or gelatin, forming small beads, thus preventing most of the vitamin from coming into contact with oxygen until it is digested in the animal intestinal tract, and (2) through use of effective antioxidants that markedly prolong the induction period that precedes active vitamin oxidation. The stabilized beadlet containing an effective antioxidant will protect these vitamins for storage periods up to 4 to 8 weeks without much loss of vitamin potency. New technology has further improved vitamin A and D_3 stability by a cross-linking process, such as the reaction between the gelatin and the sugar, that makes the beadlet insoluble in water, giving it a more resistant coating that can sustain higher pressure, friction, temperature, and humidity (Coelho, 1996). Instability of vitamin D in peroxidizing diets is sometimes overlooked. Studies have shown that very high dietary levels of vitamin D are completely destroyed in diets containing high levels of peroxidizing polyunsaturated fatty acids, and chicks suffer severe rickets by 3 weeks of age (Scott, 1973). Rickets was prevented by a normal level of vitamin D when the diet was supplemented with 57 mg of ethoxyquin per kilogram of diet.

Stress factors affecting vitamin stability during manufacture and storage of a custom premix may include heat, oxygen, moisture, oxidation, reduction, trace minerals, and pH. Stability of some vitamins is not affected (Frye, 1978). Riboflavin, niacin, d-biotin, d-pantothenic acid, vitamin B_{12}, and choline generally have excellent stability in custom premixes. Other vitamins, such as vitamin A acetate, vitamin D_3, and vitamin E acetate, are also available in stabilized forms in custom premixes. Vitamin K, unstabilized vitamin A, unstabilized vitamin D, thiamin, folacin, vitamin C, and vitamin B_6 have poor stability in custom premixes under various stress conditions (Coelho, 1996).

Most vitamins are supplemented in dry form; however, liquid vitamin supplements are useful for certain feeding operations. Their appeal is broad, the advantages being lower feed cost per kilogram of gain, convenience in handling, ready adaptation in formulation, easy control, reduced time and labor, control of feed dust, and good palatability (Perry, 1968). Liquid supplements are not without disadvantages—such as physical stability and corrosion potential—most of which are minimal with properly formulated supplements and equipment and adequate feeder use knowledge (Bauernfeind, 1969). Ready availability of the many water-soluble or water-dispersible nutrients, such as energy sources (molasses), nonprotein nitrogen (urea), trace minerals, and vitamins (A, D, and E), have permitted standard and custom formulation for ruminants in feedlots and on pasture. Special economical liquid emulsions of vitamins A, D, and E, which remain acceptably uniform in physical distribution and with adequate stability patterns, are marketed for this purpose.

When control of animal feed intake is not complete but there is good control over water consumption, special vitamin A, D, and E dry beadlet or liquid products are available to add to drinking water. They disperse in cold water into a fine emulsion with desirable physical, taste, and chemical stability characteristics for short-time use. This vitamin form is useful in drinking water for poultry and other monogastric animals. Water-soluble vitamins and drugs, in properly formulated products, can also be added to water.

Because of the high variability and unknown bioavailability of vitamins in feeds, feed manufacturers have come to rely to a large extent on commercially synthesized vitamins. In practice, feed manufacturers usually ignore to a certain degree the contribution of many vitamins in feedstuffs and provide complete vitamin supplementation. Bauernfeind (1969) summarized the advantages of synthetic vitamins in animal feeds:

1. Biological and physical characteristics are known; potency is uniform, stability is adequate with few exceptions, and supply is usually unlimited.

2. Weight added per ton to the animal diet is small; hence, adjustments upward or downward or in different ratios can be made without upsetting the remainder of the diet.

3. Ready-made combinations can be formulated in premix form for

quick addition to specific diets for a given species of animal for a defined production objective with assurance of known diet values.

4. Cost is economical, hence vitamin restrictions of individual natural feed ingredients can be removed from the computer program, thus increasing flexibility of programming for least-cost energy and protein needs and shortening computer operation time.

5. Assay costs of determining variability of natural vitamin content of feedstuffs can be decreased by supplementing with the chemically produced nutrients.

6. Assay costs of determining the vitamin content of the final mixed diet can be decreased since assay of one or two components of the premix will give confidence of the mixing adequacy of all of the premix vitamins in the final diet.

7. Use of chemically prepared vitamins eliminates unknowns existing at times in natural ingredients or seasonal nutrient variation or physiological nutrient availability.

8. Chemically prepared vitamins have versatility in form and applications—adaptability to dry feeds, liquid supplements, drinking water solutions, drenches, and parenteral and capsule forms.

FORMULATING VITAMIN PREMIXES

The custom vitamin premix is generally considered to be a concentrated mixture of vitamins added in the manufacture of complete feeds or feed supplements, and it is customized to meet vitamin specifications of the feed manufacturer.

Use of custom vitamin premixes in feed manufacturing facilitates uniform distribution of vitamins in complete feeds and ensures that specifications for vitamin fortification of feeds are met.

Vitamin premixes are mixtures of specific vitamins required in combination with some type of carrier material that is added to feeds—usually at a rate of 1 to 5 lb per ton of complete feed—at the time of mixing to ensure uniform distribution of these ingredients in mixed feeds. Commonly used carriers include soybean meal, ground grain, corn gluten meal, wheat middlings, and several other mill feeds.

Zhuge and Klopfenstein (1986) compared vitamin premix carriers and found that destruction of vitamin A was greatest when ground sorghum was used as a diluent and least when the diluent was rice hulls or ground corn. Other carriers, such as wheat middlings, corn gluten meal, and soybean meal, are less suitable than rice hulls. Most vitamin

741

premixes are delivered in 50- to 55-lb plastic-lined paper bags. This combination of materials limits recycling opportunities. A viable alternative is the use of 1-ton capacity bags or bulk bags.

Custom vitamin premixes should possess certain physical and chemical properties to ensure optimum quality and dispersion in finished feeds. The most important physicochemical properties for vitamin premixes are flowability, hydroscopicity, lumping, compression, and chargeability (BASF, 1997b).

Desirable properties suggested by Aiello (1978) and Hoffmann-La Roche (1989, 1994) are as follows:

1. Proper particle size distribution. A good standard is 100% through a #20 U.S. standard sieve.

2. Free of contaminants.

3. Minimal moisture content. Excessive moisture (> 12%) can promote destruction of certain vitamins as well as bacterial and mold growth and causes handling problems due to caking and lumping.

4. Desirable mixing properties. Free-flowing, noncaking, nondusting, nonelectrostatic, nonhygroscopic, and nonsegregating.

5. Favorable pH. Most vitamins have their own specific pH level for optimum stability; however, a pH level of 5.5 is generally considered ideal for multivitamin premixes.

6. Proper bulk density. This contributes to proper premix particle size for uniform dispersion, free-flowing properties, and ease of premix handling and packaging.

7. Storage potential. Premixes should also be formulated to ensure optimum vitamin levels and stability under practical storage conditions. This includes addition of antioxidants to improve stability of vitamins such as A, D, and E.

8. Not mixing with antagonists. To prevent vitamin destruction, it is best not to include choline and trace minerals in vitamin premixes.

■REFERENCES

Adams, C.R. (1973). *In* Effect of Processing on the Nutritional Value of Feeds, p. 142. National Academy of Sciences, Washington, D.C.
Adams, C.R. (1978). *Proc. Roche Vitam. Nutr. Update Meet.*, p. 69. Arkansas Nutrition Conference, Hot Springs.
Aiello, R. (1978). *Proc. Roche Vitam. Nutr. Update Meet.*, p. 54. Arkansas Nutrition Conference, Hot Springs.
BASF. (1991). Vitamins—One of the Most Important Discoveries of the Century,

BASF Corporation, Parsippany, New Jersey.

BASF. (1997a). Antioxidant Status and the Susceptibility of Horses to Exercise-Induced Muscle Damage, KC9618, BASF Corporation, Mount Olive, New Jersey.

BASF. (1997b). Physico-Chemical Properties of Vitamins, Trace Minerals and Carriers, KC9617, BASF Corporation, Mount Olive, New Jersey.

Bauernfeind, J.C. (1969). *World Rev. Anim. Prod. 5*, 20.

Christian, L.D. (1983). *In* Proc. AFIA Nutrition Council, p. 22. Ames, Iowa.

Coelho, M. (1994). *Feedstuffs 66*(25), 13.

Coelho, M.B. (1995). *In* Proc. Maryland Nutrition Conference for Feed Manufacturers, p. 46. College Park, Maryland.

Coelho, M.B. (1996). Impact of Vitamin Sources and Feed Processing on Vitamin Stability, p. 38. BASF Technical Symposium, Seattle, Washington.

Comben, N., Clark, R.J., and Sutherland, D.J.B. (1984). *Vet. Rec. 115*, 642.

Cunha, T.J. (1977). Swine Feeding and Nutrition. Academic Press, New York.

Cunha, T.J. (1980a). *J. Anim. Sci. 51*, 1429.

Cunha, T.J. (1980b). Horse Feeding and Nutrition. Academic Press, New York.

Cunha, T.J. (1982). Niacin in Animal Feeding and Nutrition. National Feed Ingredients Association (NFIA), Fairlawn, New Jersey.

Cunha, T.J. (1984a). *Feed Manage. 35*, 14

Cunha, T.J. (1984b). *Squibb Int. Swine Update 3*, 1.

Cunha, T.J. (1985). *Feedstuffs 57*, 37.

Cunha, T.J. (1991). Horse Feeding and Nutrition, 2nd Ed. Academic Press, New York.

Dove, C.R., and Ewan, R.C. (1986). Swine Research Report, AS-580-J. Iowa State University, Ames.

Dritz, S.S., Tokach, M.D., Nelssen, J.L., Goodband, R.D., and Lynh, G. (1995). *In* Proc. Kansas State University Swine Day, p. 7. Lawrence, Kansas.

Dubeski, P.L., d'Offay, J.M., Owens, F.N., and Gill, D.R. (1996a). *J. Anim. Sci. 74*, 1367.

Dubeski, P.L., Owens, F.N., Song, W.O., Coburn, S.P., and Mahuren, J.D. (1996b). *J. Anim. Sci. 74*, 1358.

Dudley-Cash, W.A. (1994). *Feedstuffs 66*(6), 12.

Ellis, R.P., and Vorhies, M.W. (1976). *J. Am. Vet. Med. Assoc. 168*, 231.

Friesecke, H. (1975). *In* Pantothenic Acid, No. 1533. Hoffmann-La Roche, Basel, Switzerland.

Frye, T.M. (1978). *Proc. Roche Vitam. Nutr. Update Meet.*, p. 61. Arkansas Nutrition Conference, Hot Springs.

Gadient, M. (1986). *Proc. Nutr. Conf. Feed Manuf.*, p. 73. College Park, Maryland.

Gwyther, M.J., Tillman, P.B., Frye, T.M., and Lentz, E.L. (1992). *In* 13th Annual Meeting Southern Poultry Science. Atlanta, Georgia.

Hill, C.H. (1961). *Poult. Sci. 40*, 762.

Hoffmann-La Roche. (1989). Vitamin Nutrition for Poultry, RCD 7817/689. Hoffmann-La Roche, Inc., Nutley, New Jersey.

Hoffmann-La Roche. (1991). Vitamin Nutrition for Swine, RCD 8260/191. Hoffmann-La Roche, Inc., Nutley, New Jersey.

Hoffmann-La Roche. (1994). Vitamin Nutrition for Ruminants, RCD 8775/

894. Hoffmann-La Roche, Inc., Nutley, New Jersey.

Kennedy, D.G., Rice, D.A., Bruce, D.W., Goodall, E.A., and McIlroy, S.G. (1992). *Br. Poult. Sci. 33*, 1015.

Kurnick, A.A., Hanold, F.J., and Stangeland, V.A. (1972). *Proc. Georgia Nutr. Conf.*, p. 107. Atlanta Georgia.

Livingston, A.L., Nelson, J.W., and Kohler, G.O. (1968). *J. Agric. Food Chem. 16*, 492.

Mangelson, F.L., Draper, C.I., Greenwood, D.A., and Crandall, B.H. (1949). *Poult. Sci. 28*, 603.

Marks, J. (1975). A Guide to the Vitamins. Their Role in Health and Disease, p. 73. Medical and Technical Publ., Lancaster, England.

McDowell, L.R. (2000). *Asian–Aust. J. Anim. Sci. 113*, 115.

McGinnis, C.H. (1986). Bioavailability of Nutrients to Feed Ingredients, p. 1. National Feed Ingredient Association (NFIA), Des Moines, Iowa.

McMillen, W.N., Luecke, R.W., and Thorpe, F. Jr. (1949). *J. Anim. Sci. 8*, 518.

McNaughton, J. (1990). *Feedstuffs 62*(36), 13.

Newton, G.L., and Burtle, G.J. (1992). Current Concepts in Carnitine Research, p. 59. CRC Press, Boca Raton, Florida.

Nockels, C.F. (1988). *In* Proc. 1988 Georgia Nutr. Conf. for the Feed Industry. Atlanta, Georgia.

NRC. (1973). Effect of Processing on the Nutritional Value of Feeds. National Academy of Sciences-National Research Council, Washington, D.C.

NRC. (1982). United States-Canadian Tables of Feed Composition, 3rd Ed. National Academy of Sciences-National Research Council, Washington, D.C.

NRC. (1998). Nutrient Requirements of Swine, 10th Ed., National Academy of Sciences-National Research Council, Washington, D.C.

Oldfield, J.E. (1987). *J. Nutr. 117*, 1322.

Perry, S.C. (1978). *Proc. Roche Vitam. Nutr. Update Meet.*, p. 29. Arkansas Nutrition Conference, Hot Springs.

Perry, T.W. (1968). *Feedstuffs 40*(25), 48.

Purser, K. (1981). *Anim. Nutr. Health* April, 38.

RDA. (1989). Recommended Dietary Allowances, 9th Ed. National Academy of Sciences-National Research Council, Washington, D.C.

Roche. (1979). Optimum Vitamin Nutrition. Hoffmann-La Roche, Nutley, New Jersey.

Schneider, J., and Hoppe, P.P. (1986). Bioavailability of Nutrients in Feed Ingredients, p. 1. National Feed Ingredients Association (NFIA), Des Moines, Iowa.

Scott, M.L. (1973). *In* Effect of Processing on the Nutritional Value of Feeds, p. 119. National Academy of Sciences, Washington, D.C.

Scott, M.L., Nesheim, M.C., and Young, R.J. (1982). Nutrition of the Chicken, p. 119. Scott, Ithaca, New York.

Skinner, J.T., Izat, A.L., and Waldroup, P.W. (1991). *Poult. Sci. 70*(Suppl. 1), 112.

Stahly, T.S. (1994). *In* Carolina Swine Nutrition Conference. Raleigh, North Carolina.

Stamberg, O.E., and Peterson, C.F. (1946). *Poult. Sci. 25*, 394.

Teeter, R.G., and Deyhim, F. (1996). *In* El Foro 96 de Alimentos Balanceados, p. 71. Watt Publishing Co., Mt. Morris, Illinois.

Tengerdy, R.P., and Nockels, C.F. (1975). *Poult. Sci. 54*, 1292.

Tiege, J., Saxegaard, F., and Froslie, A. (1978). *Acta Vet. Scand. 19*, 133.

Tsai, K.S., Health, H., Kumar, R., and Riggs, B.L. (1984). *Clin. Res. 32*, 411A.

Weiss, W.P. (1998). *J. Dairy Sci. 81*, 2493.

Young, L.G., Lun, A., Pos, J., Forshaw, R.P., and Edmeades, D. (1975). *J. Anim. Sci. 40*, 495.

Zhuge, G., and Klopfenstein, C.F. (1986). *Poult. Sci. 65*, 987.

Zinn, R.A., Owens, F.N., Stuart, R.L., Dunbar, J.R., and Norman, B.B. (1987). *J. Anim. Sci. 65*, 267.

VITAMIN REQUIREMENTS OF LIVESTOCK AND HUMANS; FEED COMPOSITION; METRIC CONVERSIONS

Animal	A	D	E	K	Thiamin
Beef cattle[a]	IU	IU	IU		
Feedlot	2200	275	—	MS[b]	MS
Pregnant heifers and cows	2800	275	—	MS	MS
Lactating cows and bulls	3900	275	—	MS	MS
Growing	—	—	15–60	—	MS
Dairy Cattle[c]	IU	IU	IU	—	—
Growing	2200	300	25	MS	MS
Lactating cows and bulls	3200	1000	15	MS	MS
Calf milk replacer	3800	600	40	—	6.5 ppm
Sheep[d]	IU	IU/100 kg BW			
Replacement ewes, 60 kg	1567	555	15	MS	MS
Pregnant ewes, 70 kg	3306	555	15	MS	MS
Lactating ewes, 70 kg	2380	555	15	MS	MS
Replacement ram, 70 kg	1979	555	15	MS	MS
Ewes, maintenance, 70 kg	2742	555	15	MS	MS
Goat[e]	IU	IU	IU	—	—
All classes	5000	1400	100	MS	MS
Horse[f]	IU	IU	IU	—	mg
Growing	2000	800	80	MS	3
Maintenance	2000	300	50	MS	3
Working	2000	300	80	MS	5
Pregnant	3000	600	80	MS	3
Lactating	3000	600	80	MS	3

[a]NRC (1996). Nutrient Requirements of Beef Cattle. National Academy of Sciences-National Research Council, Washington, D.C.
[b]MS = microbial synthesis.
[c]NRC (1989). Nutrient Requirements of Dairy Cattle. National Academy of Sciences-National Research Council, Washington, D.C.

100% dry basis unless otherwise specified)

Riboflavin	Niacin	B_6	Pantothenic Acid	Biotin	Folacin	B_{12}	Choline
MS	MS	MS	MS	MS	MS	MS	MS
MS	MS	MS	MS	MS	MS	MS	MS
MS	MS	MS	MS	MS	MS	MS	MS
MS	MS	MS	MS	MS	MS	MS	MS
—	—	—	—	—	—	—	—
MS	MS	MS	MS	MS	MS	MS	MS
MS	MS	MS	MS	MS	MS	MS	MS
6.5 ppm	2.6 ppm	6.5 ppm	13 ppm	0.1 ppm	0.5 ppm	0.07 ppm	0.26%
MS	MS	MS	MS	MS	MS	MS	MS
MS	MS	MS	MS	MS	MS	MS	MS
MS	MS	MS	MS	MS	MS	MS	MS
MS	MS	MS	MS	MS	MS	MS	MS
MS	MS	MS	MS	MS	MS	MS	MS
—	—	—	—	—	—	—	—
MS	MS	MS	MS	MS	MS	MS	MS
mg	—	—	—	—	—	—	—
2	MS	MS	MS	MS	MS	MS	MS
2	MS	MS	MS	MS	MS	MS	MS
2	MS	MS	MS	MS	MS	MS	MS
2	MS	MS	MS	MS	MS	MS	MS
2	MS	MS	MS	MS	MS	MS	MS

[d]NRC (1985a). Nutrient Requirements of Sheep. National Academy of Sciences-National Research Council, Washington, D.C.

[e]Morand-Fehr, P. (1981). In Goat Production. (C. Gall, ed.) p.193, Academic Press, New York.

[f]NRC (1989). Nutrient Requirements of Horses. National Academy of Sciences-National Research Council, Washington, D.C.

■ Table A1b Vitamin Requirements for Monogastric Animals (units per kg of diet,

Animal	A	D	E	K	Thiamin
	IU	IU	IU	mg	mg
Swine[a]					
Growing-finishing					
3–5 kg	2200	220	16	0.5	1.5
5–10 kg	2200	220	16	0.5	1.0
10–20 kg	1750	200	11	0.5	1.0
20–50 kg	1300	150	11	0.5	1.0
50–120 kg	1300	150	11	0.5	1.0
Breeding					
Gilts and sows	4000	200	44	0.5	1
Young and adult boars	4000	200	44	0.5	1
Lactating gilts and sows	2000	200	44	0.5	1
Poultry[b]					
Leghorn chickens					
Growing					
0–6 weeks	1500	200	10	0.5	1.0
6–12 weeks	1500	200	5	0.5	1.0
12–18 weeks	1500	200	5	0.5	0.8
18 weeks to first egg	1500	300	5	0.5	0.8
Broilers					
0–3 weeks	1500	200	10	0.5	1.8
3–6 weeks	1500	200	10	0.5	1.8
6–8 weeks	1500	200	10	0.5	1.8
Turkeys					
0–4 weeks	5000	1100	12	1.75	2
4–8 weeks	5000	1100	12	1.5	2
8–12 weeks	5000	1100	10	1.0	2
12–16 weeks	5000	1100	10	0.75	2
16–20 weeks	5000	1100	10	0.75	2
20–24 weeks	5000	1100	10	0.5	2
	IU	IU	mg	mg	mg
Breeders holding	5000	1100	10	0.5	2
Laying hens	5000	1100	25	1.0	2
Geese					
Starting 0–4 weeks	1500	200	10	0.5	1.8
Growing 4+ weeks	1500	200	5	0.5	1.3
Breeding	4000	200	10	0.5	0.8
Duck					
0–2 weeks	2500	400	10	0.5	—
Growing 2–7 weeks	2500	400	10	0.5	—
Breeding	4000	900	10	0.5	—
Pheasant					
0–4 weeks	5000	1100	12	1.75	2
4–8 weeks	5000	1100	10	1.5	2
9–17 weeks	5000	1100	10	0.75	2
Breeding	5000	1100	25	1	2

100% dry basis unless otherwise specified)

Riboflavin	Niacin	B_6	Pantothenic Acid	Biotin	Folacin	B_{12}	Choline
mg	mg	mg	mg	mg	mg	µg	mg
4.0	20.0	2.0	12	0.08	0.30	20	600
3.5	15.0	1.5	10	0.05	0.30	17.5	500
3.0	12.5	1.5	9	0.05	0.30	15	400
2.5	10.0	1.0	8	0.05	0.30	10	300
2.0	7.0	1.0	7	0.05	0.30	5	300
3.75	10	1	12	0.2	1.30	15	1250
3.75	10	1	12	0.2	1.30	15	1250
3.75	10	1	12	0.2	1.30	15	1000
3.6	27	3	10	0.15	0.55	9	1300
1.8	11	3	10	0.10	0.25	3	900
1.8	11	3	10	0.10	0.25	3	500
2.2	11	3	10	0.10	0.25	4	500
3.6	35	3.5	10	0.15	0.55	10	1300
3.6	30	3.5	10	0.15	0.55	10	1000
3.0	25	3.0	10	0.12	0.50	7	750
4.0	60	4.5	10	0.25	1.0	3	1600
3.6	60	4.5	9	0.2	1.0	3	1400
3.0	50	3.5	9	0.125	0.8	3	1100
3.0	50	3.5	9	0.125	0.8	3	1100
2.5	40	3	9	0.100	0.7	3	950
2.5	40	3	9	0.100	0.7	3	800
mg	mg	mg	mg	mg	mg	µg	mg
2.5	40	3	9	0.100	0.7	3	800
4.0	40	4	16	0.20	1.0	3	1000
3.8	65	3	15	0.15	0.55	9	1500
2.5	35	3	10	0.10	0.25	3	1000
4	20	4.5	10	0.15	0.35	4	—
4	55	2.5	11	—	—	—	—
4	55	2.5	11	—	—	—	—
4	55	3.0	11	—	—	—	—
3.4	70	4.5	10	0.25	1	3	1430
3.4	70	3.5	10	0.2	1	3	1300
3.0	40	3	10	0.1	0.7	3	1000
4.0	30	4	16	0.2	1	3	1000

Animal	A	D	E	K	Thiamin
	IU	IU	IU	mg	mg
Bobwhite quail					
Starting					
0–6 weeks	5000	1100	12	1.75	2
Growing 6+ weeks	5000	1100	10	0.75	2
Breeding	5000	1100	25	1.0	2
Japanese quail					
Starting and growing	1650	750	12	1	2
Breeding	3300	900	25	1	2
	IU/kg BW	IU/kg BW	IU/kg BW		µg/kg BW
Dog[c]					
Growth	202	22	1.2	—	54
Maintenance	75	8	0.5	—	20
	IU	IU	IU	IU	mg
Cat[d]					
Growing	3333	500	30	100	5
	IU		mg		mg
Mink[e]					
Weaning 13 weeks	5930	—	27	—	1.3
	IU				µg
Fox[e]					
Growth	2440	—	—	—	1

Riboflavin	Niacin	B_6	Pantothenic Acid	Biotin	Folacin	B_{12}	Choline
mg	mg	mg	mg	mg	mg	µg	mg
3.8	30	3.5	12	0.25	1.0	3	1500
3.0	30	3	9	0.10	0.75	3	1500
4.0	20	4	15	0.20	1.0	3	1000
4	40	3	10	0.3	1	3	2000
4	20	3	15	0.15	1	3	1500
µg/kg BW	µg/kg BW	µg/kg BW	µg/kg BW		µg/kg BW	µg/kg BW	µg/kg BW
100	450	60	400	----	8	1.0	50
50	225	22	200	----	4	0.5	25
mg	mg	mg	mg	µg	µg	µg	g
4	40	4	5	70	800	20	2.4
mg	mg	mg	mg	mg	mg	µg	
1.6	20	1.6	8	0.12	0.5	32.6	----
mg	mg	µg	mg		µg		
3.7	9.6	1.8	7.4	----	0.2	----	----

Animal	A	D	E	K	Ascorbic Acid	Thiamin
	IU	IU	IU	IU	mg	mg
Fish[f]						
Catfish	1000–2000	500	50	—	25–50	1.0
Common carp	4000	—	100	—	—	0.5
Tilapia	—	—	50	—	50	—
Trout	2500	2400	50	—	50	1
Salmon	2500	—	50	—	50	—
	IU		mg	ppm		
Rabbit[g]						
Growth, female and breeding male	580	—	40	—	—	—
Reproducing	1160	—	40	2	—	—
	mg	mg	mg	mg		mg
Laboratory animals[h]						
Rat						
Growth, gestation, or maintenance	0.7	0.025	18	1	—	4
Mouse	0.72	0.025	22	1	—	5
	IU	IU	IU	mg	mg	mg
Guinea pig						
Growing	21,960	1000	40	5	200	2
	mg	—	IU	mg	mg	mg
Hamster, golden						
Growing	2	—	27	4	—	20
	IU	IU	IU		mg	mg
Nonhuman primate[i]	10,000 –15,000	2000	50	—	100	—

Sources: All references are from the Nutrient Requirement Series, National Academy of Sciences-National Research Council, Washington, D.C.
[a]NRC (1998). (Diets are 90% dry matter.)
[b]NRC (1994). (Diets are 90% dry matter.)
[c]NRC (1985). (Requirements on body weight basis.)
[d]NRC (1986). (Diets are 100% dry matter.)

Riboflavin	Niacin	B_6	Pantothenic Acid	Biotin	Folacin	B_{12}	Choline
mg	mg	mg	mg	mg	mg	mg	mg
9	14	3	15	—	1.5	—	400
7	28	6	30	1	—	—	500
6	—	—	10	—	—	—	—
4	10	3	20	0.15	1.0	0.01	1000
7	—	6	20	—	2	—	800
	mg	µg/g					mg
—	180	39	—	—	—	—	1200
—	—	—	—	—	—	—	—
mg	mg	mg	mg	mg	mg	µg	mg
3-4	15	6	10	0.2	1	50	750
7	15	8	16	0.2	0.5	10	2000
mg	mg	mg	mg	mg	mg		mg
3	10	3	20	0.2	4	—	1800
mg	mg	mg	mg	mg	mg	µg	mg
15	—	6	10	0.2	2	10	1800
mg	mg	mg	mg	mg	mg	mg	mg
5	50	2.5	15	0.1	0.2	—	—

[e]NRC (1982a). (Diets are 100% dry matter.)
[f]NRC (1993). (Purified diets, therefore values represent near 100% bioavailability.)
[g]NRC (1977). (Diets are 90% dry matter.)
[h]NRC (1995). (Diets are 90% dry matter.)
[i]NRC (1978). (Diets are 90% dry matter.)

■ Table A.1c   Vitamin Requirements for Humans

	A	D	E	K	C
	(µgRE/day)[a]	(IU/day)	(IU/day)	(µg/day)	(mg/day)
Male	1000	400	10	65–80	60
Female	800	400	8	55–60	60
Pregnant	800	400	10	65	70
Lactating	1300	400	12	65	95
Infants					
0-6 months	375	300	3	5	30
6-12 months	375	400	4	10	35
Children and adolescents	400–700	400	7	15–30	45

Source: RDA (1989) Recommended Dietary Allowances. National Academy of Sciences-National Research Council, Washington, D.C.
[a]Retinol equivalents. 1 RE = ^{1}µg retinol or 6 µg β-carotene.

Thiamin	Riboflavin	Niacin	B_6	Pantothenic Acid	Biotin	Folacin	B_{12}
(mg/day)	(mg/day)	(mg/day)	(mg/day)	(mg/day)	(µg/day)	(µg/day)	(µg/day)
1.5	1.7	19	2.0	4–7	30–100	200	2
1.1	1.3	15	1.6	4–7	30–100	180	2
1.5	1.6	17	2.2	4–7	30–100	400	2.2
1.6	1.7	1-20	2.1	4–7	30–100	280	2.6
0.3	0.4	5	0.3	2	10	25	0.3
0.4	0.5	6	0.6	3	15	35	0.5
0.7-1.0	0.8-1.2	13	1.0-1.4	3-5	20-30	50-100	0.7-1.4

■ Table A2 Composition of Important Feeds (Vitamins Expressed at 100% Dry Matter)

Feed Name, Description	Carotene Provitamin A	A	D	E	K
	mg/kg	IU/g	IU/kg	mg/kg	mg/kg
Alfalfa hay, sun cured	58.0	—	1575	113.0	21.6
Alfalfa leaves, sun cured	88.0	—	373	—	—
Bahia grass, fresh	183	—	—	—	—
Bakery waste, dehydrated	5.0	7.0	—	45.0	—
Barley, grain	2.0	—	—	25.0	0.2
Bean, navy, seeds	—	—	—	1	—
Beet, sugar pulp, dehydrated	—	—	637	—	—
Blood, meal	—	—	—	—	—
Bluegrass, Kentucky, fresh	248	—	—	—	—
Brewer's grains, dehydrated	—	—	—	29	—
Buckwheat, common, grain	—	—	—	—	—
Buttermilk, dehydrated (cattle)	—	2.4	—	7	—
Carrot, root, fresh	678	—	—	60	—
Casein, dehydrated (cattle)	—	—	—	—	—
Cattle, liver, fresh	—	439.1	—	25	—
Cattle, spleen, fresh	—	3.0	—	56	—
Chicken broilers, whole, fresh	—	30.0	—	—	—
Chicken, hens, whole, fresh	—	—	—	310	—
Citrus, dried pulp	—	—	—	—	—
Clover, red hay, sun cured	20	—	1914	—	—
Coconut, meats,					
meal mechanically extracted	—	—	—	—	—
solvent extracted	—	—	—	—	—
Corn, dent yellow cobs, ground	1	—	—	—	—
Gluten meal	18	—	—	34	—
Grain	3	—	—	25	0.2
Silage	43	—	439	—	—
Cotton seeds, meal, mechanically extracted, 41% protein	—	—	—	35	—
Crab meal	—	—	—	—	—
Fish, anchovy meal, mechanically extracted	—	—	—	5.0	—
Fish, menhaden meal, mechanically extracted	—	—	—	13	—
Fish, sardine meal, mechanically extracted	—	—	—	—	—
Flax (linseed meal)	—	—	—	9	—
Livers, meal	—	—	—	—	—
Meat, with blood, meal rendered (tankage)	—	—	—	—	—
Milk, dehydrated (cattle)	—	12.3	353	—	—

				Water-Soluble Vitamins					
Biotin	Choline	Folic Acid	Niacin	Pantothenic Acid	Riboflavin	Thiamin	B_6	B_{12}	International Feed No.
mg/kg	mg/kg	mg/kg	mg/kg	mg/kg	mg/kg	mg/kg	mg/kg	µg/kg	
0.20	—	3.6	42	28.6	13.4	3.0	—	—	1-00-078
0.28	1062.0	5.8	47	29.0	20.6	4.6	—	—	1-00-146
—	—	—	—	—	—	—	—	—	2-00-464
0.07	1005	0.2	28	9.0	1.5	3.2	4.7	—	4-00-466
0.17	1177	0.6	94	9.1	1.8	5.0	7.3	—	4-00-549
0.12	1499	1.4	28	2.3	2.0	7.1	0.3	—	5-00-623
—	902	—	18	1.5	0.8	0.4	—	—	4-00-669
0.09	854	0.1	34	2.6	2.2	0.4	4.8	49	5-00-380
—	—	—	66	—	11.0	8.8	—	—	2-00-786
0.68	1757	7.7	47	8.9	1.6	0.7	0.8	—	5-02-141
—	501	—	21	13.1	5.4	4.2	—	—	4-00-994
0.31	1891	0.4	9	40.1	33.1	3.7	2.6	21	5-01-160
0.07	—	1.2	58	30.1	4.9	5.8	12.0	—	4-01-145
0.05	229	0.5	1	2.9	1.7	0.5	0.5	—	5-01-162
3.51	5093	8.4	269	164.9	92.2	6.3	18.0	1523	5-01-166
0.16	2036	4.8	25	8.2	15.3	3.1	1.3	247	5-07-942
—	—	—	230	—	15.6	2.9	—	—	5-07-945
0.46	6288	0.5	225	20.4	6.4	2.4	4.6	278	5-07-950
—	867	—	24	15.4	2.5	1.6	—	—	4-01-237
0.11	—	—	43	11.2	17.8	2.2	—	—	1-01-415
—	1036	1.5	26	6.8	3.4	0.8	—	—	5-01-572
—	1189	0.3	28	6.9	3.7	0.7	4.8	—	5-01-573
—	—	—	8	4.2	1.1	1.0	—	—	1-28-234
0.20	391	0.3	55	11.2	1.8	0.2	8.8	—	5-28-241
0.08	567	0.3	28	6.6	1.4	3.8	5.3	—	4-02-935
—	—	—	47	—	—	—	—	—	3-02-912
1.19	2965	2.3	38	11.2	5.7	7.0	5.4	—	5-01-617
0.07	2179	0.1	49	7.0	6.7	0.5	7.2	475	5-01-663
0.21	4036	0.2	89	10.9	8.2	0.5	5.0	233	5-01-985
0.20	3398	0.2	60	9.4	5.2	0.6	5.1	133	5-02-009
0.11	3518	—	81	11.8	5.8	0.3	—	256	5-02-015
0.36	1962	3.1	41	15.8	3.5	4.6	6.1	—	5-02-045
0.02	12,281	6.0	221	31.5	39.1	0.2	—	542	5-00-389
—	2391	1.7	40	2.8	2.4	0.4	—	147	5-00-386
0.40	—	—	9	23.8	20.6	3.9	4.9	—	5-01-167

Feed Name, Description	Fat-Soluble Vitamins				
	Carotene Provitamin A	A	D	E	K
	mg/kg	IU/g	IU/kg	mg/kg	mg/kg
Milk, skim, dehydrated	—	—	446	10	—
Millet, grain	—	—	—	—	—
Molasses, sugarcane	—	—	—	7	—
Oat, grain	—	—	—	15	—
Pangola grass, fresh	62	—	—	—	—
Pea, seeds	1	—	—	3	—
Peanut kernels, meal, mechanically extracted	—	—	—	3	—
Potato tubers, dehydrated	—	—	—	—	—
Poultry, by-products, meal, rendered	—	—	—	2	—
feathers, hydrolyzed	—	—	—	—	—
Rape, seeds, mechanically extracted	—	—	—	20	—
Rice bran with germ	—	—	—	66	—
grain, ground	—	—	—	11	—
groats, polished	—	—	—	4	—
Rye, grain	—	—	—	17	—
Ryegrass, hay, sun cured	120	—	—	211	—
Safflower, seeds, meal, mechanically extracted	—	—	—	1	—
Sesame seeds, meal, mechanically extracted	—	—	—	—	—
Sorghum					
grain	1	—	26	10	0.2
silage	15	—	662	—	—
Soybean seeds	1	—	—	37	—
meal, solvent extracted	—	—	—	3	—
Sunflower, common seeds, mechanically extracted	—	—	—	—	—
Swine livers, fresh	—	361.7	—	—	—
Timothy, fresh	179	—	—	111	—
hay, sun cured	28	—	2138	38	—
Tomato pomace, dehydrated	—	—	—	—	—
Triticale grain	—	—	—	—	—
Turnip roots, fresh	—	—	—	—	—
Wheat					
bran	3	—	—	21	—
grain	—	—	—	17	—
Whey, dehydrated (cattle)	—	0.5	—	—	—
Yeast, brewer's, dehydrated	—	—	—	2	—
Yeast, torula, dehydrated	—	—	—	—	—

Source: United States-Canadian Tables of Feed Composition (NRC, 1982b); National Academy of Sciences-National Research Council, Washington, D.C.

				Water-Soluble Vitamins					
Biotin	Choline	Folic Acid	Niacin	Pantothenic Acid	Riboflavin	Thiamin	B_6	B_{12}	International Feed No.
mg/kg	mg/kg	mg/kg	mg/kg	mg/kg	mg/kg	mg/kg	mg/kg	µg/kg	
0.35	1480	0.7	12	38.6	20.5	3.9	4.5	54	5-01-175
—	489	—	26	12.2	4.2	8.1	—	—	4-03-120
0.92	1012	0.1	49	50.3	3.8	1.2	5.7	—	4-04-696
0.31	1116	0.4	16	8.8	1.7	7.1	2.8	—	4-03-309
—	—	—	—	—	—	cc	—	—	2-03-493
0.22	662	0.3	36	21	2.0	5.2	1.7	—	5-03-600
0.35	2052	0.7	186	49.7	8.8	6.6	8.0	—	5-03-649
0.11	2879	0.7	37	22.0	1.1	—	15.5	—	4-07-850
0.09	6451	0.5	50	11.8	11.2	0.2	4.7	322	5-03-798
0.05	962	0.2	23	9.7	2.1	0.1	3.2	90	5-03-795
—	7103	—	168	9.8	3.3	1.9	—	—	5-03-870
0.47	1357	2.4	330	25.2	2.8	24.7	—	—	4-03-928
0.09	1076	0.4	39	9.1	1.2	3.2	5.0	—	4-03-938
—	1018	0.2	17	3.9	0.6	0.7	0.4	—	4-03-942
0.06	479	0.7	21	9.1	1.9	4.2	2.9	—	4-04-047
—	—	—	—	—	—	—	—	—	1-04-077
1.54	1287	0.5	—	—	—	—	—	—	5-04-109
—	1655	—	20	6.4	3.6	3.0	13.4	—	5-04-109
0.42	737	0.2	43	12.5	1.4	4.7	5.0	—	4-04-383
—	—	—	—	—	—	—	—	—	3-04-323
0.37	2939	3.9	24	17.3	3.1	10.6	—	—	5-04-610
0.36	2915	0.7	31	18.2	3.2	6.2	6.7	—	5-04-604
—	4214	—	293	33.3	3.4	3.4	12.4	—	5-09-340
2.49	—	6.9	544	77.9	90.3	7.7	10.0	935	5-04-792
—	—	—	—	—	11.5	2.9	—	—	2-04-912
0.07	811	2.3	29	7.9	10.1	1.7	—	—	2-04-912
—	—	—	—	—	6.7	12.3	—	—	1-04-893
—	514	—	—	—	0.5	—	—	—	4-20-362
—	—	2.8	72	19.0	6.5	7.1	—	—	4-05-067
0.32	1797	1.6	268	33.5	4.6	7.9	9.6	—	4-05-190
0.11	1085	0.5	64	11.4	1.6	4.8	5.6	1.0	4-05-211
0.38	1921	0.9	11	49.6	29.4	4.3	3.6	20	4-01-182
1.08	4227	10.3	482	118.4	38.1	99.2	39.8	1	7-05-527
1.47	3223	26	525	100.6	47.6	6.6	38.9	4	7-05-534

Capacity or Volume

1 cubic centimeter	=	0.061 cubic inch
1 cubic meter	=	35.315 cubic feet
	=	1.308 cubic yards
1 milliliter	=	0.0338 fluid ounce (U.S.)
1 liter	=	33.81 fluid ounces (U.S.)
	=	2.1134 pints (U.S.)
	=	1.057 quarts (U.S.)
	=	0.2642 gallon (U.S.)
1 kiloliter	=	264.18 gallons (U.S.)

Weight

1 gram	=	0.03527 ounce (advp.)
1 kilogram	=	35.274 ounces (advp.)
	=	2.205 pounds (advp.)
1 metric ton (1,000 kg)	=	0.984 ton (long)
	=	1.102 tons (short)
	=	2204.6 pounds (advp.)

Volume per unit area

1 liter/hectare	=	0.107 gallon (U.S.)/acre

Weight per unit area

1 kilogram/square centimeter	=	14.22 pounds (avdp.)/square inch
1 kilogram/hectare	=	0.892 pound (avdp.)/acre

Acre per unit weight

1 square centimeter/kilogram	=	0.0703 square inch/pound (avdp.)

Temperature conversion formulas

Centigrade (Celsius)	=	5/9 (Fahrenheit −32)
Fahrenheit	=	9/5 Centigrade (Celsius) +32

Source: Modified from J. Anim. Sci. 25 (1966), 270.

Note: When conversions are made, the results should be rounded to a meaningful number of digits relative to the accuracy of original measurements. Values for weights and volumes are based on pure water at 4°C under 760 mm of atmospheric pressure.

INDEX

PUFAs, *(cont.)*
  Essential fatty acids (EFA)
  cancer and, 688
  infections, modulating, 697–698
  vitamin E and, 161, 170–172
Pumpkins as carotene source, 45
Purine synthesis
  folacin and, 489
  vitamin B$_{12}$, 533
Pyridoxal. *See* Vitamin B$_6$
Pyridoxal phosphate (PLP), 386–393,
  396, 407–409. *See also* Vitamin B$_6$
Pyridoxamine. *See* Vitamin B$_6$
Pyridoxine-5′-β-D-glucoside (PNG),
  398–399
Pyrimidine synthesis
  folacin and, 489
  vitamin B$_{12}$, 533
Pyrithiamine, 267, 722
Pyrroloquinoline quinone (PQQ),
  666–667

Rabbits
  biotin deficiency, 469
  choline
    deficiency, 580, 586
    requirements, 577
  coprophagy, 7
  essential fatty acids (EFA) deficiency, 702
  niacin deficiency, 372
  riboflavin deficiency, 335
  thiamin deficiency, 281, 296
  vitamin A
    deficiency, 36, 62–63
    requirements, 40
  vitamin B$_6$ deficiency, 405
  vitamin B$_{12}$
    deficiency, 548
    requirements, 536
  vitamin C and, 624
  vitamin E
    deficiency, 202–203
    requirements, 171
  vitamin K
    deficiency, 251
    requirements, 241
Radioimmunoassay. *See* Analytical procedures
Rats. *See also* Laboratory animals
  carnitine deficiency, 651
  choline
    deficiency, 586
    requirements, 577

choline toxicity, 592
coprophagy, 7
essential fatty acids (EFA)
  deficiency, 701
  requirements, 690
folacin
  deficiency, 504
  requirements, 492
myo-inositol deficiency, 662
niacin
  deficiency, 372
  requirements, 358
pantothenic acid
  deficiency, 437
  requirements, 427
riboflavin
  deficiency, 334, 336
  requirements, 322
thiamin
  deficiency, 281, 295
  requirements, 277
vitamin A
  deficiency, 30, 33, 36, 62
  requirements, 40
vitamin B$_6$
  deficiency, 385–386, 404–405
  requirements, 395
vitamin B$_{12}$
  deficiency, 547
  requirements, 536
vitamin D
  deficiency, 129
  requirements, 114
vitamin E
  deficiency, 202
  requirements, 171
vitamin K
  deficiency, 251
  requirements, 241
Reproduction
  β-carotene effects on, 76–77
  biotin deficiency, 460, 464, 468
  choline deficiency, 582–583, 584
  cobalt deficiency, 541
  fatty acids and, 696–697, 699, 700–702
  folacin
    deficiency, 479, 498–499, 500–501,
      505, 506, 508
    requirements, 491, 493
    supplementation, 512–515
  pantothenic acid deficiency, 432–435,
    437
  riboflavin deficiency, 327–330, 331

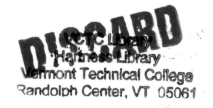